Type 1 Diabetes

http://dx.doi.org/10.5772/45927
Edited by Alan P. Escher and Alice Li

Contributors

Thomas Frese, Laura Nabors, Bashoo Naziruddin, Morihito Takita, Nigar Seven, Marlon Levy, Shereen Abdelghaffar, Aleksandar N. Jovanovic, Radojica V. Stolic, Vladan Peric, Snezana Markovic-Jovanovic, Johnny Ludvigsson, Nepton Soltani, Donovan Anthony McGrowder, Lennox Anderson-Jackson, Tazhmoye Crawford, Baqiyyah Conway, Amanda C. Peltier, Elena Matteucci, Ottavio Giampietro, Hakon Hakonarson, Marina Bakay, Rahul Pandey, Wen-Chin Lee, Huei-Jane Lee, Elina Linetsky, Camillo Ricordi, Luca Inverardi, Jixin Zhong, Mona Abbassy, Ippei Watari, Takashi Ono, Ahmed Bakry, Philip Newsholme, Kevin Keane, Mauricio Krause, Paulo Ivo Homem De Bittencourt, Jr., Werner Gurr, Mohamed Mirza Jahromi, M.Graça Pereira, Ana Cristina Almeida, Engracia Leandro, Didier Hober, Mustafa Cesur, Irmak Sayin, Chang-Qing Xia, Alan Escher

Published by InTech

Janeza Trdine 9, 51000 Rijeka, Croatia

Notice

Publishing Process Manager Iva Lipovic
Technical Editor InTech DTP team
Cover InTech Design team

Additional hard copies can be obtained from orders@intechopen.com

Type 1 Diabetes, Edited by Alan P. Escher and Alice Li
p. cm.
ISBN 978-953-51-1017-0

For EU product safety concerns:
IN TECH d.o.o., Prolaz Marije Krucifikse Kozulić 3, 51000 Rijeka, Croatia,
info@intechopen.com or visit our website at intechopen.com.

hood diabetes register [39]. Six hundred healthy children were included as controls. Viral RNA was found in 27 out of 600 (4.5%) diabetic children compared to 14 out of 600 (2.3%) control children (p=0.04).

4.1.2. Serum and plasma

The polymerase chain reaction, targeting the 5′ non coding region of enteroviral RNA was first used in an English study to detect viral genome in serum taken from 14 children at the onset of T1D and 45 control children matched for age, sex, date of specimen receipt and, as far as possible, geographic area [31]. In this study, a significant greater number of diabetic children had positive PCR results compared with controls (64% vs. 4%). Sequencing of enterovirus PCR products from six positive patients showed a significant homology with coxsackie B3 and B4 viruses, and some common patterns were observed among the sequences from infected diabetic children.

An English team investigated the relationship between enterovirus RNA and T1D in children [108]. One hundred ten children (aged 0-15 years with an average of 7.1 years) with newly diagnosed T1D were recruited. Detection of enterovirus RNA in serum collected in the week after diagnosis was based on a RT-PCR amplifying the 5′ noncoding region of enterovirus genome. Hundred and eighty-two control children were matched to cases by age (average age: 6.6 years), sex and date of serum collection at the same hospital. The number of newly diagnosed children with a positive RT-PCR was significantly higher than in the control group (27% versus 4.9%, p <0.005). Moreover, a significant proportion of diabetic children with a positive RT-PCR were of very young age. Indeed, enteroviruses were detected in 37% (20/54) of T1D children aged under 7 years, whereas only 4.6% (5/111) of corresponding control children were positive for enterovirus RNA (p <0.005). For diabetic children older than 7 years, 17.8% (10/56) were found to be positive for enterovirus RNA sequences, while viral RNA was detected in only 5.6% (4/71) of corresponding controls (p <0.05).

A French study evaluated the possible role of enteroviruses infections in the pathogenesis of T1D (Coutant et al., 2002). Sixteen newly diagnosed T1D children were included in this study. Forty nine control children matched for age, sex, date of venous collection and geographic area. A highly sensitive RT-PCR was used to investigate RNA in serum from patients and controls. Neutralzation antibodies to coxsackies viruses B1 to B6 were used to characterize the positive PCR samples. Enterovirus RNA was detected by PCR in only 2 of the 16 newly diagnosed T1D children and in only one of the 49 matched controls (p<0.1). Neutralization assay could not detect antibodies against coxsackiesviruses B1 to B6.

Two hundred and six newly diagnosed T1D children and 160 controls were included in an Australian study [37]. Enterovirus-RNA was found in either plasma or stool in 30% (62/206) of newly diagnosed T1D but only in 4 % (6/160) of controls (p<0.001). Case patients, positive for enterovirus RNA had lower C-peptide levels (p=0.04). Case children with enterovirus RNA levels were more likely to have a severe diabetic ketoacidosis (p = 0.03). Enteroviruses were detected in fewer children with HLA haplotype DRB1 * 03 DQB1 * 02 (p = 0.02) suggesting that the likely role of enteroviruses in the development of diabetes is important in some patients with specific genetic risk.

An Egyptian study included 70 diabetic children who were classified into 2 groups: the first group (I), 40 patients with newly diagnosed diabetic patients (less than one year), the second group (II), 30 children with diabetic patients with more than one year duration of disease [100]. In the control group there were 30 normal healthy children. Enterovirus infection was detected by viral culture of serum samples and confirmation of the results of tissue culture isolation was done by RT-PCR. In addition, anti-CVB IgM and IgG antibodies were searched by enzyme immuno assay. Enterovirus was isolated in group I (47.5%) and group II (23.3%). Neutralization test revealed that most of cases were coxsackievirus B4. In this study, coxsackievirus B IgM antibodies were significantly higher in diabetic patients of group I than those in group II ($p<0.01$) but there was no significant difference between group I and group II regarding IgG positivity.

A Japanese case-control study encompassed 61 patients with T1D aged 9 months to 40 years and 58 non diabetic subjects aged 1 month to 40 years whose serum was collected the same year [90]. A highly sensitive RT-PCR was used to investigate enterovirus RNA in serum samples. Moreover, neutralizing antibodies against Coxsackievirus and antibodies to GAD were measured and compared with the viral load and the enterovirus genotype. The detection of enterovirus was positive in 23 out of 61 patients (37.7%) and in 2 out of 58 controls (3.4%). The positivity of RT-PCR was decreasing by years gradually after the occurrence of T1D, there was neither gender nor age tendency. The sequence analysis of PCR amplicons displayed strong homologies with coxsackievirus B4 in 13 patients out of 23, and the level of neutralizing anti-CVB4 antibodies was significantly high in positive patients in RT-PCR. There was no relationship between the viral load in serum and antibodies against GAD.

A German group searched the enterovirus RNA by RT-PCR in the serum of diabetic children taken soon after the diagnosis of diabetes [104]. Seventeen out of 47 (36%) newly diagnosed diabetic cases were positive for enteroviral RNA whereas 2 out of 50 control subjects were positive ($p<0.001$).

Cuba is a country with a low incidence of T1D and with a high circulation of enteroviruses. In a Cuban study, the frequency of enteroviral RNA detection by RT-PCR was significantly higher in newly diagnosed T1D children whose diagnosis was made within 10 days before inclusion [26.5% (9/34)] compared to controls [2.9% (2/68)], matched for age, gender, geographic origin and date of serum collection ($p = 0.0007$) [127]. Enterovirus detection was more likely associated with severe diabetic ketoacidosis at onset (pH <7.1, $p = 0.03$) and high titres of autoantibodies against ICA ($p < 0.05$).

4.1.3. Leucocytes and other biological samples

An English study included 17 newly diagnosed patients with T1D, 38 previously diagnosed patients with T1D (the median duration of T1D was 4 years) and 43 age and sex matched non-diabetic controls [53]. Enterovirus RNA was detected by PCR in peripheral blood mononuclear cells in 41 % of newly diagnosed patients with T1D, 39% of previously diagnosed patients and 31% of non diabetic controls. This study showed no difference between diabetic patients and controls regarding the frequency of infection by enterovirus. Whether enteroviruses acted as non-specific agents with an abnormal immune response of the host, is a question raised by the authors of this study.

In a Swedish group, Yin and colleagues used RT-PCR to detect enterovirus RNA in PBMC (peripheral blood mononuclear cells) from 24 newly diagnosed children patients [171]. The 24 control children were matched for age, sex and geographical location without evidence of ongoing infection. RT-PCR was performed with primers (groups A and B) corresponding to conserved areas in the 5'non-coding region. With group A primers, 50% (12/24) of newly diagnosed patients had a positive enterovirus RT-PCR, however, control children were negative ($p<0.001$). With group B primers, enterovirus sequences were detected in 46% (11/24) of newly diagnosed patients, and in 29 % (7/24) of control children, but the difference was not statistically significant. Taking into account the results obtained with the two sets of primers, the detection of enterovirus RNA was positive in 75% (18/24) of newly diagnosed patients and only in 29% (7/24) of control children.

One hundred and twelve diabetic children and 56 healty controls have been included in an Italian study [154]. Enterovirus common capsid antigens were detected by immunofuorescence in a panel of cell lines inoculated with total leucocytes from peripheral blood, and enteroviral RNA was detected in these cultures as well. Enteroviruses were detected by RT-PCR in 93/112 case children (83%) and 4/56 control children (7%), and directly in leukocytes at lower frequency. Thirteen cases of familial enterovirus infection were observed.

Enteroviral RNA has been searched in PBMC, plasma, throat and stools of 10 newly diagnosed children and 20 control children [132]. Viral RNA was found in PBMC of 4 patients (40%), in plasma of 2 patients (20%), and in stools in 1 patient, in contrast, no sample was positive in control children. All throat swabs from patients and controls were negative. According to the authors, a prolonged enteroviral infection could be suspected in these patients in front of a positive detection of viral RNA in PBMC and/or plasma together with a negative detection of viral RNA in stool and throat swabs.

4.1.4. Pancreas

A 10 years old child with a flu-like illness within 3 days prior to admission in hospital for diabetic ketoacidosis died on the 7th day of admission [175]. The autopsy showed infiltration of the pancreas islets by lymphocytes with necrosis of beta cells. The inoculation of mouse, monkey and human cell cultures with a homogenate of the patient's pancreas had led to the isolation of a CVB4. Serology showed an 8 fold increase in titer of neutralizing antibody to this virus between the second hospital day and day of death. Inoculation of mice with this viral isolate led to hyperglycemia, inflammation of the islets of Langerhans and necrosis of beta cells. Immunoflurescence detected viral antigen in beta cells of mouse pancreatic section. The virus isolate obtained from this patient is known as CVB4 E2.

A few years later, a British group [52], did not find VP1 by immunohistochemistry in pancreas beta cells of 88 patients who had died at clinical presentation of T1D. In contrast, by using the same method VP1 protein was found in cardiac myocytes from 12 of the 20 patients whose cause of death was an acute coxsackievirus B myocarditis, and in seven of these positive cases, insulitis was observed and VP1 was detected in islet endocrine cells, but rarely in exocrine pancreas. Together, these data suggested that the beta cell destruction in patients with fatal diabetes was unlikely related to a direct cytopathic effect of coxsackievirus B, however the role of viruses in the destruction of beta cells through an autoimmune mechanism can not be excluded.

A few years later, another group investigated the presence of enteroviral RNA in the pancreas of 2 children patients with fatal acute-onset T1D and 5 controls by using RT-PCR and Southern blot hybridization [17]. The detection of Enteroviral RNA, and other viral genome (cytomegalovirus, mumps and rubella) was negative in every case.

The relationship between enterovirus and T1D and the type of pancreatic cells infected with enteroviruses has been invesigated by a finish group [172]. The study included 12 newborn infants who died of fulminant infection with enteroviruses (myocarditis in most cases). Autopsy pancreases from 65 patients with T1D and 40 control subjects matched for age and sex were also studied for presence of enteroviral RNA by in situ hybridisation. Enteroviral RNA was detected in pancreas of 58% (7/12) of the 12 newborns; the enterovirus-positive cells were detected in numerous pancreatic islets and in some duct cells but not in exocrine pancreas. In situ hybridisation identified enteroviruses in 6% (4/65) of diabetic patients. Enteroviral RNA was located exclusively in islets. None of the control subjects was positive for enteroviral RNA.

More recently, an Italian team studied the relationship between enterovirus infection, inflammation of pancreatic beta cells, autoimmunity and beta cell function [43]. Six newly diagnosed T1D patients (1 week to 9 months) and 26 control organ donors were included in this study. Immunohistochemistry, electron microscopy, RT-PCR and sequencing, and virus isolation in cell culture were used to detect enteroviruses in pancreatic autopsic tissue. Enteroviral RNA was detected in 3 out of 6 diabetic patients but not in controls. Infection was specific of beta cells with non-destructive insulitis and with naturel killer cell infiltration. There was not apparent reduction of islet beta cells in these patients. The virus isolated from one of these 3 patients, identified as CVB4 was able to infect human pancreatic beta cells of nondiabetic multiorgan donors. Viral inclusions and signs of pyknosis were observed by electronic microscopy, and a loss of beta cell function was assessed by insulin secretion response to glucose, arginine and glibenclamide. These data show that enterovirus could infect beta cells in patients with T1D and that these viruses could be responsible for inflammation and functional abnormalities of these cells.

Recently, authors raised the issue of the relevance of pancreas tissue samples to display the relationship between enterovirus infection and type 1diabetes, since no enteroviral RNA was detected by RT-PCR in samples from pancreatic organ donors with diabetes [158]. Further investigation with pancreas from additionnal donors are needed to address the issue of the persistence of enteroviruses in this organ. Whether enteroviruses are present in pancreas tissue at the time of symptom onset should be investigated but tissue samples can not be easily obtained by biopsy in the case of this organ.

The prevalence of enteroviral capsid protein (VP1) in pancreatic autopsy tissue from 72 newly diagnosed T1D children and a large cohort of controls has been studied by immunohistochemical staining by a british group [122]. The cell subtypes infected with enteroviruses were identified by immunofluorescence. The criterion of positivity was the presence of at least one intensely stained endocrine cell in an islet within any given section. According to this criterion, 61% (44/72) of diabetic children were positive in immunohistochemistry versus 7.7% (3/39) of control children ($p < 0.001$). There was no significant difference regarding age or gender between the VP1-positive and VP1-negative groups however the duration of diabetes seemed to be lower in the VP1-positive group (2.32 months vs 16.5 months; $p = 0.06$).

4.1.5. Stools

Entroviruses are present in stools of infected individuals [125]. The hypothesis of the role of enteroviruses in T1D prompted researchers to look for these viruses in stools of patients.

An Italian group investigated enteroviruses in stools from 43 newly diagnosed diabetic children and 22 control children [42]. Stools and serum samples were collected within 2 months from the beginning of diabetes symptoms. In order to isolate enterovirus, stools were inoculated to cell cultures and in suckling mice. Neutralizing antibodies to coxsackie virus B4 and anti-coxsackie viruses B1 to B6 complement fixing antibodies were measured. There was one case with high antibodies against coxsackie B4 virus but no enterovirus was isolated from stools.

A 16 month-old child with a predisposing HLA group (B18 DRw3) developed diabetes [21]. The disease outcame at hospital on the third day of steroid therapy for febrile purpura within the week of diphtheria/pertussis/tetanus and polio vaccination. Coxsackievirus B5 was isolated from stools and serologic studies showed a rise in titer of neutralizing antibodies directed to that isolate from less than 10 on the first day to 640 on the eleventh day. The sudden onset of T1D in the course an acute coxsackievirus B5 infection suggests the potential involvement of this virus in the disease in that case.

4.1.6. Intestine

Different virological methods were used in a Finnish study to evaluate whether enteroviruses can be found in small intestinal mucosa of 12 patients with T1D (age: 18 to 53, 2 out of them were male) and 10 non-diabetic subjects (age 23 to 71, 3 out of them were male) [114]. These individuals underwent gastroscopy for gastrointestinal symptoms and intestinal mucosa biopsies were taken for morphological analysis, which did not reveal any abnormality. To analyse the presence of enteroviruses in intestinal biopsy samples, immunohistochemistry was used for detecting the viral protein VP1, and in situ hybridization. RT-PCR were used for detecting viral RNA. Six out of 12 (50%) diabetic patients were positive for enteroviral RNA by in situ hybridization, whereas all control subjects were negative ($p = 0.015$). Two of these positive patients had enteroviral RNA in the cells of lamina propria; four were positive in the epithelial cells of villi, in the crypts and in the cells of lamina propria. Immunohistochemistry was positive in 9 out of 12 (75%) of diabetic patients but only in 10% (1/10) of control subjects ($p = 0.004$): the protein VP1 was mainly localized in the epithelium. Viral RNA was found by RT-PCR in a frozen sample from one of the 4 diabetic patients who were positive in both in situ hybridization and immunohistochemistry. There was no relationship between the detection of enteroviral RNA in gut mucosa of diabetic patients and duration of diabetes, gender, HLA type or hyperglycemia.

The discrepancy in results obtained by RT-PCR and in situ hybridization could be explained by the fact that intestinal biopsy samples were obtained from two sites of the intestine, and by differences in samples preparation. These results display that subjects with T1D have enteroviral components in their gut mucosa.

4.2. Enterovirus in biological samples from individuals at high-risk of diabetes

A Finnish prospective study concerned children with prediabetic state, which were derived from a previous study "Childhood Diabetes in Finland" (DiMe) [99]. The study investigated enterovirus RNA in 93 serum samples from 11 prediabetic children who progressed to T1D during the follow-up. One hundred and eight serum samples from 34 control children who participated in the same cohort but did not develop autoimmunity against beta cells or T1D were examined. In this study, serum samples from 47 children with newly diagnosed T1D were also analysed. Antibodies against islet cells (ICA), glutamic acid decarboxylase (GADA), insulin (IAA) and the protein tyrosine phosphatase-related IA-2 protein (IA2-A) were analysed. Antibodies against coxsackie viruses B1 to B6 were measured by neutralization assay. Enterovirus RNA was found in 12 %(11/93) of follow-up samples from prediabetic children compared to only 2% (2/108) of follow-up samples from matched controls ($p<0.01$). Viral RNA was detected in none (0/47) of the serum samples obtained from diabetic children. The presence of enteroviral RNA was associated with a concomitant increase in ICA ($p <0.01$) and GADA ($p <0.05$), whereas no increase was observed in the rates of IAA and IA-2A. This study suggests that enterovirus genome can be found in serum of individuals and that it is associated with the induction of autoimmunity several years before the onset of symptoms. The presence of enterovirus RNA in serum of prediabetic children has been studied in Cuba [127]. This study encompassed 32 children positive for antibodies against ICA having a first-degree relative with T1D, 31 children, negative for antibodies against ICA having a diabetic first-degree relative, and 194 controls, who were matched for age, gender, geographic origin and date of serum collection. Enterovirus RNA was found in 15.6% (5/32) of islet autoantibody-positive first-degree relatives children, whereas all controls were negative for enteroviral genome ($P = 0.003$). Enterovirus RNA was found in 3.2% of 31 children, negative for antibodies against ICA having a diabetic first-degree relative, and in 1.6% of controls.

After seroconversion for islet antibodies (against GAD, insulin, IA-2), serum and rectal swabs were collected every 3-6 months until diagnosis of diabetes in the Diabetes and Autoimmunity Study in the Young (DAISY) encompassing 2,365 american genetically predisposed children for islet autoimmunity and T1D, according to HLA, and siblings or offspring of people with T1D (regardless of their genotype) [141]. Fifty of the 140 children who seroconverted to positivity for islet autoantibodies progressed to T1D. The prevalence of enteroviral RNA in serum and rectal swabs as displayed by RT-PCR declined with age and seemed to be higher at visits positive for multiple islet autoantibodies. The risk of progression to T1D following detection of enteroviral RNA in serum, in a 4-month interval, was significantly increased compared with negative detection. In contrast, the presence of enteroviral RNA in rectal swabs did not predict progression to T1D, which is in agreement with the results of the MIDIA study including 911 Norwegian children identified at birth with a HLA genotype conferring a risk of T1D [149].

Thirty height children with an increased genetic susceptibility to diabetes followed-up from birth who have progressed to T1D and 140 control children matched for sexe, date of birth, hospital district and HLA-DQ-conferred genetic susceptibility to T1D were included in the finnish type 1 Diabetes Prediction and Prevention study (DiPP) [115]. Serum samples were analysed for enterovirus RNA by RT-PCR: 5.1% of samples were enterovirus RNA positive in case children but only 1, 9% in control children (p<0. 01). In boys, the detection of enterovirus RNA during the 6 months preceding the discovery of autoantibodies was associated with a risk of diabetes (p<0.01).

Biological samples	Number of Cases/ Controls	Children/ adults patients	Positives cases/ Controls p value	Methods of detection	Reference	country
Whole blood	24/27	0/24	6/0 p <0.01	RT-PCR	Andréoletti et al., 1997	France
Whole blood	56/37	25/31	21/0 p *	RT-PCR	Chehadeh et al., 2000	France
Woole Blood	600/600	600/0	27/14 p=0.04	RT-PCR	Dahlquist et al., 2004	Sweden
Serum	14/45	14/0	9/2 p*	RT-PCR	Clements et al., 1995	England
Serum	110/182	110/0	30/9 p<0.005	RT-PCR	Nairn et al., 1999	England
Serum	16/49	16/0	2/1 p>0.05	RT-PCR	Coutant et al., 2002	France
Serum	70/30	70/0	26/0 p <0.05	Cell culture	Maha et al., 2003	Egypt
Serum	61/58	NI	23/2 p<0.05	RT-PCR	Kawashima et al., 2004	Japan
Serum	47/50	47/0	17/2 p<0.001	RT-PCR	Moya-Suri et al., 2005	Germany
Serum	34/68	34/0	9/2 p=0.0007	RT-PCR	Sarmiento et al., 2007	Cuba
Plasma stools	206/160	206/0	62/6 plasma or stools p<0.001	RT-PCR	Craig et al., 2003	Australia

Biological samples	Number of Cases/ Controls	Children/ adults patients	Positives cases/ Controls p value	Methods of detection	Reference	country
PBMC	24/24	24/0	18/7 p*	RT-PCR	Yin et al., 2002	Sweden
leucocytes	112/56	112/0	93/4 p*	RT-PCR	Toniolo et al., 2010	Italy
PBMC plasma stools throat	10/20 10/20 10/20 10/20	10/0	4/0 p>0.05 2/0 1/0 0/0	RT-PCR	Schulte et al., 2010	Netherlands
Pancreas	149/21	NI	0/7 p*	IHC	Foulis et al., 1990	England
Pancreas	65/40	0/65	4/0 p*	HIS	Ylipaasto et al., 2004	Finland
Pancreas	6/26	2/4	3/0	IHC Electronic microscope Cell culture RT-PCR	Dotta et al., 2007	Italy
Pancreas	72/39	NI	44/3 p<0.001	IHC	Richardson et al., 2009	England
Intestine	12/10	0/12	6/0 p=0.015 9/1 p=0.004	HIS IHC	Oikarinen et al., 2007	Finland

Table 3. Detection of enterovirus and/or their components (RNA, proteins) in biological samples of patients with type 1 diabetes. PBMC: Peripheral Blood Mononuclear Cells, RT-PCR: Retrotranscription Polymerase Chain Reaction, IHC: Immunohistochemistry, HIS: Hybridization in situ, NI: Not Indicated, p*: p value not mentioned.

5. Enterovirus and type 1 diabetes: Experimental approach

In previous sections of this review, clinical studies that were conducted to assess the relationship between enteroviruses and T1D have been presented. A significant association between enterovirus infection and T1D, particularly for studies that used molecular methods, has been displayed, and when identified the most often involved enteroviruses were coxsackieviruses B. Experimental studies have been performed to understand the possible link between enterovirus and T1D. In the present section, the results of in vivo studies on one hand and those of in vitro studies on the other hand are presented and analyzed.

http://dx.doi.org/10.5772/52087

5.1. In vivo studies in animal models

In order to analyse the hypothesis that enterovirus infections enhance or elicit autoimmune disorders such as T1D, a significant body of evidence is derived from investigations using animal models. Most of them used to explore research hypotheses regarding the relationship between enteroviruses and type 1 diabetes are mouse models (NOD, C57BL/k, C57BL/6, SJL/J, DBA/2, SWR/J, BALB/c, B10, CD-1…) [83]. Despite their limitation in diseases investigations, experimental models have greatly contributed to our knowledge of human diseases. The predominance of murine models for the investigation of the relationship between enteroviruses and T1D is due, among others, to a physiology relatively similar to that of human beings and the presence of specific receptors, the more prominent of them could be the coxsackievirus and adenovirus receptor (CAR) which is a receptor for coxsackievirus B [86]. Therefore experimental datas have been obtained from models based on infection with coxsackievirus B (CVB) (figure 3).

5.1.1. Enterovirus and immune system

Experimental in vivo studies have contributed improving our understanding of genetic and immunological implications, enteroviral tropism and mechanisms of pancreatic β-cells destruction in the context of enteroviral infection [83]. Enteroviruses generally infect the exocrine pancreas, but some strains preferentially infect islets. Some studies have addressed the role of CAR, the main receptor for CVB entry into host cell, in enteroviral tropism and target organ infection. CAR is expressed by intestine, pancreas and heart epithelial cells, as well as cardiomyocytes [54]. In transgenic mice CVB3 titers were markedly reduced in CAR-deficient tissues and pancreatic CAR deletion induced a strong attenuation of pancreatic CVB3 infection and pancreatitis [86].

The development of innate and adaptive immune responses is mediated by type I interferons (IFNs) produced early during viral infection to induce an antiviral state within target cells. Experimental studies have shown that mice deficient in type I IFNs receptor are more susceptible and die more rapidly than controls when infected with CVB3 [169, 40]. An efficient immune response depends on rapid recognition of viruses by the innate immune system and this recognition is primarily achieved by pattern-recognition receptors such as toll-like receptors (TLRs), retinoid-inducible gene 1-like receptors (RIG-1) and NOD-like receptors. It is noteworthy that interactions between NOD-like receptors and enteroviruses are still poorly understood.

Toll-like receptors are transmembrane glycoproteins expressed on the cytoplasmic membrane or in intracellular vesicals of several immune and non-immune cell populations; while RIG-I-like receptors, represented by RIG-I and the interferon-induced with helicase C domain 1 (IFIH-1), also called melanoma differentiation-associated gene 5 (MDA5) are expressed in the cytosol of most cell types [91]. Among TLRs, TLR3, known to be double-stranded RNA sensor on monocytes, is known to be crucial for the survival of mice infected with CVB4 [123]; and the production of cytokines by murine plasmocytoid dendritic cells have been shown to be closely linked with CVB detection and recognition by TLR7 [168]. The MDA5 is in turn essential for type I IFNs responses to CVB, since MDA5 knockout mice are deficient to type I IFN and are prone to early death when infected with CVB (Wang et al., 2010). Thus, pattern-recognition receptors activation by enteroviruses results on IFNs and chemokines production which could lead to an inflammatory state in infected tissues. Moreover, these inflammatory factors enhance the overexpression of MHC-I molecules, which could result in an increased exposure of infected cells to the immune system and could initiate an autoimmune process that could directly contribute to islet cells damage [173]. However an activation of MDA-5 with any other factor can not initiate autoimmunity, whereas IFN-I-induced MDA-5 accelerated a preexistent autoimmune process in an animal model [38].

Some studies in animals have highlighted the potent role of antibodies and immune cells during enteroviral infection. Results on mice have shown that gammaglobulins are essential in limiting the scope and severity of enteroviral infection by preventing viral persistence in infected tissues [103] and T lymphocytes can deeply limit virus replication in CVB3-induced myocarditis and pancreatitis [63].

5.1.2. Enteroviruses can induce diabetes in mice

Experiments have been conducted to evaluate the ability of CVB4 to elicit diabetes in mice. These studies have shown that the pancreas was a predominant site of virus replication and the target of a strong immune response.

A CVB4 strain isolated by Yoon et al. from the pancreas of a 10-year-old boy who died of diabetic ketoacidosis and called CVB4E2, have induced hyperglycaemia with inflammation of the Langerhans islets and β-cell necrosis when inoculated to susceptible mice SJL/J [175]. A similar result was obtain in the same SJL/J mice strain when inoculated with a CVB5 strain isolated from stools of a diabetic patient [121]. In another study, CVB4E2 has led to hyperglycaemia and the appearance of anti-GAD antibodies in the vast majority of mice, suggesting a potent role of enteroviruses in initiating or accelerating autoimmunity against β-cells [57]. Diabetes with viral replication in β-cells has been also obtained when CVB4 JVB strain was inoculated to susceptible mice [174]. In addition, diabetes has been obtained in mice infected by CVB3 and CVB5 when animals were first treated with sub-diabetogenic doses of streptozotocin, a highly specific β-cell toxin. Findings from that study have revealed that virus-induced diabetes can be facilitated by cumulative effects induced by genetic factors or environmental insults (chemicals, drugs, toxins), since CVB strains (B3 and B5) used in that study ordinarily produce little if any β-cell damage [153]. Furthermore, CVB4-induced abnormal thymic, splenic and peripheral lymphocytes repertoire maturation has been described in mice and these lymphocyte maturation disorders have preceded the onset of hyperglycemia in animals [22].

In a study, CD-1 mice have been infected with the diabetogenic strain CVB4E2 and followed during one year. Results from this study have revealed a prolonged presence of viral RNA in pancreas tissue, a significant decrease in insulin levels and islets cells destruction by two mechanisms: directly by cytotoxic effects of IFN-γ-stimulated peritoneal macrophages and by an antibody-dependent mechanism through islet cell autoantibody (ICA) [133]. In another study, infection of mice with CVB4 has led to a rapid development of the disease mediated by bystander activation of T cells [73], which would tend to confirm early findings that have shown that infection of normal mice with CVB4 causes an overt diabetes associated with low insulin levels consistent with islet cells destruction [33].

The mechanism behind this β-cell destruction has been explored in some studies. Analysis of the results from these studies reveals that the spontaneous development of diabetes in NOD mice can be accelerated by CVB4 infection though a "bystander" effect only if a sufficient number of pre-existing autoreactive T-cells was already present [134]. This observation was in agreement with another study which has shown that the overexpression of a TCR transgene specific to an islet autoantigen has induced diabetes onset 2-4 weeks after CVB4 inoculation in mice that do not develop diabetes spontaneously [73]. Islet cell destruction by autoreactive T-cells was the result of the release of sequestered islet antigens which followed β-cell inflammation and destruction caused by CVB infection [73, 2001]. Other studies have stated that β-cells are phagocyted by antigen-presenting cells like macrophages, rather than directly destroyed by a CVB-induced process [75, 133], because antigen-presenting cells isolated from CVB4-infected mice can induce diabetes if inoculated to non-infected mice [75].

Among T1D animal models, the NOD mouse remains far the most used and studied model. The NOD mice are susceptible to spontaneous T1D that develops over several weeks and share most aspects of human T1D [83]. In NOD mice, the disease occurs after T-cell-mediated destruction of β-cells [87, 170]. Some studies have revealed that CVB infection effects in NOD mice appear to be contingent upon the precise moment at which infection occurs [134, 156]. Thus, rapid T1D induction can be obtained when older NOD mice are inoculated with CVB and the disease occurs much more rapidly when mice islets are already developing autoimmune insulitis and high islet cells lytic viral replication are observed when à virulent strain is inoculated [156]. These findings suggest that CVB replicate more readily in aged NOD mice islet cells, especially if there is inflammation, than in those of younger animals.

Another factor seems to be the magnitude of effects of CVB4 infection onto β-cells, depending on the permissiveness of target cells, which is closely related to their sensitivity to IFNs. Indeed, coxsackievirus B4-infected-NOD mice which had defective IFNs responses have developed an acute form of type 1 diabetes, similar to the one in humans following severe enteroviral infection. Interferons act by inducing an antiviral state in target cells, including pancreatic β-cells, by reducing their permissiveness to viral entry and replication. The effect of IFNs is transmitted as an intracellular signal through the Jack-STAT signaling pathway [140]. In transgenic NOD mice that express the suppressor of cytokine signaling 1 (SOCS-1), a negative regulator of IFN action which inhibit the Jack-STAT signaling pathway, CVB4 infection has resulted in β-cell loss and diabetes onset. Similar results have been obtained during the same study in transgenic NOD mice of which β-cells were lacking IFN receptors. In addition to inducing on β-cells a lower permissiveness to CVB4 infection, IFNs contributed also to deeply decrease their sensitivity to NK cell-mediated destruction [50].

5.1.3. Molecular mimicry hypothesis

Glutamic acid decarboxylase 65kD (GAD65), a candidate autoantigen in the pathogenesis of T1D, is expressed in pancreatic β-cells. Some findings from mice have shown that CTL (cytotoxic T lymphocytes) are cytotoxic to islet cells [44] and that T cell responses to GAD65 were detectable in prediabetic NOD mice spleens prior to disease onset [89, 152]. One of the mechanisms proposed to explain enterovirus-induced autoimmunity in T1D model is based on the cross-reactivity between CVB antigens and β-cell endogenous proteins through molecular mimicry. Pancreatic β-cells infection by CVB will be followed by inflammatory response resulting in β-cell destruction and increased self-antigen presentation due to their phagocytosis by antigen-presenting cells (APCs). Since P2-C protein sequence of CVB partially resembles that of human GAD65, both autoreactive and antiviral T-cells activated upon CVB infection, might act as strong enhancers that may accelerate or aggravate the ongoing autoimmune process [28, 151].

Regardless T-cells cross reactivity effects, experiments on CVB4-infected NOD mice have provided the evidence that the release of β-cell antigens followed by their presentation by APCs (antigen presentation cells) such as macrophages can initiate or promote β-cell autoimmunity [75].

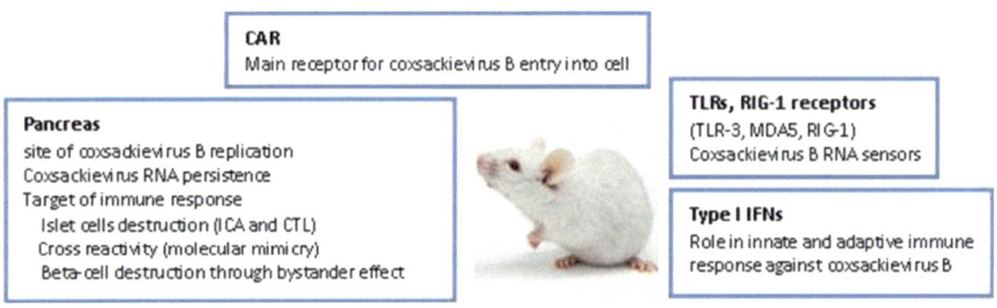

Figure 3. Information brought by animal models regarding coxsackievirus B infection and some aspects of type 1 diabetes pathogenesis

5.2. In vitro infection of β-cells and other cells with enteroviruses

Experiments have been conducted in vitro in order to analyse the hypotheses in favour of an association between enterovirus infections and T1D. Whether enteroviruses were able to infect the pancreatic tissue is a key issue concerning the relationship between enteroviruses and T1D. It has been shown that enteroviruses may be involved in the pathogenesis of T1D, either through direct β-cell infection or as triggers of the autoimmune processes. In particular, some results from in vitro experiments have suggested that enteroviruses, and especially CVB, may infect human β-cells and the infection may result in no apparent immediate effect or in functional impairment of β-cell [175, 174, 167, 124]. Most common enteroviruses in the environment can infect cultured human islets with β-cell destruction [93]. The figure 4 summarizes information brought by in vitro studies regarding coxsackievirus B infection which can be relevant for type 1 diabetes pathogenesis.

http://dx.doi.org/10.5772/52087

5.2.1. *Enterovirus infection of β-cells*

Persistent infection of human pancreatic islets by CVB associated with alpha interferon (IFN) synthesis was observed [23]. In this study conducted by our team, human pancreatic islets obtained from adult brain-dead donors and cultured in noncoated membrane inserts were infected with CVB3 and a diabetogenic (CVB4 E2) and a non-diabetogenic (CVB4 JVB) strain of CVB4. It was displayed that both α and β cells in human pancreatic islet can be persistently infected and long term CVB replication has been observed through the presence of infectious particles in culture supernatant fluids and intracellular viral negative-strand RNA up to 30 days post infection. This study showed that human islets challenged with CVB can synthesize IFN-α which is produced by infected β-cells only. These data support the hypothesis of a role of CVB in the high levels of type I IFNs that have been detected in pancreas or islets of patients with T1D [51, 76]. The viral persistence accompanied by synthesis of INF-α can enhance autoimmune processes leading to diabetes onset. The possibility that IFN-α could take part in T1D onset in genetically predisposed host have been tested in transgenic mice of which β-cells express this cytokine. It revealed that IFN-α was able to provoke the onset of the disease in transgenic animals, and that neutralizing IFN-α prevented inflammation and diabetes [142]. The expression of IFN-α in β-cells may lead to the development of diabetes in transgenic mice through the activation of autoimmune (islet-reactive) CD4+ TH1 cells [20].

Recent findings have shown that type I IFNs production can be induced in CVB infected human islet cells by intracellular viral RNA sensors such as TLR3, MDA-5 and RIG-1 genes [77]. These pattern-recognition receptors have also been told to upregulate the synthesis and production of chemokines. The sustaining of this process - IFNs and chemokines production – could be deleterious and involved in the development of autoimmunity, especially since persistent infection of islets cells in vitro by some CVB strains has been reported [23].

The infection of β-cells with CVB and the molecular pathways leading to CVB-induced β-cell death have been investigated. One study was aimed to evaluate the effects of different CVB4 strains on islets morphology and insulin release and another one compared inflammatory-related genes expression in CVB4-infected and uninfected isolated human islets. Results from these studies have revealed that even though the outcome of the infection differed, islet cells can be infected by all CVB4 strains. However, significant differences in viral titers and cell morphology were observed according to the phenotype of the strain: one with no cytopathic effect despite high virus titres (VD2921 stain), and the other with a pronounced cytopathic effect (V89-4557 strain), whereas a third one (JVB strain) have induced a significant increase of insulin release [55]. A microarray analysis of RNA from CVB4-infected human islets have shown specific induction of several inflammatory genes, some of them encoding proteins with potent biological activity such as IL-1β, IL-6, IL-8, MCP-1 and RANTES [117]. Recently, it has been reported that, except CVB1 and CVB3, all other CVB viruses induced a dose-dependent production of pro-inflammatory cytokines and chemokines in a rat insulinoma β-cell line (INS-1) [107].

The release of proinflammatory cytokines may strongly contribute to maintain a local pancreatic-islet inflammation that could result in an amplification of the immune attack against β-cells. In addition, the activation of MHC molecules in human fetal islet cells cultures infected by CVB4 could result in an increase exposure of infected cells to the immune system and support the autoimmune response against β-cells [119].

The inflammation of β-cells is supposed to be an early event in the pathogenesis of type 1diabetes [45]. An exaggerated inflammatory response to enterovirus may contribute to induce a prolonged inflammation state and β-cell loss, and could initiate or aggravate pathogenic processes of type 1 diabetes.

5.2.2. Enterovirus infection of thymus

It has been shown in mouse that CVB could infect the thymus with a disruption of organ functions that was associated with diabetes [22]. Further studies have been conducted to investigate the mechanisms and consequences of infection of thymus with CVB. The establishment of central T-cell tolerance is ensured by the thymus. Thymic epithelial cells (TEC) participate actively in the development of a biochemical environment needed for the maturation of immunocompetent T cells. Thymic epithelial cells are actively involved in the promotion of T-cell maturation by mediating negative and positive selection of thymocytes and by participating to the induction of tolerance [136].

In collaboration with Pr Vincent Geenen and his team (University of Lièges, Belgium) we investigated the hypothesis that T1D which is an autoimmune disease, can result from the disturbance of the central tolerance. Due to the role of thymus in induction and establishment of self-tolerance, enteroviral infection of TEC may result in interference and disturbance of T-cell ontogeny, which can induce or enhance the immune process leading to T1D. The infection of human TEC primary cultures with CVB4 and the resulting consequences on TEC function have been studied. Human TEC, isolated from thymus fragments obtained from children undergoing corrective surgery, were infected with CVB4 JVB and E2 strains. Findings from this study have revealed that a cytolytic virus such as CVB4 can infect persistently human TEC cultures without obvious cytopathic effect and this infection have led to a continuous increased production of cytokines IL-6, GM-CSF and LIF [14]. In order to evaluate the effect of enterovirus infection onto fetal thymus during pregnancy, intact explanted human foetal thymic organ cultures were infected with CVB4E2 strain. Results from this study have shown progressive thymocyte depletion and upregulation of MHC-I molecules expression on CD4+CD8+ double positive cells [15]. Another study was conducted on mouse to assess the effect of CVB infection on thymocytes maturation and differentiation. In this study, whole foetal thymus organ cultures obtained from 14 days foetal CD-1 mice were infected with CVB4E2 strain. Findings from that study have revealed in infected culture a disturbance of maturation and differentiation of T cells characterized by increased levels of mature CD4+ and CD8+ cells associated with decreased percentage of double positive cells [16].

Furthermore it was reported that CVB4 RNA can be found in thymus up to 70 days after per os infection of mice with CVB4E2. In vitro, CVB4 was able to infect and replicate in primary cultures of adult murine splenic and thymic cells [81].

The ability of enteroviruses such as CVB4 to infect the thymus during fetal life could have deleterious effects on thymus functions, since neonatal exposure to thymotropic virus could

http://dx.doi.org/10.5772/52087

induce a virus-specific nonresponsiveness [95]. A global analysis of all these findings suggests that thymus organ can be infected by coxsackievirus B which can disturb the organ function with possible effects on the autoimmune processes leading to T1D.

5.2.3. Antibody-dependent enhancement of enterovirus infection

The antibody-dependent enhancement (ADE) of infection is a mechanism observed in vitro with various viruses and which can intervene in pathogenic processes induced by these viruses [145]. The ADE of CVB4 infection has been discovered by our group. It is caused by enhancing antibodies devoid of neutralizing activity and has been found in serum /plasma of T1D patients and controls. These antibodies, isolated from plasma by affinity chromatography, increase the CVB4-induced synthesis of IFN-α by human peripheral blood mononuclear cells (PBMC) in vitro [25]. It has been demonstrated that IFN-α synthesis by PBMC infected with CVB4 prealably incubated with specific antibodies is a result of the infection of monocytes that occurs by a mechanism involving the receptors CAR and those for the Fc portion of IgG molecule, FcγRII (Fcγ receptor II) and FcγRIII localised at the cell surface membrane [66]. CVB4 can strongly induce the production of IFN-α by PBMCs from patients with T1D compared with PBMC from healthy controls, which is due to anti-CVB4 enhancing antibodies bound to the cell surface membrane. In addition, a higher level of IFN-α was produced by PBMC of patients inoculated with CVB4 prealably incubated with plasma of patients [67]. The target of these antibodies has been identified as the enteroviral protein VP4 and it has been shown that the prevalence and the titres of anti-VP4 antibodies were higher in patients with T1D than in control subjects [26]. Specific anti-VP4 antibodies enhance the infection of PBMC with CVB4 [129]. The sequence of VP4 recognized by these antibodies was investigated and identified in competition experiments as amino acids 11 to 30 by using synthetic overlapping peptides spanning CVB4E2 VP4 protein [130]. The VP4 protein and a VP4 peptide have been used to detect anti-CVB4 enhancing antibodies by ELISA [26, 130]. The fact that enhancing anti-CVB4 antibodies bind the viral particles through VP4 is challenging, since, according the structural analysis of frozen enteroviruses by X-ray diffraction, the capsid protein VP4 is localized along the inner virion surface, like the amino-terminal sequences of the three external proteins VP1, VP2 and VP3. The explanation lies in the dynamic character of the virus structure at 37°C that would allow an exposure of these normally internal sequences and making a piece of the VP4 protein accessible to antibodies, as it has been shown in the case of the amino-terminal part of VP1 in the poliovirus system [96].

The increased infection of monocytes with CVB4 due to enhancing antibodies could lead, in vivo, in dissemination and worsening of histological lesions that may contribute to CVB4-induced disease, as described in a model of CVB3-induced myocarditis [131, 58, 92]. Furthermore, the enterovirus –induced production of IFN-α enhanced by antibodies, can play a pathogenic role. Indeed, chronic IFN-α synthesis or its abnormal activation in response to recurrent or repeated enteroviral infections can be associated with disorders leading to autoimmune diseases [23].

Further studies are needed to investigate the role of enhancing antibodies in the CVB-induced pathogenesis of T1D.

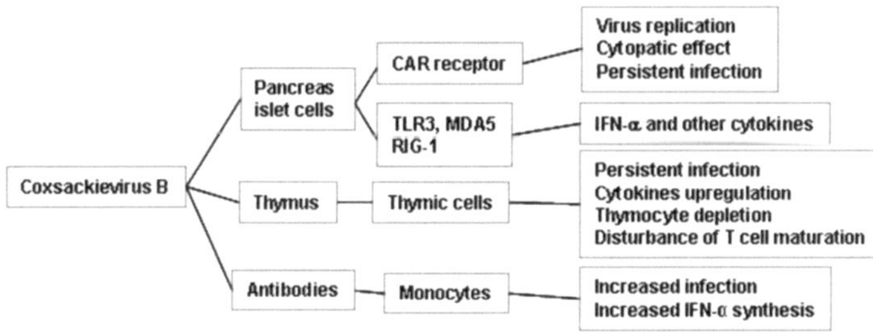

Figure 4. Information brought by in vitro studies regarding coxsackievirus B infection

5.3. Complex relationship between enteroviruses and type 1 diabetes

As mentioned above, the role of enteroviruses in T1D disease is strongly suspected. In contrast, a protective role of enteroviruses is suggested as well. Experimental data in favour of a protective role of these viruses have been reported. Indeed, some studies have shown that, rather than triggering an autoimmune process, CVB infections can provide significant protection against the development of T1D [155, 48]. Coxsackievirus B4, the human enterovirus most associated with an etiologic role in human T1D, has been reported to increase the rate of diabetes onset in older NOD mice but not in younger mice [134]. This result has been confirmed by other groups who provided evidence that disease induction required a pre-existing accumulation of β-cell specific autoreactive T cells within the pancreas, a phenomenon observed in older NOD mice, but not in younger mice [74, 156]. This protective effect may involve the virus strain, its virulence and replication rate, as well as the stage of autoimmune development, and the mechanism relies in long-term tolerance due to an increase in protective regulatory T cells with TGF-β production [49].

These findings support the concept that virus infections occurring early in childhood had a protective effect against T1D and are in agreement with the hygiene hypothesis [7, 157]. Indeed, it should be emphasized that there are significantly more enterovirus infections annually than new cases of T1D in population. The decreased enterovirus exposure rates following the increased hygiene levels might explain the high risk of developing the disease, since it has been revealed in epidemiological studies that T1D incidence is higher in developed countries than in developing ones, from less than 1 per 100,000 inhabitants in Asia to 14 in US and even more than 30 per 100,000 in Scandinavia [139].

6. Conclusion

Type 1 diabetes is a complex multifactorial disease. The involvement of enteroviruses as a major non-genetic etiological factor is a topic of reflexion for several research teams worldwide. Studies from these teams have shown that enteroviral infections, especially coxsackievirus B infections, are closely linked with T1D. Findings from experimental in vitro and in vivo studies have lightened the potent role that can play enteroviruses in inducing and/or worsening the disease. However, in certain particular conditions, enteroviruses can induce a protective effect in mouse model. Therefore, further studies are needed to understand the mechanisms behind this complex relationship between enteroviruses and T1D.

Declaration of interest

No conflict of interest

Acknowledgements

The authors thank Delphine Caloone for technical assistance and all their collaborators. The studies performed by the authors or in progress have been or are supported by EU FP5 VIR-DIAB Project (Contract QLK 2-CT-2001-01910), EU FP6 Integrated Project EURO-THY-MAIDE, (Contract LSHB-CT-2003-503410), EU FP7 PEVNET Project (FP7-HEALTH-2010-single-stage N° 261441), grants from Nord-Pas-de-Calais Région (ArCir convention 2004/018; BBS 2006), CHRU Lille, the ministère de l'Education nationale de la recherche et de la technologie, Université de Lille 2, France, and the comité mixte de coopération universitaire franco-tunisien (CMCU 2004 N○ 04/G0810 and CMCU 2008N808/G0808). Didier Hober was Fondation pour la Recherche Médicale 2008 prize winner. Didier Hober is a member of the VIrus in Diabetes International Study group (VIDIS group).

Author details

Didier Hober[1*], Famara Sané[1], Karena Riedweg[1], Ilham Moumna[1], Anne Goffard[1], Laura Choteau[1], Enagnon Kazali Alidjinou[1] and Rachel Desailloud[2]

*Address all correspondence to: didier.hober@chru-lille.fr

1 Université Lille 2, CHRU, Laboratoire de Virologie/ EA3610, 59037 Lille, France

2 UPJV CHU, Service d'Endocrinologie-Diabétologie-Nutrition, 80054 Amiens, France

References

[1] Aarnisalo, J., Veijola, R., Vainionpaa, R., Simell, O., Knip, M., & Ilonen, J. (2008). Cytomegalovirus infection in early infancy: risk of induction and progression of autoimmunity associated with type 1 diabetes. *Diabetologia* 51(5), 769-72.

[2] Acharya, R., Fry, E., Stuart, D., Fox, G., Rowlands, D., & Brown, F. (1989). The three-dimensional structure of foot-and-mouth disease virus at 2.9 A resolution. *Nature* 337(6209), 709-16.

[3] Ahmad, N., & Abraham, A. A. (1982). Pancreatic isleitis with coxsackie virus B5 infection. *Hum Pathol.* 13(7), 661-2.

[4] Andino, R., Boddeker, N., Silvera, D., & Gamarnik, A. V. (1999). Intracellular determinants of picornavirus replication. *Trends Microbiol.* 7(2), 76-82.

[5] Andreoletti, L., Hober, D., Hober-Vandenberghe, C., Belaich, S., Vantyghem, M. C., Lefebvre, J., & Wattre, P. (1997). Detection of coxsackie B virus RNA sequences in whole blood samples from adult patients at the onset of type I diabetes mellitus. *J Med Virol.* 52(2), 121-7.

[6] Bach, J.F. (2002). The effect of infections on susceptibility to autoimmune and allergic diseases. N *Engl J Med.* 347(12), , 911 EOF-20 EOF.

[7] Bach, J.F. (2005). Infections and autoimmune diseases. *J Autoimmun 25 Suppl.*, 74-80.

[8] Baek, H. S., & Yoon, J. W. (1990). Role of macrophages in the pathogenesis of encephalomyocarditis virus-induced diabetes in mice. *J Virol* 64(12), 5708-15.

[9] Baek, H. S., & Yoon, J. W. (1991). Direct involvement of macrophages in destruction of beta-cells leading to development of diabetes in virus-infected mice. *Diabetes* 40(12), 1586-97.

[10] Balada, E., Vilardell-Tarres, M., & Ordi-Ros, J. (2010). Implication of human endogenous retroviruses in the development of autoimmune diseases. *Int Rev Immunol* 29(4), 351-70.

[11] Beyan, H., Drexhage, R. C., van der Heul, Nieuwenhuijsen. L., de Wit, H., Padmos, R. C., Schloot, N. C., Drexhage, H. A., & Leslie, R. D. (2010). Monocyte gene-expression profiles associated with childhood-onset type 1 diabetes and disease risk: a study of identical twins. *Diabetes* 59(7), 1751-5.

[12] Blixt, M., Niklasson, B., & Sandler, S. (2007). Characterization of beta-cell function of pancreatic islets isolated from bank voles developing glucose intolerance/diabetes: an animal model showing features of both type 1 and type 2 diabetes mellitus, and a possible role of the Ljungan virus. *Gen Comp Endocrinol* 154(1-3), 41-7.

[13] Bortell, R., Pino, S. C., Greiner, D. L., Zipris, D., & Rossini, A. A. (2008). Closing the circle between the bedside and the bench: Toll-like receptors in models of virally induced diabetes. *Ann N Y Acad Sci*, 1150, 112-22.

[14] Brilot, F., Chehadeh, W., Charlet-Renard, C., Martens, H., Geenen, V., & Hober, D. (2002). Persistent infection of human thymic epithelial cells by coxsackievirus B4. *J Virol.* 76(10), 5260-5.

[15] Brilot, F., Geenen, V., Hober, D., & Stoddart, C. A. (2004). Coxsackievirus B4 infection of human fetal thymus cells. *J Virol.* 78(18), 9854-61.

[16] Brilot, F., Jaidane, H., Geenen, V., & Hober, D. (2008). Coxsackievirus B4 infection of murine foetal thymus organ cultures. *J Med Virol.* 80(4), 659-66.

[17] Buesa-Gomez, J., de la Torre, J. C., Dyrberg, T., Landin-Olsson, M., Mauseth, R. S., Lernmark, A., & Oldstone, M. B. (1994). Failure to detect genomic viral sequences in pancreatic tissues from two children with acute-onset diabetes mellitus. *J Med Virol.* 42(2), 193-7.

[18] Burgess, M. A., & Forrest, J. M. (2009). Congenital rubella and diabetes mellitus. *Diabetologia* 52(2), 369-70; author reply 373.

[19] Cameron, C. E., Suk, Oh. H., & Moustafa, I. M. (2010). Expanding knowledge of 3proteins in the poliovirus lifecycle. *Future Microbiol.* 5(6), 867-81.

[20] Chakrabarti, D., Hultgren, B., & Stewart, T. A. (1996). IFN-alpha induces autoimmune T cells through the induction of intracellular adhesion molecule-1 and B7.2. *J Immunol.* 157(2), 522-8.

[21] Champsaur, H., Dussaix, E., Samolyk, D., Fabre, M., Bach, C., & Assan, R. (1980). Diabetes and Coxsackie virus B5 infection. *Lancet* 1(8162), 251.

[22] Chatterjee, N. K., Hou, J., Dockstader, P., & Charbonneau, T. (1992). Coxsackievirus B4 infection alters thymic, splenic, and peripheral lymphocyte repertoire preceding onset of hyperglycemia in mice. *J Med Virol.* 38(2), 124-31.

[23] Chehadeh, W., Kerr-Conte, J., Pattou, F., Alm, G., Lefebvre, J., Wattre, P., & Hober, D. (2000a). Persistent infection of human pancreatic islets by coxsackievirus B is associated with alpha interferon synthesis in beta cells. *J Virol.* 74(21), 10153-64.

[24] Chehadeh, W., Weill, J., Vantyghem, M. C., Alm, G., Lefebvre, J., Wattre, P., & Hober, D. (2000b). Increased level of interferon-alpha in blood of patients with insulin-dependent diabetes mellitus: relationship with coxsackievirus B infection. *J Infect Dis.* 181(6), 1929-39.

[25] Chehadeh, W., Bouzidi, A., Alm, G., Wattre, P., & Hober, D. (2001). Human antibodies isolated from plasma by affinity chromatography increase the coxsackievirus B4induced synthesis of interferon-alpha by human peripheral blood mononuclear cells in vitro. *J Gen Virol.* 82(Pt 8), 1899-907.

[26] Chehadeh, W., Lobert, P. E., Sauter, P., Goffard, A., Lucas, B., Weill, J., Vantyghem, M. C., Alm, G., Pigny, P., & Hober, D. (2005). Viral protein VP4 is a target of human antibodies enhancing coxsackievirus B4and B3-induced synthesis of alpha interferon. *J Virol.* 79(22), 13882-91.

[27] Chiou, C. C., Chung, W. H., Hung, S. I., Yang, L. C., & Hong, H. S. (2006). Fulminant type 1 diabetes mellitus caused by drug hypersensitivity syndrome with human herpesvirus 6 infection. *J Am Acad Dermatol.* 54 (2 Suppl), S, 14-7.

[28] Christen, U., Edelmann, K. H., Mc Gavern, D. B., Wolfe, T., Coon, B., Teague, M. K., Miller, S. D., Oldstone, M. B., & von Herrath, M. G. (2004). A viral epitope that mimics a self antigen can accelerate but not initiate autoimmune diabetes. *J Clin Invest.* 114(9), 1290-8.

[29] Chung, Y. H., Jun, H. S., Kang, Y., Hirasawa, K., Lee, B. R., Van Rooijen, N., & Yoon, J. W. (1997). Role of macrophages and macrophage-derived cytokines in the pathogenesis of Kilham rat virus-induced autoimmune diabetes in diabetes-resistant Bio-Breeding rats. *J Immunol.* 159(1), 466-71.

[30] Chung, Y. H., Jun, H. S., Son, M., Bao, M., Bae, H. Y., Kang, Y., & Yoon, J. W. (2000). Cellular and molecular mechanism for Kilham rat virus-induced autoimmune diabetes in DR-BB rats. *J. Immunol* 165(5), 2866-76.

[31] Clements, G. B., Galbraith, D. N., & Taylor, K. W. (1995). Coxsackie B virus infection and onset of childhood diabetes. *Lancet* 346(8969), 221-3.

[32] Colbere-Garapin, F., Christodoulou, C., Crainic, R., & Pelletier, I. (1989). Persistent poliovirus infection of human neuroblastoma cells. *Proc Natl Acad Sci U S A* 86(19), 7590-4.

[33] Coleman, T. J., Gamble, D. R., & Taylor, K. W. (1973). Diabetes in mice after Coxsackie B 4 virus infection. *Br Med J.* 3(5870), 25-7.

[34] Concannon, P., Rich, S. S., & Nepom, G. T. (2009). Genetics of type 1A diabetes. *N Engl J Med.* 360(16), 1646-54.

[35] Coulson, B. S., Witterick, P. D., Tan, Y., Hewish, M. J., Mountford, J. N., Harrison, L. C., & Honeyman, M. C. (2002). Growth of rotaviruses in primary pancreatic cells. *J Virol* 76(18), 9537-44.

[36] Coutant, R., Carel, J. C., Lebon, P., Bougnères, P. F., Palmer, P., & Cantero-Aguilar, L. (2000). Detection of enterovirus RNA sequences in serum samples from autoantibody-positive subjects at risk for diabetes. *Diabet Med.* 19(11), 968-9.

[37] Craig, M. E., Howard, N. J., Silink, M., & Rawlinson, W. D. (2003). Reduced frequency of HLA DRB1*03DQB1*02 in children with type 1 diabetes associated with enterovirus RNA. *J Infect Dis.* 187(10), 1562-70.

[38] Crampton, S. P., Deane, J. A., Feigenbaum, L., & Bolland, S. (2011). IFIH1 gene dose effect reveals MDA-5 mediated chronic type I IFN gene signature, viral resistance and accelerated autoimmunity. *J Immunol, DOI:In Press.*

[39] Dahlquist, G. G., Forsberg, J., Hagenfeldt, L., Boman, J., & Juto, P. (2004). Increased prevalence of enteroviral RNA in blood spots from newborn children who later developed type 1 diabetes: a population-based case-control study. *Diabetes Care* 27(1), 285-6.

[40] Deonarain, R., Cerullo, D., Fuse, K., Liu, P. P., & Fish, E. N. (2004). Protective role for interferon-beta in coxsackievirus B3 infection. *Circulation* 110(23), 3540-3.

[41] De Stefano, F., Mullooly, J. P., Okoro, C. A., Chen, R. T., Marcy, S. M., Ward, J. I., Vadheim, C. M., Black, S. B., Shinefield, H. R., Davis, R. L., & Bohlke, K. (2001). Childhood vaccinations, vaccination timing, and risk of type 1 diabetes mellitus. *Pediatrics* 108(6), E112.

[42] Di Pietro, C., Del Guercio, M. J., Paolino, G. P., Barbi, M., Ferrante, P., & Chiumello, G. (1979). Type 1 diabetes and Coxsackie virus infection. *Helv Paediatr Acta* 34(6), 557-61.

[43] Dotta, F., Censini, S., van Halteren, A. G., Marselli, L., Masini, M., Dionisi, S., Mosca, F., Boggi, U., Muda, A. O., Prato, S. D., Elliott, J. F., Covacci, A., Rappuoli, R., Roep, B. O., & Marchetti, P. (2007). Coxsackie B4 virus infection of beta cells and natural killer cell insulitis in recent-onset type 1 diabetic patients. *Proc Natl Acad Sci U S A* 104(12), 5115-20.

[44] Dudek, N. L., Thomas, H. E., Mariana, L., Sutherland, R. M., Allison, J., Estella, E., Angstetra, E., Trapani, J. A., Santamaria, P., Lew, A. M., & Kay, T. W. (2006). Cytotoxic T-cells from T-cell receptor transgenic NOD8.3 mice destroy beta-cells via the perforin and Fas pathways. *Diabetes* 55(9), 2412-8.

[45] Eizirik, D. L., Colli, M. L., & Ortis, F. (2009). The role of inflammation in insulitis and beta-cell loss in type 1 diabetes. *Nat Rev Endocrinol.* 5(4), 219-26.

[46] Ejrnaes, M., von, Herrath. M. G., & Christen, U. (2006). Cure of chronic viral infection and virus-induced type 1 diabetes by neutralizing antibodies. *Clin Dev Immunol.* 13(2-4), 337-47.

[47] Ellerman, K. E., Richards, C. A., Guberski, D. L., Shek, W. R., & Like, A. A. (1996). Kilham rat triggers T-cell-dependent autoimmune diabetes in multiple strains of rat. *Diabetes* 45(5), 557-62.

[48] Filippi, C.M., & von Herrath, M.G. (2008). Viral trigger for type 1 diabetes: pros and cons. *Diabetes* 57(11), 2863-71.

[49] Filippi, C. M., Estes, E. A., Oldham, J. E., & von Herrath, M. G. (2009). Immunoregulatory mechanisms triggered by viral infections protect from type 1 diabetes in mice. *J Clin Invest* 119(6), 1515-23.

[50] Flodstrom, M., Maday, A., Balakrishna, D., Cleary, M. M., Yoshimura, A., & Sarvetnick, N. (2002). Target cell defense prevents the development of diabetes after viral infection. *Nat Immunol.* 3(4), 373-82.

[51] Foulis, A. K., Farquharson, M. A., & Meager, A. (1987). Immunoreactive alpha-interferon in insulin-secreting beta cells in type 1 diabetes mellitus. *Lancet* 2 (8573), 1423-7.

[52] Foulis, A. K., Farquharson, M. A., Cameron, S. O., Mc Gill, M., Schonke, H., & Kandolf, R. (1990). A search for the presence of the enteroviral capsid protein VP1 in pancreases of patients with type 1 (insulin-dependent) diabetes and pancreases and hearts of infants who died of coxsackieviral myocarditis. *Diabetologia* 33(5), 290-8.

[53] Foy, C. A., Quirke, P., Lewis, F. A., Futers, T. S., & Bodansky, H. J. (1995). Detection of common viruses using the polymerase chain reaction to assess levels of viral presence in type 1 (insulin-dependent) diabetic patients. *Diabet Med.* 12(11), 1002-8.

[54] Freimuth, P., Philipson, L., & Carson, S. D. (2008). The coxsackievirus and adenovirus receptor. *Curr Top Microbiol Immunol.* , 323, 67-87.

[55] Frisk, G., & Diderholm, H. (2000). Tissue culture of isolated human pancreatic islets infected with different strains of coxsackievirus B4: assessment of virus replication and effects on islet morphology and insulin release. *Int J Exp Diabetes Res.* 1(3), 165-75.

[56] Gale, E.A. (2008). Congenital rubella: citation virus or viral cause of type 1 diabetes? *Diabetologia* 51(9), 1559-66.

[57] Gerling, I., Chatterjee, N. K., & Nejman, C. (1991). Coxsackievirus B4-induced development of antibodies to 64000Mr islet autoantigen and hyperglycemia in mice. *Autoimmunity* 10(1), 49-56.

[58] Girn, J., Kavoosi, M., & Chantler, J. (2002). Enhancement of coxsackievirus B3 infection by antibody to a different coxsackievirus strain. *J Gen Virol.* 83(Pt 2), 351-8.

[59] Goto, A., Takahashi, Y., Kishimoto, M., Nakajima, Y., Nakanishi, K., Kajio, H., & Noda, M. (2008). A case of fulminant type 1 diabetes associated with significant elevation of mumps titers. *Endocr J.* 55(3), 561-4.

[60] Graham, K. L., Sanders, N., Tan, Y., Allison, J., Kay, T. W., & Coulson, B. S. (2008). Rotavirus infection accelerates type 1 diabetes in mice with established insulitis. *J Virol.* 82(13), 6139-49.

[61] Hanafusa, T., & Imagawa, A. (2007). Fulminant type 1 diabetes: a novel clinical entity requiring special attention by all medical practitioners. *Nat Clin Pract Endocrinol Metab* 3(1), 36-45; quiz 2p following 69.

[62] Helmke, K., Otten, A., & Willems, W. (1980). Islet cell antibodies in children with mumps infection. *Lancet* 2(8187), 211-2.

[63] Henke, A., Huber, S., Stelzner, A., & Whitton, J. L. (1995). The role of CD8+ T lymphocytes in coxsackievirus B3induced myocarditis. *J Virol.* 69(11), 6720-8.

[64] Hiemstra, H. S., Schloot, N. C., van Veelen, P. A., Willemen, S. J., Franken, K. L., van Rood, J. J., de Vries, R. R., Chaudhuri, A., Behan, P. O., Drijfhout, J. W., & Roep, B. O. (2001). Cytomegalovirus in autoimmunity: T cell crossreactivity to viral antigen and autoantigen glutamic acid decarboxylase. *Proc Natl Acad Sci U S A* 98(7), 3988-91.

[65] Hillebrands, J. L., van der Werf, N., Klatter, F. A., Bruggeman, C. A., & Rozing, J. (2003). Role of peritoneal macrophages in cytomegalovirus-induced acceleration of autoimmune diabetes in BB-rats. *Clin Dev Immunol.* 10(2-4), 133-9.

[66] Hober, D., Chehadeh, W., Bouzidi, A., & Wattre, P. (2001). Antibody-dependent enhancement of coxsackievirus B4 infectivity of human peripheral blood mononuclear cells results in increased interferon-alpha synthesis. *J Infect Dis.* 184(9), 1098-108.

[67] Hober, D., Chehadeh, W., Weill, J., Hober, C., Vantyghem, M. C., Gronnier, P., & Wattre, P. (2002). Circulating and cell-bound antibodies increase coxsackievirus B4in-

duced production of IFN-alpha by peripheral blood mononuclear cells from patients with type 1 diabetes. *J Gen Virol.* 83(Pt 9), 2169-76.

[68] Hogle, J.M. (2002). Poliovirus cell entry: common structural themes in viral cell entry pathways. *Annu Rev Microbiol.*, 56, 677-702.

[69] Hogle, J. M., Chow, M., & Filman, D. J. (1985). Three-dimensional structure of poliovirus at 2.9 A resolution. *Science* 229(4720), 1358-65.

[70] Honeyman, M. C., Coulson, B. S., Stone, N. L., Gellert, S. A., Goldwater, P. N., Steele, C. E., Couper, J. J., Tait, B. D., Colman, P. G., & Harrison, L. C. (2000). Association between rotavirus infection and pancreatic islet autoimmunity in children at risk of developing type 1 diabetes. *Diabetes* 49(8), 1319-24.

[71] Honeyman, M. C., & Harrison, L. C. (2009). Congenital rubella, diabetes and HLA. *Diabetologia* 52(2), 371-2; author reply 373.

[72] Honeyman, M. C., Stone, N. L., Falk, B. A., Nepom, G., & Harrison, L. C. (2010). Evidence for molecular mimicry between human T cell epitopes in rotavirus and pancreatic islet autoantigens. *J Immunol.* 184(4), 2204-10.

[73] Horwitz, M. S., Bradley, L. M., Harbertson, J., Krahl, T., Lee, J., & Sarvetnick, N. (1998). Diabetes induced by Coxsackie virus: initiation by bystander damage and not molecular mimicry. *Nat Med.* 4(7), 781-5.

[74] Horwitz, M. S., Fine, C., Ilic, A., & Sarvetnick, N. (2001). Requirements for viral-mediated autoimmune diabetes: beta-cell damage and immune infiltration. *J Autoimmun.* 16(3), 211-7.

[75] Horwitz, M. S., Ilic, A., Fine, C., Balasa, B., & Sarvetnick, N. (2004). Coxsackieviral-mediated diabetes: induction requires antigen-presenting cells and is accompanied by phagocytosis of beta cells. *Clin Immunol.* 110(2), 134-44.

[76] Huang, X., Yuang, J., Goddard, A., Foulis, A., James, R. F., Lernmark, A., Pujol-Borrell, R., Rabinovitch, A., Somoza, N., & Stewart, T. A. (1995). Interferon expression in the pancreases of patients with type I diabetes. *Diabetes* 44(6),658-64.

[77] Hultcrantz, M., Huhn, M. H., Wolf, M., Olsson, A., Jacobson, S., Williams, B. R., Korsgren, O., & Flodstrom-Tullberg, M. (2007). Interferons induce an antiviral state in human pancreatic islet cells. *Virology* 367(1), 92-101.

[78] Hviid, A., Stellfeld, M., Wohlfahrt, J., & Melbye, M. (2004). Childhood vaccination and type 1 diabetes. *N Engl J Med.* 350(14), 1398-404.

[79] Hyoty, H., Hiltunen, M., Reunanen, A., Leinikki, P., Vesikari, T., Lounamaa, R., Tuomilehto, J., & Akerblom, H. K. (1993a). Decline of mumps antibodies in type 1 (insulin-dependent) diabetic children and a plateau in the rising incidence of type 1 diabetes after introduction of the mumps-measles-rubella vaccine in Finland. Childhood Diabetes in Finland Study Group. *Diabetologia* 36(12), 1303-8.

[80] Hyoty, H., Parkkonen, P., Rode, M., Bakke, O., & Leinikki, P. (1993b). Common peptide epitope in mumps virus nucleocapsid protein and MHC class II-associated invariant chain. *Scand J Immunol.* 37(5), 550-8.

[81] Jaidane, H., Gharbi, J., Lobert, P. E., Caloone, D., Lucas, B., Sane, F., Idziorek, T., Romond, M. B., Aouni, M., & Hober, D. (2008). Infection of primary cultures of murine splenic and thymic cells with coxsackievirus B4. *Microbiol Immunol.* 52(1), 40-6.

[82] Jaidane, H., & Hober, D. (2008). Role of coxsackievirus B4 in the pathogenesis of type 1 diabetes. *Diabetes Metab.* 34(6 Pt 1), 537-48.

[83] Jaidane, H., Sane, F., Gharbi, J., Aouni, M., Romond, M. B., & Hober, D. (2009). Coxsackievirus B4 and type 1 diabetes pathogenesis: contribution of animal models. *Diabetes Metab Res Rev.* 25(7), 591-603.

[84] Jun, H. S., Kang, Y., Notkins, A. L., & Yoon, J. W. (1997). Gain or loss of diabetogenicity resulting from a single point mutation in recombinant encephalomyocarditis virus. *J Virol.* 71(12), 9782-5.

[85] Jun, H. S., Kang, Y., Yoon, H. S., Kim, K. H., Notkins, A. L., & Yoon, J. W. (1998). Determination of encephalomyocarditis viral diabetogenicity by a putative binding site of the viral capsid protein. *Diabetes* 47(4), 576-82.

[86] Kallewaard, N. L., Zhang, L., Chen, J. W., Guttenberg, M., Sanchez, M. D., & Bergelson, J. M. (2009). Tissue-specific deletion of the coxsackievirus and adenovirus receptor protects mice from virus-induced pancreatitis and myocarditis. *Cell Host Microbe* 6(1), 91-8.

[87] Kanazawa, Y., Komeda, K., Sato, S., Mori, S., Akanuma, K., & Takaku, F. (1984). Non-obese-diabetic mice: immune mechanisms of pancreatic beta-cell destruction. *Diabetologia* 27 Suppl,, 113-5.

[88] Kasuga, A., Harada, R., & Saruta, T. (1996). Insulin-dependent diabetes mellitus associated with parvovirus B19 infection. *Ann Intern Med.* 125(8), 700-1.

[89] Kaufman, D. L., Clare-Salzler, M., Tian, J., Forsthuber, T., Ting, G. S., Robinson, P., Atkinson, M. A., Sercarz, E. E., Tobin, A. J., & Lehmann, P. V. (1993). Spontaneous loss of T-cell tolerance to glutamic acid decarboxylase in murine insulin-dependent diabetes. *Nature*, 69-72.

[90] Kawashima, H., Ihara, T., Ioi, H., Oana, S., Sato, S., Kato, N., Takami, T., Kashiwagi, Y., Takekuma, K., Hoshika, A., & Mori, T. (2004). Enterovirus-related type 1 diabetes mellitus and antibodies to glutamic acid decarboxylase in Japan. *J Infect.* 49(2), 147-51.

[91] Kemball, C. C., Alirezaei, M., & Whitton, J. L. (2010). Type B coxsackieviruses and their interactions with the innate and adaptive immune systems. *Future Microbiol.* 5(9),, 1329-1347.

[92] Kishimoto, C., Kurokawa, M., & Ochiai, H. (2002). Antibody-mediated immune enhancement in coxsackievirus B3 myocarditis. *J Mol Cell Cardiol* 34(9),, 1227 -1238 .

[93] Klemola, P., Kaijalainen, S., Ylipaasto, P., & Roivainen, M. (2008). Diabetogenic effects of the most prevalent enteroviruses in Finnish sewage. *Ann N Y Acad Sci.*, 1150, 210-2.

[94] Kondrashova, A., Reunanen, A., Romanov, A., Karvonen, A., Viskari, H., Vesikari, T., Ilonen, J., Knip, M., & Hyoty, H. (2005). A six-fold gradient in the incidence of type 1 diabetes at the eastern border of Finland. *Ann Med.* 37(1),, 67 -72 .

[95] Korostoff, J. M., Nakada, M. T., Faas, S. J., Blank, K. J., & Gaulton, G. N. (1990). Neonatal exposure to thymotropic gross murine leukemia virus induces virus-specific immunologic nonresponsiveness. *J Exp Med.* 172(6), 1765-75.

[96] Li, Q., Yafal, A. G., Lee, Y. M., Hogle, J., & Chow, M. (1994). Poliovirus neutralization by antibodies to internal epitopes of VP4 and VP1 results from reversible exposure of these sequences at physiological temperature. *J Virol.* 68(6), 3965-70.

[97] Lin, J. Y., Chen, T. C., Weng, K. F., Chang, S. C., Chen, L. L., & Shih, S. R. (2009). Viral and host proteins involved in picornavirus life cycle. *J Biomed Sci.* 16, 103.

[98] Lindberg, B., Ahlfors, K., Carlsson, A., Ericsson, U. B., Landin-Olsson, M., Lernmark, A., Ludvigsson, J., Sundkvist, G., & Ivarsson, S. A. (1999). Previous exposure to measles, mumps, and rubella--but not vaccination during adolescence--correlates to the prevalence of pancreatic and thyroid autoantibodies. *Pediatrics* 104(1), e12.

[99] Lonnrot, M., Salminen, K., Knip, M., Savola, K., Kulmala, P., Leinikki, P., Hyypia, T., Akerblom, H. K., & Hyoty, H. (2000). Enterovirus RNA in serum is a risk factor for beta-cell autoimmunity and clinical type 1 diabetes: a prospective study. Childhood Diabetes in Finland (DiMe) Study Group. *J Med Virol.* 61(2), 214-20.

[100] Maha, M. M., Ali, M. A., Abdel-Rehim, S. E., Abu-Shady, E. A., El -Naggar, B. M., & Maha, Y. Z. (2003). The role of coxsackieviruses infection in the children of insulin dependent diabetes mellitus. *J Egypt Public Health Assoc.* 78(3-4), 305-18.

[101] Marguerat, S., Wang, W. Y., Todd, J. A., & Conrad, B. (2004). Association of human endogenous retrovirus K-18 polymorphisms with type 1 diabetes. *Diabetes* 53(3), 852-4.

[102] Mc Cartney, S. A., Vermi, W., Lonardi, S., Rossini, C., Otero, K., Calderon, B., Gilfillan, S., Diamond, M. S., Unanue, E. R., & Colonna, M. (2011). RNA sensor-induced type I IFN prevents diabetes caused by a beta cell-tropic virus in mice. *J Clin Invest.*

[103] Mena, I., Perry, C. M., Harkins, S., Rodriguez, F., Gebhard, J., & Whitton, J. L. (1999). The role of B lymphocytes in coxsackievirus B3 infection. *Am J Pathol.* 155(4), 1205-15.

[104] Moya-Suri, V., Schlosser, M., Zimmermann, K., Rjasanowski, I., Gurtler, L., & Mentel, R. (2005). Enterovirus RNA sequences in sera of schoolchildren in the general popu-

lation and their association with type 1diabetes-associated autoantibodies. *J Med Microbiol.* 54(Pt 9), 879-83.

[105] Muckelbauer, J. K., Kremer, M., Minor, I., Diana, G., Dutko, F. J., Groarke, J., Pevear, D. C., & Rossmann, M. G. (1995). The structure of coxsackievirus B3 at 3.5 A resolution. *Structure* 3(7), 653-67.

[106] Munakata, Y., Kodera, T., Saito, T., & Sasaki, T. (2005). Rheumatoid arthritis, type 1 diabetes, and Graves' disease after acute parvovirus B19 infection. *Lancet* 366(9487), 780.

[107] Nair, S., Leung, K. C., Rawlinson, W. D., Naing, Z., & Craig, M. E. (2010). Enterovirus infection induces cytokine and chemokine expression in insulin-producing cells. *J Med Virol.* 82(11), 1950-7.

[108] Nairn, C., Galbraith, D. N., Taylor, K. W., & Clements, G. B. (1999). Enterovirus variants in the serum of children at the onset of Type 1 diabetes mellitus. *Diabet Med.* 16(6), 509-13.

[109] Niklasson, B., Heller, K. E., Schonecker, B., Bildsoe, M., Daniels, T., Hampe, C. S., Widlund, P., Simonson, W. T., Schaefer, J. B., Rutledge, E., Bekris, L., Lindberg, A. M., Johansson, S., Ortqvist, E., Persson, B., & Lernmark, A. (2003). Development of type 1 diabetes in wild bank voles associated with islet autoantibodies and the novel ljungan virus. *Int J Exp Diabesity Res.* 4(1), 35-44.

[110] Niklasson, B., Samsioe, A., Blixt, M., Sandler, S., Sjoholm, A., Lagerquist, E., Lernmark, A., & Klitz, W. (2006). Prenatal viral exposure followed by adult stress produces glucose intolerance in a mouse model. *Diabetologia* 49(9), 2192-9.

[111] Nugent, C. I., Johnson, K. L., Sarnow, P., & Kirkegaard, K. (1999). Functional coupling between replication and packaging of poliovirus replicon RNA. *J Virol,* 73(1), 427-35.

[112] Numazaki, K., Goldman, H., Wong, I., & Wainberg, M. A. (1988). Viral infection of human fetal islets of Langerhans. Replication of human cytomegalovirus in cultured human fetal pancreatic islets. *Am J Clin Pathol.* 90(1), 52-7.

[113] O'Brayan, T. A., Beck, M. J., Demers, L. M., & Naides, S. J. (2005). Human parvovirus B19 infection in children with new onset Type 1 diabetes mellitus. *Diabet Med.* 22(12), 1778-9.

[114] Oikarinen, M., Tauriainen, S., Honkanen, T., Oikarinen, S., Vuori, K., Kaukinen, K., Rantala, I., Maki, M., & Hyoty, H. (2008). Detection of enteroviruses in the intestine of type 1 diabetic patients.*Clin Exp Immunol.* 151(1), 71-5.

[115] Oikarinen, S., Martiskainen, M., Tauriainen, S., Huhtala, H., Ilonen, J., Veijola, R., Simell, O., Knip, M., & Hyoty, H. (2011). Enterovirus RNA in blood is linked to the development of type 1 diabetes. *Diabetes* 60(1), 276-9.

[116] Oldstone, M. B., Nerenberg, M., Southern, P., Price, J., & Lewicki, H. (1991). Virus infection triggers insulin-dependent diabetes mellitus in a transgenic model: role of anti-self (virus) immune response. *Cell* 65(2), 319-31.

[117] Olsson, A., Johansson, U., Korsgren, O., & Frisk, G. (2005). Inflammatory gene expression in Coxsackievirus B-4infected human islets of Langerhans. *Biochem Biophys Res Commun* 330(2), 571-6.

[118] Ou, D., Mitchell, L. A., Metzger, D. L., Gillam, S., & Tingle, A. J. (2000). Cross-reactive rubella virus and glutamic acid decarboxylase (65 and 67) protein determinants recognised by T cells of patients with type I diabetes mellitus. *Diabetologia* 43(6), 750-62.

[119] Parkkonen, P., Hyoty, H., Koskinen, L., & Leinikki, P. (1992). Mumps virus infects beta cells in human fetal islet cell cultures upregulating the expression of HLA class I molecules. *Diabetologia* 35(1), 63-9.

[120] Ramondetti, F., Sacco, S., Comelli, M., Bruno, G., Falorni, A., Iannilli, A., D'Annunzio, G., Iafusco, D., Songini, M., Toni, S., Cherubini, V., & Carle, F. (2011). RIDI study group. Type 1 diabetes and measles, mumps and rubella chilhood infections within the Italian Insulin-dependent diabetes Regitstry. *Diabet Med*, 1464-5491.

[121] Rayfield, E. J., Kelly, K. J., & Yoon, J. W. (1986). Rubella virus-induced diabetes in the hamster. *Diabetes* 35(11), 1278-81.

[122] Richardson, S. J., Willcox, A., Bone, A. J., Foulis, A. K., & Morgan, N. G. (2009). The prevalence of enteroviral capsid protein vp1 immunostaining in pancreatic islets in human type 1 diabetes. *Diabetologia* 52(6), 1143-51.

[123] Richer, M. J., Lavallee, D. J., Shanina, I., & Horwitz, M. S. (2009). Toll-like receptor 3 signaling on macrophages is required for survival following coxsackievirus B4 infection. *PLoS One* 4(1), e4127.

[124] Roivainen, M., Rasilainen, S., Ylipaasto, P., Nissinen, R., Ustinov, J., Bouwens, L., Eizirik, D. L., Hovi, T., & Otonkoski, T. (2000). Mechanisms of coxsackievirus-induced damage to human pancreatic beta-cells. *J Clin Endocrinol Metab* 85(1), 432-40.

[125] Salminen, K. K., Vuorinen, T., Oikarinen, S., Helminen, M., Simell, S., Knip, M., Ilonen, J., Simell, O., & Hyoty, H. (2004). Isolation of enterovirus strains from children with preclinical Type 1 diabetes. *Diabet Med.* 21(2), 156-64.

[126] Sano, H., Terasaki, J., Tsutsumi, C., Imagawa, A., & Hanafusa, T. (2008). A case of fulminant type 1 diabetes mellitus after influenza B infection. *Diabetes Res Clin Pract.* 79(3), e, 8-9.

[127] Sarmiento, L., Cabrera-Rode, E., Lekuleni, L., Cuba, I., Molina, G., Fonseca, M., Heng-Hung, L., Borroto, A. D., Gonzalez, P., Mas-Lago, P., & Diaz-Horta, O. (2007). Occurrence of enterovirus RNA in serum of children with newly diagnosed type 1 diabetes and islet cell autoantibody-positive subjects in a population with a low incidence of type 1 diabetes. *Autoimmunity* 40(7), 540-5.

[128] Sato, K., Inaba, Y., Shinozaki, T., Fujii, R., & Matumoto, M. (1981). Isolation of human rotavirus in cell cultures: brief report. *Arch Virol.* 69(2), 155-60.

[129] Sauter, P., Lobert, P. E., Lucas, B., Varela-Calvino, R., Alm, G., Wattre, P., & Hober, D. (2007). Role of the capsid protein VP4 in the plasma-dependent enhancement of the Coxsackievirus B4E2infection of human peripheral blood cells. *Virus Res.* 125(2), 183-90.

[130] Sauter, P., Chehadeh, W., Lobert, P. E., Lazrek, M., Goffard, A., Soumillon, M., Caloone, D., Vantyghem, M. C., Weill, J., Fajardy, I., Alm, G., Lucas, B., & Hober, D. (2008). A part of the VP4 capsid protein exhibited by coxsackievirus B4 E2 is the target of antibodies contained in plasma from patients with type 1 diabetes. *J Med Virol.* 80(5), 866-78.

[131] Sauter, P., & Hober, D. (2009). Mechanisms and results of the antibody-dependent enhancement of viral infections and role in the pathogenesis of coxsackievirus B-induced diseases. *Microbes Infect.* 11(4), 443-51.

[132] Schulte, B. M., Bakkers, J., Lanke, K. H., Melchers, W. J., Westerlaken, C., Allebes, W., Aanstoot, H. J., Bruining, G. J., Adema, G. J., Van Kuppeveld, F. J., & Galama, J. M. (2010). Detection of enterovirus RNA in peripheral blood mononuclear cells of type 1 diabetic patients beyond the stage of acute infection. *Viral Immunol.* 23(1), 99-104.

[133] See, D. M., & Tilles, J. G. (1995). Pathogenesis of virus-induced diabetes in mice. *J Infect Dis.* 171(5), 1131-8.

[134] Serreze, D. V., Ottendorfer, E. W., Ellis, T. M., Gauntt, C. J., & Atkinson, M. A. (2000). Acceleration of type 1 diabetes by a coxsackievirus infection requires a preexisting critical mass of autoreactive T-cells in pancreatic islets. *Diabetes* 49(5), 708-11.

[135] Shimada, A., & Maruyama, T. (2004). Encephalomyocarditis-virus-induced diabetes model resembles "fulminant" type 1 diabetes in humans. *Diabetologia* 47(10), 1854-5.

[136] Singer, K. H., & Haynes, B. F. (1987). Epithelial-thymocyte interactions in human thymus. *Hum Immunol* 20(2), 127-44.

[137] Smelt, M. J., Faas, M. M., de Haan, B. J., Hofstede, J., Cheung, C. W., van der Iest, H., de Haan, A., & de Vos, P. (2010). Rat pancreatic beta cells and cytomegalovirus infection. *Pancreas* 39(1), 47-56.

[138] Smyth, M.S., & Martin, J.H. (2002). Picornavirus uncoating. *Mol Pathol.* 55(4), 214-9.

[139] Soltesz, G., Patterson, C. C., & Dahlquist, G. (2007). Worldwide childhood type 1 diabetes incidence--what can we learn from epidemiology? *Pediatr Diabetes 8 Suppl.*, 6, 6-14.

[140] Stark, G.R. (2007). How cells respond to interferons revisited: from early history to current complexity. *Cytokine Growth Factor Rev.* 18(5-6),, 419 -423 .

[141] Stene, L. C., Oikarinen, S., Hyoty, H., Barriga, K. J., Norris, J. M., Klingensmith, G., Hutton, J. C., Erlich, H. A., Eisenbarth, G. S., & Rewers, M. (2010). Enterovirus infec-

tion and progression from islet autoimmunity to type 1 diabetes: the Diabetes and Autoimmunity Study in the Young (DAISY). *Diabetes* 59(12), 3174-80.

[142] Stewart, T. A., Hultgren, B., Huang, X., Pitts-Meek, S., Hully, J., & Mac, Lachlan. N. J. (1993). Induction of type I diabetes by interferon-alpha in transgenic mice. *Science* 260(5116), 1942-6.

[143] Sutkowski, N., Conrad, B., Thorley-Lawson, D. A., & Huber, B. T. (2001). Epstein-Barr virus transactivates the human endogenous retrovirus HERV-K18 that encodes a superantigen. *Immunity* 15(4), 579-89.

[144] Tai, A. K., Luka, J., Ablashi, D., & Huber, B. T. (2009). HHV-6A infection induces expression of HERV-K18encoded superantigen. *J Clin Virol.* 46(1), 47-8.

[145] Takada, A., & Kawaoka, Y. (2003). Antibody-dependent enhancement of viral infection: molecular mechanisms and in vivo implications. *Rev Med Virol.* 13(6), 387-98.

[146] Takeuchi, O., & Akira, S. (2008). MDA5/RIG-I and virus recognition. *Curr Opin Immunol.* 20(1), 17-22.

[147] Taniguchi, T., Okazaki, K., Okamoto, M., Seko, S., Nagashima, K., Yamada, Y., Iwakura, T., & Seino, Y. (2005). Autoantibodies against the exocrine pancreas in fulminant type 1 diabetes. *Pancreas* 30(2), 191-2.

[148] Tapia, G., Cinek, O., Rasmussen, T., Grinde, B., Stene, L. C., & Ronningen, K. S. (2011a). Longitudinal study of parechovirus infection in infancy and risk of repeated positivity for multiple islet autoantibodies: the MIDIA study. *Pediatr Diabetes* 12(1), 58-62.

[149] Tapia, G., Cinek, O., Rasmussen, T., Witso, E., Grinde, B., Stene, L. C., & Ronningen, K. S. (2011b). Human enterovirus RNA in monthly fecal samples and islet autoimmunity in Norwegian children with high genetic risk for type 1 diabetes: the MIDIA study. *Diabetes Care* 34(1), 151-5.

[150] The Juvenile Diabetes Research Foundation: The Network for Pancreatic Organ Donors with Diabetes. www.jdrfnpod.org.

[151] Tian, J., Lehmann, P. V., & Kaufman, D. L. (1994). T cell cross-reactivity between coxsackievirus and glutamate decarboxylase is associated with a murine diabetes susceptibility allele. *J Exp Med.* 180(5), 1979-84.

[152] Tisch, R., Yang, X. D., Singer, S. M., Liblau, R. S., Fugger, L., & Mc Devitt, H. O. (1993). Immune response to glutamic acid decarboxylase correlates with insulitis in non-obese diabetic mice. *Nature* 366(6450), 72-5.

[153] Toniolo, A., Onodera, T., Yoon, J. W., & Notkins, A. L. (1980). Induction of diabetes by cumulative environmental insults from viruses and chemicals. *Nature* 288(5789), 383-5.

[154] Toniolo, A., Maccari, G., Federico, G., Salvatoni, A., Bianchi, G., & Baj, A. (2010). Are enterovirus infections linked to the early stages of type 1 diabetes? *American Society for Microbiology Meeting, San Diego, CA.*

[155] Tracy, S., Drescher, K. M., Chapman, N. M., Kim, K. S., Carson, S. D., Pirruccello, S., Lane, P. H., Romero, J. R., & Leser, J. S. (2002). Toward testing the hypothesis that group B coxsackieviruses (CVB) trigger insulin-dependent diabetes: inoculating non-obese diabetic mice with CVB markedly lowers diabetes incidence. *J Virol.* 76(23), 12097-111.

[156] Tracy, S., & Drescher, K. M. (2007). Coxsackievirus infections and NOD mice: relevant models of protection from, and induction of, type 1 diabetes. *Ann N Y Acad Sci.*, 1103, 143-51.

[157] Tracy, S., Drescher, K. M., Jackson, J. D., Kim, K., & Kono, K. (2010). Enteroviruses, type 1 diabetes and hygiene: a complex relationship. *Rev Med Virol.* 20(2), 106-16.

[158] Tracy, S., Drescher, K. M., & Chapman, N. M. (2011). Enteroviruses and type 1 diabetes. *Diabetes metab Res rev.* 27(8), 820-3.

[159] Tuthill, T. J., Groppelli, E., Hogle, J. M., & Rowlands, D. J. (2010). Picornaviruses. *Curr Top Microbiol Immunol*, 343, 43-89.

[160] van Belle, T.L., Coppieters, K.T., & von Herrath, M.G. (2011). Type 1 diabetes: etiology, immunology, and therapeutic strategies. *Physiol Rev.* 91(1), 79-118.

[161] van der Werf, N., Hillebrands, J. L., Klatter, F. A., Bos, I., Bruggeman, C. A., & Rozing, J. (2003). Cytomegalovirus infection modulates cellular immunity in an experimental model for autoimmune diabetes. *Clin Dev Immunol.* 10(2-4), 153-60.

[162] van der Werf, N., Kroese, F. G. M., Rozing, J., & Hillebrands, J. L. (2007). Viral infections as potential triggers of type 1 diabetes. *Diabetes Metab Res Rev.* (23), 169-83.

[163] Vehik, K., & Dabelea, D. (2011). The changing epidemiology of type 1 diabetes: why is it going through the roof? *Diabetes Metab Res Rev.* 27(1), 3-13.

[164] Vigeant, P., Menard, H. A., & Boire, G. (1994). Chronic modulation of the autoimmune response following parvovirus B19 infection. *J Rheumatol* 21(6), 1165-7.

[165] Viskari, H., Paronen, J., Keskinen, P., Simell, S., Zawilinska, B., Zgorniak-Nowosielska, I., Korhonen, S., Ilonen, J., Simell, O., Haapala, A. M., Knip, M., & Hyoty, H. (2003). Humoral beta-cell autoimmunity is rare in patients with the congenital rubella syndrome. *Clin Exp Immunol.* 133(3), 378-83.

[166] von, Poblotzki. A., Gerdes, C., Reischl, U., Wolf, H., & Modrow, S. (1996). Lymphoproliferative responses after infection with human parvovirus B19. *J Virol* 70(10), 7327-30.

[167] Vuorinen, T., Nikolakaros, G., Simell, O., Hyypia, T., & Vainionpaa, R. (1992). Mumps and Coxsackie B3 virus infection of human fetal pancreatic islet-like cell clusters. *Pancreas* 7(4), 460-4.

[168] Wang, J. P., Asher, D. R., Chan, M., Kurt-Jones, E. A., & Finberg, R. W. (2007). Cutting Edge: Antibody-mediated TLR7dependent recognition of viral RNA. *J Immunol.* 178(6), 3363-7.

[169] Wessely, R., Klingel, K., Knowlton, K. U., & Kandolf, R. (2001). Cardioselective infection with coxsackievirus B3 requires intact type I interferon signaling: implications for mortality and early viral replication. *Circulation* 103(5), 756-61.

[170] Wicker, L. S., Todd, J. A., & Peterson, L. B. (1995). Genetic control of autoimmune diabetes in the NOD mouse. *Annu Rev Immunol.*, 13, 179-200.

[171] Yin, H., Berg, A. K., Tuvemo, T., & Frisk, G. (2002). Enterovirus RNA is found in peripheral blood mononuclear cells in a majority of type 1 diabetic children at onset. *Diabetes* 51(6), 1964-71.

[172] Ylipaasto, P., Klingel, K., Lindberg, A. M., Otonkoski, T., Kandolf, R., Hovi, T., & Roivainen, M. (2004). Enterovirus infection in human pancreatic islet cells, islet tropism in vivo and receptor involvement in cultured islet beta cells. *Diabetologia* 47(2), 225-39.

[173] Ylipaasto, P., Kutlu, B., Rasilainen, S., Rasschaert, J., Salmela, K., Teerijoki, H., Korsgren, O., Lahesmaa, R., Hovi, T., Eizirik, D. L., Otonkoski, T., & Roivainen, M. (2005). Global profiling of coxsackievirus- and cytokine-induced gene expression in human pancreatic islets. *Diabetologia* 48(8), 1510-22.

[174] Yoon, J. W., Onodera, T., & Notkins, A. L. (1978). Virus-induced diabetes mellitus. XV. Beta cell damage and insulin-dependent hyperglycemia in mice infected with coxsackie virus B4. *J Exp Med.* 148(4), 1068-80.

[175] Yoon, J. W., Austin, M., Onodera, T., & Notkins, A. L. (1979). Isolation of a virus from the pancreas of a child with diabetic ketoacidosis. *N Engl J Med.* 300(21), 1173-9.

[176] Yoon, J. W., & Jun, H. S. (2006). Viruses cause type 1 diabetes in animals. *Ann N Y Acad Sci.*, 1079, 138-46.

[177] Zanone, M. M., Favaro, E., Quadri, R., Miceli, I., Giaretta, F., Romagnoli, R., David, E., Perin, P. C., Salizzoni, M., & Camussi, G. (2010). Association of cytomegalovirus infections with recurrence of humoral and cellular autoimmunity to islet autoantigens and of type 1 diabetes in a pancreas transplanted patient. *Transpl Int.* 23(3), 333-7.

[178] Zipris, D., Hillebrands, J. L., Welsh, R. M., Rozing, J., Xie, J. X., Mordes, J. P., Greiner, D. L., & Rossini, A. A. (2003). Infections that induce autoimmune diabetes in BBDR rats modulate CD4+CD25+ T cell populations. *J Immunol.* 170(7), 3592-602.

[179] Zipris, D., Lien, E., Nair, A., Xie, J. X., Greiner, D. L., Mordes, J. P., & Rossini, A. A. (2007). TLR9signaling pathways are involved in Kilham rat virus-induced autoimmune diabetes in the biobreeding diabetes-resistant rat. *J Immunol.* 178(2), 693-701.

Section 2

Genetics

Chapter 3

Update of Type 1 Diabetes

Mohamed M. Jahromi

Additional information is available at the end of the chapter

http://dx.doi.org/10.5772/55960

1. Introduction

Diabetes is one of the fastest growing diseases. World health organization estimates that approximately 340 million people have type 1 diabetes and this number increases by 3-5% each year so the type 1 diabetes population reached 25 million by 2010. Type 1 diabetes is an autoimmune disease that is caused as a result of destruction of pancreatic β-cells. Several factors may contribute to the pathogenesis of type 1 diabetes. Genetic susceptibility of type 1 diabetes is determined by polymorphisms/mutations in multiple genes in both human and animal models.

The Major Histocomapatibility Complex (MHC) accounts for approximately 40% of the familial aggregation of type 1 diabetes and the insulin gene for only 10 % suggesting the existence of additional loci. The gene for "Protein Tyrosine Phosphatase, Non-receptor type 22 (lymphoid)."PTPN22, the lymphocyte signaling molecule, on chromosome 1p13.3–p13.1 is a confirmed locus that contributes to multiple autoimmune disorders, including type 1 diabetes. Diabetes associated Cytotoxic T - Lymphocyte Antigen 4 (CTLA-4) locus polymorphisms in most populations have relative risks less than 1.5. A fundamental question is whether there are genetic polymorphisms that confer major risk for type 1 diabetes, other than the Human Leukocyte Antigen (HLA) DR and DQ alleles (class II HLA alleles). Recently, genes outside MHC region have considered playing an important role in the onset of diabetes.

As accumulative report suggest the role of olfactory receptor in the pathogenesis of diabetic microvascular and other diabetic complications, undoubtedly, this haplotype specific alteration of type 1 diabetes risk is an independent risk for the disease and can address the promising MHC-linked gene other than DR/DQ. Moreover, there is nothing to hinder for that this might be a signal that identify the role of olfactory receptor gene in the pathogenesis of type 1 diabetes in patients who are prone to diabetic complications.

Diabetes is one of the fastest growing diseases. Diabetes affects today an estimated 371 million people world-wide compared to 366 million by the end of 2011. Of course this includes 20 million to 40 million of patients with type 1 diabetes. While type 1 diabetes accounts for 5% to 20% of those with diabetes, it is associated with higher morbidity, mortality and health care cost than the more prevalent type 2 diabetes. Overall, 4.8 million people died and $ 471 billion were spent due to diabetes in 2012 [1-2].

New figures indicate that the number of people living with diabetes is expected to rise from 371 million in 2012 to 552 million by 2030, if no urgent action is taken. This equates to approximately three new cases every ten seconds or almost ten million per year. International diabetes federation also estimated that almost half of the people with diabetes are unaware that they have diabetes [2].

In some of the poorest regions in the world such as Africa, where infectious diseases have traditionally been the focus of health care systems, diabetes cases are expected to increase by 90% by 2030. At least 78% of people in Africa are undiagnosed and do not know they are living with diabetes (Figure 1):

- 80% of people with diabetes live in low and middle income countries.
- 78,000 children develop type 1 diabetes every year
- The greatest number of people with diabetes is between 40-59 years of age [2].

2. Why is there an increasing trend in the incidence of diabetes?

In the past, most diabetics were known to have a genetic tendency towards the disease. However, that trend has rapidly given way in the past few decades to other causes, at least from a statistical perspective. These genetically-independent trends that explain the growth in the incidence of diabetes can be summarized as follows: (a) overall growth in population, (b) increased life expectancy resulting in a higher ratio of aged population more prone to diabetes, (c) increasing obesity trends, (d) unhealthy diets and (e) sedentary lifestyles.

In other words, diabetes has increasingly become a lifestyle-related disease as it afflicts young and old, in developed and developing nations, around the world. As the number of patients grows across the globe, there has never been a stronger and more urgent need for therapeutic measures that arrest the growth of the disease and alleviate its secondary manifestations.

Middle East & North Africa: 1 in 9 adults in this region have diabetes; More than half of people with diabetes in this region don't know they have it. Europe: 1 out of every 3 dollars spent on diabetes healthcare was spent in this region; 21.2 million people in this region have diabetes and don't know it. Western Pacific: 1 in 3 adults with diabetes lives in this region; 6 of the top 10 countries for diabetes prevalence are Pacific Islands. South & Central America: Only 5% of all healthcare dollars for diabetes were spent in this region; 1 in 11 adults in this region has diabetes. Africa: Over the next 20 years, the number of people with diabetes in the region will almost double; This region has the highest mortality rate due to diabetes. South East Asia: 1

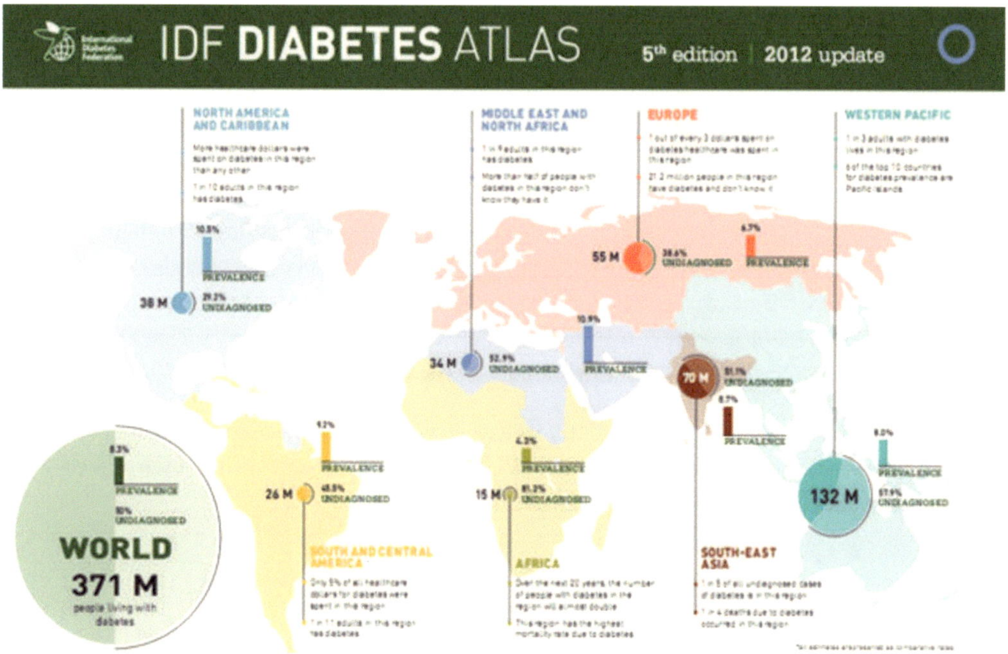

Figure 1. According to international diabetes federation5th edition; 2012the number of diabetes increases to 371 million. North America & Caribean: More healthcare dollars were spent on diabetes in this region than any other; 1 in 10 adults in this region has diabetes.

in 5 of all undiagnosed cases of diabetes is in this region; 1 in 4 deaths due to diabetes occurred in this region [2]

2.1. Pathogenesis

Type 1 diabetes develops slowly and progressive abnormalities in beta cell-function herald what appears to be a sudden development of hyperglycemia. Rising the hemoglobin A1c test (HbA1c) in the normal range[3], impaired fasting or glucose tolerance, as well as loss of first phase insulin secretion usually precede overt diabetes. The exact beta cell mass remaining at diagnosis is poorly defined and there are almost no studies of insulitis prior to diabetes onset [4]. For patients with long-term type 1 diabetes there is evidence of some beta cell function remaining (C-peptide secretion) though beta cell mass is usually decreased to less than 1% of normal [5]. At present methods to image/quantitate beta cell mass and insulitis are only beginning to be developed. In particular Positron Emission Tomography (PET) scanning utilizing a labeled amine (dihydrotetrabenazine) may provide the first method to image islet mass [6] and this is now being evaluated in man. A number of techniques are being evaluated to image insulitis [7].

A large body of evidence indicates that the development of type 1 diabetes is determined by a balance between pathogenic and regulatory T lymphocytes [8]. A fundamental question is whether there is a primary autoantigen for initial T cell autoreactivity with subsequent recognition of multiple islet antigens. A number of investigators have addressed in the Non-Obese Diabetic (NOD) mouse (spontaneously develops type 1 diabetes) the importance of immune reactivity to insulin with the dramatic finding that eliminating immune responses to insulin blocks development of diabetes and insulitis, and importantly immune responses to downstream autoantigens such as the Islet specific molecule Glucose-6-phosphatase catalytic subunit-Related Protein(IGRP) [9]. Knocking out both insulin genes (mice in contrast to humans have two insulin genes) with introduction of a mutated insulin with alanine rather than tyrosine at position 16 of the insulin B chain prevents development of diabetes [10]. Recognition of this B-chain peptide of insulin by T lymphocytes depends upon a "non-stringent" T cell receptor with conservation of only the alpha chain sequence (Valpha and Jalpha) and not the N-region of the alpha chain, or the Beta chain [11].

As in other immune diseases both genetic factors as well as environmental factors contribute in the pathogenesis of the disease (Figure 2). Environmental factors exert their effects ones genetic susceptibility factors already exist.

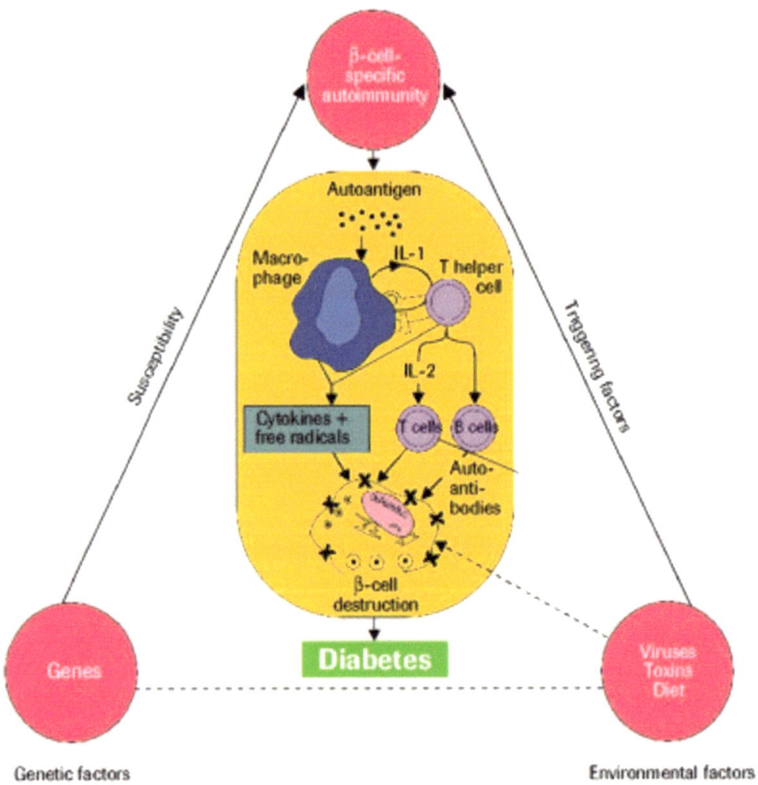

Figure 2. A schematic figure shows how environmental factors trigger TYPE 1 DIABETES onset in genetically susceptible persons which ends to the process of β-cell-specific autoimmunity processes which lead to the destruction of pancreatic β-cell. As antigen presenting cell is triggered by auto antigens it releases intiinfalmatory cytokines eg IL-1 that signals T-helper 1 class to activate B-cell and T cell in order to release autoantibodies to attach pancreatic β-cell.

3. Genetic factors

A mutation of the Forkhead bOX Protein 3 (FOXP3 gene, a transcription factor that controls the development of regulatory T cells is a cause of neonatal diabetes [12]. The syndrome is termed IPEX (Immune dysregulation, Polyendocrinopathy, Enteropathy, X-linked) syndrome. As reflected in the name, children with disorder suffer from overwhelming autoimmunity and usually die as infants. Of note bone marrow transplantation can reverse disease. IPEX syndrome is rare, as is neonatal diabetes. In the differential diagnosis of neonatal diabetes it must be recognized that half of children developing permanent neonatal diabetes have a mutation of the Kir6.2 molecule of the sulfonylurea receptor. These children with their non-autoimmune form of diabetes can be treated with oral sulfonylurea therapy.

Though more common than IPEX syndrome, the Autoimmune Polyendocrine Syndrome Type 1 (APS-1) syndrome is also rare. It results from a mutation of the "autoimmune regulator" AIRE gene, another transcription factor [13]. Approximately 15% of patients with this syndrome develop autoimmune diabetes. The leading hypothesis as to etiology (e.g. Addison's disease, mucocutaneous candidiasis, and hypoparathyroidism) is that AIRE controls expression of autoantigens and negative selection of autoreactive T lymphocytes within the thymus. A very recent dramatic discovery is the demonstration that essentially 100% of patients with Autoimmune Polyendocrine Syndrome type 1 (APS-1) have autoantibodies reacting with interferon alpha and other interferons. Such autoantibodies are extremely rare and essentially not found in patients with type 1 diabetes or Addison's disease outside of the syndrome.

Patients with type 1 diabetes and their relatives are at risk for development of thyroid autoimmunity, celiac disease, Addison's disease, pernicious anemia and a series of other autoimmune disorders [14]. Approximately 1/20 patients with type 1 diabetes have celiac disease by biopsy though the majority have no symptoms [15]. These asymptomatic individuals are usually detected with screening for transglutaminase autoantibodies. The level of transglutaminase autoantibodies relates to the probability of a positive biopsy and it is important for clinicians to know the threshold for likely positive biopsy for the assay they employ [16]. There remains controversy as to whether asymptomatic celiac disease when detected should be treated with a gluten free diet and large clinical trials are needed to address this question.

3.1. MHC genes

Type 1 diabetes has become one of the most intensively studied polygenic disorders. There are MHC as well as non-MHC genes or loci candidate to contribute in the genetic susceptibility to type 1 diabetes pathogenesis. According to the recent version of the National Center for Biotechnology Information (NCBI) map viewer these genes are located on all human chromosomes [17] (Figure 3). The strongest associations with both susceptibility and protection from type 1 diabetes are HLA DR and DQ molecules. For instance DQB1*0602 alleles are associated with dominant protection and DR3-DQ2 molecules (DQB1*0201) and DR4-DQ8 (DQB1*0302) with susceptibility [18].

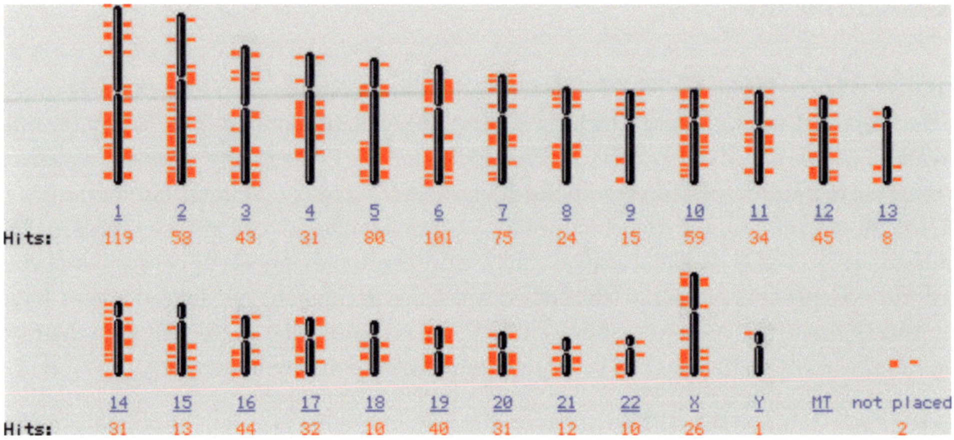

Figure 3. A schematic projection of type 1 diabetes susceptible genes location according to 2012 version of NCBI map viewer. Type 1 diabetes susceptible genes were reported on all chromosome of human[17].

Type 1 diabetes is a T cell organ specific autoimmune disease [19] with approximately 40% of the familial aggregation accounted for by the MHC region [20-21]. Nevertheless, it is generally assumed that the positive predictive value of MHC alleles is relatively low given the complex genetics and potential multiple environmental factors hypothesized to contribute to diabetes risk. However, approximately 1/2 to 1/3 of U.S. children who develop type 1 diabetes prior to age 15 have the highest risk DR/DQ genotype (HLA-DRB1*03-DQA1*0501-DQB1*0201/ DRB1*04-DQA1*0301-DQB1*0302, DR3-DQB1*02-01/DR4-DQB1*0302) [22-25]. Pursuing the hypothesis that additional major determinants of Type 1 diabetes risk (in addition to DR/ DQ genes) are within or close to the MHC region, highly conserved HLA-F [24-32].

Recently, OR gene have been associated with different diseases which support the hypothesis of the importance of OR in CNS in addition to smell [33]. Increasing studies suggest significant association among SNP in OR genes that link autoimmunity, psychiatric disorders, and smell impairment [33-36].

Interestingly, a large cluster of the human OR family 14, subfamily J and member 1gene (OR14J1) were found in proximity to the HLA-F, and so they were called "MHC-linked" OR-genes [1, 37-38]. Olfactory Receptor (OR) is our Central Nervous System (CNS) external messenger which translates the information from the odorant into neural pulses, a window for our mind. In addition, the important role of CNS in the pathogenesis of type 1 diabetes any variation in the genetic make-up of the OR might lead to the destruction of its function and notably malfunction of the CNS. The OR14J1C allele of OR gene in the conserved region of HLA-F showed a significant association with type 1 diabetes, except the known diabetogenic DQ/DR genes [39].

3.2. Non–MHC genes

Although important, the MHC susceptibility genes are not sufficient to induce type 1 diabetes, suggesting polygenic inheritance in most cases [40]. An important component of the susceptibility to type 1 diabetes resides in certain non-MHC genes that have an effect only in the presence of the appropriate MHC alleles.

In particular, polymorphisms of a promoter of the insulin gene and an amino acid change of PTPN22 are associated with the risk of TYPE 1 DIABETES in multiple populations [4-6]. A repeat sequence in the 5' region of the insulin gene is associated with greater insulin expression in the thymus and it is hypothesized that this contributes to decreasing the development of diabetes [7]. The polymorphism of the lymphocyte-specific tyrosine phosphatase gene influences T cell receptor signaling, and the same polymorphism is a major risk factor for multiple autoimmune disorders [8].

A polymorphism in the cytotoxic T-lymphocyte-associated antigen-4 gene was shown to be associated with the risk of type 1 diabetes in a meta-analysis of 33 studies involving over 5000 patients [9]. Other genes are implicated in risk for type 1 diabetes (eg, CTLA-4) [10] and other genetic loci, but their influence is very small, or so small that replication has been difficult.

Additional evidence for the role of non-MHC genes comes from studies in NOD (nonobese diabetic) mice. These mice develop spontaneous autoimmune diabetes with striking similarities to type 1 diabetes in humans [11]. Autoimmune infiltration of the islets of Langerhans (insulitis) begins at about 50 days of age and clinical diabetes appears at about 120 days.

Interferon (IFN-γ)+ T cells (Th1 cells) appear to be an important mediator of the insulitis in NOD mice, and destruction of the islet cells can be slowed by the administration of anti- IFN-γ antibodies. IFN-γ -inducing factor (IGIF; also called interleukin (IL)-18) and IL-12 are potent inducers of IFN-γ, and the progression of insulitis begins in parallel with increased release of these two cytokines(kent et al 2005). IGIF gene expression is upregulated in NOD mice, and the location of the IGIF gene suggests that it is a candidate gene for susceptibility to type 1 diabetes [41].Genetically altered (knockout) mice deficient in IL-18 had hyperphagia, obesity, hyperinsulinemia, and hyperglycemia; intracerebral administration of recombinant IL-18 decreased food intake and reversed hyperglycemia (Bach 2002). A new locus associated with type 1 diabetes, has been identified near the gene encoding the p40 subunit of IL12B in NOD mice [42].

It was initially thought that, in contrast to Th1 cells, Th2 cells (which produce IL-4, -5, -10, and -13) protected against the onset and progression of type 1 diabetes. However, Th2 cells also are capable of inducing islet-cell destruction, and therefore the onset and progression of type 1 diabetes are probably under the control of both Th1 and Th2 cells [1,43].

In our extensive cytokine gene polymorphisms effect on type 1 diabetes immunogenetics (44-46]we have shown clearly that a single nucleotide polymorphism (SNP) in the genetic of IL-4 gene, however, would contribute to the domination of T-h-1 cell to Th2 (IL-4) [46], lack of action of IL-4, the th2 cytokine initiator. Further, a Single Nucleotide Polymorphism (SNP) in the Transforming Growth Factor (TGF)-β gene ends up to lower production of TGF- β protein level. That may contribute to the lack of immunosuppressive effect of TGF- β in the pathogenesis of type 1 diabetes [47].

4. Environmental factors

During the last decades, the incidence of type 1 diabetes has increased significantly, reaching percentages of 3% annually worldwide. This increase suggests that besides genetic factors environmental perturbations (including viral infections) are also involved in the pathogenesis of type 1 diabetes.

There is a number of environmental factors contribute to the marked global variation in the incidence of type 1 diabetes. Evidence suggests that the incidence is lower in the tropics compared with further north or south of the equator.

Assuming that the observation that there is a direct relationship between incidence of type 1 diabetes and equatorial distance, a number of environmental factors appear to be protective against the development of an autoimmune pathological process. Ultra violet radiation results in increased levels of vitamin D, which is an important modulator of the immune system. Detailed studies have shown not only that lower levels of circulating vitamin D predispose to autoimmunity, but that vitamin D supplementation may also reduce the risk of developing type 1 diabetes (vitamin D). Further data are required to establish the clinical utility and cost-effectiveness of such interventions, including the demonstration of these positive effects over a longer period of time.

Other dietary considerations may also be important, with avoidance of cow's milk at an early age seemingly providing protection against autoimmunity. Again, it is unclear as to whether or not use of hydrolysed infant formulae instead of cow's milk for weaning will be of significant clinical benefit, as long-term prospective data of this type are lacking. However, the fact that cereal exposure at a young age may also provoke increased autoimmune activity reinforces the notion that antigen ingestion may affect immune system function.

The role for infectious agents in type 1 diabetes remains unclear, as there are variations on the hygiene hypothesis which suggest that certain infections may prove protective whereas others may be pathogenic. Certainly, evidence in animal models convincingly demonstrates an association between viral antigens and autoimmunity and human biopsies have shown viral particles in the pancreas of type 1 diabetes patients. However, there is a lack of data demonstrating a causal effect for viral infections. Furthermore, the intriguing prospect that parasitic infections may protect against type 1 diabetes requires further study, so that molecular mechanisms may be elucidated for therapeutic purposes.

Future research needs to be conducted on a large scale, with the inclusion of both randomised and prospective studies in order to establish the link between environmental factors and type 1 diabetes pathogenesis. In particular, long-term follow-up of infants is required to assess the true benefits of interventional trials. In addition, consideration of the interaction of genetics with environmental factors is necessary to complete the picture, as it is likely that both mechanisms are involved in determining geographical variation of disease [18, 48].

Environmental influences are another important factor in the development of type 1 diabetes. This has been illustrated in twin studies; less than 50 percent of monozygotic twins of probands with type 1 diabetes develop diabetes [49-50]. These observations are most likely explained by environmental factors such as viruses and dietary antigens.

5. Autoimmunity

Islet Cell Autoantibodies (ICAs) were first detected in serum from patients with autoimmune polyendocrine deficiency; they have subsequently been identified in 70 to 80 percent of patients with newly diagnosed type 1 diabetes and in prediabetic subjects (American Diabetic Association 1997). Measurement of serum ICA by staining of frozen sections of human pancreas was the major screening test used to identify subjects at risk for clinical diabetes but currently, large studies utilize a series of radioassays for autoantibodies reacting with specific islet autoantigens.

Children with type 1 diabetes who do not have islet-cell or other autoantibodies at presentation have a similar degree of metabolic decompensation as do children who have these antibodies, although those with more of the different types of antibodies appear to have the most accelerated islet destruction and a higher requirement for exogenous insulin during the second year of clinical disease [51]. A few patients without obvious evidence of islet autoimmunity have been described in whom the onset of hyperglycemia was abrupt, glycosylated hemoglobin values were normal, and serum pancreatic enzyme concentrations were high [52].

Autoantibodies to biochemically characterized beta-cell autoantigens: Insulin Autoantibodies (IAA), Auto-antibodies to the tyrosine phosphatases IA-2, Glutamic Acid Decarboxylase Autoantibodies (GADA), and zinc transporter 8 autoantibody (ZnT8A) [53] help to define type 1 diabetes a, if measured prior to or shortly after initiation of insulin therapy. IAA are masked by antibodies induced by exogenous insulin and become very hard to measure after just 10 to 14 days of insulin therapy. ZnT8A tend to disappear quickly after diagnosis of diabetes, while GADA and IA-2A tend to persist longer, but are rarely seen more than 5 years after diagnosis. Testing for at least two of these autoantibodies at diagnosis is now considered standard of care in type 1 diabetes. Good commercial assays exist for IA-2A, GADA, and ZnT8A, with the former two recently harmonized [54]. IAA are low-affinity antibodies and harder to measure; however, high-quality non-radioactive assays for IAA are close to being commercially available [55]. The search for additional islet autoantibodies and assay that would reliably detect autoreactive T-lymphocytes are active areas of research.

6. Complications

The management of type 1 diabetes and modalities for prevention of complications has evolved, such that the majority of patients with excellent care and education should avoid major microvascular complications. The finding from the Diabetes Control and Complications Trial (DCCT) follow-up study of "metabolic memory", namely long term benefit from early intensive glucose management is very encouraging [56]. Intensive management and strict guidelines for lipid lowering and early introduction of renoprotective medications are the norm. Laser therapy for advanced retinal disease is also the norm and "anti- Vascular endothelial growth factor (VEGF)" ocular therapy for macular edema is being extensively studied. Effective prevention of microvascular complications requires detection of early lesions, including determination of lipids, blood pressure, microalbuminuria, retinal exams. Preventative foot care and cardiovascular evaluation are also essential, with macrovascular disease a major problem for patients with long-term diabetes. Patients with type 1 diabetes have more severe progressive coronary artery atherosclerosis for any level of Low-density lipoprotein (LDL) cholesterol (57-586-57). Neuropathy remains difficult to treat [59] despite introduction of several newer medications.

Patients with diabetes and renal failure have a particularly poor prognosis when on dialysis. Every effort should be directed toward "early" renal transplantation in patients with type 1 diabetes and renal failure.

Genetic factors and key gene mutations have been implicated in the pathogenesis of diabetes. However, increasing evidence suggests that complex interactions between genes and the environment may play a major role in many common human diseases such as diabetes and its complications [39, 59-73]. Furthermore, the increased risk for both type 1 diabetes and type 2 diabetes can be controlled through medications, changes in dietary habits and increased exercise; subjects with diabetes continue to be plagued with numerous life-threatening complications. This continued development of diabetic complications even after achieving glucose control suggests a metabolic memory of prior glycemic exposure and indicates a missing link in diabetes etiology which recent studies have suggested may be attributed to epigenetic changes in target cells without alterations in gene coding sequences. Exploring a role for epigenetics in diabetic complications could allow for new insights clarifying the interplay between the environment and gene regulation and identify much needed new therapeutic targets.

Diabetic microvascular complications have been reported to be encountered with impairment in the olfactory system. Recently we have shown that polymorphism in the olfactory receptor, OR14J1C, may lead to an olfactory impairment that could be due to presence of microvascular diseases or other complication directly related to type 1 diabetes. The genetic alteration in the OR14J1 gene, A to C, could be linked to epigenetic processes [39].

6.1. What are common consequences of diabetes?

Over time, diabetes can damage the heart, blood vessels, eyes, kidneys, and nerves.

- Diabetes increases the risk of heart disease and stroke. 50% of people with diabetes die of cardiovascular disease (primarily heart disease and stroke).

- Combined with reduced blood flow, neuropathy in the feet increases the chance of foot ulcers and eventual limb amputation.

- Diabetic retinopathy is an important cause of blindness, and occurs as a result of long-term accumulated damage to the small blood vessels in the retina. After 15 years of diabetes, approximately 2% of people become blind, and about 10% develop severe visual impairment.

http://dx.doi.org/10.5772/55960

- Diabetes is among the leading causes of kidney failure. 10-20% of people with diabetes die of kidney failure.
- Diabetic neuropathy is damage to the nerves as a result of diabetes, and affects up to 50% of people with diabetes. Although many different problems can occur as a result of diabetic neuropathy, common symptoms are tingling, pain, numbness, or weakness in the feet and hands.
- The overall risk of dying among people with diabetes is at least double the risk of their peers without diabetes.

7. Conclusion

Type 1 diabetes has become perhaps the most intensively studied autoimmune illness results from autoimmune destruction of the insulin-producing ß-cells in the islets of Langerhans. This process occurs in genetically susceptible subjects, is probably triggered by one or more environmental agents, and usually progresses over many months or years during which the subject is asymptomatic and euglycemic. This long latent period is a reflection of the large number of functioning β-cells that must be lost before hyperglycemia occurs.

Polymorphisms in MHC genes and Non-MHC genes account for genetic susceptibility of the diseases. Genes in both the MHC and elsewhere in the genome have influence risk, but only HLA alleles have a large effect.

There are a number of autoantigens within the pancreatic ß-cells that may play important roles in the initiation or progression of autoimmune islet injury and its autoimmunity which might be a good prediction factor. Environmental factors that may affect risk include pregnancy-related and perinatal influences, viruses, and ingestion of cows' milk and cereals.

Author details

Mohamed M. Jahromi*

Address all correspondence to: mjahromi@yahoo.com

Pathology Department, Salmaniya Medical Complex, Ministry of Health, Manama, Kingdom of Bahrain

References

[1] Marian RowersChallenges in Diagnosing Type 1 diabetes in Different Populations. Diabetes Metab J. (2012). , 36, 90-97.

[2] http://wwwidf.org/diabetesatlas

[3] Stene, L. C, Barriga, K, Hoffman, M, et al. Normal but increasing hemoglobin A1c levels predict progression from islet autoimmunity to overt type 1 diabetes: Diabetes Autoimmunity Study in the Young (DAISY). Pediatr Diabetes (2006). , 7(5), 247-253.

[4] Gianani, R, Putnam, A, Still, T, et al. Initial results of screening of non- diabetic organ donors for expression of islet autoantibodies. J Clin Endocrinol Metab (2006). , 91, 1855-1861.

[5] Meier, J. J, Bhushan, A, Butler, A. E, Rizza, R. A, & Butler, P. C. Sustained beta cell apoptosis in patients with long-standing type 1 diabetes: indirect evidence for islet regeneration? Diabetologia (2005). , 48(11), 2221-2228.

[6] Souza, F, Simpson, N, Raffo, A, et al. Longitudinal noninvasive PET-based beta cell mass estimates in a spontaneous diabetes rat model. J Clin Invest (2006). , 116(6), 1506-1513.

[7] Turvey, S. E, Swart, E, Denis, M. C, et al. Noninvasive imaging of pancreatic inflammation and its reversal in type 1 diabetes. J Clin Invest (2005). , 115(9), 2454-2461.

[8] Chatenoud, L, & Bach, J. F. Regulatory T cells in the control of autoimmune diabetes: the case of the NOD mouse. Int Rev Immunol (2005).

[9] Krishnamurthy, B, Dudek, N. L, Mckenzie, M. D, et al. Responses against islet antigens in NOD mice are prevented by tolerance to proinsulin but not IGRP. J Clin Invest (2006). , 116(12), 3258-3265.

[10] Nakayama, M, Abiru, N, Moriyama, H, et al. Prime role for an insulin epitope in the development of type 1 diabetes in NOD mice. Nature (2005). , 435(7039), 220-223.

[11] Homann, D, & Eisenbarth, G. S. An immunologic homunculus for type 1 diabetes. Journal of Clinical Investigation (2006). , 116(5), 1212-1215.

[12] Wildin, R. S, & Freitas, A. IPEX and FOXP3: Clinical and research perspectives. J Autoimmun (2005). Suppl: , 56-62.

[13] Su, M. A, & Anderson, M. S. Aire: an update. Curr Opin Immunol (2004). , 16(6), 746-752.

[14] wwwncbi.nlm.nih.gov

[15] Barker, J. M, Yu, J, Yu, L, et al. Autoantibody "sub-specificity" in type 1 diabetes: Risk for organ specific autoimmunity clusters in distinct groups. Diab care (2005). , 28, 850-855.

[16] Hoffenberg, E. J, Emery, L. M, Barriga, K. J, et al. Clinical features of children with screening-identified evidence of celiac disease. peds (2004). , 113(5), 1254-1259.

[17] Liu, E, Li, M, Bao, F, et al. Need for quantitative assessment of transglutaminase autoantibodies for celiac disease in screening-identified children. J Pediatr (2005). , 146(4), 494-499.

[18] Jahromi, M. M, & Eisenbarth, G. S. Genetic Determinants of type 1 diabetes Across Populations. Ann NY Acad Sci (2006). , 289-299.

[19] Kornete, J. M, & Piccirillo, C. A. Critical co-stimulatory pathways in the stability of Foxp3+ Treg cell homeostasis in Type I diabetes. Autoimmun Rev. (2011). , 11, 104-111.

[20] Noble, J. A, Valdes, A. M, Cook, M, Klitz, W, Thomson, g, & Erlich, H. A. The role of HLA class II genes in insulin-dependent diabetes mellitus: molecular analysis of 180 Caucasian, multiplex families.Am. J. Hum. Genet (1996). , 59, 1134-1148.

[21] Lambert, A. P, Gillespie, K. M, Thomson, G, Cordell, H. J, Todd, J. A, & Gale, E. A. and Bingley PJ. Absolute risk of childhood-onset type 1 diabetes defined by human leukocyte antigen class II genotype: a population-based study in the United Kingdom. J. Clin. Endocrinol. Metab (2004). , 89, 4037-4043.

[22] Rewers, M, Bugawan, T. L, Norris, J. M, Blair, A, Beaty, B, Hoffman, M, et al. Newborn screening for HLA markers associated with IDDM: diabetes autoimmunity study in the young (DAISY). Diabetologia (1996). , 39, 807-812.

[23] Johansson, S, Lie, B. A, Todd, J. A J. A, Pociot, F, Nerup, J, & Cambon-thomsen, A. et al. Evidence of at least two type 1 diabetes susceptibility genes in the HLA complex distinct from HLA-DQB1,-DQA1 and-DRB1. Genes Immun (2003). , 4, 46-53.

[24] Aly, T. A, Ide, A, Jahromi, M. M, Barker, J. M, Fernando, M. S, Babu, S. R, et al. Extreme Genetic Risk for Type 1A Diabetes. Proc Natl Acad Sci U S A (2006). , 103, 14074-14079.

[25] Cheung, Y. H, Watkinson, J, & Anastassiou, D. Conditional meta-analysis stratifying on detailed HLA genotypes identifies a novel type 1 diabetes locus around TCF19 in the MHC. Hum Genet (2011). , 129, 161-176.

[26] Nejentsev, S, Howson, J. M, Walker, N. M, Szeszko, J, Field, S. F, Stevens, H. E, et al. The Wellcome Trust Case Control Consortium, Clayton DG, and Todd JA. Localization of type 1 diabetes susceptibility to the MHC class I genes HLA-B and HLA-A. Nature (2007). , 450, 887-892.

[27] Erlich, H, Valdes, A. M, Noble, J, Carlson, J. A, Varney, M, Concannon, P, et al. HLA DR-DQ haplotypes and genotypes and type 1 diabetes risk: analysis of the type 1 diabetes genetics consortium families. Diabetes. (2008). , 57, 1084-1092.

[28] Aly, T. A, Baschal, E. E, Jahromi, M. M, Fernando, M. S, Babu, S. R, Fingerlin, T. E, et al. Analysis of Single Nucleotide Polymorphisms Identifies Major Type 1A Diabetes Locus Telomeric of the Major Histocompatibility Complex.Diabetes (2008). , 57, 770-776.

[29] Baschal, E. E, Aly, T. A, Jasinski, J. M, Steck, A. K, Johnson, K. N, Noble, J. A, et al. The frequent and conserved DR3-B8-A1 extended haplotype confers less diabetes risk than other DR3 haplotypes. Diabetes Obes Metab (2009)., 11, 25-30.

[30] Concannon, P, Chen, W. M, Julier, C, Morahan, G, Akolkar, B, Erlich, H. A, et al. Genome-wide scan for linkage to TYPE 1 DIABETES in 2,496 multiplex families from the TYPE 1 DIABETES Genetics Consortium. Diabetes (2009)., 58, 1018-1022.

[31] Pociot, F, Akolkar, B, Concannon, P, Erlich, H. A, Julier, C, Morahan, G, et al. Genetics of TYPE 1 DIABETES: what's next? Diabetes (2010)., 59, 1561-1571.

[32] Zhang, B. Y, Zhang, J, & Liu, J. S. Block-Based Bayesian Epistasis Association Mapping With Application To Wtccc Type 1 Diabetes Data. Ann Appl Stat (2011). , 5, 2052-2077.

[33] Orozco, G, Barton, A, Eyre, S, Din, B, Worthington, J, Ke, X, Thomson, W, & Hla-dpb1-col, A. and three additional xMHC loci are independently associated with RA in a UK cohort. Genes and Immunity (2011)., 12, 169-175.

[34] NakaokaCui T, Tajima A, Oka A, Mitsunaga S, Kashiwase K, Homma Y, Sato S, Suzuki Y, Inoko H, Inoue I. A Systems Genetics Approach Provides a Bridge from Discovered Genetic Variants to Biological Pathways in Rheumatoid Arthritis. PLoS ONE ;(2011). e25389.

[35] Zhao, Y, Jiang, Z, & Guo, C. New hope for type 2 diabetics: targeting insulin resistance through the immune modulation of stem cells. Autoimmun Rev. (2011). , 11, 137-42.

[36] Takabatake, N, Toriyama, S, Takeishi, Y, Shibata, Y, Konta, T, Inoue, S, et al. A non-functioning single nucleotide polymorphism in olfactory receptor gene family is associated with the forced expiratory volume in the first second/the forced vital capacity values of pulmonary function test in a Japanese population. Biochem Biophys Res Commun. (2007)., 364, 662-667.

[37] Younger, R. M, Amadou, C, Bethel, G, Ehlers, A, Lindahl, K. F, Forbes, S, et al. Characterization of clustered MHC-linked olfactory receptor-genes in human and mouse. Genome Res (2001)., 11, 519-530.

[38] Santos, C. J, Uehara, S, Ziegler, A, & Uchanska-ziegler, B. Bicalho Mda G. Variation and linkage disequilibrium within odorant receptor gene clusters linked to the human major histocompatibility complex. Hum Immunol (2010)., 719, 843-850.

[39] Jahromi, M. M. HAPLOTYPE SPECIFIC ALTERATION OF DIABETES MHC RISK BY OLFACTORY RECEPTOR GENE POLYMORPHISM. Autoimmun Rev. (2012). May 8.

[40] Field, S. F, Howson, J. M, Smyth, D. J, Walker, N. M, Dunger, D. B, & Todd, J. A. Analysis of the type 2 diabetes gene, TCF7L2, in 13,795 TYPE 1 DIABETES cases and control subjects. Diabetologia (2007)., 2007, 212-213.

[41] Kent, S. C, Chen, Y, Bregoli, L, et al. Expanded T cells from pancreatic lymph nodes of type 1 diabetic subjects recognize an insulin epitope. Nature (2005). , 435(7039), 224-228.

[42] Ouyang, Q, Standifer, N. E, Qin, H, et al. Recognition of HLA Class I-Restricted {beta}-Cell Epitopes in TYPE 1 DIABETES. Diabetes (2006). , 55(11), 3068-3074.

[43] Achenbach, P, Warncke, K, Reiter, J, et al. TYPE 1 DIABETES risk assessment: improvement by follow-up measurements in young islet autoantibody-positive relatives. Diabetologia (2006). , 49(12), 2969-2976.

[44] Jahromi, M. M, Millward, B. A, & Demaine, A. G. The 5′ flanking G (-174) C region of the IL-6 gene polymorphism is highly associated with TYPE 1 DIABETES millitus. J Interferon and Cytokine Research; (2000). , 2000, 885-888.

[45] Cartwright, N, Demaine, A, Jahromi, M, Sanders, H, & Kaminski, E. A study of cytokine protein secretion, frequencies of cytokine expressing cells and IFN-G gene polymorphisms in normal individuals. J Transplantation (1999). , 10, 1546-1552.

[46] Jahromi, M. M, Millward, B. A, & Demaine, A. G. A CA repeat polymorphism of the interfron-γ gene is highly associated with TYPE 1 DIABETES: IFNG and IL-4 gene polymorphism and TYPE 1 DIABETES. J Interferon and Cytokine Research; (2000). , 20, 187-190.

[47] Jahromi, M. M, Millward, B. A, & Demaine, A. G. Significant Correlation between Association of Polymorphism in Codon 10 of the TGF-β1 T (29) C with TYPE 1 DIABETES and Patients with Nephropathy Disorder.J Interferon and Cytokine Research (2010).

[48] Alruhaili, M. Type 1 diabetes in the tropics: the protective effects of environmental factors. AJDM(2010). , 18, 1-8.

[49] American Diabetes AssociationReport of the Expert Committee on the Diagnosis and Classification of Diabetes Mellitus. Diab care (1997). , 20(7), 1183-1197.

[50] Wang, J, Miao, D, Babu, S, et al. Autoantibody negative diabetes is not rare at all ages and increases with older age and obesity. J Clin Endocrinol Metab (2007). , 92(11), 88-92.

[51] Gale, E. A. Latent autoimmune diabetes in adults: a guide for the perplexed. Diabetologia (2005). , 48(11), 2195-2199.

[52] Barker, J. M, Goehrig, S. H, Barriga, K, et al. Clinical characteristics of children diagnosed with TYPE 1 DIABETES through intensive screening and follow-up. Diab care (2004). , 27(6), 1399-1404.

[53] Fariba Vaziri-SaniAhmed J. Delli, Helena Elding-Larsson, Bengt Lindblad, Annelie Carlsson, Gun Forsander, Sten A. Ivarsson, Johnny Ludvigsson, Claude Marcus, and Åke Lernmark, on behalf of the Swedish Better Diabetes Diagnosis Study Group. A novel triple mix radiobinding assay for the three ZnT8 (ZnT8-RWQ) autoantibody

variants in children with newly diagnosed diabetes. J Immuno Methods (2011). , 371, 25-37.

[54] Bonifacio, E, Yu, L, Williams, A. K, Eisenbarth, G. S, Bingley, P. J, Marcovina, S. M, Adler, K, Ziegler, A. G, Mueller, P. W, Schatz, D. A, Krischer, J. P, Steffes, M. W, & Akolkar, B. Harmonization of glutamic acid decarboxylase and islet antigen-2 autoantibody assays for national institute of diabetes and digestive and kidney diseases consortia. J Clin Endocrinol Metab. (2010). , 95, 3360-3367.

[55] Yu, L, Miao, D, Scrimgeour, L, Johnson, K, Rewers, M, & Eisenbarth, G. S. Distinguishing persistent insulin autoantibodies with differential risk: nonradioactive bivalent proinsulin/insulin autoantibody assay. Diabetes. (2012). , 61, 179-186.

[56] Patricia, A. Cleary, Trevor J. Orchard, Saul Genuth, Nathan D. Wong, Robert Detrano, Jye-Yu C. Backlund, Bernard Zinman, Alan Jacobson, Wanjie Sun, John M. Lachin, and David M. Nathan, for the DCCT/EDIC Research Group. The Effect of Intensive Glycemic Treatment on Coronary Artery Calcification in Type 1 Diabetic Participants of the Diabetes Control and Complications Trial/Epidemiology of Diabetes Interventions and Complications (DCCT/EDIC) Study. Diabetes (2006). , 55, 3556-3565.

[57] Herold, K. C, Gitelman, S. E, Masharani, U, et al. A Single Course of Anti-CD3 Monoclonal Antibody hOKT3{gamma}1(Ala-Ala) Results in Improvement in C-Peptide Responses and Clinical Parameters for at Least 2 Years after Onset of TYPE 1 DIABETES. diab (2005). , 54(6), 1763-1769.

[58] Sustained effect of intensive treatment of TYPE 1 DIABETES mellitus on development and progression of diabetic nephropathy: the Epidemiology of Diabetes Interventions and Complications (EDIC) studyJAMA (2003). , 290(16), 2159-2167.

[59] Genuth, S. Insights from the diabetes control and complications trial/epidemiology of diabetes interventions and complications study on the use of intensive glycemic treatment to reduce the risk of complications of TYPE 1 DIABETES. Endocr Pract (2006). Suppl , 1, 34-41.

[60] Cleary, P. A, Orchard, T. J, Genuth, S, et al. The Effect of Intensive Glycemic Treatment on Coronary Artery Calcification in Type 1 Diabetic Participants of the Diabetes Control and Complications Trial/Epidemiology of Diabetes Interventions and Complications (DCCT/EDIC) Study. Diabetes (2006). , 55(12), 3556-3565.

[61] Nathan, D. M, Cleary, P. A, Backlund, J. Y, et al. Intensive diabetes treatment and cardiovascular disease in patients with TYPE 1 DIABETES. N Engl J Med (2005). , 353(25), 2643-2653.

[62] Martin, C. L, Albers, J, Herman, W. H, et al. Neuropathy among the diabetes control and complications trial cohort 8 years after trial completion. Diabetes Care (2006). , 29(2), 340-344.

[63] King, G. L, & Loeken, M. R. Hyperglycemia-induced oxidative stress in diabetic complications. Histochem Cell Biol. (2004). , 122, 333-338.

[64] Hoeldtke, R. D, Bryner, K. D, & Vandyke, K. Oxidative stress and autonomic nerve function in early type 1 diabetes. Clin Auton Res (2011). , 21, 19-28.

[65] Brands, A. M, Kessels, R. P, De Haan, E. H, Kappelle, L. J, & Biessels, G. J. Cerebral dysfunction in type 1 diabetes: effects of insulin, vascular risk factors and blood-glucose levels. Eur J Pharmacol. (2004). , 490, 159-168.

[66] Sima, A. A, Zhang, W, Muzik, O, Kreipke, C. W, Rafols, J. A, & Hoffman, W. H. Sequential abnormalities in type 1 diabetic encephalopathy and the effects of C-Peptide. Rev Diabet Stud (2009). , 6, 211-222.

[67] Sima, A. A. Encephalopathies: the emerging diabetic complications. Acta Diabetol (2010). , 47, 279-293.

[68] Hoffman, W. H, Andjelkovic, A. V, Zhang, W, Passmore, G. G, & Sima, A. A. Insulin and IGF-1 receptors, nitrotyrosin and cerebral neuronal deficits in two young patients with diabetic ketoacidosis and fatal brain edema. Brain Res (2010). , 1343, 168-177.

[69] Mira, A. D, & Ward, H. Encephalopathy following diabetic ketoacidosis in a type 1 diabetes patient. Pract Diab Int (2010). , 27, 76-78.

[70] Guven, A, Cebeci, N, Dursun, A, Aktekin, E, Baumgartner, M, & Fowler, B. Methylmalonic acidemia mimicking diabetic ketoacidosis in an infant. Pediatr Diabetes (2011). May 5. doi:j. x., 1399-5448.

[71] Fritsch, M, Rosenbauer, J, Schober, E, Neu, A, Placzek, K, & Holl, R. W. German Competence Network Diabetes Mellitus and the DPV Initiative. Predictors of diabetic ketoacidosis in children and adolescents with type 1 diabetes. Experience from a large multicentre database. Pediatr Diabetes (2011). , 12, 307-312.

[72] Hawkins, K. A, & Pearlson, G. D. Age and gender but not common chronic illnesses predict odor identification in older African Americans. Am J Geriatr Psychiatry (2011). , 19, 777-782.

[73] Grassi, M. A, Tikhomirov, A, Ramalingam, S, Below, J. E, Cox, N. J, & Nicolae, D. L. Genome-wide Meta-analysis for Severe Diabetic Retinopathy". Human Molecular Genetics (2011). , 20, 2472-2481.

Chapter 4

Genes Involved in Type 1 Diabetes

Marina Bakay, Rahul Pandey and
Hakon Hakonarson

Additional information is available at the end of the chapter

http://dx.doi.org/10.5772/52435

1. Introduction

The prevalence of diabetes is increasing worldwide and to date it impacts the lives of approximately 200 million people (Steyn et al., 2009). It is estimated that by 2030, there will be 439 million adults affected by diabetes (International Diabetes Federation/diabetes prevalence: www.idf.org). Type 1 diabetes (T1D) represents approximately 10% of these patients and is most prevalent in populations of European ancestry, where there is ample evidence of increased annual incidence during the past five decades (Onkamo et al., 1999; EURODIAB ACE Study Group, 2000).

T1D is a complex trait that results from the interplay between environmental and genetic factors. Much evidence supports a strong genetic component associated with T1D. The epidemiological data showing differences in geographic prevalence is one clear indicator, with populations of European ancestry having the highest presentation rate. T1D has high concordance among monozygotic twins (33 to 42%) (Redondo et al., 2001) and runs strongly in families with sibling risk being approximately 10 times greater than in the general population (Clayton, 2009); this is in clear contrast to the "less genetic" type 2 diabetes, where the sibling risk ratio is relatively modest at 3.5 (Rich, 1990).

T1D develops at all ages and occurs through the autoimmune destruction of pancreatic β-cells with resulting lack of insulin production. The immune system participates in β-cell destruction through several of its components including natural killer (NK) cells, B lymphocytes, macrophages, dendritic cells (DC), and antigen-presenting cells (APCs). Studies in human and animal models have shown that both innate and adaptive immune responses participate in disease pathogenesis, possibly reflecting the multifactorial nature of this autoimmune disorder.

In this review, we provide an update on genome-wide association studies (GWAS) discoveries to date and discuss the latest associated regions added to the growing repertoire of gene networks predisposing to T1D.

2. Genetic component in Type 1 diabetes

2.1. Before genome-wide association studies

Historically, prior to GWAS, only six loci had been fully established to be associated with T1D. The human leukocyte antigen (HLA) region on chromosome 6p21 was the first known candidate to be strongly associated with T1D in 1970s (Singal & Blajchman, 1973; Nerup et al., 1974; Cudworth & Woodrow, 1975). This cluster of homologous cell-surface proteins is divided into class I (A, B, C) and class II (DP, DQ, RD). The HLA genes encode highly polymorphic proteins, which are essential in self versus non-self immune recognition. The class I molecules are ubiquitously expressed and present intracellular antigen to $CD8^+$ T cells. Class II molecules are expressed mainly on professional APCs: DCs, macrophages, B-lymphocytes and thymus epithelium. Class II molecules are composed of A and B chains, and present antigens to $CD4^+$ T cells, which promote inflammation by secreting cytokines upon recognition of their specific targets. Approximately half of the genetic risk for T1D is conferred by the genomic region harboring the HLA class II genes primarily HLA-DRB1, -DQA1 and -DQB1 genes). In 1984, insulin (INS) gene encoded on chromosome 11p15 was identified as second loci linked with T1D (Bell et al., 1984). In 1996, the cytotoxic T-lymphocyte-associated protein 4 (CTLA4) gene encoded on chromosome 2q33 was recognized as third loci (Nistico et al., 1996). In 2004, a protein tyrosine phosphatase, non-receptor type 22 (PTPN22) gene encoded on chromosome 1p13, was found to be associated with susceptibility to T1D in another case-control study (Bottini et al., 2004). Vella et al., 2005 reported interleukin 2 receptor alpha (IL2RA) gene as fifth T1D loci on chromosome 10p15. In 2006, Smyth et al. identified the interferon-induced with helicase C domain 1 (IFIH1) gene on chromosome 2q24.3 as the sixth gene to be strongly associated with T1D.

2.2. GWAS of T1D

The advent of GWAS in the mid-2000s has changed the situation dramatically, increasing the pace and efficiency of discovery for the T1D associated loci, by a factor of ten. The critical platform for this work was laid by the HapMap project (International HapMap Consortium, 2003, 2005). The GWAS approach has been made possible by the development of high-density genotyping arrays. The genome is laid out in discrete linkage disequilibrium (LD) blocks with limited haplotype diversity within each of these blocks. Therefore, a minimal set of single nucleotide polymorphisms (SNPs) can detect almost all common haplotypes present, thus improving genotyping accuracy and reducing cost.

The first full-scale GWAS for T1D were published in 2007 by our group (Hakonarson et al., 2007) and The Wellcome Trust Case-Control Consortium (WTCCC, 2007). We examined a large pediatric cohort of European descent using the Illumina HumanHap 550 BeadChip platform.

The design involved 561 cases, 1,143 controls and 467 triads in the discovery stage, followed by a replication effort in 939 nuclear families. In addition to finding the "usual" suspects, including an impressive 392 SNPs capturing the very strong association across the major histocompatibility complex (MHC), we identified significant association with variation at the KIAA0350 gene, which we replicated in an additional cohort. The WTCCC study investigated seven common complex diseases including T1D by genotyping 2,000 cases and 3,000 controls with ~500,000 SNPs using the Affymetrix GeneChip, and reported a number of novel T1D loci, including the KIAA0350 genomic region (WTCCC, 2007). Todd et al., 2007 confirmed these findings, using 4,000 cases, 5,000 controls and 3,000 T1D families as well as association reported in the WTCCC study to the 12q13 region. In a separate effort we fast-tracked 24 SNPs at 23 distinct loci from our original study and established association to the 12q13 region with a combined *P*-value of 9.13×10^{-10} (Hakonarson et al., 2008); this was the same locus as reported by the WTCCC and Todd et al., 2007. The 12q13 region harbors several genes, including ERBB3, RAB5B, SUOX, RPS26 and CDK2. However, the causative variants at this locus remain unknown. Concannon et al., 2008 reported an association between SNP at the UBASH3A locus on 21q22.3 and T1D by using SNP genotyping data from a linkage study of affected sib pairs in nearly 2,500 multiplex families, a finding also corroborated by our efforts as well as association to the BACH2 gene (Grant et al., 2009).

2.3. Meta-analyses of T1D GWAS datasets

In order to get the most from GWAS and to increase the statistical power, several independent research groups carried out meta-analyses using datasets from different investigative groups. Cooper et al., 2008 performed the first meta-analysis by using T1D datasets from the WTCCC, 2007 and the Genetics of Kidneys in Diabetes (GoKind) study (Mueller et al, 2006; Manolio et al., 2007), and confirmed associations for PTPN22, CTLA4, MHC, IL2RA, 12q13, 12q24, CLEC16A and PTPN2. The SNPs with lowest nominal *P*-values were taken forward for further genotyping in an additional British cohort of 6,000 cases, 7,000 controls and 2,800 families. As a result, the IL2-IL21 association strengthened further and they found strong evidence for four additional loci: BACH2; a 10p15 region harboring the protein kinase C, theta gene (PRKCQ); a 15q24 region harboring nine genes including cathepsin H (CTSH) and a 22q13 region harboring tumor necrosis factor related protein 6 (C1QTNF6). Additional studies are required to elucidate the culprit genes and their mechanism at the 15q24 and 22q13 loci.

Barrett et al., 2009 meta-analysis uncovered in excess of 40 loci, including 18 novel regions, plus they confirmed a number of previously reported (Smyth et al., 2008; Fung et al., 2009; Cooper et al., 2009). The study included samples from WTCCC, 20070, the GoKind study (Mueller et al., 2006) and controls and family sets from Type 1 Diabetes Genetics Consortium (T1DGC). The meta-analysis observed association to 1q32.1 (which harbors the immunoregulatory interleukin genes IL10, IL19 and IL20), 9p24.2 contains only Glis family zinc finger protein 3 (GLIS3; first suggested by us in Grant et al., 2009), 12p13.31 which harbors a number of immunoregulatory genes including CD69 and 16p11.2 harboring IL27. These findings were further supported by our *in silico* replication efforts (Qu et al., 2010).

To identify additional genetic loci for T1D susceptibility, we examined associations in the largest meta-analysis to date between the disease and ~2.54 million genotyped and imputed SNPs in a combined cohort of 9,934 cases and 16,956 controls (Bradfield et al., 2011). Targeted follow-up of 53 SNPs in 1,120 affected trios uncovered three new loci associated with T1D that reached genome wide significance. The most significantly associated SNP (rs539514, $P = 5.66x10^{-11}$) resided in an intronic region of the LMO7 (LIM domain only 7) gene on 13q22. The second most significantly associated SNP (rs478222, $P = 3.50x10^{-9}$) resided in an intronic region of the EFR3B (protein EFR3 homolog B) gene on 2p23; however the region of linkage disequilibrium is approximately 800kb and harbors additional multiple genes, including NCOA1, C2orf79, CENPO, ADCY3, DNAJC27, POMC, and DNMT3A. The third most significantly associated SNP (rs924043, $P = 8.06x10^{-9}$) was in an intergenic region on 6q27, where the region of association is approximately 900kb and harbors additional genes including WDR27, C6orf120, PHF10, TCTE3, C6orf208, LOC154449, DLL1, FAM120B, PSMB1, TBP and PCD2. These latest associations add to the growing repertoire of gene networks predisposing to T1D. Table 1 summarizes all T1D associated loci reported to date.

Reference	Sample Size	Replication Sample Size	Ethnic Group	Study Type	Main Findings
Hakonarson et al., 2007	467 trios, 561 cases, 1,143 controls	2,350 individuals in 549 families; 390 trios	European ancestry	GWAS	HLA-DRB1, HLA-DQA2, CLEC16A, INS, PTPN22
WTCCC 2007	1,963 cases, 2,938 controls	see Todd et al., 2007	European, British	GWAS	HLA-DRB1, INS, CTLA4, PTPN22, IL2RA, IFIH1, PPARG, KCNJ11, TCF7L2
Todd et al., 2007	see WTCCC 2007	2997 trios, 4,000 cases, 5,000 controls	European British	GWAS	PHTF1-PTPN22, ERBB3, CLEC16A, C12orf30
Hakonarson et al., 2008	467 trios, 561 cases, 1,143 controls	549 families, 364 trios	European ancestry	GWAS	SUOX - IKZF4
Concannon et al., 2008	2,496 families	2,214 trios, 7,721 cases, 9,679 controls	European ancestry	GWAS	INS, IFIH1, CLEC16A, UBASH3A
Cooper et al., 2008	3,561 cases, 4,646 controls	6,225 cases, 6,946 controls, 3,064 trios	European ancestry	GWAS meta-analysis	PTPN22, CTLA4, HLA, IL2RA, ERRB3, C12orf30, CLEC16A, PTPN2
Grant et al., 2009	563 cases, 1,146 controls, 483 case-parents trios	636 families, 3,303 cases, 4,673 controls	European ancestry	GWAS	EDG7, BACH2, GLIS3, UBASH3A, RASGRP1

Reference	Sample Size	Replication Sample Size	Ethnic Group	Study Type	Main Findings
Awata et al., 2009	735 cases, 621 controls	-	Japanese	TaqMan genotyping	ERBB3, CLEC16A
Zoledziewska et al., 2009	1037 cases, 1706 controls	-	European, Sardinian	TaqMan genotyping	CLEC16A
Fung et al., 2009	8010 cases, 9733 controls	-	European, British	TaqMan genotyping	STAT4, STAT3, ERAP1, TNFAIP3, KIF5A/ PIP4K2C
Wu et al., 2009	205 cases, 422 controls	-	Han Chinese	TaqMan genotyping	CLEC16A
Barrett et al., 2009	7,514 cases, 9,045 controls	4,267 cases, 4,670 controls, 4,342 trios	European	GWAS meta-analysis	MHC, PTPN22, INS, C10orf59, SH2B3, ERBB3, CLEC16A, CTLA4, PTPN2, IL2RA, IL27, C6orf173, IL2, ORMDL3, GLIS3, CD69, IL10, IFIH1, UBASH3A, COBL, BACH2, CTSH, PRKCQ, C1QTNF6, PGM1
Wallace et al., 2010	7,514 cases, 9,045 controls	4,840 cases, 2,670 controls, 4,152 trios	European ancestry	GWAS meta-analysis	DLK1, TYK2
Wang et al., 2010	989 cases, 6197 controls	-	European ancestry	GWAS	PTPN22, IL10, IFIH1, KIAA0746, BACH2, C6orf173, TAGAP, GLIS3, L2R, INS, ERBB3, C14orf181, IL27, PRKD2, HERC2, CLEC16A, IFNG, IL26,
Reddy et al., 2011	1434 cases, 1864 controls	-	European ancestry, southeast USA	TaqMan genotyping	PTPN22, INS, IFIH1, SH2B3, ERBB3, CTLA4, C14orf181, CTSH, CLEC16A, CD69, ITPR3, C6orf173, SKAP2, PRKCQ, RNLS, IL27, SIRPG, CTRB2
Bradfield et al., 2011	9,934 cases, 16,956 controls	1,120 trios	European ancestry	GWAS meta-analysis	LMO7, EFR3B, 6q27, TNFRSF11B,

Reference	Sample Size	Replication Sample Size	Ethnic Group	Study Type	Main Findings
					LOC100128081, FOSL2
Asad et al., 2012	424 families, 3078 cases, 1363 controls	-	European, Scandinavians	Genotyping and sequencing	HTR1A, RFN180
Huang et al., 2012	16,179 individuals	-	European ancestry	Genomes-based imputation	CUX2, IL2RA

Table 1. T1D susceptibility loci identified to date.

2.4. Immune components in T1D

The immune system is well organized and well regulated with a basic function of protecting the host against pathogens. This places the immune system in a vital position between healthy and diseased states of the host. Its protective task is regulated by a complex regulatory mechanism involving a diverse army of cells and molecules of humoral and cellular factors working in concert to protect the body against invaders. The human immune system has two components: innate and adaptive. Innate immunity is comprised of physical, chemical, and microbiological barriers to the entry of antigen, and the elements of immune system (DC, macrophages, mast cells, NK cells, neutrophils, monocytes, complements, cytokines and acute phase proteins), which provide immediate host defense. Adaptive immunity is the hallmark of the immune system of higher animals with T and B cells as the key cellular players that provide more specific life-long immunity.

In T1D this system breaks down: insulin-producing β-cells are subjected to specific attack by the host immune system. To better understand the etiology of T1D, a plethora of research has been done to link the systematic destruction of β-cells and the role of the immune system. Linkage studies in 1970s revealed MHC as the first key contributor to T1D susceptibility. Further linkage analysis and candidate gene association studies revealed additional loci associated with T1D. Starting in 2007, GWAS have increased the number of loci be associated with T1D to almost 60. In Figure 1 we present 59 T1D susceptibility loci as where we have classified them into loci harboring non-immune (14) vs. immune (45) genes. Functional aspects of some genes are discussed below.

The complex crosstalk between innate and adaptive immune cells has major impact on the pathogenesis and development of T1D as illustrated in Figure 2. The initiation phase (Phase I) of T1D development takes place in the pancreas where conventional dendritic cells (cDCs) capture and process β-cell antigens. Apoptosis ('natural cell death') or viral infection can lead to β-cell death. Antiviral responses are mediated by invariant natural killer T (iNKT) cells; crossplay between iNKT and plasmacytoid DCs (pDCs) controls viral replication thus prevents subsequent inflammation, tissue damage, and downregulating T1D pathogenesis.

Migration of activated cDCs to the draining lymph node primes pathogenic islet antigen-specific T cells. This activation is promoted by macrophages through IL12 secretion. B cells present β-cell antigen to diabetogenic T cells and secrete autoantibodies in response. The activation of islet antigen-specific T cells can be inhibited by cDCs through engagement of programmed cell death ligand 1 (PDL1). The expansion phase (Phase II): iNKT cells can further promote the recruitment of tolerogenic cDCs and pDCs. These DCs promote expansion of regulatory T (TReg) cells through the production of indoleamine 2,3-dioxygenase (IDO), IL10, transforming growth factor-β (TGFβ) and inducible T cell co-stimulator ligand (ICOSL). Phase III: In the pancreas, β-cell can be killed by diabetogenic T cells and NK cells through the release of interferon-γ (IFNγ), granzymes and perforin, as well as by macrophages through the production of tumour necrosis factor (TNF), IL-1β and nitric oxide (NO). IL12 produced by cDCs sustains the effector functions of activated diabetogenic T cells and NK cells. TReg cells that inhibit diabetogenic T cells and innate immune cells through IL10 and TGFβ can prevent β-cell damage. Tolerogenic pDCs stimulated by iNKT cells could also control diabetogenic T cells through IDO production. Lastly, β-cells can inhibit diabetogenic T cells by expressing PDL1 and escape the cell death.

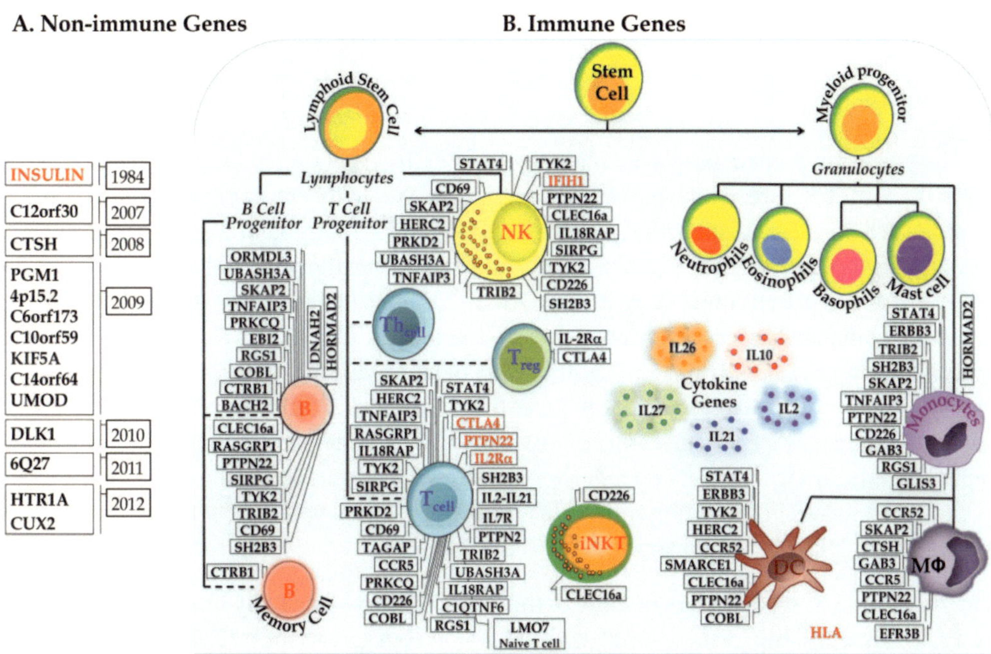

Figure 1. Immune and Non-immune T1D genes are depicted in a concept map representing the components of the immune system. The discovery of T1D susceptibility genes started as early as 1974 with just six genes identified by 2006 shown in red. The advent of GWAS led to flurry of novel genes associated with T1D reaching the excess of 40 by 2009 and almost 60 by 2012.

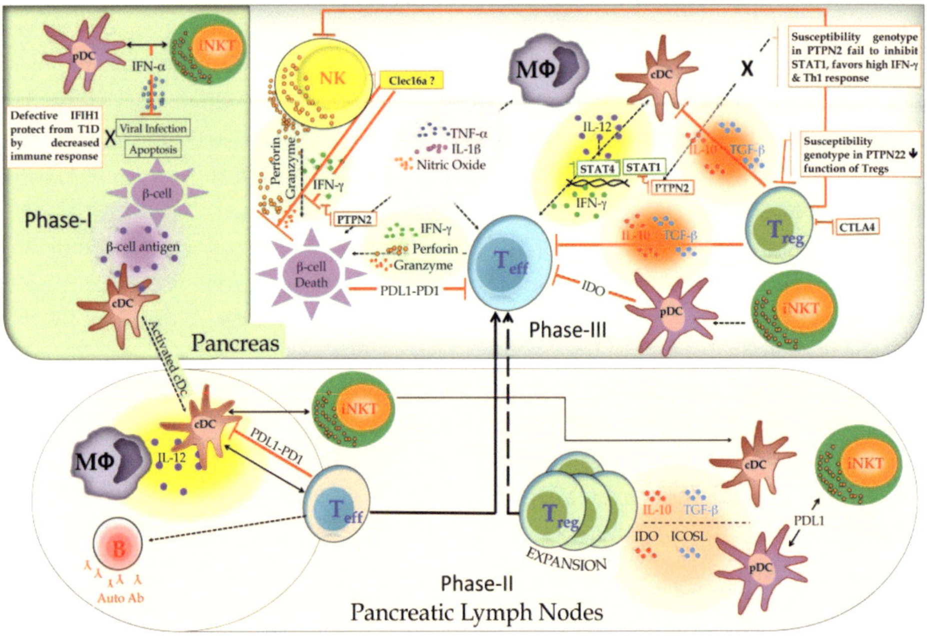

Figure 2. Pathogenesis model of T1D involves complex interactions between innate and adaptive immune cell types.

2.5. CLEC16A (16p13)

The C-type lectin domain family 16, member A (CLEC16A) gene encodes protein with C-type lectin domain structure, which makes it potentially related to the immune response (Robinson et al., 2006). It is established that C-type lectins function both as adhesion and pathogen recognition receptors (PPRs) (Cambi & Figdor, 2003). In addition, CLEC16A is almost exclusively expressed in immune cells including DCs, B-lymphocytes and NK cells. Our 2007 GWAS in a large pediatric cohort of European descent identified CLEC16A as a novel T1D susceptibility gene within a 233-kb linkage disequilibrium block on chromosome 16p13. Three common non-coding variants of the CLEC16A gene (rs2903692, rs725613 and rs17673553) reached genome-wide significance for association with T1D (Hakonarson et al., 2007). Subsequent replication studies in an independent cohort confirmed the association. Importantly, the allele of CLEC16A linked to protection from T1D was also associated with higher levels of CLEC16A expression in NK cells (Hakonarson et al., 2007).

The 2007 WTCCC study independently discovered CLEC16A (formally known as KIAA0350) as a T1D susceptibility locus associated with the non-coding variant rs12708716. This finding was confirmed immediately for T1D in populations of European descent (Todd et al., 2007, Cooper et al., 2008). To date, several SNPs (rs2903692, rs17673553, rs725613, rs12708716, rs12921922, rs12931878) within the CLEC16A gene have been reported to be associated with T1D in several populations: Sardinian (Zoledziewska et al., 2009), Spanish (Martinez et al., 2010), southeast USA (Reddy et al., 2011), Chinese (Wu et al., 2009; Sang et al., 2012), and

Japanese (Yamashita et al., 2011). Recently CLEC16A was also associated with adult-onset of autoimmune diabetes (Howson et al., 2011).

Several GWAS in different autoimmune diseases such as multiple sclerosis (MS) (Zuvich, 2011; Nischwitz et al., 2011), Addison's disease (Skinningsrud et al., 2008), systemic lupus erythematosus (SLE) (Gateva et al., 2009; Zhang et al., 2011), Celiac disease (Dubois et al., 2010), Crohn's disease (Márquez et al., 2009), selective immunoglobulin A deficiency (Jagielska et al., 2012), alopecia areata (Jagielska et al., 2012), rheumatoid arthritis (Martinez et al., 2010) and primary biliary cirrhosis (Mells et al., 2011; Hirschfield et al., 2012) also demonstrated association of the 16p13 loci with disease risk, implying that the 16p13 region contains a key regulator of the self-reactive immune response.

Recently, Davison et al., 2012 reported intron 19 of the CLEC16A gene behaves as a regulatory sequence, which affects the expression of a neighboring gene dexamethasone-induced (DEXI). While it is clear that intron 19 of CLEC16A is highly enriched for transcription-factor-binding events, more functional studies are needed to advance from GWAS to candidate causal genes and their biological functions.

To find causal variant of CLEC16A gene we sequenced the 16p13 region in 96 T1D patients and found 10 new non-synonymous SNPs resulting in one stop-codon, two splice site mutations, and 7 amino acid changes (unpublished data). The studies are under way to examine if these changes are correlated with CLEC16A expression and if these SPNs are present in control group.

Little is yet proven about CLEC16A functions. Kim et al., 2010 characterized ema as an endosomal membrane protein is required for endosomal trafficking and promotes endosomal maturation. Expression of human orthologue of ema 'CLEC16A' rescued the Drosophila mutant demonstrating conserved function of the protein. A recent study by the same group also reported its requirement for the growth of autophagosomes and proposed that the Golgi is a membrane source for autophagosomal growth, and that ema facilitates this process (Kim et al., 2012). Expression of CLEC16A rescued the autophagosome size defect in the ema mutant, suggesting that regulation of autophagosome morphogenesis may be one of the fundamental functions of CLEC16A. Another recent study elucidated the dynamic expression changes and localization of CLEC16A in lipopolysaccharide (LPS) induced neuroinflammatory processes in adult rats. CLEC16A expression was strongly induced in active astrocytes in inflamed cerebral cortex. *In vitro* studies indicated that the up-regulation of CLEC16A might be involved in astrocyte activation following LPS challenge (Wu et al., 2012).

2.6. Other novel T1D susceptibility loci (2011-2012)

In our latest effort to identify additional genetic loci for T1D, we examined associations in the largest meta-analysis to date between T1D and ~2.54 million SNPs in a combined cohort of 9,934 cases and 16,956 controls. Targeted follow-up of 53 SNPs in 1,120 affected trios uncovered three novel loci associated with T1D that reached genome-wide significance (Bradfield et al., 2011).

LMO7 (13q22): The most significantly associated SNP (rs539514, $P = 5.66 \times 10^{-11}$) resides in an intronic region of the LMO7 (LIM domain only 7) gene on 13q22 (Bradfield et al., 2011). LMO7 is a multi-domain mammalian protein with a calponin homology (CH) domain, a discs-large homologous regions (DHR) domain, and a LIM domain. Proteins of this family are involved in protein-protein interactions, regulation of cell adhesion and signaling (Ooshio et al., 2004; Yamada et al., 2004). The expression of LMO7 is cell type specific (Furuya et al., 2002; Kang et al., 2000; Lindvall et al., 2005; Bradfield et al., 2011; Rozenblum et al., 2002; Sasaki et al., 2003) and is essential for the development of muscle and heart tissues. Mice with homozygous deletions of LMO7 display retinal, muscular, and growth retardation (Semenova et al., 2003). LMO7 is upregulated in multiple cancers, especially at the metastatic stage; however under normal conditions its expression is low and limited to very few tissues (Furuya et al., 2002; Kang et al., 2000; Sasaki et al., 2003; Perou et al., 2000). In cultured rat ascites hepatoma cells, the upregulation of LMO7 correlates with the ability of transforming growth factor β (TGFβ) to enhance the invasiveness of these cells (Nakamura et al., 2005). Recent GWAS meta-analysis by Bradfield et al., 2011 identified LMO7 association with T1D. Although the function of LMO7 does not clearly relate to the etiology of T1D, LMO7 is expressed in pancreatic islets and thus is a possible biological candidate at this locus (Kutlu et al., 2009).

EFR3B (2q23): The second most significantly associated SNP among the new loci (rs478222, P=3.50x10^{-9}) resides in an intronic region of the EFR3B (protein EFR3 homolog B) gene on 2p23; however, the region of linkage disequilibrium is approximately 800 kb and harbors additional multiple genes, including NCOA1, C2orf79, CENPO, ADCY3, DNAJC27, POMC, and DNMT3A. EFR3B is an 817 amino acid protein that exists as three alternatively spliced isoforms and belongs to the EFR3 family. The gene encoding EFR3B maps to human chromosome 2p23.3. A number of genetic diseases have been linked to genes on chromosome 2 including Harlequin icthyosis, lipid metabolic disorder sitosterolemia, and Alstrom syndrome. Our recent study shows novel association of 2q23 locus with T1D risk. Location of SNP rs478222 in the intronic region of EFR3B gene makes it a good candidate, however the 2q23 region harbors additional multiple genes, including NCOA1, C2orf79, CENPO, ADCY3, DNAJC27, POMC, and DNMT3A.

Nuclear receptor coactivator 1 (NCOA1) protein is a member of the p160/steroid receptor coactivator (SRC) family. The product of this gene binds to a variety of nuclear hormone receptors in a ligand-dependent manner, suggesting that NCOA1 may play a role as a bridging molecule between nuclear hormone receptors and general transcription factors (Onate et al., 1995; Torchia et al., 1997).

C2orf79 is peptidyl-tRNA hydrolase domain containing 1 (PTRHD1) predicted protein with unknown function.

Centromere protein O (CENPO) gene encodes a component of the interphase centromere complex. The protein is localized to the centromere throughout cell division and is required for bipolar spindle assembly, chromosome segregation and checkpoint signaling during mitosis (Okada et al., 2006).

Adenylate cyclase 3 (ADCY3) gene encodes a membrane-associated enzyme. This protein catalyzes the formation of the secondary messenger cyclic adenosine monophosphate (cAMP) and is highly expressed in human placenta, testis, ovary, and colon (Ludwig & Seuwen,

[11] Clayton, D. G. (2009). Prediction and interaction in complex disease genetics: experience in type 1 diabetes. PLoS genetics. 2009 Jul; 5(7):e1000540.

[12] Cohen, D. R, Ferreira, P. C, Gentz, R, & Curran, T. (1989). The product of a fos- related gene, Fra-1, binds cooperatively to the AP-1 site with Jun: transcription factor AP-1 is comprised of multiple protein complexes. Genes Dev. 1989 Feb; , 3(2), 173-184.

[13] Concannon, P, Onengut-gumuscu, S, & Todd, J. A. Type 1 Diabetes Genetics Consortium. ((2008). A human type 1 diabetes susceptibility locus maps to chromosome 21q22.3. Diabetes. 2008 Oct; , 57(10), 2858-2861.

[14] Cooper, J. D, Smyth, D. J, Smiles, A. M, & Todd, J. A. (2008). Meta-analysis of genome-wide association study data identifies additional type 1 diabetes risk loci. Nature genetics. 2008 Dec; , 40(12), 1399-401.

[15] Cooper, J. D, Walker, N. M, & Healy, B. C. Type I Diabetes Genetics Consortium. ((2009). Analysis of 55 autoimmune disease and type II diabetes loci: further confirmation of chromosomes 4q27, 12q13.2 and 12q24.13 as type I diabetes loci, and support for a new locus, 12q13.q14.1. Genes and immunity. 2009 Dec ;10 Suppl 1:S95-120., 3.

[16] Coulie, B, Tack, J, Bouillon, R, & Janssens, J. (1998). Hydroxytryptamine-1 receptor activation inhibits endocrine pancreatic secretion in humans. Am J Physiol 1998 Feb: 274(2 Pt 1): E, 317-320.

[17] Cudworth AG & Woodrow JC(1975). Evidence for HL-A-linked genes in "juvenile" diabetes mellitus. Br Med J. 1975 Jul 19; , 3(5976), 133-5.

[18] Davison, L. J, Wallace, C, Cooper, J. D, & Wallace, C. (2012). Long-range DNA looping and gene expression analyses identify DEXI as an autoimmune disease candidate gene. Hum Mol Genet. 2012 Jan 15; , 21(2), 322-33.

[19] Dontje, W, Schotte, R, Cupedo, T, & Blom, B. (2006). Delta-like1-induced Notch 1 signaling regulates the human plasmacytoid dendritic cell versus T cell lineage decision through control of GATA-3 and Spi-B. Blood 2006 Mar; , 107(6), 2446-2452.

[20] Dubois, P. C, Trynka, G, Franke, L, & Van Heel, D. A. (2010). Multiple common variants for celiac disease influencing immune gene expression. Nat Genet. 2010 Apr; , 42(4), 295-302.

[21] EURODIAB ACE Study Group(2000). Variation and trends in incidence of childhood diabetes in Europe. EURODIAB ACE Study Group. Lancet. 2000 Mar; , 355(9207), 873-876.

[22] Fung, E. Y, Smyth, D. J, Howson, J. M, & Todd, J. A. (2009). Analysis of 17 autoimmune disease-associated variants in type 1 diabetes identifies 6q23/TNFAIP3 as a susceptibility locus. Genes and immunity. 2009 Mar; , 10(2), 188-91.

[23] Furuya, M, Tsuji, N, Endoh, T, & Watanabe, N. (2002). A novel gene containing PDZ and LIM domains, PCD1, is overexpressed in human colorectal cancer. Anticancer Res. 2002 Nov-Dec; 22(6C): , 4183-4186.

[24] Gateva, V, Sandling, J. K, Hom, G, & Graham, R. R. replication study identifies TNIP1, PRDM1, JAZF1, UHRF1BP1 and IL10 as risk loci for systemic lupus erythematosus. Nat. Genet. 2009 Nov; , 41(11), 1228-1233.

[25] Gingras, H, Cases, O, Krasilnikova, M, & Nepveu, A. (2005). Biochemical characterization of the mammalian Cux2 protein. Gene 2005 Jan; , 344, 273-285.

[26] Grant, S. F, Qu, H. Q, Bradfield, J. P, & Hakonarson, H. (2009). Follow-up analysis of genome-wide association data identifies novel loci for type 1 diabetes. Diabetes. 2009 Jan; , 58(1), 290-295.

[27] Hakonarson, H, Grant, S. F, Bradfield, J. P, & Polychronakos, C. association study identifies KIAA0350 as a type 1 diabetes gene. Nature. 2007 Aug 2; , 448(7153), 591-594.

[28] Hakonarson, H, Qu, H. Q, Bradfield, J. P, & Polychronakos, C. (2008). A novel susceptibility locus for type 1 diabetes on Chr12q13 identified by a genome-wide association study. Diabetes. 2008 Apr; , 57(4), 1143-1146.

[29] Hirschfield, G. M, Xie, G, Lu, E, & Siminovitch, K. A. (2012). Association of primary biliary cirrhosis with variants in the CLEC16A, SOCS1, SPIB and SIAE immunomodulatory genes. Genes Immun. 2012 Jun; , 13(4), 328-335.

[30] Howson, J. M, Rosinger, S, Smyth, D. J, & Todd, J. A. (2011). Genetic analysis of adult-onset autoimmune diabetes. Diabetes. 2011 Oct; , 60(10), 2645-2653.

[31] Huang, J, Ellinghaus, D, Franke, A, & Li, Y. (2012). Genomes-based imputation identifies novel and refined associations for the Wellcome Trust Case Control Consortium phase 1 Data. Eur J Hum Genet. 2012 Jul; , 20(7), 801-805.

[32] Hung, C. N, Poon, W. T, Lee, C. Y, & Chan, A. Y. (2012). A case of early-onset obesity, hypocortisolism, and skin pigmentation problem due to a novel homozygous mutation in the proopiomelanocortin (POMC) gene in an Indian boy. J Pediatr Endocrinol Metab. 25(1-2): 175-179.

[33] International HapMap Consortium(2003). The International HapMap Project. Nature. 2003 Dec; , 426(6968), 789-796.

[34] International HapMap Consortium(2005). A haplotype map of the human genome. Nature. 2005 Oct 27; , 437(7063), 1299-1320.

[35] Iulianella, A, Sharma, M, Durnin, M, & Trainor, P. A. (2008). Cux2 (Cutl2) integrates neural progenitor development with cell-cycle progression during spinal cord neurogenesis. Development 2008 Feb; , 135(4), 729-741.

[36] Iwata, I, Nagafuchi, S, Nakashima, H, & Niho, Y. (1999). Association of polymorphism in the NeuroD/BETA2 gene with type 1 diabetes in the Japanese. Diabetes. 1999 Feb; , 48(2), 416-419.

[37] Jagielska, D, Redler, S, Brockschmidt, F. F, & Betz, R. C. (2012). Follow-Up Study of the First Genome-Wide Association Scan in Alopecia Areata: IL13 and KIAA0350 as

Susceptibility Loci Supported with Genome-Wide Significance. J Invest Dermatol. 2012 Apr.

[38] Kang, S, Xu, H, Duan, X, & Kennedy, G. C. (2000). PCD1, a novel gene containing PDZ and LIM domains, is overexpressed in several human cancers. Cancer Res. 2000 Sep; , 60(18), 5296-5302.

[39] Kavvoura FK & Ioannidis JP(2005). Ala45Thr polymorphism of the NEUROD1 gene and diabetes susceptibility: a meta-analysis. Hum Genet. 2005 Feb; , 116(3), 192-199.

[40] Keutgens, A, Zhang, X, Shostak, K, & Chariot, A. (2010). BCL-3 degradation involves its polyubiquitination through a FBW7-independent pathway and its binding to the proteasome subunit PSMB1. J Biol Chem. 2010 Aug 13; , 285(33), 25831-25840.

[41] Kim, S, Wairkar, Y. P, & Daniels, R. W. DiAntonio A. ((2010). The novel endosomal membrane protein Ema interacts with the class C Vps-HOPS complex to promote endosomal maturation. Cell Biol. 2010 Mar; , 188(5), 717-734.

[42] Kim, S, & Naylor, S. A. DiAntonio A. ((2012). Drosophila Golgi membrane protein Ema promotes autophagosomal growth and function. Proc Natl Acad Sci USA 2012 May; 109(18): E, 1072-1081.

[43] Krude, H, Biebermann, H, Luck, W, & Gruters, A. (1998). Severe early-onset obesity, adrenal insufficiency and red hair pigmentation caused by POMC mutations in humans. Nat Genet. 1998 Jun; , 19(2), 155-157.

[44] Kutlu, B, Burdick, D, Baxter, D, & Hood, L. (2009). Detailed transcriptome atlas of the pancreatic beta cell. BMC Med Genomics 2009 Jan; 2:3.

[45] Lesurtel, M, Soll, C, Graf, R, & Clavien, P. A. (2008). Role of serotonin in the hepato-gastro- Intestinal tract: an old molecule for new perspectives. Cell Mol Life Sci 2008 Mar; , 65(6), 940-952.

[46] Li, D. Kang Q & Wang DM. ((2007). Constitutive coactivator of peroxisome proliferator-activated receptor (PPAR-gamma), a novel coactivator of PPAR-gamma that promotes adipogenesis. Molec. Endocr. 2007 Oct; , 21(10), 2320-2333.

[47] Lindvall, J. M, Blomberg, K. E, Wennborg, A, & Smith, C. I. (2005). Differential expression and molecular characterisation of Lmo7, Myo1e, Sash1, and Mcoln2 genes in Btk-defective B-cells. Cell Immunol. 2005 May; , 235(1), 46-55.

[48] Ludwig, M, & Seuwen, K. (2002). Characterization of the human adenylyl cyclase gene family: cDNA, gene structure, and tissue distribution of the nine isoforms. J. Recept. Signal Transduct. Res. 2002 Feb-Nov; 22(1-4): 79-110.

[49] Manolio, T. A, Rodriguez, L. L, Brooks, L, & Collins, F. S. (2007). New models of collaboration in genome-wide association studies: the Genetic Association Information Network. Nature genetics. 2007 Sep; , 39(9), 1045-1051.

[50] Marquez, A, Varade, J, Robledo, G, & Urcelay, E. (2009). Specific association of a CLEC16A/KIAA0350 polymorphism with NOD2/CARD15(-) Crohn's disease patients. Eur J Hum Genet. 2009 Oct; , 17(10), 1304-1308.

[51] Martinez, A, Perdigones, N, Cénit, M. C, & Urcelay, E. (2010). Chromosomal region 16further evidence of increased predisposition to immune diseases. Ann Rheum Dis. 2010 Jan; 69(1): 309-311., 13.

[52] Mells, G. F, Floyd, J. A, Morley, K. I, & Anderson, C. A. (2011). Genome-wide association study identifies 12 new susceptibility loci for primary biliary cirrhosis. Nat. Genet. 2011 Mar; , 43(4), 329-332.

[53] Mohanan, V. V, Khan, R, & Paulose, C. S. (2006). Hypothalamic 5-HT functional regulation through 5-HT1A and 5-HT2C receptors during pancreatic regeneration. Life Sci 2006 Feb; , 78(14), 1603-1609.

[54] Mueller, P. W, Rogus, J. J, Cleary, P. A, & Warram, J. H. (2006). Genetics of Kidneys in Diabetes (GoKinD) study: a genetics collection available for identifying genetic susceptibility factors for diabetic nephropathy in type 1 diabetes. J Am Soc Nephrol. 2006 Jul; , 17(7), 1782-1790.

[55] Nakamura, H, Mukai, M, Komatsu, K, & Miyoshi, J. (2005). Transforming growth factor-beta1 induces LMO7 while enhancing the invasiveness of rat ascites hepatoma cells. Cancer Lett. 2005 Mar; , 220(1), 95-99.

[56] Nepomuceno-silva, J. L, De Melo, L. D, Mendonçã, S. M, & Lopes, U. G. (2004). RJLs: a new family of Ras-related GTP-binding proteins. Gene 2004 Mar; , 327(2), 221-232.

[57] Nerup, J, Platz, P, Andersen, O. O, & Svejgaard, A. (1974). HLA antigens and diabetes mellitus. Lancet. 1974 Oct; , 2(7885), 864-866.

[58] Nerup, J. Pociot F & European Consortium for IDDM Studies. ((2001). A genomewide scan for type 1-diabetes susceptibility in Scandinavian families: identification of new loci with evidence of interactions. Am J Hum Genet 2001 Dec; , 69(6), 1301-1313.

[59] Nischwitz, S, Cepok, S, Kroner, A, & Weber, F. (2011). More CLEC16A gene variants associated with multiple sclerosis. Acta Neurol Scand 2011 Jun; , 123(6), 400-406.

[60] Nistico, L, Buzzetti, R, Pritchard, L. E, & Todd, J. A. (1996). The CTLA-4 gene region of chromosome 2q33 is linked to, and associated with, type 1 diabetes. Belgian Diabetes Registry. Human molecular genetics. 1996 Jul; , 5(7), 1075-1080.

[61] Okada, M, Cheeseman, I. M, Hori, T, & Fukagawa, T. (2006). The CENP-H-I complex is required for the efficient incorporation of newly synthesized CENP-A into centromeres. Nature Cell Biol. 2006 May; , 8(5), 446-457.

[62] Onate, S. A, & Tsai, S. Y. Tsai MJ. & O'Malley BW. ((1995). Sequence and characterization of a coactivator for the steroid hormone receptor superfamily. Science 1995 Nov; , 270(5240), 1354-1357.

[63] Onkamo, P, Vaananen, S, Karvonen, M, & Tuomilehto, J. (1999). Worldwide increase in incidence of Type I diabetes--the analysis of the data on published incidence trends. Diabetologia. 1999 Dec; , 42(12), 1395-1403.

[64] Ooshio, T, Irie, K, Morimoto, K, & Takai, Y. (2004). Involvement of LMO7 in the association of two cell-cell adhesion molecules, nectin and E-cadherin, through afadin and alpha-actinin in epithelial cells. J. Biol. Chem. 2004 Jul; , 279(30), 31365-31373.

[65] Perou, C. M, Sørlie, T, Eisen, M. B, & Botstein, D. (2000). Molecular portraits of human breast tumours. Nature. 2000 Aug; , 406(6797), 747-752.

[66] Qu, H. Q, Bradfield, J. P, Li, Q, & Polychronakos, C. (2010). In silico replication of the genome-wide association results of the Type 1 Diabetes Genetics Consortium. Human molecular genetics. 2010 Jun 15; , 19(12), 2534-2538.

[67] Reddy, M. V, Wang, H, Liu, S, & She, J. X. (2011). Association between type 1 diabetes and GWAS SNPs in the southeast US Caucasian population. Genes Immun. 2011 Apr; , 12(3), 208-212.

[68] Redondo, M. J, Yu, L, Hawa, M, & Leslie, R. D. (2001). Heterogeneity of type I diabetes: analysis of monozygotic twins in Great Britain and the United States. Diabetologia. 2001 Mar; , 44(3), 354-362.

[69] Rozenblum, E, Vahteristo, P, Sandberg, T, & Kallioniemi, O. P. (2002). A genomic map of a 6-Mb region at 13q21-q22 implicated in cancer development: identification and characterization of candidate genes. Hum. Genet. 2002 Feb; , 110(2), 111-121.

[70] Rich, S. S. (1990). Mapping genes in diabetes. Genetic epidemiological perspective. Diabetes. 1990 Nov; , 39(11), 1315-1319.

[71] Robinson, M. J, Sancho, D, & Slack, E. C. Reis e Sousa C. ((2006). Myeloid C-type lectins in innate immunity. Nat Immunol. 2006 Dec; , 7(12), 1258-1265.

[72] Sang, Y, & Zong, W. Yan J & Liu M. ((2012). The Correlation between the CLEC16A Gene and Genetic Susceptibility to Type 1 Diabetes in Chinese Children. Int J Endocrinol. 2012:245384.

[73] Santos, M. A, Sarmento, L. M, Rebelo, M, & Demengeot, J. (2007). Notch1 engagement by Delta-like-1 promotes differentiation of B lymphocytes to antibody-secreting cells. Proc. Natl. Acad. Sci. USA 2007 Sep; , 104(39), 15454-15459.

[74] Sasaki, M, Tsuji, N, Furuya, M, & Watanabe, N. (2003). PCD1, a novel gene containing PDZ and LIM domains, is overexpressed in human breast cancer and linked to lymph node metastasis. Anticancer Res. 2003 May; 23(3B): , 2717-2721.

[75] Semenova, E, Wang, X, Jablonski, M. M, & Tilghman, S. M. (2003). An engineered 800 kilobase deletion of Uchl3 and Lmo7 on mouse chromosome 14 causes defects in viability, postnatal growth and degeneration of muscle and retina. Hum Mol Genet 2003 Jun; , 12(11), 1301-1312.

[76] Singal DP & Blajchman MA(1973). Histocompatibility (HL-A) antigens, lymphocytotoxic antibodies and tissue antibodies in patients with diabetes mellitus. Diabetes. 1973 Jun; , 22(6), 429-432.

[77] Skinningsrud, B, Husebye, E. S, Pearce, S. H, & Undlien, D. E. (2008). Polymorphisms in CLEC16A and CIITA at 16are associated with primary adrenal insufficiency. J. Clin. Endocrinol. Metab., 2008 Sep; 93(9): 3310-3317., 13.

[78] Smyth, D. J, Cooper, J. D, Bailey, R, & Todd, J. A. association study of nonsynonymous SNPs identifies a type 1 diabetes locus in the interferon-induced helicase (IFIH1) region. Nature genetics. 2006 Jun; , 38(6), 617-619.

[79] Smyth, D. J, Plagnol, V, Walker, N. M, & Todd, J. A. (2008). Shared and distinct genetic variants in type 1 diabetes and celiac disease. The New England journal of medicine. 2008 Dec 25; , 359(26), 2767-2777.

[80] Steyn, N. P, Lambert, E. V, & Tabana, H. (2009). Conference on "Multidisciplinary approaches to nutritional problems". Symposium on "Diabetes and health". Nutrition interventions for the prevention of type 2 diabetes. Proc. Nutr. Soc. 2009 Feb; , 68(1), 55-70.

[81] Su, Y, Büchler, P, Gazdhar, A, & Friess, H. (2006). Pancreatic regeneration in chronic pancreatitis requires activation of the notch signaling pathway. J. Gastrointest. Surg. 2006 Nov; , 10(9), 1230-1241.

[82] Sundler, F, Hakanson, R, Loren, I, & Lundquist, I. (1980). Amine storage and function in peptide hormone-producing cells. Invest Cell Pathol. 1980 Jan-Mar; , 3(1), 87-103.

[83] Todd, J. A, Walker, N. M, Cooper, J. D, & Clayton, D. G. (2007). Robust associations of four new chromosome regions from genome-wide analyses of type 1 diabetes. Nature genetics. 2007 Jul; , 39(7), 857-864.

[84] Torchia, J, Rose, D. W, Inostroza, J, & Rosenfeld, M. G. (1997). The transcriptional coactivator p/CIP binds CBP and mediates nuclear-receptor function. Nature. 1997 Jun 12; , 387(6634), 677-684.

[85] Trachtulec, Z, Hamvas, R. M, Forejt, J, & Klein, J. (1997). Linkage of TATA-binding protein and proteasome subunit C5 genes in mice and humans reveals synteny conserved between mammals and invertebrates. Genomics. 1997 Aug; , 44(1), 1-7.

[86] Vella, A, Cooper, J. D, Lowe, C. E, & Todd, J. A. (2005). Localization of a type 1 diabetes locus in the IL2RA/CD25 region by use of tag single-nucleotide polymorphisms. Am J Hum Genet. 2005 May; , 76(5), 773-779.

[87] Wallace, C, Smyth, D. J, Maisuria-armer, M, & Clayton, D. G. (2010). The imprinted DLK1-MEG3 gene region on chromosome 14q32.2 alters susceptibility to type 1 diabetes. Nat Genet. 2010 Jan; , 42(1), 68-71.

[88] Wellcome Trust Case Control Consortium: WTCCC ((2007). Genome-wide association study of 14,000 cases of seven common diseases and 3,000 shared controls. Nature. 2007 Jun; , 447(7145), 661-678.

[89] Wang, K, Baldassano, R, Zhang, H, & Hakanarson, H. (2010). Comparative genetic analysis of inflammatory bowel disease and type 1 diabetes implicates multiple loci with opposite effects. Human molecular genetics. 2010 May; , 19(10), 2059-2067.

[90] Wong, S. T, Trinh, K, Hacker, B, & Storm, D. R. (2000). Disruption of the type III adenylyl cyclase gene leads to peripheral and behavioral anosmia in transgenic mice. Neuron. 2000 Sep; , 27(3), 487-497.

[91] Wu, X, Zhu, X, Wang, X, & Liu, Y. (2009). Intron polymorphism in the KIAA0350 gene is reproducibly associated with susceptibility to type 1 diabetes (T1D) in the Han Chinese population. Clin Endocrinol (Oxf). 2009 Jul; , 71(1), 46-49.

[92] Wu, X, Li, J, Chen, C, & Gao, Y. (2012). Involvement of CLEC16A in activation of astrocytes after LPS treated. Neurochem Res. 2012 Jan; , 37(1), 5-14.

[93] Yamada, A, Irie, K, Fukuhara, A, & Takai, Y. (2004). Requirement of the actin cytoskeleton for the association of nectins with other cell adhesion molecules at adherens and tight junctions in MDCK cells. Genes Cells 2004 Sep; , 9(9), 843-855.

[94] Yamashita, H, Awata, T, & Kawasaki, E. Japanese Study Group on Type 1 Diabetes Genetics. ((2011). Analysis of the HLA and non-HLA susceptibility loci in Japanese type 1 diabetes. Diabetes Metab Res Rev. 2011 Nov; , 27(8), 844-848.

[95] Yanagisawa, Y, & Ito, E. Yuasa Y & Maruyama K ((2002). The human DNA methyltransferases DNMT3A and DNMT3B have two types of promoters with different CpG contents. Biochim. Biophys. Acta 2002 Sep; , 1577(3), 457-465.

[96] Yoo, A. S, Staahl, B. T, Chen, L, & Crabtree, G. R. (2009). MicroRNA-mediated switching of chromatin-remodelling complexes in neural development. Nature. 2009 Jul; , 460(7255), 642-646.

[97] Zawalich, W. S, Tesz, G. J, & Zawalich, K. C. (2004). Effects of prior 5-hydroxytryptamine exposure on rat islet insulin secretory and phospholipase C responses. Endocrine. 2004 Feb; , 23(1), 11-16.

[98] Zhang, Z, Cheng, Y, Zhou, X, & Zhang, X. (2011). Polymorphisms at 16are associated with systemic lupus erythematosus in the Chinese population. J Med. Genet. 2011 Jan; 48(1): 69-72., 13.

[99] Zoledziewska, M, Costa, G, Pitzalis, M, & Marrosu, M. G. (2009). Variation within the CLEC16A gene shows consistent disease association with both multiple sclerosis and type 1 diabetes in Sardinia. Genes Immun. 2009 Jan; , 10(1), 15-17.

[100] Zuvich, R. L, Bush, W. S, Mccauley, J. L, & Haines, J. L. (2011). Interrogating the complex role of chromosome 16in multiple sclerosis susceptibility: independent genetic signals in the CIITA-CLEC16A-SOCS1 gene complex. Hum. Mol. Genet., 2011 Sep; 20(17): 3517-3524., 13.

Section 3

Beta-Cell Function and Dysfunction

Chapter 5

Beta-Cell Function and Failure

Soltani Nepton

Additional information is available at the end of the chapter

http://dx.doi.org/10.5772/52153

1. Introduction

1.1. Beta cells (β-cells)

Beta cells are a type of cell in the pancreas located in the so-called islets of Langerhans. They make up 65-80% of the cells in the islets.

The Islets diameter is about 50 to 300 micrometers. They are composed of several types of cells. At least 70 percent are beta cells, which are localized in the core of the islet. These cells are surrounded by alpha cells that secrete glucagon, smaller numbers of delta cells that secrete somatostatin, and PP cells or F cells that secrete pancreatic polypeptide. All of the cells communicate with each other through extracellular spaces and through gap junctions. This arrangement allows cellular products secreted from one cell type to influence the function of downstream cells. As an example, insulin secreted from beta cells can suppress glucagon secretion.

A neurovascular bundle containing arterioles and sympathetic and parasympathetic nerves enters each islet through the central core of beta cells. The arterioles branch to form capillaries that pass between the cells to the periphery of the islet and then enter the portal venous circulation.

2. Beta cells functions

Insulin is synthesized as preproinsulin in the ribosomes of the rough endoplasmic reticulum in the beta cells (fig 1). Preproinsulin is then cleaved to proinsulin, which is transported to the Golgi apparatus where it is packaged into secretory granules located close to the cell membrane. Proinsulin is cleaved into equimolar amounts of insulin and C-peptide in the secretory granules. The process of insulin secretion involves fusion of the secretory granules with the cell membrane and exocytosis of insulin, C-peptide, and proinsulin

Insulin is a hormone that controls the blood glucose concentration. The liver maintains the base-line glucose level, but the beta cells can respond quickly to spikes in blood glucose by releasing some of its stored insulin while simultaneously producing more. The response time is very quick.

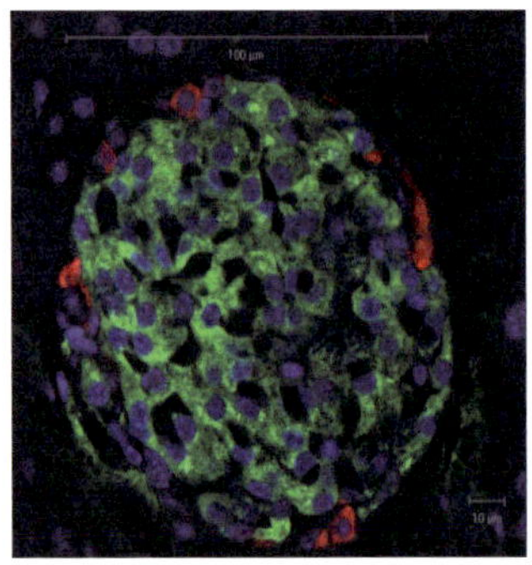

Figure 1 Mouse pancreatic islet as seen by light microscopy. Beta cells can be recognized by the green insulin staining. Glucagon is labeled in red and the nuclei in blue

Apart from insulin, beta cells release C-peptide, a consequence of insulin production, into the bloodstream in equimolar amounts. C-peptide helps to prevent neuropathy and other symptoms of diabetes related to vascular deterioration.Measuring the levels of C-peptide can give a practitioner an idea of the viable beta cell mass.

Beta-cells also produce amylin, also known as IAPP, islet amyloid polypeptide. Amylin functions as part of the endocrine pancreas and contributes to glycemic control. Amylin's metabolic function is now somewhat well characterized as an inhibitor of the appearance of nutrient [especially glucose] in the plasma. Thus, it functions as a synergistic partner to insulin. Whereas insulin regulates long-term food intake, increased amylin decreases food intake in the short term.

GABA (γ amino butyric acid) is produced by pancreatic beta cell. GABA released from beta cells can act on GABA $_A$receptor in the α cells, causing membrane hyperpolarization and hence suppressing glucagon secretion. An impaired insulin-Akt-GABA$_A$ receptors glucagon secretory pathway in the islet may be an underlying mechanism for unsuppressed glucagon secretion, despite hyperglycemia, in diabetic subjects. Some studies demonstrated that beta cells also express GABA $_A$ receptors, forming an autocrine GABA signaling system. However, the role of this autocrine GABA signaling in the regulation of beta cell functions remains largely unknown.

Zinc is needed by over 300 enzyme systems.Some of those are involved with the metabolism of blood sugar and are so important that a lack of zinc, in and of itself, can cause type I or type II diabetes.

Zinc is highly concentrated in the insulin-secreting beta cells of our pancreas. Zinc can keep insulin molecules together in the beta cells.Beta cells must have zinc to function. In fact, beta cells

http://dx.doi.org/10.5772/52153

contain their own special zinc transporter called zinc transporter 8 that enables beta cells to take up zinc.Gene alterations in this zinc transporter are now known to cause type II diabetes while type I diabetes is associated with antibodies against this zinc transporter (meaning the immune system knocks out function of beta cells so they can't produce insulin).

Zinc directly influences how insulin is produced and secreted by our beta cells. So the people with zinc deficiency can't store and release insulin.Furthermore, zinc is self-protecting to the beta cells.It has now been shown that zinc directly reduces the inflammatory signals that damage the beta cells, a process that leads to type I diabetes.

3. Mechanisms of insulin secretion from beta cells

The secretion of insulin from pancreatic beta cells is a complex process involving the integration and interaction of multiple external and internal stimuli. Thus, nutrients, hormones, neurotransmitters, and drugs all activate or inhibit insulin secretion. The primary stimulus for insulin release is the beta-cell response to changes in glucose concentration. Normally, glucose induces a biphasic pattern of insulin release. First-phase insulin release occurs within the first few minutes after exposure to an elevated glucose level; this is followed by a more permanent second phase of insulin release. Of particular importance is the observation that first-phase insulin secretion is lost in patients with type 2 diabetes. Thus, molecular mechanisms involved in phasic insulin secretion are important. This processes discussed as follow (fig 2).

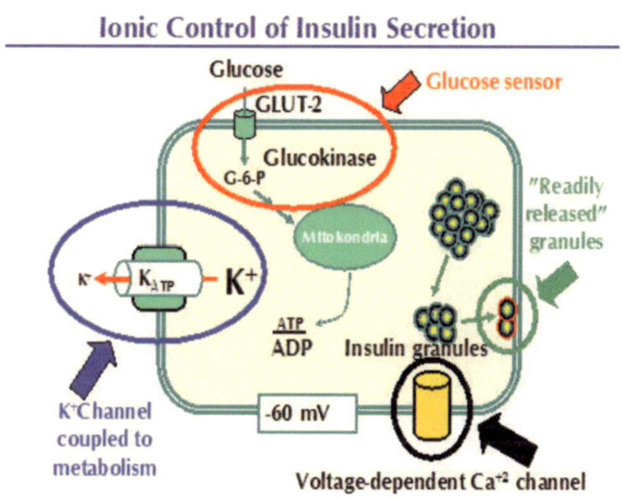

Figure 2. The beta cell structure

A widely accepted sequence of events involved in glucose-induced insulin secretion is as follows:

1. Glucose is transported into beta cells through facilitated diffusion of GLUT2 glucose transporters.
2. Intracellular glucose is metabolized to ATP.
3. Elevation in the ATP/ADP ratio induces closure of cell-surface ATP-sensitive K+ (KATP) channels, leading to cell membrane depolarization.
4. Cell-surface voltage-dependent Ca2+ channels (VDCC) are opened, facilitating extracellular Ca2+ influx into the beta cell.
5. A rise in free cytosolic Ca2+ triggers the exocytosis of insulin.

It is understood that glucose stimulates insulin secretion in the pancreatic beta cell by means of a synergistic interaction between at least two signaling pathways. In the K (ATP) channel-dependent pathway, glucose stimulation increases the entry of extrinsic Ca2+ through voltage-gated channels by closure of the K (ATP) channels and depolarization of the beta cell membrane. The resulting increase in intracellular Ca2+ stimulates insulin exocytosis. While in the GTP-dependent pathway, intracellular Ca2+ is elevated by GTP-dependent proteins and augments the Ca2+-stimulated release. Secretagogues and insulin secretion inhibitors act at intermediate steps of these signaling pathways and influence the process of insulin exocytosis. Several researchers have investigated this intricate mode of known secretagogue action using isolated islets as an *in vitro* model. To quote a few; imidazoline antagonists of alpha 2-adrenoreceptors increase insulin release *in vitro* by inhibiting ATP-sensitive K+ channels in pancreatic beta cells. Some researchers have evaluated the properties of sulphonylurea receptors (SUR) of human islets of Langerhans. They studied the binding affinity of various oral hypoglycaemic agents to the receptor and also tested insulinotropic action of the drugs on intact human islets. This binding potency order was parallel with the insulinotropic potency of the evaluated compounds. Some investigators have shown an insulinotropic effect of Triglitazone (CS-045) and have shown its mode of action to be distinct from glibenclamide (a sulphonylurea drug). A-4166, a derivative of D-phenylalanine, evokes a rapid and short-lived hypoglycaemic action *in vivo*. It has been shown to act via the tolbutamide binding sites14. Some studies showed S21403, a meglitinide analogue to be a novel insulinotropic tool in the treatment of type 2 diabetes, as it affected cationic fluxes and the drugs secretary responses displayed favourable time course of prompt, and not unduly prolonged, activation of beta cells. Some studies demonstrated that tetracaine (an anaesthetic) stimulates insulin secretion by release of intracellular calcium and for the first time elucidated the role of intracellular calcium stores in stimulus-secretion coupling in the pancreatic beta cells. JTT-608, is a nonsulphonylurea oral hypoglycaemic agent which stimulates insulin release at elevated but not low glucose concentrations by evoking PKA-mediated Ca2+ influx.

4. The importance of KATP channels

The KATP channels play an integral role in glucose-stimulated insulin secretion by serving as the transducer of a glucose-generated metabolic signal (ie, ATP) to cell electrical activity (membrane depolarization). Thus, like neurons, beta cells are electrically excitable and capable of generating Ca2+ action potentials that are important in synchronizing islet cell activity and insulin release. In addition to being signal targets for glucose, KATP channels are the targets for sulfonylureas, which are commonly prescribed oral agents in the treatment of type 2 diabetes. The sulfonylureas, like glucose, induce closure of KATP channels and stimulate insulin secretion.

The beta-cell KATP channel is a complex octameric unit of 2 different proteins: the sulfonylurea receptor (SUR-1) and an inward rectifier (Kir6.2). The sulfonylurea receptor belongs to a superfamily of ATP-binding cassette proteins and contains the binding site for sulfonylurea drugs and nucleotides. The inward rectifier represents the K+ conducting pore and is also regulated by ATP. It is interesting that KATP channels are present in other tissues of the body, including heart (SUR-2A/Kir 6.2), smooth muscle (SUR-2B/Kir 6.2), and brain (SUR-1/Kir 6.2). Recently, Mark L. Evans, MD, Yale University Medical School, New Haven, Connecticut, and colleagues have suggested that glucose sensing in the brain during hypoglycemia may be mediated by KATP channels located in brain hypothalamic neurons. Thus, these molecules may also serve as new therapeutic targets for the restoration of impaired hypoglycemia awareness and glucose counterregulation in type 1 diabetes.

5. Voltage-dependent Ca2+ channels: Novel regulators

Extracellular Ca2+ influx through L-type voltage-dependent Ca2+ channels (VDCC) raises free cytoplasmic Ca2+ levels and triggers insulin secretion. The structure of the VDCC is complex and consists of 5 subunits: alpha1, alpha2, beta, gamma, and delta units. The alpha subunit constitutes the ion-conducting pore, whereas the other units serve a regulatory role. Previous work has identified that isoforms of alpha1 subunits interact with exocytotic proteins. More recently, using the yeast hybrid screening method, a novel protein, Kir-GEM, interacting with the beta3 isoform of the VDCC, has been identified by Seino and colleagues. Furthermore, it has been determined that Kir-GEM inhibits alpha ionic activity and prevents cell-surface expression of alpha subunits. The investigators have proposed that in the presence of Ca2+, Kir-GEM binds to the beta isoform, and this interaction interferes in the trafficking or translocation of alpha subunits to the plasma membrane. The relevance of Kir-GEM in insulin secretion was made evident by its attenuation of glucose-stimulated Ca2+ increases and C-peptide secretion in an insulin-secreting cell line.

The potential therapeutic role of Kir-GEM lies in the inhibitory effects on VDCC activity that may serve to protect beta cells from overstimulation and subsequent failure, which is part of the disease etiology of type 2 diabetes.

6. Novel cAMP signaling pathways of insulin release

The incretins are another set of factors that are important hormonal regulators of insulin secretion. The incretins are polypeptide hormones released in the gut after a meal that potentiate insulin secretion in a glucose-dependent manner. Due to their dependence on ambient glucose for action, they are emerging as important new therapeutic agents to promote insulin secretion without accompanying hypoglycemia (a common complication of sulfonylurea treatment).

Unlike sulfonylureas, incretins act by activating Gs (a G-protein that activates adenylyl cyclase) to increase cAMP in beta cells. cAmp, like ATP, is an important signal that regulates insulin release. Typically, the main mechanism of action of cAMP is by activation of an enzyme called protein kinase A (PKA) that, in turn, phosphorylates other substrates to turn on (or off) vital cell functions. Using a biochemical assay called the yeast hybrid screening method to identify and isolate new proteins, some researchers identified a novel protein, cAMP-GEF II, a cAMP sensor (cAMPS) that forms a complex with other intracellular proteins (Rim2 and Rab3) to directly regulate insulin exocytosis. Then, using molecular reagents that antagonize the effects of cAMPS, they observed that incretin-potentiated insulin secretion is attenuated. These results provide a mechanism whereby cAMP can directly promote exocytosis of insulin granules without activation of PKA (ie, a PKA-independent pathway), and thereby provide additional molecular targets for therapeutic intervention.

7. Beta cell dysfunction and apoptosis

Type one diabetes: Islet beta-cells are almost completely destroyed when patients with type 1 diabetes are diagnosed. Type 1 diabetes occurs when the bodies own immune system destroys the beta cells. Some people develop a type of diabetes – called secondary diabetes -- which is similar to type 1 diabetes, but the beta cells are not destroyed by the immune system but by some other factor, such as cystic fibrosis or pancreatic surgery.

Type two diabetes: Defects in insulin action and insulin secretion are both present in type 2 diabetes, and both are believed to be genetically predetermined. In the absence of a defect in beta-cell function, individuals can compensate indefinitely for insulin resistance with appropriate hyperinsulinemia, as observed even in obese populations. Both insulin secretion and insulin action are impaired in type 2 diabetes. However, when allowance is made for the hyperglycaemia and the fact that glucose stimulates insulin secretion, it becomes apparent that the insulin levels in diabetic patients are lower than in healthy controls and inadequate beta-cell function therefore represents a key feature of the disease. Theoretically, the insulin secretory defect could result from either defects of beta-cell function or a reduction in beta-cell mass. Most quantitative estimates indicate that type 2 diabetes associates with either no change or $< 30\%$ reduction in beta-cell mass. Moreover, the secretion defect is more severe than can be accounted for solely by the reduction in beta-cell mass. It therefore appears that the insulin secretory defect in type 2 diabetes does not primarily result from insufficient beta-cell mass but rather from an impairment of insulin secretion.

8. Prevention of beta cell dysfunction and apoptosis

Islet beta-cells are almost completely destroyed when patients with type 1 diabetes are diagnosed. To date, insulin substitute therapy is still one of the main treatments. The cure of type 1 diabetes requires beta-cell regeneration from islet cell precursors and prevention of recurring autoimmunity. Therefore, beta-cell replacement, regeneration and proliferation emerge as a new research focus on therapy for type 1 diabetes; however, its application is limited by the shortage of pancreas donors. In-vitro expansion of human cadaveric islet beta cells represents an attractive strategy for generation of abundant beta-like cells. Human beta cells patent a very low proliferation capacity in vivo, and intact isolated islets cultured in suspension do not proliferate, although they remain functional for months. When islets are allowed to attach, limited replication of beta cells can be induced by growth factors or extracellular matrix components before the beta-cell phenotype is lost. Previous accepting of the determinants of tissue mass during adult life is still rudimentary. Insights into this problem may suggest novel approaches for the treatment of neoplastic as well as degenerative diseases. In the case of the pancreas, elucidating the mechanisms that govern β cell mass will be important for the design of regenerative therapy for both type 1 and type 2 diabetes, diseases characterized by an insufficient mass of β cells. It is clear that β cell mass increase during pregnancy and in insulin-resistant states, but evidence on the ability of β cells to regenerate from a severe, diabetogenic injury is conflicting. Whereas autoimmune diabetes is normally irreversible, recent evidence from both humans and rodents suggests that β cell function (i.e., insulin production and the maintenance of glucose homeostasis) can partly recover if autoimmunity is blocked.

Islet beta-cell regeneration and development are controlled by many growth factors, especially insulin-like growth factor-1 (IGF-1). Pancreatic islets produce Igf1 and Igf2, which bind to specific receptors on β-cells. Igf1 has been shown to influence β-cell apoptosis, and both Igf1 and Igf2 increase islet growth; Igf2 does so in a manner additive with fibroblast growth factor 2. Some study showed that IGF-1 can protect beta-cells from the destruction of apoptosis factors and promoting beta-cell survival and proliferation. Interleukin-1beta (IL-1 beta) is a potent pro-inflammatory cytokine that has been shown to inhibit islet beta cell function as well as to activate Fas-mediated apoptosis in a nitric oxide-dependent manner. Furthermore, this cytokine is effective in recruiting lymphocytes that mediate beta cell destruction in type one diabetes. IGF-I has been shown to block IL-1beta actions in vitro.

Glucagon like peptide 1 (GLP-1) is a potent insulin secretagogue released by L-cells of the distal large intestine in response to meal ingestion and, together with glucose-dependent insulinotropic polypeptide (GIP), account for 90% of the incretin effect. Type 2 diabetic patients are characterized by severely impaired β-cell function, reduced plasma GLP-1 response to meal/glucose ingestion that correlates with reduced insulin secretion, and severe β-cell resistance to the stimulatory effect of GLP-1 on insulin secretion. GLP-1 also inhibits glucagon secretion, delays gastric emptying, and promotes weight loss by its appetite-suppressant effect. GLP-1 analogs also stimulate islet neogenesis and β-cell replication and inhibit islet apoptosis. The gluco-incretin hormones GLP-1 and GIP can protect beta-cell against apoptosis induced by cytokines or glucose and free fatty acids. Both hormones bind to specific Gs-coupled receptors, which trigger cAMPformation. In beta-cells, basal cAMP levels controls glucose competence, i.e., the magnitude of the insulin secretion response to a given increase in extracellular glucose concentration. Increases in cAMP levels, for instance as stimulated by GLP-1 or GIP action, potentiate glucose-stimulated insulin secretion by both protein kinase A (PKA)-dependent and independent mechanisms; they also stimulate gene transcription through PKA dependent phosphorylation of the transcription factor CREB. In beta-cells, increased cAMP levels also activate the MAP kinase cascade, leading to rapid phosphorylation of Erk1/2. An activation of the PI3Kinase/Akt pathway is also observed. PI3kinase may be directly activated by the ßγ subunit of Gs, be secondary to transactivation of the EGF receptor by betacellulin, or may follow transcriptional induction of IRS-2 through the PKA/CREB pathway. The IRS- 2/PI3kinase/Akt pathway is known to have anti-apoptotic effects; however, it is unclear why increased expression of IRS-2 leads to activation of its signaling pathway. IRS-2 may be downstream of the insulin (IR) or IGF-1 (IGF-1R) receptors. Studies of mice with beta-cell specific inactivation of either receptor indicated that the insulin receptor was important for compensatory growth of the beta-cells in response to insulin resistance whereas the IGF-1 receptor was involved in the control of glucose competence. Although these properties make GLP-1 an ideal antidiabetic agent, it is rapidly cleaved ($T_{1/2}$ = 1–2 min) by dipeptidyl peptidase-4. GLP-1 enhances beta cell function with an increase in the ability to secrete insulin and restore first phase insulin release. Our pervious study showed that a novel GLP-1 analogue consisting of the fusion of active GLP-1 and IgG heavy chain constant regions (GLP-1/IgG-fc) therapy can enhances beta cell mass. It also could increase insulin secretion. Within the pancreas, GLP-1 expands β-cell mass via promotion of β-cell growth and reduction of β-cell death.

γ-Aminobutyric acid (GABA), a prominent inhibitory neurotransmitter, is present in high concentrations in β-cells of islets of Langerhans. The GABA shunt enzymes, glutamate decarboxylase (GAD) and GABA transaminase (GABA-T) have also been localized in islet β-cells. With the recent demonstration that the 64,000-Mr antigen associated with insulin-dependent diabetes mellitus is GAD, there isincreased interest in understanding the role of GABA in islet functions. Only a small component of β-cell GABA is contained in insulin secretory granules, making it unlikely that GABA, co-released with insulin, is physiologically significant. Our immunohistochemical study of GABA in β-cells of intact islets indicates that GABA is associated with a vesicular compartment distinctly different from insulin secretory granules. Whether this compartment represents a releasable pool of GABA has yet to be determined. GAD in β-cells is associated with a vesicular compartment, similar to the GABA vesicles. In addition, GAD is found in a unique extensive tubular cisternal complex (GAD complex). It is likely that the GABA-GAD vesicles are derived from this GAD-containing complex. Physiological studies on the effect of extracellular GABA on islet hormonal secretion have had variable results. Effects of GABA on insulin, glucagon, and somatostatin secretion have been proposed. The most compelling evidence for GABA regulation of islet hormone secretion comes from studies on somatostatin secretion, where it has an inhibitory effect. Some researchers present new evidence demonstrating the presence of GABAergic nerve cell bodies at the periphery of islets with numerous GABA-containing processes extending into the islet mantle. This close association between GABAergic neurons and islet α- and δ-cells strongly suggests that GABA inhibition of somatostatin and glucagon secretionis mediated by these neurons. Intracellular β-cell GABAA and its metabolismmay have a role in β-cell function. New evidence indicates that GABA shunt activity is involved in regulation of insulin secretion. In addition, GABA or its metabolites may regulate proinsulin synthesis. These new observations provide insight into the complex nature of GABAergic neurons and β-cell GABA in regulation of islet function. Our study showed that GABA exerts has protective and regenerative effects on islet beta cells and reverses diabetes. GABA therapy increased beta cell proliferation and decreased beta cell apoptosis, which in turn increase beta cell mass and induced the reversal of hyperglycemia in the different kind of mice. Our data suggest that GABA exerts has ani-inflammatory effects, and is directly inhibitory to T cells and macrophages.

Magnesium deficiency has recently been proposed as a novel factor implicated in the pathogenesis of the diabetic complications. In our previous study we showed that oral chronic Mg administration could improve islet structure and decrease the blood glucose.

Another potential treatment is the combination of two growth factors called gastrin and epidermal growth factor (EGF), which has been shown to promote beta-cell regeneration in rats.

Many traditional treatments have been recommended in the alternative system of medicine for treatment of diabetes mellitus and regeneration of beta cells such as Garlic, Teucriumpolium, Cinnamon and Psidium guava leaves. Photochemical analysis of those herbs have revealed the presence of flavonoids, which include quercetin and its derivatives. It is concluded that quercetin, a flavonoid with antioxidant properties brings about the regeneration of the pancreatic islets and probably increases insulin release in streptozocin-induced diabetic rats.

Connective tissue growth factor (CTGF), to induce adult β cell mass expansion. Some study showed that CTGF is required for embryonic β cell proliferation3, and that CTGF overexpression in embryonic cells increases β cell proliferation and β cell mass.

The mouse pancreas develops from ventral and dorsal evaginations of the posterior foregut endoderm at embryonic day, a process dependent on the transcription factors Pdx1 and Ptf1. Differentiation of all pancreatic endocrine cell types (α, β, Δ and PP) is dependent on the transcription factor, neurogenin 3 (Ngn3). *Ngn3* expression is controlled by a variety of factors, including the Notch signaling pathway and the transcriptional regulators pancreatic and duodenal homeobox 1 (Pdx1), SRY-box 9 (Sox9) and hepatic nuclear factor 6 (Hnf6). Although β cell neogenesis begins, these early insulin-positive cells do not contribute to mature islets. Instead, endocrine cells that will go on to contribute to the mature islets begin to differentiate period known as the secondary transition. Some transcription factors critically involved in β cell differentiation include NK2 homeobox 2 (Nkx2.2), Nkx6.1, islet 1 (Isl-1), neuronal differentiation 1 (NeuroD1), motor neuron and pancreas homeobox 1(Mnx1), paired box gene 4 (Pax4) and Pdx1.

In adults, physiological stimuli can enhance β cell proliferation during development. Although several factors have been identified that play a role in the regulation of embryonic and neonatal β cell proliferation. One cell cycle regulator that does play a role in embryonic β cell proliferation is the cell cycle inhibitor, p27Kip1. Inactivation of *p27Kip1* during embryogenesis results in an increase in β cell proliferation and subsequently β cell mass. There was no change, however, in early postnatal β cell proliferation, suggesting that p27Kip1 is not crucial to postnatal proliferation.

As mentioned above Pdx1expressed in multipotent pancreatic progenitors in the early stages of pancreas development, but, Pdx1 expression becomes enhanced in insulin-positive cells and is found at only low levels in exocrine cells. This expression pattern is maintained into adulthood and Pdx1 plays a critical rolein maintenance of the mature β cell phenotype. Inactivation of *Pdx1* in embryonic insulin-expressing cells results in a dramatic decrease in β cell proliferation at late gestation, leading to decreased β cell mass at birth and early onset diabetes. Two large Maf (musculoaponeuroticfibrosarcoma oncogene homolog) transcription factors that are closely related to one another, MafA and MafB, are critical for β cell differentiation and embryonic *Pdx1* expression22 and therefore may have an indirect effect on embryonic β cell replication.

Inactivation of the eIF2α endoplasmic reticulum resident kinase, PERK (proteinkinase RNA-like endoplasmic reticulum kinase), specifically in embryonic β cells (PERKΔbeta) results in a 2-fold decrease in β cell proliferation, which persists through postnatal day (P).

Author details

Soltani Nepton

Physiology Department, Faculty of Medicine, Hormozgan University of Medical Science, Iran

References

[1] Beguin P, Nagashima K, Gonoi T, et al. Regulation of Ca2+ channel expression at the cell surface by the small G-protein kir/Gem. Nature. 411:701-706, 2001.

[2] Bhonde R, Shukla RC, Kanitkar M, Shukla R, Banerjee M, Datar S. Isolated islets in diabetes research. Indian J Med Res 125: 425-440, 2007

[3] Butler AE, Janson J, Bonner-Weir S, et al. Decreased B-cell mass in patients with type 2 diabetes. Program and abstracts of the 62nd Scientific Sessions of the American Diabetes Association, 14(18), 2002; San Francisco, California. Poster 1502-P. Diabetes, Volume 51, Supplement 2.

[4] Chang-Chen KJ, Mullur R, Bernal-Mizrachi E. Beta-cell failure as a complication of diabetes. Rev EndocrMetabDisord. 9(4): 329-43, 2008.

[5] Chen ZH, Li T, Chen ZB, Luo B, Sun RP. Prevention of beta cell dysfunction and apoptosis by adenoviral gene transfer of rat insulin-like growth factor 1. Chin Med J. 20;122(18): 2159-64, 2009

[6] Cornu M, Thorens B. GLP-1 protects beta-cells against apoptosis by enhancing the activity of an IGF-2/IGF1-receptor autocrine loop. Islets 1(3): 280-282, 2009

[7] Cornu M, Yang GY, Jaccard E, Poussin C, Widmann C, Thorens B. Glp-1 Protects Beta-Cells Against Apoptosis By Increasing The ActivtiyOfAn Igf-2/Igf1-Receptor Autocrine Loop. Diabetes. 28, 2009

[8] DeFronzo RA, Abdul-Ghani M. Type 2 Diabetes Can Be Prevented With Early Pharmacological Intervention. Diabetes Care. 34(2): S202-S209, 2011

[9] Evans ML, Keshavarz T, Flanagan DV, et al. ICV brain glibenclamide suppresses counterregulatory responses to brain glucopenia in rats: evidence for a role for brain KATP channels in hypoglycemia sensing. Program and abstracts of the 62nd Scientific Sessions of the American Diabetes Association, 17, 2002; San Francisco, California. Abstract 293-OR. Diabetes, Volume 51, Supplement 2.

[10] Fisher TE, Bourque CW. The function of CA(2+) channel subtypes in exocytic secretion: new perspectives from synaptic and non-synaptic release. ProgBiophysMol Biol. 77:269-303, 2001

[11] Giannoukakis N, Mi Z, Rudert WA, Gambotto A, Trucco M, Robbins P. Prevention of beta cell dysfunction and apoptosis activation in human islets by adenoviral gene transfer of the insulin-like growth factor I. Gene Ther. 7(23):2015-22, 2000.

[12] Gunasekaran U, Hudgens CW, Wright BT, Maulis MF, Gannon M. Differential regulation of embryonic and adult β cell replication.Cell Cycle. 11(13), 2012

[13] Holst J. State of the art lecture. GLP-1 based therapy of diabetes: facts and expectations. Program and abstracts of the 62nd Scientific Sessions of the American Diabetes Association; 14(18), 2002, San Francisco, California.

[14] Kashima Y, Shibasaki T, Miki T, Seino S. Importance of the cAMP-GEFII/Rim2 complex in incretin-potentiated insulin secretion. Program and abstracts of the 62nd Scientific Sessions of the American Diabetes Association, 14(18), 2002, San Francisco, California. 265-OR. Diabetes, Volume 51, Supplement 2.

[15] LeRoith D. Beta-cell dysfunction and insulin resistance in type 2 diabetes: role of metabolic and genetic abnormalities. Am J Med, 28(113): 6A:3S-11S, 2002

[16] Mansoori A, Zaheri H, Soltani N, Kharazmi F, Keshavarz M, Kamalinajad M. Effect of the administration of Psidium guava leaves on lipid profiles and sensitivity of the vascular mesenteric bed to phenylephrine in STZ-induced diabetic rats. JMD, 2(1): 138-145, 2012

[17] Mikhailov MV, Mikhailova EA, Ashcroft SJ. Structure-function relationships in the beta-cell K (ATP) channel.BiochemSoc Trans. 30(2):323-7, 2002

[18] Miki T, Liss B, Minami K, et al. KATP channels in the maintenance of glucose homeostasis. Program and abstracts of the 62nd Scientific Sessions of the American Diabetes Association, 14(18), 2002, San Francisco, California. Poster 1492-P. Diabetes, Volume 51, Supplement 2.

[19] Mirghazanfari SM, Keshavarz M, Nabavizadeh F, Soltani N, Kamalinejad M. 2010. The effect of Teucriumpolium L. Extracts on insulin release from in situ isolated per-

fused rat pancrease in newly modified isolation method: the role of Ca and K channels. Iranian Biomedical Journal. 14(4):178-185

[20] Russ HA, Sintov E, Anker-Kitai L, Friedman O, Lenz A, Toren G, Farhy C, Pasmanik-Chor M, Oron-Karni V, Ravassard P, Efrat S. Insulin-Producing Cells Generated from Dedifferentiated Human Pancreatic Beta Cells Expanded In Vitro. PLoS ONE 6(9): e25566, 2011

[21] Seino S. Plenary Lecture: Molecular mechanisms of insulin secretion. Program and abstracts of the 62nd Scientific Sessions of the American Diabetes Association, 14(18), 2002, San Francisco, California. Diabetes, Volume 51, Supplement 2.

[22] Soltani N, Keshavarz M, Dehpour AR. 2007. Effect of oral magnesium sulfate administration on blood pressure and lipid profile in streptozocin diabetic rat.Eur J Pharmacol. 560(2-3):201-5

[23] Soltani N, Kumar M, Glinka Y, Prud'homme GJ, Wang Q. 2007. Gene therapy of diabetes using a novel GLP-1/IgG1-Fc fusion construct normalizes glucose levels in db/db mice.Gene Ther. 14(2):162-72

[24] Soltani N, Qiu H, Aleksic M, Glinka Y, Zhao F, Liu R, Li Y, Zhang N, Chakrabarti R, Ng T, Jin T, Zhang H, Lu WY, Feng ZP, Prud'homme GJ, Wang Q. GABA exerts protective and regenerative effects on islet beta cells and reverses diabetes. ProcNatlAcadSci U S A. Jun 27, 2011

The Impact of Inflammation on Pancreatic β-Cell Metabolism, Function and Failure in T1DM and T2DM: Commonalities and Differences

Philip Newsholme, Kevin Keane,
Paulo I Homem de Bittencourt Jr. and
Mauricio Krause

Additional information is available at the end of the chapter

http://dx.doi.org/10.5772/55349

1. Introduction

Type 1 diabetes mellitus (T1DM) is a chronically progressive autoimmune disease that affects approximately 1% of the population in the developed world. This adverse immune response is induced and promoted by the interaction of both genetic and environmental factors. In contrast, in type 2 diabetes mellitus (T2DM), insulin-resistance coupled with reduced insulin output appears to be the major cause of hyperglycaemia (affecting approximately 6% of the population). Although the aetiology of diabetes may differ from T1DM to T2DM, a common feature associated with both types is the failure of pancreatic β-cells in the islets of Langerhans, thus causing a reduction in insulin secretion, cell mass and ultimately apoptotic death. However, the impact and time-course of pancreatic β-cell death, which may appear very different in T1 and T2DM, may be related through common molecular mechanisms.

Glucose-stimulated insulin secretion (GSIS) is central to the physiological control of metabolic fuel homeostasis, and its impairment is a hallmark of pancreatic β-cell failure in T2DM. β-Cells are often referred to as "fuel sensors" as they continually monitor and respond to dietary nutrients, under the modulation of additional neuro-hormonal and immunological signals, in order to secrete insulin to best meet the needs of the organism. Therefore, β-cell dysfunction and death in diabetes leads to hyperglycaemia and its complications. An intriguing characteristic of the pancreatic β-cells is their similarity to immune cells: 1) they can release cytokines; 2) they strongly respond to cytokines from other cells and tissues; 3) their function is dependent on the production of reactive oxygen (ROS) and nitrogen species (RNS); 4) they express high levels of pro-inflammatory proteins such as nuclear transcription factor κB (NFκB), inducible nitric oxide synthase (iNOS), NADPH oxidase (NOX), Toll-like receptors (TLR) and other proteins in response to immune signals, but also to metabolic challenge. However and in contrast to professional immunoinflammatory cells, such as macrophages or neutrophils, the β-cell is fragile when subjected to immune attack and is highly vulnerable to oxidative stress.

In this chapter, we intend to review the mechanisms of insulin secretion in response to a wide variety of metabolic stimuli, the 'immune-like' characteristics of the pancreatic β-cells with respect to metabolism, secretion and cell defence, the similarities between β-cell failure/death in T1DM and T2DM and finally, to suggest novel targets for the treatment of diabetes.

2. Regulation of β-cell function and insulin secretion

Control of energy metabolism is essential in maintaining cellular homeostasis in all animals across the metazoan (all animals with differentiated tissues). Insulin and glucagon are hormones produced by vertebrate organisms to regulate glycaemic homeostasis. In addition, insulin-like and glucagon-like peptide genes have been detected in invertebrate organisms including, insects, molluscs and nematodes, thus inferring a similar metabolic control that is conserved among most species [1,2]. However, in the case of vertebrates, insulin and glucagon are produced by cells located in the islets of Langerhans of the animal pancreas. Under normal physiological conditions, blood glucose concentration is maintained within narrow limits by an alternate release of these powerful proteins, regardless of nutrient intake or expenditure (*e.g.* exercise). There are four main cell types that contribute to the regulation of this pancreatic function and they include, α-cells, β-cells, δ-cells and pancreatic peptide (PP)-cells [3]. The role of α-cells is to synthesise and secrete glucagon in response to low extracellular glucose concentrations, thus replenishing the plasma carbohydrate level [3]. δ-Cells secrete somatostatin that has an inhibitory effect on insulin and glucagon release, while PP-cells secrete pancreatic peptide whose physiological function has not been fully elucidated [3]. Conversely, the function of β-cells has been extensively studied and they are responsible for the biosynthesis and release of insulin in response to elevated plasma glucose, amino acid and saturated fatty acid levels [3]. These cells represent the most abundant cell type in pancreatic islets and are the primary source of dysfunction in DM.

β-Cell responsiveness and subsequent insulin secretion is subject to a plethora of cellular regulatory mechanisms. Insulin biosynthesis and secretion is a highly controlled system that has many influencing extracellular and intracellular factors including, glucose, fatty acids, amino acids, nucleotides, calcium/potassium electrochemical gradient, metabolic coupling factors (MCFs), and level of ROS and RNS. Furthermore, the fact that cellular insulin secretion is achieved by the physical release of vesicles or granules containing the protein, suggests that the process acquires a greater degree of complexity and control, and is subject to vesicle manufacture, recruitment and finally plasma membrane docking.

Glucose-Stimulated Insulin Secretion (GSIS) is fundamental to insulin exocytosis as glucose is the most potent insulin secretagogue [4]. In an environment of excess extracellular glucose,

http://dx.doi.org/10.5772/55349

β-cell plasma membrane transporter proteins GLUT1 and GLUT2, actively transport free glucose molecules inside the cell where glycolysis can be initiated to create the nucleotide ATP (Fig. 1). Consequently, intracellular metabolism of glucose by glycolysis, and further metabolism of pyruvate via the downstream tricarboxylic acid (TCA) cycle, leads to elevated NADH, $FADH_2$ and ultimately ATP levels [4]. The increased intracellular ATP:ADP ratio closes membrane-bound ATP-sensitive K^+ channels, resulting in plasma membrane depolarisation and a subsequent opening of membrane-bound voltage activated Ca^{2+} channels. A rapid influx of calcium ions is promoted, causing the exocytosis of insulin through fusion of the insulin containing vesicles with the plasma membrane via VAMP (vesicle-associated membrane protein) and SNARE (soluble NH2-ethylmaleimide-sensitive fusion protein attachment protein receptor) association [5]. This specific process of insulin secretion is known as K_{ATP}-dependent GSIS, and since ATP generation is critical, the metabolic control points of glycolysis, the TCA cycle and oxidative phosphorylation (*i.e.* activity of metabolic enzymes such as hexokinase, phosphofructokinase, pyruvate kinase, pyruvate dehydrogenase, pyruvate carboxylase, glutamate dehydrogenase and mitochondrial redox-shuttles) have a significant impact on regulation of insulin release.

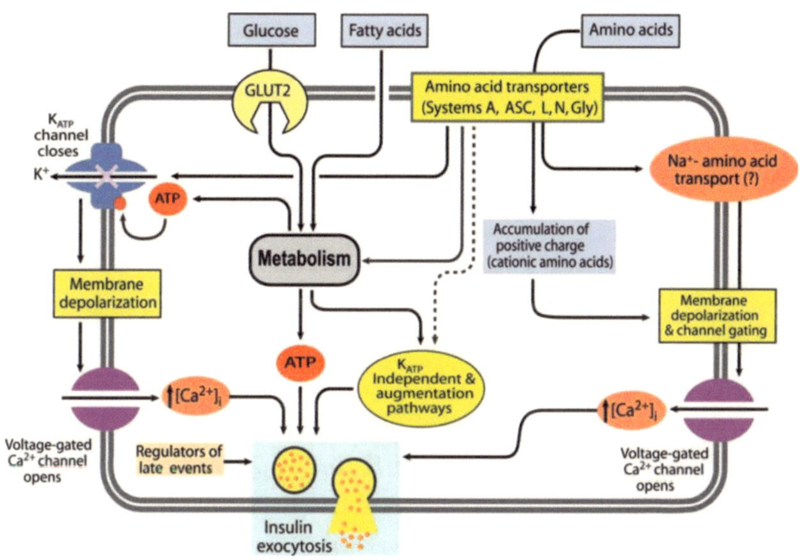

Figure 1. Mechanisms of nutrient and amino acid stimulated insulin secretion. Glucose metabolism is essential for stimulation of insulin secretion. The mechanisms by which amino acids enhance insulin secretion are understood to primarily rely on (a) direct depolarization of the plasma membrane (e.g. cationic amino acid, L-arginine); (b) metabolism (e.g. alanine, glutamine, leucine); and (c) co-transport with Na^+ and cell membrane depolarization (e.g. alanine). Notably, rapid partial oxidation may also initially increase both the cellular content of ATP (impacting on K^+ATP channel closure prompting membrane depolarization) and other stimulus secretion coupling factors. In the absence of glucose, fatty acids may be metabolised to generate ATP and maintain basal levels of insulin secretion. Adapted from [3].

However, there also remains the possibility that K_{ATP}-independent GSIS can occur in the β-cell, although the exact methodology is still not fully understood. K_{ATP}-independent GSIS has been illustrated in studies utilising diazoxide to maintain K^+ channels in the open position [6] and in mice with disrupted/deleted K^+ channels [7, 8]. GSIS was subsequently shown to be possible in a K_{ATP}-independent manner and it is believed that these two co-ordinate mechanisms of insulin secretion (*i.e.* K_{ATP}-dependent & K_{ATP}-independent GSIS), are responsible for the bi-phasic insulin response in animals. It is thought that the initial rise in insulin secretion is K_{ATP}-dependent, while the second phase is mediated through K_{ATP}-independent interactions dependent on mitochondrial activity [4,9].

Mitochondrial, lipid and amino acid metabolism plays a significant role in regulation of insulin secretion and GSIS. Lipid and amino acid metabolites can generate, or can directly become MCFs that enhance or inhibit GSIS. While individual amino acids alone at physiological concentrations do not enhance GSIS, some specific amino acids at higher concentrations, or in combination with others, can cause increments in GSIS [10]. Arginine, alanine, leucine and glutamine can increase GSIS, while homocysteine and cysteine at elevated concentration can inhibit GSIS [10]. The effect of amino acids is also dependent on whether β-cells are exposed acutely or chronically, as chronic exposure may influence the expression of genes involved in the control of insulin secretion [10,11]. In addition, another nutrient source, fatty acids, can also regulate GSIS in both a positive or negative manner depending on the level of saturation, carbon chain length, and whether exposure is under acute or chronic conditions. Saturated fatty acids like palmitic and stearic acid are known to chronically decrease GSIS *in vitro*, but palmitic acid can acutely enhance GSIS [12-14]. Conversely, chronic exposure to monounsaturated oleic acid and polyunsaturated arachidonic acid can increase insulin production in β-cells [13,15]. Fatty acids can amplify β-cell GSIS, and it is likely that they elevate insulin levels by causing changes in calcium influx and proteins associated with ion channel activity [16]. Mitochondrial metabolism of amino and fatty acid is at the hub of the reported effects on insulin secretion and GSIS, mainly because TCA-mediated metabolism of both leads to increased ATP production and protein biosynthesis, which is a prerequisite for insulin secretion (Fig. 1). The intricacies of mitochondrial-mediated metabolism of amino and fatty acids will be discussed below.

3. Pancreatic β-cell metabolism and influencing factors

Pancreatic β-cells are unique and can be distinguished from other cell types by their metabolic profile. Several key characteristics of β-cells include the ability to utilise glucose in the physiological range of 2-20mmol/L, express low levels of lactate dehydrogenase (LDH) and plasma membrane monocarboxylate pyruvate/lactate transporter, have a corresponding high activity of glycerol-3-phosphate and malate/aspartate redox shuttles, and finally possess an elevated level of pyruvate dehydrogenase (PDH) and pyruvate carboxylase (PC) activity, ensuring that both oxidative and anaplerotic metabolism of glucose and pyruvate can occur preferentially in the near absence of lactate generation (Fig. 2) (further details can be found in [4,10,11,17-21]). These adaptions are designed to specifically accelerate oxidative phosphorylation and TCA activity as a means to increase ATP output and consequently insulin exocytosis.

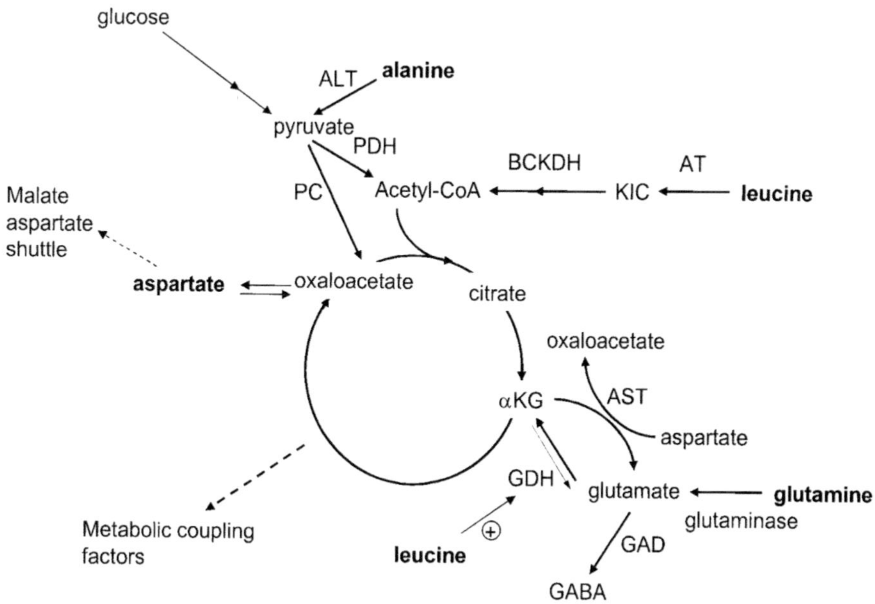

Figure 2. Schematic diagram representing the metabolism of selected amino acids, highlighting related metabolic stimulus-secretion coupling factors involved in insulin release. The pathway of glutamine metabolism via glutaminase, GDH, and entry into the TCA cycle (glutaminolysis) is shown along with key points of amino acid interaction with glutamine and glucose metabolism. KG, -ketoglutarate; ALT, alanine aminotransferase; AST, aspartate aminotransferase; AT, aminotransferase; BCKDH, branched-chain-keto-acid dehydrogenase; PC, pyruvate carboxylase; PDH, pyruvate dehydrogenase; KIC, ketoisocaproic acid. Adapted from [21].

Pancreatic β-cells regenerate NAD^+ for glycolysis primarily through high expression of mitochondrial NADH shuttles like glycerol-3-phosphate and the malate/aspartate shuttle (Fig. 3), for specific details refer to [11,22]. Briefly, the glycerol-3-phosphate shuttle consists of cytosolic and mitochondrial glycerol-3-phosphate dehydrogenase that operate in unison to convert dihydroxyacetone phosphate to glycerol-3-phosphate and NAD^+, with a subsequent generation of $FADH_2$ from NAD^+ [4]. In contrast, the malate/aspartate shuttle is the main shuttle responsible for transferring glycolytic reducing equivalents to the mitochondria in the β-cell [11]. Here, cytosolic malate dehydrogenase reduces oxaloacetate to malate and NAD^+, with a subsequent generation of NADH inside the mitochondria. Using an amino group provided by glutamate, mitochondrial oxaloacetate can be converted back to aspartate maintaining this cyclic event. The malate/aspartate shuttle is dominantly expressed in β-cells, eloquently linking glycolysis to mitochondrial & amino acid metabolism.

As alluded to previously, amino acid metabolism is essential for nutrient- and glucose-stimulated insulin secretion, and the effects of several amino acids have been reviewed extensively [3,10, 11]. To summarise these findings briefly, both arginine and alanine have been shown to promote insulin release through changes in electrogenic transport, progressing to activation of Ca^{2+} ion channels [10,23,24]. It has also been demonstrated that they enhance glutamate production and consequently may play a role in malate/aspartate shuttle-mediated generation of NADH, and/or in glutathione synthesis and antioxidant defence [25]. Therefore, both arginine and alanine may

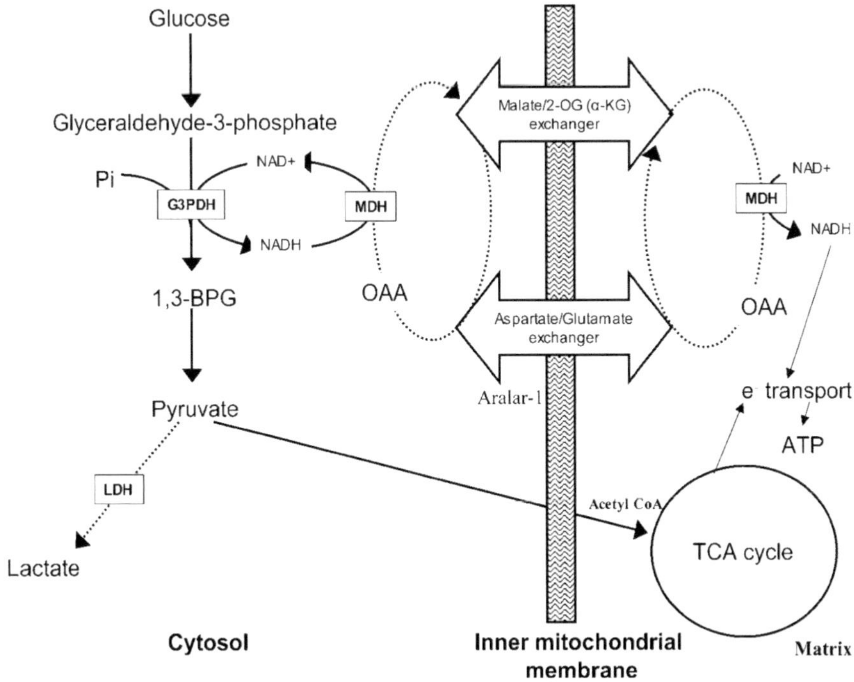

Figure 3. The malate–aspartate shuttle is the principal mechanism for the movement of reducing equivalents in the form of NADH from the cytoplasm to the mitochondrion in β-cells. Cytoplasmic malate dehydrogenase (MDH) reduces oxaloacetate (OAA) to malate while oxidizing NADH to NAD+. Malate then enters the mitochondrion where the reverse reaction is performed by mitochondrial malate dehydrogenase. Movement of mitochondrial oxaloacetate to the cytoplasm to maintain this cycle is achieved by transamination to aspartate with the amino group being donated by glutamate. The 2-oxoglutarate (α-ketoglutarate) generated leaves the mitochondrion for the cytoplasm. Adapted from [11].

protect β-cells from oxidative insult in addition to promoting insulin secretion. However, prolonged exposure of β-cells to alanine results in decreased alanine-induced insulin secretion, while reaction of arginine with inducible nitric oxide synthase (iNOS) can promote nitric oxide (NO) production [10,19]. NO is an important signalling molecule, which is essential for β-cell glucose uptake at low levels, but at high concentration may be toxic [26]. Interaction of NO with superoxide (O^-) can also lead to the formation of peroxynitrite ($ONOO^-$), a damaging free radical that can disrupt mitochondrial function [27]. In fact, $ONOO^-$, which is in equilibrium with its conjugate peroxynitrous acid (ONOOH, $pK_a \approx 6.8$) [28], is a highly reactive oxidant species produced by the combination of the oxygen free radical O_2^- and NO [29] and has been demonstrated to be a more potent oxidant and cytotoxic mediator than NO or O_2^- individually, in a variety of inflammatory conditions [30]. $ONOO^-$ is extremely cytotoxic to rat and human islet cells *in vitro* [31] and its *in vivo* formation has been reported in pancreatic islets where it has been associated with β-cell destruction and development of T1DM in NOD mice [32].

High levels of homocysteine and cysteine have also been shown to elicit a negative effect on β-cell function. In obese hyperinsulinaemic T2DM patients, homocysteine levels are increased, while they are increased in T1DM patients, but only following disease-related complications

http://dx.doi.org/10.5772/55349

such as diabetic nephropathy [11,33]. It has been suggested that homocysteine can decrease GSIS in rat pancreatic β-cells [34], although the inhibitory mechanism is still not fully understood. It may decrease insulin secretion by altering enzyme and/or protein activity, or by causing oxidative stress [35,36]. In addition, homocysteine can be converted to asymmetric dimethylarginine, which is inhibitor of neuronal NOS and can also inhibit iNOS to a lesser extent and therefore may reduce NO production, which is important for β-cell insulin secretion and function [10,37]. In contrast, cysteine has been shown to increase β-cell GSIS at low concentrations [38] and is essential for antioxidant defence and glutathione synthesis, along with glycine and glutamate. Cysteine supplementation was found to protect β-cells from hydrogen peroxide (H_2O_2)-induced cell death and prevented glucotoxicity in mouse β-cells [39,40]. However, at elevated concentrations, it impaired GSIS through excessive hydrogen sulphide (H_2S) formation [41].

Glutamine is required for β-cell metabolism and function, and is consumed at rapid rates [10]. Glutamine supplementation does not induce insulin release [10], but co-treatment with leucine significantly enhances GSIS via activation of glutamate dehydrogenase (GDH), allowing entry of glutamine into the TCA cycle (Fig. 2) [42]. It has been suggested that glutamine alone does not induce insulin secretion because it is not oxidised during its metabolism. Instead, metabolism of glutamine may yield aspartate and GABA (γ-aminobutyric acid), a potent inhibitor of glucagon secretion (Fig. 2) [3]. However, using NMR studies, we found that the major products of glutamine metabolism were aspartate and glutamate. Here, glutamate entered the γ-glutamyl cycle and increased the synthesis of the antioxidant, glutathione [43]. Formation of glutamate from glutamine also has important implications in activation of the aspartate/glutamate shuttles and in ATP production from the TCA cycle, via glutamate metabolism to α-ketoglutarate. Consequently, glutamine may function to enhance ATP production and insulin release by changes in down-stream metabolism, most notably via glutamine-derived glutamate. Alternatively, glutamate can be transported externally from the cell and into the surrounding matrix, which may cause glutamate receptor activation and desensitisation if the rate of release is over extended periods [44]. Since glucagon secretion from pancreatic α-cells is sensitive to glutamate exposure, its release may represent a novel paracrine control mechanism for modulation of blood carbohydrate levels [44]. Some groups have reported that total intracellular glutamate levels increased in response to glucose, while others reported no significant change [25,45,46]. Recently, it has been suggested that glutamate is transported into insulin-containing vesicles, thereby promoting Ca^{2+}-dependent insulin secretion [47]. However, the role of glutamate in mediating insulin secretion remains hotly debated.

Taken together, this evidence suggests that a variety of amino acids may contribute significantly to regulation of pancreatic β-cell insulin secretion. However, other β-cell metabolic processes are important to insulin secretion and must be considered. These include four key metabolic shunts that divert glucose from being utilised by TCA cycle (*i.e.*, aldose reductase, pentose-phosphate, glycogen synthesis and hexosamine pathways; please, see Fig. 4) as well as down-stream glycolytic enzymes such as PC and PDH, and also enzymes involved in fatty acid metabolism like acetyl CoA carboxylase (ACC) and fatty acid synthase.

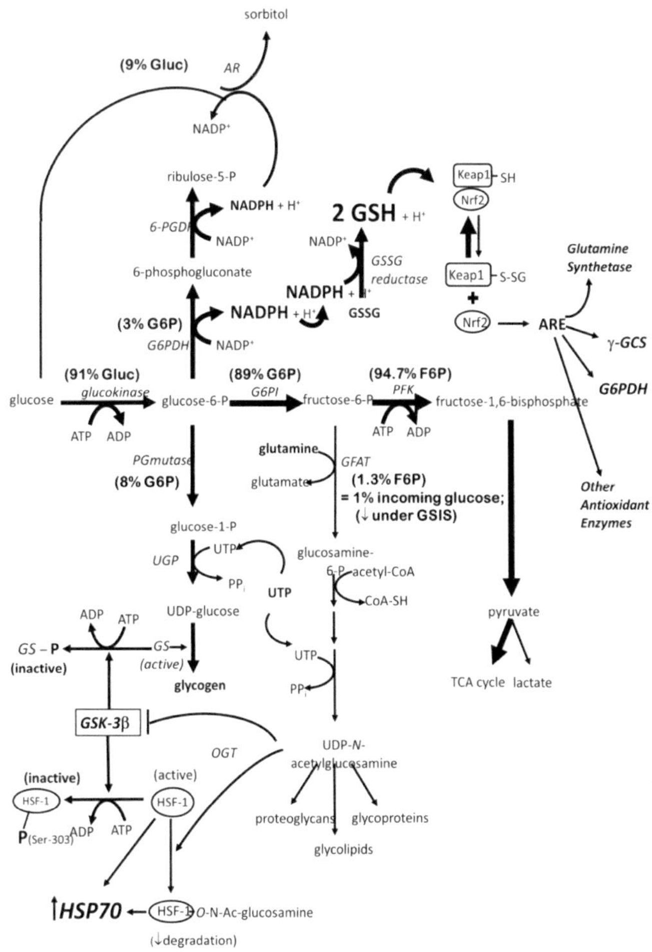

Figure 4. Flux balance analysis of glucose utilisation in β-cells. The fluxes through the biochemical pathways shown here were calculated by using Michaelis-Menten function, intracellular metabolite concentrations estimated from different works. Percentages in parentheses refer to the proportional amount of the metabolite consumed through that step. AR, aldose reductase; ARE, antioxidant response (ARE) elements in the promoter regions of target genes; F6P, fructose-6-phosphate; G6P, glucose-6-phosphate; G6PDH, glucose-6-phosphate dehydrogenase; G6PI, glucose-6-phosphate isomerase (a.k. as phosphoglucoisomerase); γ-GCS, glutamate cysteine ligase, a.k. as γ-glutamylcysteine synthetase; GFAT, glutamine:fructose-6-phosphate amidotransferase a.k. as GFPT, for glutamine-fructose-6-phosphate transaminase; Gluc, glucose; GS, glycogen synthase; GSIS, glucose-stimulated insulin secretion; GSK-3β, glycogen synthase kinase-3β; HSF-1, heat shock transcription factor-1; HSP70, the 70-kDa family of heat shock proteins (includes both hsp72, encoded by the HSPA1A gene, and hsp73, a.k. as hsc70, encoded by the HSPA8 gene); Keap1, Kelch-like ECH-associated protein 1; Nrf2, Nuclear factor erythroid 2-related transcription factor 2; OGT, *O-N*-acetylglucosamine transferase, a.k. as UDP-*N*-acetyl-D-glucosamine:protein-*O*-β-*N*-acetyl-D-glucosaminyl transferase and uridine diphospho-*N*-acetylglucosamine:polypeptide β-*N*-acetylglucosaminyl transferase; PFK, phosphofructokinase; PGmutase, phosphoglucomutase; UGP, UDP-glucose pyrophosphorylase.

Highlighting the peculiarities of β-cell metabolism in a coordinated effort to increase the activity of a number of metabolic pathways in response to glucose, Huang & Joseph (2012) have shown, by using metabolomic analysis, during GSIS in clonal β-cells, a conspicuous accumulation of pyruvate, succinate, fumarate, malate, α-ketoglutarate, dihydroxyacetone phosphate (DHAP), (iso)citrate, palmitate, glucose-6-phosphate and 6-phosphogluconate whereas aspartate was consumed in response to glucose [48]. Here, the authors have clearly demonstrated that under glucose stimulus, β-cells strongly enhance metabolic flux towards glycolysis and TCA cycle. Indeed, there is a very delicate poise to coordinately regulate the flux of glucose towards the formation of NADPH (through the pentose-phosphate shunt) avoiding excessive formation of sorbitol (via the polyol-aldose reductase shunt) which would empty glycolytic flux (Fig. 4). It has long been recognised, for instance, that overexpression of the aldose reductase gene is able to induce apoptosis in pancreatic β-cells by causing a redox imbalance [49] while, on the contrary, pharmacological blockage of aldose reductase may impair GSIS, thus suggesting that the conversion of free intracellular glucose to sorbitol in the β-cell is an essential step in the glucose-induced release mechanism (Fig.4) [50].

Although the physiological significance is still under debate, glucose 6-phosphate may also be targeted towards glycogen synthesis in pancreatic islets, which is enhanced during GSIS and impaired in STZ-diabetic rats (Fig. 4) [51,52]. Finally, glucose may be deviated from ultimate metabolism through further glycolytic steps via the reaction of fructose-6-phosphate with glutamine through the hexosamine biochemical pathway (HBP) (Fig. 4). Increased fluxes through HBP may, on the one hand, block glycogen synthase kinase-3β (GSK-3β), thus liberating glycogen synthesis by glycogen synthase and, on the other, may reduce heat shock factor-1 (HSF-1) degradation thus allowing enhanced expression of the 70-kDa heat shock protein (HSP70), which is cytoprotective to β-cells (Fig. 4) [53,54]. Over-enhanced flux through HBP is an inducer of endoplasmic reticulum (ER) stress, while being associated with insulin-resistance [55].

PC and PDH are both highly expressed in β-cells and allow conversion of pyruvate to oxaloacetate (PC) and acetyl-CoA (PDH), with subsequent entry into the TCA cycle [4]. Interestingly, siRNA inhibition of PC reduces cell proliferation and GSIS in insulinoma cells and rat islets, while overexpression in rat islets could enhance GSIS and cell proliferation [56, 57]. The role of PDH is less understood and it is thought to support PC activity by providing acetyl-CoA for citrate production. Both enzymes are important regulators of the pyruvate/malate and pyruvate/citrate shuttles. Common to each pathway is the conversion of glycolytic-derived pyruvate to oxaloacetate by PC, as described above. In the case of the pyruvate/malate shuttle, oxaloacetate is then converted to malate and translocated to the cytosol, where malic enzyme1 (ME1) converts malate back to pyruvate along with generation of NADPH. Pyruvate can re-enter the mitochondria to repeat the cycle with further generation of NADPH [4]. However, for the pyruvate/citrate shuttle, PC-mediated oxaloacetate leads to condensation with acetyl CoA (possibly generated by PDH), and the subsequent formation of citrate. Translocation of citrate to the cytosol results in oxaloacetate and acetyl CoA regeneration from citrate by ATP-citrate lyase (ACL). Oxaloacetate re-enters the pyruvate/malate cycle with generation of NADPH as outlined previously, while acetyl CoA is carboxylated to malonyl CoA by acetyl CoA carboxylase (ACC). Malonyl CoA is then converted to long chain acyl CoA by fatty acid synthase leading to fatty acid production. Additionally, malonyl CoA can also inhibit carnitine palmitoyl transferase 1 (CPT-1), which in a low glucose state, transports fatty acids into the mitochondria to generate ATP by oxidation [4,10]. However, in high glucose situations, inhibition of CPT-1 leads to fatty acid accumulation in the cytosol and this accumulation may increase insulin exocytosis by augmenting calcium influx and ion channel proteins [10,16]. Interestingly, formation of malonyl CoA from acetyl CoA by ACC is positively regulated by the glutamine-sensitive protein phosphatase type 2A (PP2A), while it is negatively regulated by the amino acid-sensitive AMP-activated kinase (AMPK) [11,58,59]. These concepts again fully illustrate the inherent relationship between β-cell metabolism of glucose, amino acids and lipids with insulin exocytosis [11,58,59].

AMPK is crucial in lipid metabolism control and can chronically regulate β-cell function by altering the expression of vital transcription factors that govern lipogenic and glycolytic enzymes [10]. Chronic exposure of β-cells to high circulatory lipid levels, as occurs in T2DM, can inhibit glucose oxidation and result in a decreased ATP/AMP ratio along with a subsequent activation of AMPK, which inhibits fatty acid synthesis, while enhancing fatty acid oxidation, and impairing GSIS [10]. The exact metabolic mechanisms of how lipids can augment GSIS are still not fully understood but are believed to involve modulation of Ca^{2+} mobilisation via interaction with G-protein coupled receptors [60]. Recent evidence has shown that these G-protein coupled receptors are highly expressed in β-cells and correlated with insulinogenic index [10,61]. It has also been demonstrated that interaction of omega-3 fatty acids and the GPR120 receptor, plays an instrumental role in mediating insulin-sensitisation and anti-inflammatory effects in obese mice models [62].

AMPK also occupies a central position in metabolic regulation in order to avoid inflammatory dysregulation. Accordingly, in different cell types, AMPK phosphorylates and inhibit glutamine:fructose-6-phosphate amidotransferase-1 (GFAT-1), the flux-generating step of HBP (Fig. 4), thus allowing for the down-regulation of such a shunt from glycolysis under low glucose situations [63], while chronic hexosamine flux stimulates fatty acid oxidation by activating AMPK [64]. However, regulatory pathways under AMPK control are not solely intended to divert metabolic fluxes. Rather, AMPK regulation of GSK-3β allows the concomitant regulation of inflammatory cytokine production, since the inhibition of GSK-3β elicits the deinhibition of HSF-1, thus triggering the expression of HSP70, which is an intracellular anti-inflammatory protein.

It is of note that, besides the now classical molecular chaperone action, the most remarkable intracellular effect of HSP70 is the inhibition of NF- κB activation, which has profound implications for immunity, inflammation, cell survival and apoptosis. HSP70 blocks nuclear factor κB (NF—κB) activation at different levels. For instance, HSP70 inhibits the phosphorylation of inhibitor of κB (IκBs), while heat-induced HSP70 protein molecules are able to directly bind to IκB kinase gamma (IKKγ) thus inhibiting tumor necrosis factor- α (TNFα)-induced apoptosis [65]. In fact, the supposition that HSP70 might act intracellularly as a suppressor of NF- κB pathways has been raised after a number of seminal discoveries in which HSP70 was intentionally induced, such as the inhibition of TNFα-induced activation of phospholipase A_2 in murine fibrosarcoma cells [66], the suppression of astroglial iNOS expression paralleled by decreased NF— κB activation [67] and the protection of rat hepatocytes from TNFα-induced apoptosis by treating cells with the nitric oxide (NO)-donor SNAP, which reacts with intracellular glutathione molecules generating S-nitrosoglutathione (SNOG) that induces HSP70, and, consequently, HSP70 expression [68].

HSP70 confers protection against sepsis-related circulatory fatality via inhibition of iNOS (NOS-2) gene expression in the rostral ventrolateral medulla through the prevention of NF-κB activation, inhibition of IκB kinase activation and consequent inhibition of IκB degradation [69]. This is corroborated by the finding that HSP70 assembles with liver NF-κB/IκB complex in the cytosol thus impeding further transcription of NF-κB-dependent TNF-α and NOS-2 genes that worsen sepsis [70]. This may also be unequivocally demonstrated by treating cells or tissues with HSP70 antisense oligonucleotides that completely reverse the beneficial NF-κB-inhibiting effect of HSP70 and inducible HSP70 expression (see [68,69]). Hence, HSP70 is anti-inflammatory per se, when intracellularly located, which also explains why cyclopentenone prostaglandins (cp-PGs), which are the most powerful physiological inducers of HSP70 by activating HSF-1, are at the same time powerful anti-inflammatory autacoids [71-73].

Another striking effect of HSP70 is the inhibition of apoptosis. The intrinsic apoptotic pathway is characterized by the release of mitochondrial pro-apoptotic factors and activation of caspase enzymes, while stimulation of cell surface receptors triggers the extrinsic death-pathway. The inhibitory potential of HSP70 over apoptosis occurs via many intracellular downstream pathways (e.g. JNK, NF-κB and Akt), which are both directly and indirectly blocked by HSP70, or through inhibition of mitochondrial Bcl-2 release. Together, these mechanisms are responsible for HSP70's anti-apoptotic function in stressed-cells [74].

In conclusion, intracellularly activated HSPs of the 70-kDa family are cytoprotective and anti-inflammatory by avoiding protein denaturation and excessive NF-κB activation which may be damaging to the cells [75]. These observations link energy sensing (AMPK) to anti-inflammation (HSP70) and points out to the complexity of the impact of metabolic regulation for cell survival and function. In addition, expression of cytokines such as interleukin-1β (IL-1β), tumour necrosis factorα (TNFα), and interferon-γ (INF-γ) in pancreatic islets is important in inflammation and progression of both T1 and T2DM, and is associated with β-cell dysfunction and death. Therefore, agents or nutrients that promote anti-inflammatory responses may be beneficial as anti-diabetic therapies. Since interaction of the immune system with pancreatic islets is central to T1DM and is becoming increasing linked to T2DM, the precise mechanisms of pancreatic cell death in relation to immunological function will now be discussed.

4. Immune-like characteristics of β-cells and response to cytokines

The pathophysiology of pancreatic islets in T1 and T2DM is characterised by an inflammatory process that includes immune cell infiltration, presence of apoptotic cells, expression of cytokines or adipokines and even amyloid deposits [76]. Although the aetiology of T1DM differs from T2DM, a common feature of both is an immune system-mediated destruction of pancreatic β-cells, ultimately leading to pancreatic dysfunction and reduced β-cell mass. However, the immunological-mediated attack does not solely originate from invading macrophages and/or cytokines produced by T-lymphocytes, as initially occurs in early stage T1DM. In fact, it also stems from local production of pro-inflammatory cytokines by the pancreatic β-cells themselves. The similarity between pancreatic β-cells and immune cells is an intriguing characteristic. Both can release and respond to cytokines; their function is dependent on changes in concentration of ROS/RNS and they both express high levels of pro-inflammatory proteins such as NFκB, iNOS, NOX and TLR's. Pancreatic β-cells have been shown to express biologically active cytokines like the pro-inflammatory cytokine IL-1β in hyperglycaemic conditions [77,78]. Due to their potent effects, cytokine production is stringently regulated. Control mechanisms include down-stream activation/processing (conversion of pro-IL-1β to IL-1β by inflammasomes), and co-expression of binding proteins/antagonists (like the IL-1 receptor antagonist, IL-1Ra), that regulate cytokine bio-reactivity [76]. However, expression of the biologically active form of IL-1β was evident in pancreatic β-cells, indicating that similar to immune cells, these cells possess the necessary cellular machinery to allow expression of immunologically active cytokines [77]. Autocrine production of IL-1β, has been correlated with autoimmune destruction of β-cells in T1DM and is also associated with glucotoxicity in the pathogenesis of T2DM patients [76,79]. IL-1β elicits its potent cytotoxic effects through activation of NFκB, and a subsequent initiation of the extrinsic cell-death pathway [78]. Additionally, chronic exposure to IL-1β results in increased iNOS expression, and consequently excess NO production. High levels of NO inhibit mitochondrial ATP synthesis and up-regulate the expression of pro-inflammatory genes in β-cells, which may potentiate β-cell failure [78].

Similar to macrophages and dendritic cells, β-cells also express TLR's that normally function to regulate the immune system [80]. TLR's interact with a wide variety of pathogen-related molecules, including lipopolysaccharide (LPS), a component of bacterial cell walls. This allows phagocytosis of microbes before infection can be established. However, in β-cells, it is believed that TLR's play a role in insulin-resistance and inflammation in T2DM. TLR2 and TLR4 have been suggested as receptors for fatty acids, and may alter insulin signalling during dyslipidaemia. We have shown that β-cells express a range of TLR's and could indeed respond to LPS via TLR's, and this interaction decreased insulin exocytosis accordingly [80]. However, glutamine restored insulin release. Glutamine can also regulate pro-inflammatory gene expression in mononuclear cells [11,80]. Glutamine also up-regulates nuclear factor of activated T cells (NFAT), and thus promotes β-cell growth, while suppressing β-cell death. Mutations in NFAT-dependent genes have been demonstrated to result in hereditary forms of T2DM [11]. Moreover, as discussed above, glutamine can enter HBP thus regulating GSK-3β activity and HSP70 expression which promotes anti-inflammation and cytoprotection [53,54].

Pancreatic β-cells are also reported to express other cytokines, including IL-6, IL-8, granulocyte colony-stimulating factor (G-CSP) and MIP-1 (macrophage inflammatory protein-1) that not only induce apoptotic β-cell death, but also signal patrolling macrophages, enhancing islet immune cell infiltration [76]. Macrophages, monocytes, neutrophils and dendritic cells perform their function by engulfing invading foreign matter including bacteria or dead cells, and degrade them using super oxide (O_2^-) generated from plasma membrane-bound NOX [27].

http://dx.doi.org/10.5772/55349

β-Cells also express NOX in large quantities, and utilise controlled NOX-derived ROS to drive mitogenic signalling and proliferation [27]. However, during hyperglycaemia or dyslipidaemia as occurs in T2DM, levels of NOX-derived ROS may increase and overwhelm antioxidant defences, leading to mitochondrial dysfunction, DNA oxidation, lipid peroxidation and β-cell death.

These reports illustrate the immune-like characteristics of pancreatic β-cells and clearly demonstrate the ability of these cells to not only respond to cytokines, but to be capable of producing endogenous cytokines in an autocrine fashion. This suggests that the immune system plays an integral part in progression of DM and may offer potential therapeutic targets. However, to develop immune-related treatments, more research is required into understanding the mechanisms of islet inflammation in both T1 and T2DM.

5. Islet inflammation in T1DM and T2DM

T1DM is exclusively an autoimmune form of DM, and islet inflammation is characterised by the presence of leukocyte infiltrates that include B-cells, T-cells, macrophages and Natural Killer (NK) cells [81]. Macrophages play a critical role since they phagocytose apoptotic and necrotic β-cells, as well as produce ROS and cytokines (TNFα, INF-γ and IL-1β), that can promote β-cell death, which leads to patient insulin-dependence. However, effector CD4-helper and CD8-cytotoxic T-cells represent the predominant pancreatic infiltrate for this disease, and recent evidence has suggested that T1DM progression may be dependent on a precarious equilibrium between migration and activation of effector and regulatory T-cells (Treg) [82]. An important element in T1DM disease development is the generation of autoreactive effector T-cells that kill pancreatic β-cells through expression of Fas, lytic granules and cytokines such as INF-γ [82]. Research into formation of these autoimmune cell types is still at an early stage, and it was only definitively shown in 2012, that autoreactive effector cytotoxic-CD8 T-cells were indeed present in T1DM human pancreatic islets [81]. Furthermore, the means by which these "homicidal" immune cells are generated and go on to attack β-cells is still not fully understood. However, part of the process is believed to involve dendritic cell migration to draining lymph nodes following antigen presentation, and stimulation of autoreactive T-cell differentiation [82,83]. T-cells sub-sets such as T_h1, T_h2 and T_h17 are thus formed and they express the necessary weaponry that is responsible for β-cell death in T1DM [82], this being exacerbated by strong psychological stress [84], one of the possible triggering factors for the onset of T1DM (for review, please see [85]). Additionally, T-cell–mediated release of INF-γ and TNFα can up-regulate expression of pro-apoptotic proteins (Bim and PUMA) leading to β-cell death, along with promoting recruitment and clearance of damaged-cells by macrophages [77,86]. On the other hand, in normal individuals, activity of these autoimmune cells is normally controlled by Treg cells and it is the failure to control the action of effector T-cells that result in autoimmune disease. The mechanisms by which Treg cells prevent autoimmune attack is also not fully elucidated, but they are thought to prevent cytotoxic action of T-cells by use of contact inhibition and release of soluble signalling factors, such as IL-10 and TGFβ (transforming growth factorβ) [82]. It is also unclear whether the precise causes of inflammation in T1DM are a consequence of T-cell failure to respond to Treg, or whether defective or low Treg numbers are to blame for disease progression. Nonetheless, the interplay between these cell populations offers a potential therapeutic strategy for T1DM treatment [82].

Interestingly, an autoimmune element has also been reported in patients with T2DM, along with the accepted thesis of insulin-resistance [76,87]. Hyperglycaemia, dyslipidaemia and low-grade inflammation (consisting of circulating inflammatory cytokines or adipokines released by adipocyte expansion), are considered important factors in the progression of T2DM and are generally present in obese individuals who are at risk of T2DM development [77]. These conditions lead to β-cell stress through a variety of processes that mainly include uncontrolled generation of ROS/RNS and cytokine-dependent initiation of death signals. Both processes combine to reduce β-cell function and decrease β-cell mass by inducing apoptotic cell death, leading to further hyperglycaemic and dyslipidaemic complications, and causing amplification of ROS/RNS generation, cytokine release and cytokine-mediated recruitment of the immune system (i.e. inflammation). These inflammatory factors are all detrimental for β-cell survival. As mentioned previously, IL-1β is elevated in the hyperglycaemic state, is increased in T1DM and is also expressed by β-cells in T2DM [77-79,88]. Moreover, concomitant down-regulation of the receptor antagonist IL-1Ra was also observed in β-cells cultured in hyperglycaemic conditions [76]. β-Cells are similar to immune cells and dysregulated expression of IL-1β in islets can cause auto-stimulation and subsequent release of IL-1β by other β-cells, via NFκB activation [76,88]. In addition, IL-1β can promote the local expression of other cytokines, for example IL-6 and IL-8. These cytokines aid in the recruitment of patrolling macrophages, which may subsequently become activated by high microenvironment levels of IL-1β and amplify IL-1β content in their own right [76]. In terms of islet inflammation, IL-1β expression and its effects on β-cell death appears to be a uniting factor, in both T1 and T2DM and is being considered a possible therapeutic target [77,89].

While inflammation is essential to maintain tissue homeostasis, it is also beneficial and allows repair of damaged organs. However, it is the presence of chronic, out of control and unchecked inflammatory factors that contribute to β-cell death and ensuing DM. Ultimately, increased local microenvironment cytokine production in islets is detrimental and understanding the mechanisms of cytokine release and regulation, and also suppression of β-cell function, will allow the development of new treatment regimens.

6. Inflammatory mediators and suppression of β-cell function

Since inflammation and β-cell death is common to both T1 and T2DM, it is reasonable to assume that shared inflammatory mediators may exist between the two conditions. It is these mediators that promote infiltration of immune cells, suppression of β-cell function, culminating in reduced insulin exocytosis and increased β-cell apoptosis. These mediators can be loosely classified into four categories, cytokines, chemokines, ROS/RNS and other inflammatory products. However, it must be noted that the activity of these modulators can be heavily influenced by nutrient availability, such as in hyperglycaemia and dyslipidaemia conditions. Further to this, there is significant crossover between the molecules in these categories, and several can significantly impact on the others, indicating a complex role in both T1 and T2DM.

T1DM is an autoimmune disease and it comes as no surprise that cytokine expression is elevated in these patients [79]. Interestingly, it is becoming more evident that cytokines also play a critical role in T2DM progression, and increased levels have been reported in T2DM patients [76,87]. The most obvious source of cytokine production is from islet invading immune cells, although other researchers have illustrated that islet β-cells could also express cytokines [76,79]. Cytokine and adipokine release also occurs from adipose tissue since it expands rapidly in obese patients. Here, hypoxia also plays a key part in cytokine release due to an inflammatory response to lack of vasculature in rapidly growing adipose tissue [90,91]. Recent evidence has suggested that adipocyte invading macrophages are a significant supplier of TNFα to the circulation in obese T2DM patients, and this could be a contributing-factor that modulates inflammation in disease progression [92,93]. It is likely that all sources contribute in some way or another to elevate cytokine levels, and consequently compound inflammation in DM patients.

The main cytokines that are responsible for inflammation in T1 and T2DM, include IL-1β, TNFα, INF-γ, IL-6 and IL-8. Central to the inflammatory role of each is stimulation of stress-induced kinases, IKKβ (inhibitor of nuclear factor kappaB kinase subunit β) and/or c-JNK (c-Jun-N-terminal kinase) [90]. Activation of IKKβ leads to translocation and activation of the NFκB. This factor targets transcription of genes associated with inflammation, and can cause subsequent up-regulation and release of IL-1β, TNFα, IL-6 and IL-8 [94,95]. Therefore, the aforementioned cytokines can initiate an auto-stimulatory or feed-forward inflammatory effect through NFκB-signalling in β-cells, resulting in amplification of inflammation. IL-1β and TNFα initiate NFκB-signalling directly via association with their relative receptors (IL-1R and TNFR) [96] and can also activate the apoptotic JNK pathway indirectly by intracellular interaction of TNF receptor associated factor (TRAF) with the cytoplasmic portion of IL-1R or TNFR [97]. NFκB can play either a pro-survival or pro-death role given the correct circumstances [98]. Both NFκB and JNK are intrinsically connected, and NFκB can prevent JNK-mediated cell death, the regulatory interactions of which have been reviewed expertly elsewhere [99]. An important component of NFκB activation and function is the presence/absence of ROS/RNS. Therefore, ROS/RNS can influence NFκB-dependent cytokine expression and consequently immune response [98].

ROS/RNS can activate nuclear translocation of NFκB which promotes gene expression. However, ROS/RNS can also have an inhibitory effect when NFκB has already translocated to the nucleus [98]. The process by which ROS/RNS affects NFκB function is not entirely known but is believed to involve alteration of the NFκB catalytic site through interaction with cysteine residues, or by inhibiting specific kinase enzymes such as IκBα, that results in phosphorylation of NFκB [98]. Cellular ROS can be generated from Electron Transport Chain (ETC) respiratory complexes or from specific enzymes (e.g. NOX-mediated production for phagocytosis) [27,98]. Most notably, in hyperglycaemic/glucotoxic conditions (in T1 or T2DM), mitochondria are the major source of ROS/RNS primarily because of high oxidative phosphorylation and ATP production [100]. As a result of unavoidable oxidative chemistry and prolonged ETC activity, superoxide (O_2^-) anions can be formed and may "leak" from the mitochondria and elicit cellular damage [100]. Additionally, excess glucose can cause increased intracellular calcium, which may enhance mitochondrial O_2^- output, but also activate NOX-derived ROS via protein kinase C (PKC) [100]. High glucose can also induce NOX activity through NADPH production from the conversion of glucose-6-phosphate to pentose leading to increased O_2^- [100]. Superoxide is a precursor reactive species and can be converted to other forms of strong oxidants including H_2O_2, and free radicals such as hydroxyl radicals and also peroxynitrite following reaction with NO [27,100]. These reactive species can cause DNA, lipid and protein damage and can also activate/regulate NFκB, who in turn can promote cytokine release and increased NO/O_2^- production by activation of iNOS and NOX expression [100,101]. Thus, ROS/RNS can exacerbate the immunological response and lead to cell death in a cyclic fashion (Fig. 5).

Lipid- and adipose-derived factors are considered other inflammatory mediators. In T2DM patients, dyslipidaemia occurs along with hyperglycaemia and consequently vascular circulation and intracellular accumulation of lipids can have a profound effect on the inflammatory response. Excess fatty acids can induced ROS generation through increased TCA metabolite production, increased NADH/NAD+ ratio and elevated intracellular Ca^{2+} [100]. They can also increase O_2^- and NO production via activation of NOX and iNOS, respectively, all potentially activating the NFκB pathway [97,100,102]. Formation of ceramide from long chain fatty acids also contributes to precipitation of lipotoxicity in β-cells and results in ROS generation and apoptotic death [97,100]. Ceramide, synthesised by serine palmitoyltransferase from long chain fatty acids like palmitic acid [100], is capable of inhibiting the pro-survival PI3K pathway, activating caspase-9 [100]. Like other fatty acids, ceramide can associate with and activate TLR's, which may elicit an immune response [90].

Since adipose tissue expands in obese patients, increased adipose-derived factors have been detected in patient serum, including leptin, TNFα and IL-6. Leptin and adiponectin can play a role in the immune reaction in DM patients. Leptin, an appetite control endocrine factor, inhibits feeding by interaction with receptors in the hypothalamus and a subsequent stimulation of neurotransmitter release, for example norepinephrine [103]. It is considered a cytokine due to its homology in structure with IL-6, and its receptor-mediated effects [77,103,104]. It has been shown to induce β-cell death by up-regulating IL-1β, and has also been implicated in exacerbation of T1DM in animal models [77,105]. Conversely, adiponectin is considered an anti-inflammatory protein, and enhances IL-1Ra and IL-10 expression [90,106], leading to reduced IL-1β and enhanced suppression of T-cell mediated inflammation.

Chemokines can also be secreted from adipose tissue and are elevated in the adipose tissue of obese mice and humans [90,107]. CC-chemokine ligand-2 (CCL-2) functions to recruit monocytes to adipose tissue resulting in differentiation into activated macrophages [108]. Others such as CCL-3, CCL-6, CCL-7, CCL-8 and CCL-9, have also been reported to be elevated in high-fat fed mice, suggesting they may play a role in immune cell recruitment and inflammation [90].

Several mechanisms and modulators may contribute to the inflammatory response observed in T1 and T2DM. Cytokines, ROS and NFκB-signalling appear to be critical in mediating immune cell infiltration and further cytokine production. The balance between β-cell survival

http://dx.doi.org/10.5772/55349

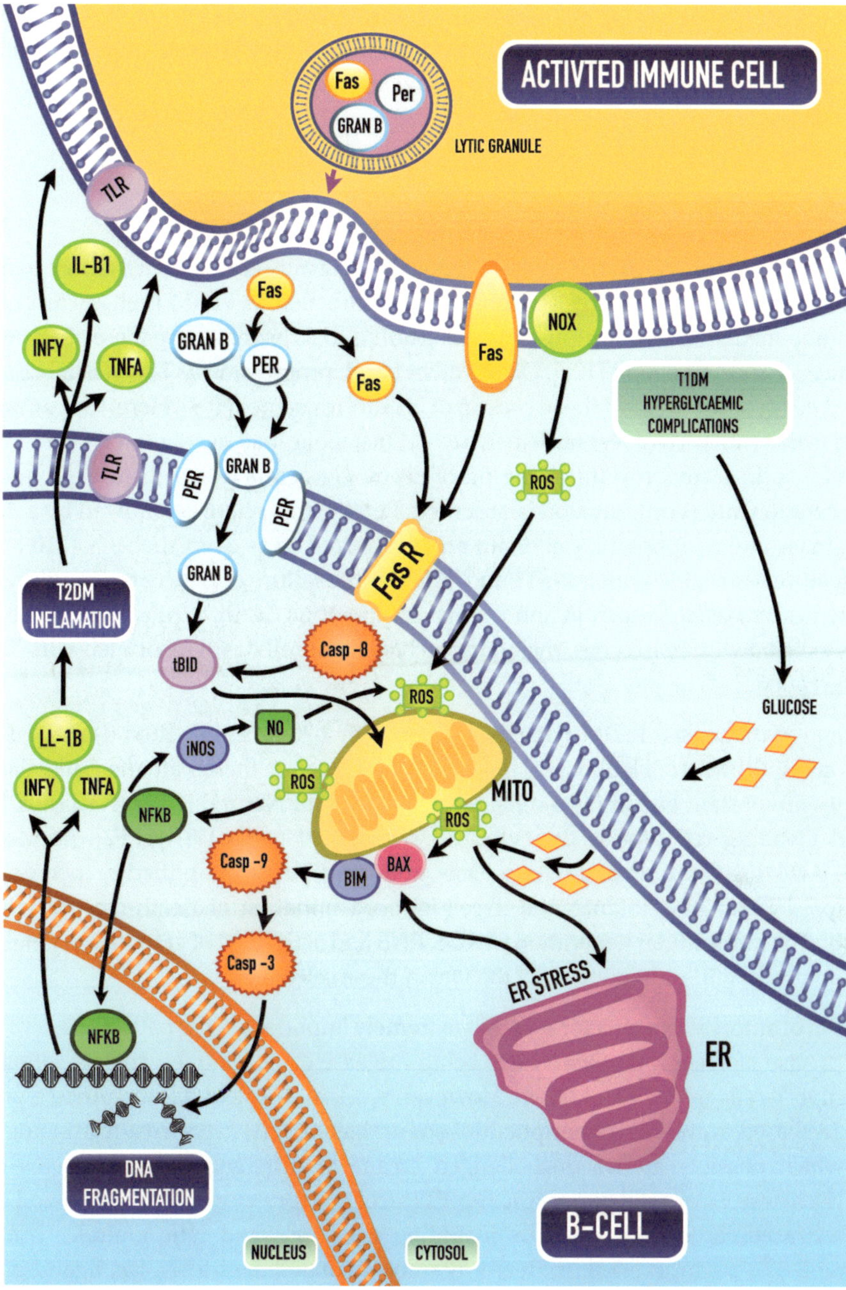

Figure 5. Illustration depicting the potential convergence points of the immunological NFκB and the metabolic ROS/ER stress pathways in pancreatic β-cells. Islet inflammation is characterised by the presence of leukocyte infiltrates that mediate the destruction of β-cells by release of cytokines, generation of ROS (NO, cytokine-NFκB-dependent]) and by activating the granzyme b- and death-receptor-mediated death pathways. Also shown is the effect of excess glucose on ROS production and ER stress that ultimately activates caspase enzymes via mitochondrial- and ER-mediated death pathways. ROS/RNS can also activate and regulate the NFκB stress pathway, which may lead to expression of cytokines that promotes immune cell infiltration exacerbating β-cell death.

and death is dependent on the interactions of these mediators, but also on the glycaemic and lipidaemic environment. We will now discuss the precise mechanisms of β-cell death in T1 and T2DM, and examine the commonalities between both.

7. Pancreatic β-cell failure and death in T1DM

Pancreatic β-cell failure can be defined as a reduction in insulin secretion or a failure to respond to plasma glucose (i.e. insulin-resistance). β-cell dysfunction in T1DM is characterised by an autoimmune-mediated destruction of β-cells leading to a decrease in pancreatic β-cell mass and reduced insulin secretion [109]. On the other hand, progression of T2DM is more variable and β-cell death occurs against the backdrop of insulin-resistance [109]. Here, the pathogenesis of T2DM usually involves a response to increased metabolic load by increased β-cell mass and enhanced insulin secretion [110]. A period of normoglycaemia ensues before a reduction in insulin secretion and β-cell function is observed. Finally, this phase is followed by a decrease in β-cell mass due to apoptotic cell death and is referred to as overt diabetes [110,111]. The shared feature associated with both T1 and T2DM is the failure of pancreatic β-cells resulting in reduced cell mass, dysfunction and ultimately apoptotic death. While there are commonalities associated with both types, the main mechanism of cell death associated with T1DM is immune-related.

At the time of diagnosis, T1DM patients present with a 70-80% reduction β-cell mass [109]. Insulitis and infiltration of leukocytes into islets is common in these patients. Several types of leukocytes are present including B-cells, macrophages and Natural Killer (NK) cells, but the principal invading cell type is the cytotoxic T-cell (CD4 and CD8) [81,82]. Immune cells promote β-cell death via several mechanisms, and these can be simplified to include phagocytosis, production of cytokines and T-cell-induced initiation of death-receptor-mediated apoptosis. The intracellular generation of ROS/RNS and activation of caspase enzymes occurs inside target cells and ultimately seals the fate of these cells.

Generation of autoreactive effector T-cells is extremely important in the pathogenesis of T1DM, but the precise biochemical mechanisms behind release of self-antigen and development of autoreactive T-cells remains unknown. However, work in this field has identified a potential role for decreased expression of peripheral tissue antigens (PTA) in pancreatic draining lymph nodes, which possibly allows unchallenged escape of differentiated autoreactive T-cells [82,83,112]. These T-cells kill pancreatic β-cells through expression of Fas ligand and expression of extracellular cytotoxic factors including cytokines, and lytic granules containing granzyme B and perforin [113]. In death-receptor-mediated apoptosis, Fas ligand or TNFα initiates death signals through association with FasR (Fas receptor) or TNFR (tumour necrosis factor receptor). An intracellular conformational change occurs that results in activation of caspase-8 [114,115]. This in turn serves to activate caspase-3 downstream promoting the apoptotic cascade [116].

T-cell-mediated release of granzyme B and perforin also leads to caspase activation in target cells. Here, perforin creates pores in the plasma membrane of the target cell, while granzyme

B is released into the cytosol and activates caspase-3 [113,117]. Interestingly, in order to yield activation of caspase-3, both caspase-8 from the death-receptor pathway outlined above, and granzyme B converge and initiate the mitochondrial-mediated death pathway via cleavage of BID [a member of the B-cell lymphoma-2 (Bcl-2) family of proteins], to truncated BID (tBID). In this process, cytosolic tBID translocates to the mitochondrial membrane and activates other Bcl-2-related proteins, such as BAX. Release of cytochrome *c* is then stimulated, which acts as the trigger for mitochondrial-mediated activation of caspase -9 and -3 [118,119,120]. Therefore, both the death-receptor and granzyme B-mediated death pathways activate the mitochondrial-mediated death pathway.

Conversely, macrophages induce β-cell death through production of ROS, cytokines and eventually phagocytosis. Macrophages express high levels of NOX, and use O_2^- to kill invading organisms or possibly damaged β-cells. Expression of high amounts of ROS/RNS or reduced antioxidant defences, results in mitochondrial dysfunction, which can culminate in mitochondrial-mediated apoptosis. Briefly, this involves major structural changes caused by ROS/RNS-mediated lipid/protein oxidation on both the inner and outer mitochondrial membranes, thus increasing the membrane permeability to proteins [121]. This is regulated by the interaction of pro- and anti-apoptotic Bcl-2 family proteins (Bcl-2, Bcl-X_L, BAX, BAK, BIM, BID and BAD) [122]. The release of cytochrome *c* to the cytosol and its association with apoptosis protease activation factor-1 (Apaf-1) and pro-caspase-9, forms a heptameric wheel-like caspase-activating complex, known as the apoptosome, which subsequently leads to activation of caspase-9 and effector caspase-3, further down-stream [123]. Caspase activation promotes cell death by degradation of DNA and cytoskeletal proteins [124].

In addition, immune cells release cytokines (e.g. TNFα, INF-γ and IL-1β) that also promote up-regulation of ROS/RNS via activation of NFκB (e.g. NO), who in turn can be regulated by ROS [100,101]. Induction of NO expression can cause activation of tumour suppressor protein (p53) leading to inhibition of cell cycle and death [109]. Cytokines can also inflict cell death via stimulation of the JNK pathway [97]. Here, IL-1β and TNFα activate mitochondrial translocation of JNK, who is a regulator of Bcl-2 proteins. JNK phosphorylates BIM, which results in the release of BAX-dependent cytochrome *c* and initiation of mitochondrial-mediated apoptosis [125,126]. Additionally, release of INF-γ by T-cells, can also phosphorylate BIM in β-cells, promoting cell death in a similar manner [77,86].

A variety of biochemical signalling pathways are available by which autoimmune cells utilise to initiate β-cell destruction. Consequently, due to a complete lack of insulin secretion and subsequent diminished glucose-uptake by muscle and adipose tissue, hyperglycaemia ensues in T1DM patients. High levels of blood glucose leads to further complications including, glucotoxicity, lipotoxicity and glucolipotoxicity and these are key players in exacerbation of the disease, and can lead to the clinical complications of T2DM [108]. Therefore, the precise way in which these factors affect β-cell turnover and survival will be discussed in the next section. Nonetheless, β-cell death in T1DM is based on classical immune-related death processes, but also relies on involvement of ROS and mitochondrial mediated which may occur in a sub-population of beta cells in T2DM.

8. Pancreatic β-cell failure and death in T2DM

Failure of pancreatic β-cells is essential in the progression of both T1 and T2DM. The development of T2DM is more gradual than T1, and appears to occur in specific stages. It is dependent on the establishment of insulin-resistance and displays increased degrees of variability in comparison with T1DM. Therefore, determination of the precise mechanisms of T2DM-related cell death remains difficult and, these are still not fully understood.

T2DM patients have a 30-50% reduction in β-cell mass on average post-mortem and the primary candidate pathways leading to β-cell apoptosis are oxidative stress, ER stress, amyloid accumulation, ectopic lipid deposition, lipotoxicity and glucotoxicity [127]. These stresses can all be caused by over-nutrition and neatly connects T2DM to obesity [90]. Glucose, the most important insulin secretatogue, is also the most important regulator of β-cell mass and function [128]. Impaired glucose-tolerance and hyperglycaemia are hallmarks of T2DM and prolonged glucose exposure can promote glucose-desensitisation, decreased insulin secretion and generation of oxidative stress in β-cells [128]. Consequently, glucotoxicity plays a significant part in pancreatic β-cell death in T2DM.

Understandably, excess glucose increases β-cell glucose metabolism and oxidative phosphorylation. Elevated ETC activity promotes increased superoxide (O_2^-) anion leakage from the mitochondria and may cause oxidative cellular damage [100]. Furthermore, high glucose levels induces NOX activity via NADPH production from metabolism of glucose to pentose, and through the TCA cycle, both leading to increased O_2^- output [100]. O_2^- can be converted to the less reactive H_2O_2 via superoxide dismutase, to the highly reactive hydroxyl anion by the iron-catalysed Fenton reaction, or to peroxynitrite ($ONOO^-$) via reaction with iNOS-derived NO [27,129]. β-cells are considered vulnerable to ROS/RNS generation because they express relatively low levels of antioxidant enzymes, like glutathione and catalase [27,128,129]. These enzymes immediately convert H_2O_2 to molecular oxygen and water. However, the detrimental combination of reduced activity of antioxidant enzymes, along with ROS/RNS generation can result in oxidative damage to DNA, lipids and proteins, thereby promoting mitochondrial-mediated apoptosis. In addition, ROS/RNS can also activate and regulate biochemical stress pathways, such as the NFκB, leading to further negative effects in β-cells [100,101].

Excess glucose can cause increased intracellular calcium, as outlined previously, which may enhance mitochondrial O_2^- production, but also deplete ER Ca^{2+}, promoting activation of the ER-stress-mediated death pathway [111,128] alongside unfolded protein response (UPR) (for review, please see [130]). In normal conditions, proteins are synthesised in the ER and are subsequently secreted or routed into a variety of sub-cellular compartments. However, accumulation of native or unfolded proteins within the lumen of the ER can activate caspase enzymes and ultimately promote cell death [131,132]. Reaction of ROS with the ER leads to protein accumulation via dysregulation of the ER oxidative folding pathway [111]. It also results in oxidative activation of Ca^{2+} release channels in the ER membrane, thereby depleting the ER of Ca^{2+} [111]. This ER stress activates pro-caspase-12, located on the cytoplasmic side of the ER, in a manner similar to caspase-9 [133,134]. Caspase-12 apoptosomes also causes translocation of JNK to the mitochondrial membrane inducing BIM phosphorylation, ultimately leading to cytochrome *c* release and initiation of mitochondrial-dependent apoptosis [111,135,136].

Lipid accumulation (lipotoxicity) in the ER may also play a significant function in mediating ER stress in β-cells. Obesity is a primary risk factor associated with T2DM, and is accompanied with increased plasma glucose and lipid levels due to high carbohydrate- and fat-based diets [137]. The process by which free fatty acids modulate ER stress is not entirely known [111] but, it has been shown that palmitic acid could deplete ER Ca^{2+} levels and augment ER morphology and integrity, which may cause activation of ER stress by the mechanisms mentioned above [137,138]. Furthermore, excess fatty acid esterification in the ER, may divert ER machinery and delay the processing and export of proteins in the ER [137]. Since there is a large demand for protein/insulin production in pancreatic islets, β-cells have a highly active and well developed ER. This suggests that β-cells may be more susceptible to ER stress during protein synthesis [109,137]. Given the effects of elevated plasma glucose and lipids in T2DM patients, ER stress could be a vital mechanism facilitating glucotoxicity-, lipotoxicity- or glucolipotoxicity-mediated β-cell failure and death [137].

Moreover, accumulation of islet amyloid polypeptide (IAPP) may also contribute to β-cell dysfunction and death in a manner similar to that described above [110,111,139]. IAPP precipitates into lethal oligomers inside the ER and like unfolded proteins, activates the ER stress-mediated death pathway [139]. IAPP deposits are present in over 90% of T2DM islets, post-mortem, indicating a substantial participation in T2DM progression [109,111].

In summary, several biochemical mechanisms have been suggested to be responsible for pancreatic β-cell failure and death in T2DM. However, there appears to be significant interplay between the purported pathways and conditions of glucotoxicity-, lipotoxicity- and glucolipotoxicity, which are common in the aetiology of T2DM and require further investigation. Interestingly, from this review there are noteworthy commonalities associated with T1 and T2DM mechanisms of β-cell failure and death. In the following section we will attempt to summarise these, with a view to identifying the potential therapeutic targets that are of interest to the research community.

9. Similarities between β-cell failure and death in T1DM and T2DM

T1DM is considered a chronic autoimmune disease and the major mechanisms responsible β-cell death and dysfunction are immune-related. In contrast, the main mechanisms responsible β-cell death and dysfunction in T2DM are related to metabolism. Thus, the convergence points of these two aetiologically-different disorders appear to be the immunological NFκB pathway and, the metabolic ROS/ER stress pathways (Fig. 5).

Islet inflammation in T1DM is characterised by the presence of leukocyte infiltrates [81]. In particular, macrophages and T-cells mediate the destruction of β-cells by phagocytosis, release of cytokines, generating ROS (NO, cytokine-NFκB-dependent [82]) and by activating the granzyme b- and death-receptor-mediated death pathways (Fig. 5). At the biochemical level, production of cytokines such as INF-γ, TNFα and IL-1β act in synergy to promote expression of iNOS and consequently NO, via stimulation of NFκB in mouse islet β-cells [82]. If not regulated, this generation of ROS may impact on ER stress and possibly promote cell death, which has been shown to be an import cell death process in T2DM (Fig. 5). Furthermore, cytokine–mediated activation of β-cell NFκB may result in an autocrine production of similar cytokines by β-cells, amplifying these death signals [76,79]. Another complication that arises with T1DM and immune-mediated reduction of β-cell mass is impaired insulin secretion, which may possibly promote additional hyperglycaemia and dyslipidaemia in these patients. Therefore, and as explained earlier, glucolipotoxicity may follow, along with further cell death that is achieved through mitochondrial- and/or ER-mediated death processes (Fig. 5).

In T2DM, hyperglycaemia and dyslipidaemia are critical factors and are generally present in obese individuals with the disease [77]. Consequently, excess glucose and circulating free fatty acids may promote increased ROS production and ER stress by enhancing oxidative phosphorylation and causing a build-up of unfolded proteins in the ER. Elevated ROS and ER stress will activate caspase enzymes via mitochondrial- and ER-mediated death pathways, respectively (Fig. 5). Interestingly, ROS/RNS can also activate and regulate the NFκB stress pathway, which may possibly lead to transcription of genes coding either cytokines or immune cell chemo-attractants (Fig. 5) [98]. Given the spontaneous reactivity of ROS, it is not clear yet exactly how it influences NFκB activation. However, it has been shown to react in a variety of ways promoting stimulation or inhibition of NFκB, with effects dependent on context [98]. For example, if ROS does promote expression of NFκB-derived cytokines or immune cell chemo-attractants, these signals may alert nearby macrophages and T-cells to the elevated level of β-cell ROS, and initiate the removal of these damaged cells. Consequently, this could result in immune cell infiltration into pancreatic islets of T2DM patients and possibly β-cell death (Fig. 5).

Interestingly, an autoimmune element has been reported in obese patients with T2DM, who have presented with elevated circulatory cytokine and acute-phase protein levels [77,87]. A common denominator that may link both T1 and T2DM is IL-1β. Autocrine production of IL-1β by β-cells has been observed in T1DM and in T2DM patients [76,79]. Furthermore, *in vitro* culture of islets from non-diabetic doners in high glucose, caused increased production and secretion of IL-1β, along with subsequent NFκB activation, Fas up-regulation, reduced insulin secretion and β-cell DNA fragmentation [77,78]. Chronic exposure to IL-1β also increases expression of iNOS, and consequently may up-regulate ROS generation and the expression of other pro-inflammatory cytokines like IL-6 and IL-8, which may further potentiate β-cell failure [78]. These reports clearly demonstrate the inherent link between glucotoxicity and the inflammatory processes [77]. In addition, investigators took a step further and showed that exogenous addition of IL-1Ra, the IL-1 receptor antagonist (Anakinra), protected the islets from IL-1β, but also reduced glycated haemoglobin in a small clinical trial of T2DM patients [77,140]. Clinical trials utilising IL-1Ra, still continue [90].

In conclusion, T1 and T2DM are different diseases, but do appear to share some common biochemical ground in terms of disease development. Although T1DM is mostly an autoimmune-related syndrome, elements of metabolic dysregulation are evident. Likewise, even though T2DM is very much a metabolic disease, there are also immunological-related factors that may exacerbate disease progression. NFκB, IL-1β, ER-stress and generation of ROS/RNS are instrumental players in both diseases, and may warrant further investigation with regard to development of novel therapies.

10. β-cell therapies and possible targets for prevention of β-cell failure

The traditionalistic concept of separate T1 and T2DM syndromes has become clouded with knowledge of the involvement of inflammation in T2DM and the metabolic syndrome in T1DM [108]. It is now apparent that treatment modalities that were specifically designed for one form of diabetes may have application in the other. Exercise, weight loss and diet are the most effective strategies to delay T2DM disease development, but similar strategies have shown significant efficacy in T1DM [108,128].

Researchers have targeted TNFα in children with newly diagnosed T1DM and showed that a recombinant TNFR fusion protein preserved c-peptide function, along with enhancing insulin production [82,141]. However, to date, anti-TNFα treatment has failed to improve blood glucose in T2DM patients [90]. Infiltration of cytotoxic T-cells in T1DM has been well characterised [82]. Therefore, some developing treatment strategies for this precise component of T1DM disease is the generation of T-cell targeted therapy to prevent the destruction of transplanted islets, some of which include introduction of anti-inflammatory Tregs that regulate T-cell activation [89]. Since inflammation has been detected in T2DM, these approaches may have similar applications. Directing treatment towards the immunological pathways is quite attractive and recent evidence has suggested that the most promising results involve blockade of IL-1β or NFκB activation [90]. Again, it is noteworthy to highlight that enhanced HSP70 expression has been convincingly demonstrated to protect against obesity-induced insulin-resistance [142], while low HSP70 contents in skeletal muscle of T2DM patients are associated with insulin-resistance [143,144]. Hence, pharmacological (e.g. the hydroxylamine derivative BGP-15, now under clinical trial) as well as physiological (hyperthermic, hot tube) treatments have started to be cogitated as promising therapeutic approaches in T2DM [142,145]. Moreover, physical exercise, which is a powerful antidiabetic intervention, is one of the strongest ways to increase intracellular HSP70 expression in many tissues (for reviews, please see [75,146]), including in pancreatic β-cells (A. Bittencourt et al., manuscript in preparation).

Elevated IL-1β and reduced IL-1Ra is known to correlate with T1DM, but the recent identification of inflammation in T2DM has meant that the IL-1 receptor antagonist (Anakinra), has been trialed in both T2DM and T1DM patients with successful results [77,140,147]. Here, the agent lowered blood glucose, reduced inflammation, improved insulin-sensitivity and secretion. These reports again illustrate the pivotal role played by IL-1β in mediating DM development, and thus clinical trials continue [90].

Salicylate-derivatives, such as salsalate, are also being used in an anti-inflammatory capacity to inhibit the activation of NFκB, although the precise mechanisms of action are not fully understood. These agents have the clear advantages of being orally available and well tolerated. Salsalate has been shown to improve insulin sensitivity and production, increase secretion of the anti-inflammatory cytokine adiponectin, reduce blood glucose and C-reactive protein (CRP) and decrease fatty acid and triglyceride levels [90].

From our own studies we have shown how different amino and fatty acid combinations may affect β-cell metabolism. This proposes the concept of diet manipulation as an additional treatment for hyperglycaemia and lipidaemia in T2 and even T1DM patients. We demonstrated the antioxidant activities of arachidonic acid, arginine and glutamine, and this data may suggests that dietary supplementation, high in specific amino or fatty acids, may have favourable effects in DM patients. Given the role of ROS and ER stress in β-cell death, dietary or pharmacological agents that target these pathways may also represent novel treatments for the delay or prevention of DM.

11. Conclusions and perspectives

Over-nutrition and diminished physical activity in the modern lifestyle has led to a staggering increase in T2DM onset in Western cultures [108]. However, the epidemic is also progressing into the developing world, indicating that T2DM has become a major global health issue [108]. Since the 1990's, T1DM has more than doubled in number and is expected to double again before 2020 [108,148]. The traditional classification of distinct criteria for T1 and T2DM syndromes has become blurred due to the global increase in obese individuals and the incidence of obesity-related insulin-resistance [108]. Currently the paradigm of T1 and T2DM treatment appears to be changing in line with the clarification of dysfunctional pathways that are common to both disease types. Although diet-and-exercise still remains the most effective (and cheapest) treatment, new therapies will be required going into the future. Consequently, an increased understanding of the molecular and biochemical mechanisms that lead to disease onset and progression are mandatory.

In this manuscript, we have examined some of the key pathways that are essential in the pathogenesis of both T1 and T2DM, and we have reviewed some of the novel treatments that are currently being developed to counteract these dysfunctional processes. It is clear that inflammation, generation of ROS/RNS and ER stress leads to significant damage to pancreatic β-cells, culminating in cell dysfunction, and ultimately cell death. It is hoped that further study of the NFκB and the ER stress-mediated pathways, will reveal novel therapeutic targets that can be developed into a new generation of anti-diabetic treatments, that will improve β-cell function, survival and regeneration in T1 and T2DM.

Acknowledgements

The authors would like to thank Mr. Peter McEvoy for assistance with design and illustration of Figure 5.

http://dx.doi.org/10.5772/55349

Abbreviations

ACC - Acetyl coA carboxylase

ACL - ATP-citrate lyase

AMPK - AMP-activated kinase

Apaf-1 - Apoptosis protease activation factor-1

Bcl-2 - B-cell lymphoma-2

Cp-PGs - Cyclopentenone prostaglandins

CPT-1 - Carnitine palmitoyl transferase 1

DHAP - Dihydroxyacetone phosphate

ER - Endoplasmic reticulum

ETC - Electron transport chain

FasR - Fas receptor

GABA - γ-aminobutyric acid

G-CSP - Granulocyte colony-stimulating factor

GDH - Glutamate dehydrogenase

GFAT-1 - Glutamine:fructose-6-phosphate amidotransferase-1

GSIS - Glucose-stimulated insulin secretion

GSK3β - Glycogen synthase kinase-3β

HBP - Hexosamine biochemical pathway

HSF-1 - Heat shock factor-1

HSP70 - Heat shock protein-70

iNOS - Inducible nitric oxide synthase

JNK - c-Jun-N-terminal kinase

LDH - Lactate dehydrogenase

MCFs - Metabolic coupling factors

ME1 - Malic enzyme1

MIP-1 - Macrophage inflammatory protein-1

NFAT - Nuclear factor of activated T cells

NFκB - Nuclear factor κB

NOD - Non-obese diabetic

NOX - NADPH oxidase

PC - Pyruvate carboxylase

PDH - Pyruvate dehydrogenase

PP2A - Protein phosphatase type 2A

PTA - Peripheral tissue antigens

RNS - Reactive nitrogen species

ROS - Reactive oxygen species

SNARE -Soluble NH2-ethylmaleimide-sensitive fusion protein attachment protein receptor

SNOG - S-nitrosoglutathione

T1DM - Type 1 diabetes mellitus

T2DM - Type 2 diabetes mellitus

TCA - Tricarboxylic acid

TGFβ − Transforming growth factorβ

TLR - Toll-like receptors

TNFR - TNFα receptor

TRAF - TNF receptor associated factor

Tregs - Regulatory T-cells

VAMP - Vesicle-associated membrane protein

Author details

Philip Newsholme[1], Kevin Keane[1], Paulo I Homem de Bittencourt Jr.[2,3] and Mauricio Krause[4,5]

1 School of Biomedical Sciences, Curtin University, Western Australia

2 Department of Physiology, Institute of Basic Health Sciences, Federal University of Rio Grande do Sul, Porto Alegre, Brazil

3 National Institute of Hormones and Women's Health, Brazil

4 Institute of Technology Tallaght and Institute for Sport and Health UCD Dublin, Ireland

5 School of Public Health and Physiotherapy, UCD Dublin, Ireland

References

[1] Chan, S. J, & Steiner, D. F. Insulin Through the Ages: Phylogeny of a growth promoting and metabolic regulatory hormone. American Zoologist (2000). , 40, 213-22.

[2] Irwin, D. M, Humer, O, & Youson, J. H. Lamprey Proglucagon and the origin of glucagon-like peptides. Molecular Biology and Evolution (1999). , 16(11), 1548-57.

[3] Newsholme, P, Abdulkader, F, Rebelato, E, Romanatto, T, Pinheiro, C. H, Vitzel, K. F, Silva, E. P, Bazotte, R. B, Procopio, J, Curi, R, Gorjao, R, & Pithon-curi, T. C. Amino acids and diabetes: implications for endocrine, metabolic and immune functions. Frontiers in Bioscience (2011). , 16, 315-39.

[4] Jitrapakdee, S, Wutthisathapornchai, A, Wallace, J. C, & MacDonald, M.J. Regulation of insulin secretion: role of mitochondrial signalling. Diabetologia (2010). , 53(6), 1019-32.

[5] Rutter, G. A, & Hill, E. V. Insulin vesicle release: walk, kiss, pause…then run. Physiology (Bethesda, Md.) (2006). , 21, 189-96.

[6] Gembal, M, Gilon, P, & Henquin, J. C. Evidence that glucose can control insulin release independently from its action on ATP-sensitive K+ channels in mouse B cells. Journal of Clinical Investigations (1992). , 89(4), 1288-95.

[7] Remedi, M. S, Rocheleau, J. V, Tong, A, Patton, B. L, Mcdaniel, M. L, Piston, D. W, Koster, J. C, & Nichols, C. G. Hyperinsulinism in mice with heterozygous loss of K(ATP) channels. Diabetologia (2006). , 49(10), 2368-78.

[8] Miki, T, Nagashima, K, Tashiro, F, Kotake, K, Yoshitomi, H, Tammamoto, A, Gonoi, T, Iwanaga, T, Miyazaki, J. I, & Seino, S. Defective insulin secretion and enhanced insulin action in KATP channel-deficient mice. Proceedings of the National Academy of Sciences (1998). , 95, 10402-06.

[9] Straub, S. G, & Sharp, G. W. G. Glucose-stimulated signalling pathways in biphasic insulin secretion. Diabetes and Metabolism Research and Reviews (2002). , 18(6), 451-63.

[10] Newsholme, P, & Krause, M. Nutritional Regulation of Insulin Secretion: Implications for Diabetes. The Clinical Biochemist Reviews (2012). , 33(2), 35-47.

[11] Newsholme, P, Bender, K, Kiely, A, & Brennan, L. Amino acid metabolism, insulin secretion and diabetes. The Biochemical Society Transactions (2007). Pt 5): 1180-6.

[12] Opara, E. C, Garfinkel, M, Hubbard, V. S, Burch, W. M, & Akwari, O. E. Effect of fatty acids on insulin release; role of chain length and degree of unsaturation. The American Journal of Physiology (1994). Pt 1): E, 635-9.

[13] Keane, D. C, Takahashi, H. K, Dhayal, S, Morgan, N. G, Curi, R, & Newsholme, P. Arachidonic acid actions on functional integrity and attenuation of the negative ef-

fects of palmitic acid in a clonal pancreatic β-cell line. Clinical Science (London) (2011). , 120(5), 195-206.

[14] Hosokawa, H, Corkey, B. E, & Leahy, J. L. Beta-cell hypersensitivity to glucose following 24-h exposure of rat islets to fatty acids. Diabetologia (1997). , 40(4), 392-7.

[15] Vassiliou, E. K, Gonzalez, A, Garcia, C, Tadros, J. H, Chakraborty, G, & Toney, J. H. Oleic acid and peanut oil high in oleic acid reverse the inhibitory effect of insulin production of the inflammatory cytokine TNF-α both *in vitro* and *in vivo* systems. Lipids in Health and Disease (2009).

[16] Keane, D, & Newsholme, P. Saturate and unsaturated (including arachidonic acid) non-esterified fatty acid modulation of insulin secretion from pancreatic β-cells. The Biochemical Society Transactions (2008). Pt 5): 955-8.

[17] Jensen, M. V, Joseph, J. W, Ronnebaum, S. M, Burgess, S. C, Sherry, A. D, & Newgard, C. B. Metabolic cycling in control of glucose-stimulated insulin secretion. The American Journal of Physiological Endocrinology and Metabolism (2008). E, 1287-97.

[18] Newsholme, P, Keane, D, Welters, H. J, & Morgan, N. G. Life and death decisions of the pancreatic beta-cell: the role of fatty acids. Clinical Science (London) (2007). , 112(1), 27-42.

[19] Mcclenaghan, N. H, Scullion, S. M, Mion, B, Hewage, C, Malthouse, J. P, Flatt, P. R, Newsholme, P, & Brennan, L. Prolonged L-alanine exposure induces changes in metabolism, Ca2+ handling and desensitisation of insulin secretion clonal pancreatic beta-cells. Clinical Science (London) (2009). , 116(4), 341-51.

[20] Bender, K, Maechler, P, Mcclenaghan, N. H, Flatt, P. R, & Newsholme, P. Overexpression of malate-aspartate NADH shuttle member Aralar1 in the clonal beta-cell line BRIN-BD11 enhances amino-acid-stimulated insulin secretion and cell metabolism. Clinical Science (London) (2009). , 117(9), 321-30.

[21] Newsholme, P, Brennan, L, & Bender, K. Amino acid metabolism, β-cell function and diabetes. Diabetes (2006). S, 39-47.

[22] Maassen, J. A, Hart, t, Janssen, L. M, Reiling, G. M, Romijn, EJ. A, & Lemkes, . Mitochondrial diabetes and its lesson for common type 2 diabetes. The Biochemical Society Transactions (2006). Pt 5): 819-23.

[23] Sener, A, Best, L. C, Yates, A. P, Kadiata, M. M, Oliveares, E, Louchami, K, Jijakli, H, Ladriere, L, & Malaisse, W. J. Stimulus-secretion coupling of arginine-induced insulin-release: comparison between the cationic amino acid and its methyl ester. Endocrine (2000). , 13(3), 329-40.

[24] Mcclenaghan, N. H, Barnett, C. R, & Flatt, P. R. Na^+ cotransport by metabolizable and nonmetabolizable amino acids stimulates a glucose-regulated insulin-secretory response. Biochemical and Biophysical Research Communications (1998). , 249(2), 299-303.

[25] Broca, C, Brennan, L, Petit, P, Newsholme, P, & Maechler, P. Mitochondria-derived glutamate at the interplay between branched-chain amino acid and glucose-induced insulin secretion. FEBS Letters (2003).

[26] Krause, M, Rodrigues-krause, J, Hagan, O, De Vito, C, Boreham, G, Susta, C, Newsholme, D, & Murphy, P. C. Differential nitric oxide levels in the blood and skeletal muscle of type 2 diabetic subjects may be a consequence of adiposity: a preliminary study. Metabolism: Clinical and Experimental (2012). , 61(11), 1528-37.

[27] Newsholme, P, Rebelato, E, Abdulkader, F, Krause, M, Carpinelli, A, & Curi, R. Reactive oxygen and nitrogen species generation, antioxidant defences and β-cell function: a critical role for amino acids. The Journal of Endocrinology (2012). , 214(1), 11-20.

[28] Pryor, W. A, & Squadrito, G. L. The chemistry of peroxynitrite: a product from the reaction of nitric oxide with superoxide. American Journal of Physiology (1995). Pt 1): L, 699-722.

[29] Beckman, J. S, Beckman, T. W, Chen, J, Marshall, P. A, & Freeman, B. A. Apparent hydroxyl radical production by peroxynitrite: implications for endothelial injury from nitric oxide and superoxide. Proceedings of the National Academy of Sciences (1990). , 87(4), 1620-24.

[30] Crow, J. P, & Beckman, J. S. The role of peroxynitrite in nitric oxide-mediated toxicity. Current Topics in Microbiology and Immunology (1995). , 196(1), 57-73.

[31] Delaney, C. A, Tyrberg, B, Bouwens, L, Vaghef, H, Hellman, B, & Eizirik, D. L. Sensitivity of human pancreatic islets to peroxynitrite-induced cell dysfunction and death. FEBS Letters (1996). , 394(3), 300-6.

[32] Rabinovitch, A, & Suarez-pinzon, W. L. Role of cytokines in the pathogenesis of autoimmune diabetes mellitus. Reviews in Endocrine and Metabolic Disorders (2003). , 4(3), 291-9.

[33] Sancez-margalet, V, Valle, M, Ruz, F. J, Gascon, F, Mateo, J, & Goberna, R. Elevated plasma total homocysteine levels in hyperinsulinaemic obese subjects. The Journal of Nutritional Biochemistry (2002). , 13(2), 75-79.

[34] Patterson, S, Flatt, P. R, & Mcclenaghan, N. H. Homocysteine and other structurally-diverse amino thiols can alter pancreatic beta cell function without evoking cellular damage. (2006). Biochemica et Biophysica Acta 2006; , 1760(7), 1109-14.

[35] Medina, M, Urdiales, J. L, & Amores-sanchez, M. I. Roles of homocysteine in cell metabolism: old and new functions. The European Journal of Biochemistry (2001). , 268(14), 3871-82.

[36] Patterson, S, Flatt, P. R, & Mcclenaghan, N. H. Homocysteine-induced impairment of insulin secretion from clonal pancreatic BRIN-BD11 beta-cells is not prevented by catalase. Pancreas (2007). , 34(1), 144-51.

[37] Baylis, C. Nitric oxide deficiency in chronic kidney disease. The American Journal of Physiology: Renal Physiology (2008). F, 1-9.

[38] Ammon, H. P, Hehl, G, Enz, G, Setaidi-ranti, A, & Verspohl, J. Cysteine analogues potentiate glucose-induced insulin release in vitro. Diabetes (1986). , 35(12), 1390-6.

[39] Rasilainen, S, Nieminen, J. M, Levonen, A. L, Otonkoski, T, & Lapatto, R. Dose-dependent cysteine-mediated protection of insulin-producing cells from damage by hydrogen peroxide. Biochemical Pharmacology (2002). , 63(7), 1297-304.

[40] Kaneko, Y, Kimura, T, Taniquchi, S, Souma, M, Kojima, Y, Kimura, Y, Kimura, H, & Niki, I. Glucose-induced production of hydrogen sulphide may protect the pancreatic beta-cells from apoptotic cell death by high glucose. FEBS Letters (2009). , 538(2), 377-82.

[41] Kaneko, Y, Kimura, T, & Kimura, H. and Niki I. L-cysteine inhibits insulin release from pancreatic beta-cells: possible involvement of metabolic production of hydrogen sulphide, a novel gasotransmitter. Diabetes (2006). , 55(5), 1391-7.

[42] Sener, A, & Malaisse, W. J. L-l. e. u. c. i. n. e. and a nonmetabolized analogue activate pancreatic islet glutamate dehydrogenase. Nature (1980). , 288(5787), 187-9.

[43] Brennan, L, Corless, M, Hewage, C, Malthouse, J. P, Mcclenaghan, N. H, Flatt, P. R, & Newsholme, P. C NMR analysis reveals a link between L-glutamine metabolism, D-glucose metabolism and gamma-glutamyl cycle activity in a clonal pancreatic beta-cell line. Diabetologia (2007). , 46(11), 1512-21.

[44] Corless, M, Kiely, A, Mcclenaghan, N. H, Flatt, P. R, & Newsholme, P. Glutamine regulates expression of key transcription factor, signal transduction, metabolic gene, and protein expression in a clonal pancreatic beta-cell line. The Journal of Endocrinology (2006). , 190(3), 719-27.

[45] Brennan, L, Shine, A, Hewage, C, Malthouse, J. P, Brindle, K. M, Mcclenaghan, N. H, Flatt, P. R, & Newsholme, P. A nuclear magnetic resonance-based demonstration of substantial oxidative L-alanine metabolism and L-alanine-enhanced glucose metabolism in a clonal pancreatic beta-cell line: metabolism of L-alanine is important to the regulation of insulin secretion. Diabetes (2002). , 51(6), 1714-21.

[46] MacDonald MJ. and Fahien L.A. Glutamate is not a messenger in insulin secretion. The Journal of Biological Chemistry (2000). , 275(44), 34025-7.

[47] Gammelsaeter, R, Coppola, T, Marcaggi, P, Storm-mathisen, J, Chaudry, F. A, Attwell, D, Regazzi, R, & Gundersen, V. A role for glutamate transporters in the regulation of insulin secretion. PLoS One (2011). e22960.

[48] Huang, M, & Joseph, J. W. Metabolomic analysis of pancreatic β-cell insulin release in response to glucose. Islets (2012). , 4(3), 210-22.

[49] Hamaoka, R, Fujii, J, Miyagawa, J, Takahashi, M, Kishimoto, M, Moriwaki, M, Yamamoto, K, Kajimoto, Y, Yamasaki, Y, Hanafusa, T, Matsuzawa, Y, & Taniguchi, N.

Overexpression of the aldose reductase gene induces apoptosis in pancreatic beta-cells by causing a redox imbalance. The Journal of Biochemistry. (1999)., 126(1), 41-7.

[50] Gabbay, K. H, & Tze, W. J. Inhibition of glucose-induced release of insulin by aldose reductase inhibitors. Proceedings of the National Academy of Sciences (1972)., 69(6), 1435-9.

[51] Ladrière, L, Louchami, K, Laghmich, A, Malaisse-lagae, F, & Malaisse, W. J. Labeling of pancreatic glycogen by D-[U-14c]glucose in hyperglycemic rats. Endocrine (2001)., 14(3), 383-97.

[52] Doherty, M, & Malaisse, W. J. Glycogen accumulation in rat pancreatic islets: in vitro experiments. Endocrine (2001)., 14(3), 303-9.

[53] He, B, Meng, Y. H, & Mivechi, N. F. Glycogen synthase kinase 3beta and extracellular signal-regulated kinase inactivate heat shock transcription factor 1 by facilitating the disappearance of transcriptionally active granules after heat shock. Molecular and Cellular Biology (1998)., 18(11), 6624-33.

[54] Kazemi, Z, Chang, H, Haserodt, S, & Mcken, C. and Zachara NE. O-linked beta-N-acetylglucosamine (O-GlcNAc) regulates stress-induced heat shock protein expression in a GSK-3beta-dependent manner. The Journal of Biological Chemistry (2010)., 285(50), 39096-107.

[55] Srinivasan, V, Tatu, U, Mohan, V, & Balasubramanyam, M. Molecular convergence of hexosamine biosynthetic pathway and ER stress leading to insulin-resistance in L6 skeletal muscle cells. Molecular and Cellular Biochemistry (2009).

[56] Hasan, N. M, Longacre, M. J, Stoker, S. W, Boonsaen, T, Jitrapakdee, S, Kendrick, M. A, & Wallace, J. C. and MacDonald M.J. Impaired anaplerosis and insulin secretion in insulinoma cells caused by small interfering RNA-mediated suppression of pyruvate carboxylase. The Journal of Biological Chemistry (2008)., 283(42), 28048-59.

[57] Xu, J, Han, J, Long, Y. S, Epstein, P. N, & Liu, Y. Q. The role of pyruvate carboxylase in insulin secretion and proliferation in rat pancreatic beta-cells. Diabetologia (2008)., 51(11), 2022-30.

[58] Gaussin, V, Hue, L, Stalmans, W, & Bollen, M. Activation of hepatic acetyl-CoA carboxylase by glutamate and Mg^{2+} is mediated by protein phosphatase-2A. The Biochemical Journal (1996). Pt 1): 217-24.

[59] Xiang, X, Saha, A. K, Wen, R, Ruderman, N. B, & Luo, Z. AMP-activated protein kinase activators can inhibit the growth of prostate cancer cells by multiple mechanisms. Biochemical and Biophysical Research Communications (2004)., 321(1), 161-7.

[60] Shapiro, H, Shachar, S, Sekler, I, Hershfinkel, M, & Walker, M. D. Role of GPR40 in fatty acid action on the beta-cell line INS-1E. Biochemical and Biophysical Research Communications (2005)., 335(1), 97-104.

[61] Tomita, T, Masuzaki, H, Iwakura, H, Fujikura, J, Noquchi, M, Tanaka, T, Ebihara, K, Kawamura, J, Komoto, I, Kawaquchi, Y, Fujimoto, K, Doi, R, Shimada, Y, Hosoda, K, Imamura, M, & Nakao, K. Expression of the gene for a membrane-bound fatty acid receptor in the pancreas and islet cell tumours in humans: evidence for GPR40 expression in pancreatic beta-cells and implications for insulin secretion. Diabetologia (2006). , 49(5), 962-8.

[62] Krause, M. S, Mcclenaghan, N. H, & Flatt, P. R. Homem de Bittencourt P.I., Murphy C. and Newsholme P. L-arginine is essential for pancreatic b-cell functional integrity, metabolism and defence from inflammatory challenge. The Journal of Endocrinology (2011). , 211(1), 87-97.

[63] Eguchi, S, Oshiro, N, Miyamoto, T, Yoshino, K, Okamoto, S, Ono, T, Kikkawa, U, & Yonezawa, K. AMP-activated protein kinase phosphorylates glutamine : fructose-6-phosphate amidotransferase 1 at Ser243 to modulate its enzymatic activity. Genes to Cells (2009). , 14(2), 179-89.

[64] Luo, B, Parker, G. J, Cooksey, R. C, Soesanto, Y, Evans, M, Jones, D, & Mcclain, D. A. Chronic hexosamine flux stimulates fatty acid oxidation by activating AMP-activated protein kinase in adipocytes. The Journal of Biological Chemistry (2007). , 282(10), 7172-80.

[65] Ran, R, Lu, A, Zhang, L, Tang, Y, Zhu, H, Xu, H, Feng, Y, Han, C, Zhou, G, Rigby, A. C, & Sharp, F. R. Hsp70 promotes TNF-mediated apoptosis by binding IKK gamma and impairing NF-kappa B survival signaling. Genes and Development (2004). , 18(12), 1466-81.

[66] Jaattela, M. Overexpression of major heat shock protein hsp70 inhibits tumor necrosis factor-induced activation of phospholipase A2. The Journal of Immunology (1993). , 151(8), 4286-94.

[67] Feinstein, D. L, Galea, E, Aquino, D. A, Li, G. C, Xu, H, & Reis, D. J. Heat shock protein 70 suppresses astroglial-inducible nitric-oxide synthase expression by decreasing NFkappaB activation. The Journal of Biological Chemistry (1996). , 271(30), 17724-32.

[68] Kim, Y. M, De Vera, M. E, Watkins, S. C, & Billiar, T. R. Nitric oxide protects cultured rat hepatocytes from tumor necrosis factor-alpha-induced apoptosis by inducing heat shock protein 70 expression. The Journal of Biological Chemistry (1997). , 272(2), 1402-11.

[69] Chan, J. Y, Ou, C. C, Wang, L. L, & Chan, S. H. Heat shock protein 70 confers cardiovascular protection during endotoxemia via inhibition of nuclear factor-kappaB activation and inducible nitric oxide synthase expression in the rostral ventrolateral medulla. Circulation (2004). , 110(23), 3560-66.

[70] Chen, H. W, Kuo, H. T, Wang, S. J, Lu, T. S, & Yang, R. C. In vivo heat shock protein assembles with septic liver NF-kappaB/I-kappaB complex regulating NF-kappaB activity. Shock (2005). , 24(3), 232-8.

[71] Rossi, A, Kapahi, P, Natoli, G, Takahashi, T, Chen, Y, Karin, M, & Santoro, M. G. Anti-inflammatory cyclopentenone prostaglandins are direct inhibitors of IkappaB kinase. Nature (2000). , 403(6765), 103-18.

[72] Homem de Bittencourt P.I. Jr. and Curi R. Antiproliferative prostaglandins and the MRP/GS-X pump role in cancer immunosuppression and insight into new strategies in cancer gene therapy. Biochemical Pharmacology (2001). , 62(7), 811-19.

[73] Gutierrez, L. L, Maslinkiewicz, A, & Curi, R. and Homem de Bittencourt P.I. Jr. Atherosclerosis: a redox-sensitive lipid imbalance suppressible by cyclopentenone prostaglandins. Biochemical Pharmacology (2008). , 75(12), 2245-62.

[74] Beere, H. M. The stress of dying": the role of heat shock proteins in the regulation of apoptosis. The Journal of Cell Science (2004). Pt 13): 2641-51.

[75] Heck, T. G, & Schöler, C. M. and Homem de Bittencourt P.I. HSP70 expression: does it a novel fatigue signalling factor from immune system to the brain? Cell Biochemistry and Function (2011). , 29(3), 215-26.

[76] Ehses, J. A, Boni-schnetzler, M, Faulenbach, M, & Donath, M. Y. Macrophages, cytokines and b-cell death in type 2 diabetes. The Biochemical Society Transactions (2008). Pt 3): 340-2.

[77] Donath, M. Y, Schumann, D. M, Faulenbach, M, Ellingsgaard, H, Perren, A, & Ehses, J. A. Islet inflammation in type 2 diabetes. Diabetes Care (2008). Suppl 2): S, 161-4.

[78] Wang, C, Guan, Y, & Yang, J. Cytokines in the progression of pancreatic β-cell dysfunction. The International Journal of Endocrinology (2010). , 1, 1-10.

[79] Mandrup-poulsen, T. The role of interleukin-1 in the pathogenesis of IDDM. Diabetologia (1996). , 39(9), 1005-29.

[80] Kiely, A, Robinson, A, Mcclenaghan, N. H, Flatt, P. R, & Newsholme, P. Toll-like receptor agonist induced changes in clonal rat BRIN-BD11 β-cell insulin secretion and signal transduction. The Journal of Endocrinology (2009). , 202(3), 365-73.

[81] Coppieters, K. T, Dotta, F, Amirian, N, Campbell, P. D, Kay, T. W, Atkinson, M. A, Roep, B. O, & Von Herrath, M. G. Demonstration of islet-autoreactive CD8 T cells in insulitic lesions from recent onset and long-term type 1 diabetes patients. The Journal of Experimental Medicine (2012). , 209(1), 51-60.

[82] Bending, D, Zaccone, P, & Cooke, A. Inflammation and type one diabetes. International Immunology (2012). , 24(6), 339-46.

[83] Turley, S, Poirot, L, Hattori, M, Benoist, C, & Mathis, D. Physiological beta-cell death triggers priming of self-reactive T cells by dendritic cells in type-2 diabetes model. The Journal of Experimental Medicine (2003). , 198(10), 1527-37.

[84] Elenkov, I. J, & Chrousos, G. P. Stress Hormones, Th1/Th2 patterns, Pro/Anti-inflammatory Cytokines and Susceptibility to Disease. Trends in Endocrinology and Metabolism (1999). , 10(9), 359-68.

[85] Homem de Bittencourt Jr, P.I. and Newsholme P. A novel L-arginine/L-glutamine coupling hypothesis: implications for type 1 diabetes, Type 1 Diabetes- Complications, Pathogenesis, and Alternative Treatments, Chih-Pin Liu (Ed.), 978-9-53307-756-7InTech (2011). Available from: http://www.intechopen.com/books/type-1 diabetes-complications-pathogenesis-and-alternative-treatments/a-novel-l-arginine-l-glutamine-coupling-hypothesis-implications-for-type-1-diabetes

[86] Barthson, J, Germano, C. M, Moore, F, Maida, A, Drucker, D. J, Marchetti, P, Gysemans, C, Mathieu, C, Nunez, G, Juriscova, A, Eizirik, D. L, & Gurzov, E. N. Cytokines tumour necrosis factor-(alpha) and interferon-(gamma) induce pancreatic (beta)-cell apoptosis through STAT1-mediated Bim activation. The Journal of Biological Chemistry (2011). , 286(45), 39632-43.

[87] Ehses, J. A, Perren, A, Eppler, E, Ribaux, P, Pospisilik, J. A, Maor-cahn, R, Gueripel, X, Ellingsgaard, H, Schneider, M. K, Biollaz, G, Fontana, A, Reinecke, M, Homo-delarche, F, & Donath, M. Y. Increased cell number of islet associated macrophages in type 2 diabetes. Diabetes (2007). , 56(9), 2356-70.

[88] Boni-schnetzler, M. M. L, Ehses, J. A, Weir, G. C, & Donath, M. Y. (2007). IL-1beta expression is induced by glucose and IL-1beta auto-stimulation, and increased in beta cells of type 2 diabetics. Diabetes 2007; 56(Suppl 1): A413.

[89] Ryan, A, Murphy, M, Godson, C, & Hickey, F. B. Diabetes mellitus and apoptosis: inflammatory cells. Diabetes and Apoptosis (2009). , 14(12), 1435-50.

[90] Donath, M. Y, & Shoelson, S. E. Type 2 diabetes as an inflammatory disease. Nature Reviews Immunology (2011). , 11(2), 98-107.

[91] Pasarica, M, Rood, J, Ravussin, E, Schwarz, J. M, Smith, S. R, & Redman, L. M. Reduced oxygenation in human obese adipose tissue is associated with impaired insulin suppression of lipolysis. The Journal of Clinical Endocrinology and Metabolism (2010). , 95(8), 4052-5.

[92] Weisberg, S. P, Mccann, D, Desai, M, Rosenbaum, M, Leibel, R. L, & Ferrante Jr., A. W. Obesity is associated with macrophage accumulation in adipose tissue. The Journal of Clinical Investigations (2003). , 112(12), 1796-808.

[93] Xu, H, Barnes, G. T, Yang, Q, Tan, G, Yang, D, Chou, C. J, Sole, J, Nichols, A, Ross, J. S, Tartaglia, L. A, & Chen, H. Chronic inflammation in fat plays a crucial role in the development of obesity-related insulin-resistance. The Journal of Clinical Investigations (2003). , 112(12), 1821-30.

[94] Arkan, M. C, Hevener, A. L, Greten, F. R, Maeda, S, Li, Z. W, Long, J. M, Wynshaw-boris, A, Poli, G, Olefsky, J, & Karin, M. IKK-β links inflammation to obesity-induced insulin-resistance. Nature Medicine (2005). , 11(2), 191-8.

[95] Bowie, A, & O Neill, L.A.J. The interleukin-1 receptor/toll-like receptor superfamily: signal generators for pro-inflammatory interleukins and microbial products. Journal of Leukocyte Biology (2000).

[96] Nishikori, M. Classical and alternative NFκB activation pathways and their role in lymphoid malignancies. The Journal of Clinical and Experimental Hematopathology (2005). , 45(1), 15-24.

[97] Donath, M. Y, Storling, J, Maedler, K, & Mandrup-poulsen, T. Inflammatory mediators and islet β-cell failure: a link between type 1 and type 2 diabetes. The Journal of Molecular Medicine (Berlin) (2003). , 81(8), 455-70.

[98] Morgan, M. J, & Liu, Z. G. Crosstalk of reactive oxygen species and NFκB signalling. Cell Research (2011). , 21(1), 103-15.

[99] Wullaert, A, Heyninck, K, & Bayaert, R. Mechanisms of crosstalk between TNF-induced NFκB and JNK activation in hepatocytes. Biochemical Pharmacology (2006). , 72(9), 1090-101.

[100] Newsholme, P, Haber, E. P, Hirabara, S. M, Rebelato, E. L. O, Procopio, J, Morgan, D, Oliveira-emilio, H. C, Carpinelli, A. R, & Curi, R. Diabetes associated cell stress and dysfunction: role of mitochondria and non-mitochondrial ROS production and activity. The Journal of Physiology (2007). Pt 1): 9-24.

[101] Schoonbroodt, S, & Piette, J. Oxidative stress interference with nuclear factor-κ B activation pathways. Biochemical Pharmacology (2000). , 60(8), 1075-83.

[102] Shimabukuro, M, Zhou, Y. T, Levi, M, & Unger, R. H. Fatty acid-induced beta-cell apoptosis: a link between obesity and diabetes. Proceedings of the National Academy of Sciences (1998). , 95(5), 2498-502.

[103] Otero, M, Lago, R, Lago, F, Casanueva, F. F, Dieguez, C, Gomez-reino, J. J, & Gualillo, O. Leptin, from fat to inflammation: old questions and new insights. FEBS Letters (2005). , 579(2), 295-301.

[104] Zhang, F, Basinski, M. B, Beals, J. M, Briggs, S. L, Churgay, J. M, & Clawson, D. K. DiMarchi R.D., Furman T.C., Hale J.E., Hsiung H.M., Schoner B.E., Smith D.P., Zhang X.Y., Wery J.P. and Schevitz R.W. Crystal structure of the obese protein leptin-E100. Nature (1997). , 387(6629), 206-9.

[105] Matarese, G, Sanna, V, Lechler, R. I, Sarvet-nick, N, Fontana, S, & Zappacosta, S. and La Cava A. Leptin accelerates autoimmune diabetes in female NOD mice. Diabetes (2002). , 51(5), 1356-61.

[106] Wolf, A. M, Wolf, D, Rumpold, H, Enrich, B, & Tilg, H. Adiponectin induces the anti-inflammatory cytokines IL-10 and IL-1RA in human leukocytes. Biochemical and Biophysical Research Communications (2004). , 323(2), 630-5.

[107] Harman-boehm, I, Bluher, M, Redel, H, Sion-vardy, N, Ovadia, S, Avinoach, E, Shai, I, Kloting, N, Stumvoll, M, Bashan, N, & Rudich, A. Macrophage infiltration into omental versus subcutaneous fat across different populations: effects of regional adiposity and the comorbidities of obesity. The Journal of Clinical Endocrinology and Metabolism (2007). , 92(6), 2240-7.

[108] Odegaard, J. I, & Chawla, A. Connecting type 1 and type 2 diabetes through innate immunity. Cold Spring Harbour Perspectives in Medicine (2012). a007724.

[109] Cnop, M, Welsh, N, Jonas, J. C, Jorns, A, Lenzen, S, & Eizirik, D. L. Mechanisms of pancreatic β-cell death in type 1 and type 2 diabetes: Many differences, few similarities. Diabetes (2005). Suppl 2): S, 97-107.

[110] Lee, S. C, & Pervaiz, S. Apoptosis in the pathophysiology of diabetes mellitus. The International Journal of Biochemistry and Cell Biology (2007). , 39(3), 497-504.

[111] Back, S. H, Kang, S. W, Han, J, & Chung, H. T. Endoplasmic reticulum stress in the β-cell pathogenesis of type 2 diabetes. Experimental Diabetes Research (2012).

[112] Yip, L, Su, L, & Sheng, D. Deaf1 isoforms control the expression of genes encoding peripheral tissue antigens in the pancreatic lymph nodes during type 1 diabetes. Nature Immunology (2009). , 10(9), 1026-33.

[113] Clark, R, & Griffiths, G. M. Lytic granules, secretory lysosome and disease. Current Opinion in Immunology (2003). , 15(5), 516-21.

[114] Ashkenazi, A, & Dixit, V. M. Death receptors: signalling and modulation. Science (1998). , 281(5381), 1305-8.

[115] Sakamoto, S, & Kyprianou, N. Targeting anoikis-resistance in prostate cancer metastasis. Molecular Aspects of Medicine (2010). , 31(2), 205-14.

[116] Chang, H. Y, & Yang, X. Proteases for cell suicide: functions and regulation of caspases. Microbiology & Molecular Biology Reviews (2007). , 64(4), 821-46.

[117] Batinac, T, Zamolo, G, Coklo, M, & Hadzisejdic, I. Possible key role of granzyme B in keratoacanthoma regression. Medical Hypotheses (2006). , 66(6), 1129-32.

[118] Sutton, V. R, Wowk, M. E, Cancilla, M, & Trapani, J. Caspase activation by granzyme B is indirect, and caspase autoprocessing requires the release of pro-apoptotic mitochondrial factors. Immunity (2003). , 18(3), 319-29.

[119] Li, H, Zhu, H, Xu, C. J, & Yuan, J. Cleavage of Bid by caspase-8 mediates the mitochondrial damage in the Fas pathway of apoptosis. Cell (1998). , 94(4), 494-501.

[120] Yang, S. H, Chein, C. M, Lu, M. C, Hu, X. W, & Lin, S. R. Up-regulation of Bax and endonuclease G, and down-modulation of Bcl-XL involved in cardiotoxin III-induced apoptosis in K562 cells. Experimental and Molecular Medicine (2006). , 38(4), 435-44.

[121] Green, D. R, & Reed, J. C. Mitochondria and apoptosis. Science (1998). , 281(5381), 1309-12.

[122] Breckenridge, D. G, & Xue, D. Regulation of mitochondrial membrane permeabilization by BCL-2 family proteins and caspases. Current Opinion in Cell Biology (2004). , 16(6), 647-52.

[123] Wang, Z. B, Liu, Y. Q, & Cui, Y. F. Pathways to caspase activation. Cell Biology International (2005). , 29(7), 489-96.

[124] Portt, L, Norman, G, Clapp, C, Greenwood, M, & Greenwood, M. T. Anti-apoptosis and cell survival: A review. Biochimica et Biophysica Acta (2011). , 1813(1), 238-59.

[125] Ferri, K. F, & Kroemer, G. Organelle-specific initiation of cell death pathways. Nature Cell Biology (2001). E, 255-63.

[126] Brandt, B, Abou-eladab, E. F, Tiedge, M, & Walzel, H. Role of the JNK/c-Jun/AP-1 signalling pathway in galectin-induced T-cell death. Cell Death and Disease (2010). e23., 1.

[127] Rahier, J, Guiot, Y, Goebbels, R. M, Sempoux, C, & Henquin, J. C. Pancreatic beta-cell mass in European subjects with type 2 diabetes. Diabetes, Obesity and Metabolism (2008). Suppl 4): 32-42.

[128] Chang-chen, K. J, Mullur, R, & Bernal-mizrachi, E. cell failure as a complication of diabetes. Reviews in Endocrine Metabolic Disorders (2008). , 9(4), 329-43.

[129] Gehrmann, W, Elsner, M, & Lenzen, S. Role of metabolically generated reactive oxygen species for lipotoxicity in pancreatic β-cells. Diabetes, Obesity and Metabolism (2010). Suppl 2): 149-58.

[130] Chakrabarti, A, Chen, A. W, & Varner, J. D. A review of the mammalian unfolded protein response. Biotechnology and Bioengineering (2011). , 108(12), 2777-93.

[131] Kaufman, R. J Stress signalling from the lumen of the endoplasmic reticulum: coordination of gene transcriptional and translational controls. Genes & Development (1999). , 13(10), 1211-33.

[132] Szegezedi, E, Logue, S. E, Gorman, A. M, & Samali, A. Mediators of endoplasmic reticulum stress-induced apoptosis. EMBO Reports (2006). , 7(9), 880-5.

[133] Nakagawa, T, & Yuan, J. Cross-talk between two cysteine protease families. Activation of caspase-12 by calpain in apoptosis. Journal of Cell Biology (2000). , 150(4), 887-94.

[134] Rao, R. V, Peel, A, & Loqvinova, A. del Rio G., Hermel E., Yokota T., Goldsmith P.C., Ellerby L.M., Ellerby H.M. and Bredesen D.E. Coupling endoplasmic reticulum stress to the cell death program: role of the ER chaperone GRP78. FEBS Letters (2002).

[135] Putcha, G. V, Le, S, Frank, S, Besirli, C. G, Clark, K, Chu, B, Alix, S, & Youle, R. J. LaMarche A., Maroney A.C. and Johnson E.M. Jr. JNK-mediated BIM phosphorylation potentiates BAX-dependent apoptosis. Neuron (2003). , 38(6), 899-914.

[136] Donath, M. Y, Ehses, J. A, Maedler, K, Schumann, D. M, Ellingsgaard, H, Eppler, E, & Reinecke, M. Mechanisms of β-cell death in type 2 diabetes. Diabetes (2005). Suppl 2): S, 108-13.

[137] Cunha, D. A, Hekerman, P, Ladriere, L, Bazarra-castro, A, Ortis, F, Wakeham, M. C, Moore, F, Rasschaert, J, Cardozo, A. K, Bellomo, E, Overbergh, L, Mathieu, C, Lupi, R, Hai, T, Herchuelz, A, Marchetti, P, Rutter, G. A, Eizirik, D. L, & Cnop, M. Initiation and execution of lipotoxic ER stress in pancreatic β-cells. The Journal of Cell Science (2008). Pt 14): 2308-18.

[138] Cnop, M. Fatty acids and glucolipotoxicity in the pathogenesis of type 2 diabetes. The Biochemical Society Transactions (2008). Pt 3): 1180-6.

[139] Haataja, L, Gurlo, T, Huang, C. J, & Butler, P. C. Islet amyloid in type 2 diabetes, and the toxic oligomer hypothesis. Endocrine Reviews (2008). , 29(3), 303-16.

[140] Larsen, C. M, Faulenbach, M, Vaag, A, Volund, A, Ehses, J. A, Seifert, B, Mandrup-poulsen, T, & Donath, M. Y. Interleukin-1-receptor antagonist in type 2 diabetes mellitus. New England Journal of Medicine (2007). , 356(15), 1517-26.

[141] Mastrandrea, L, Yu, J, Behrens, T, Buchlis, J, Albini, C, Fourtner, S, & Quattrin, T. Etanercept treatment in children with new-onset type 1 diabetes: pilot randomised, placebo-controlled, double blind study. Diabetes Care (2009). , 32(7), 1244-9.

[142] Chung, J, Nguyen, A. K, Henstridge, D. C, Holmes, A. G, Chan, M. H, Mesa, J. L, Lancaster, G. I, Southgate, R. J, Bruce, C. R, Duffy, S. J, Horvath, I, Mestril, R, Watt, M. J, Hooper, P. L, Kingwell, B. A, Vigh, L, Hevener, A, & Febbraio, M. A. HSP72 protects against obesity-induced insulin-resistance. Proceedings of the National Academy of Sciences (2008). , 105(5), 1739-44.

[143] Kurucz, I, Morva, A, Vaag, A, Eriksson, K. F, Huang, X, Groop, L, & Koranyi, L. Decreased expression of heat shock protein 72 in skeletal muscle of patients with type 2 diabetes correlates with insulin-resistance. Diabetes (2002). , 51(4), 1102-9.

[144] Rodrigues-krause, J, Krause, M, Hagan, O, De Vito, C, Boreham, G, Murphy, C, Newsholme, C, & Colleran, P. G. Divergence of intracellular and extracellular HSP72 in type 2 diabetes: does fat matter? Cell Stress Chaperones. (2012). , 17(3), 293-302.

[145] Gupte, A. A, Bomhoff, G. L, Swerdlow, R. H, & Geiger, P. C. Heat treatment improves glucose tolerance and prevents skeletal muscle insulin-resistance in rats fed a high-fat diet. Diabetes (2009). , 58(3), 567-78.

[146] Krause, M. S. and Homem de Bittencourt P.I. Jr. Type 1 diabetes: can exercise impair the autoimmune event? The L-arginine/glutamine coupling hypothesis. Cell Biochemistry and Function (2008). , 26(4), 406-33.

[147] Mandrup-poulsen, T, Pickersgill, L, & Donath, M. Y. (2010). Blockade of interleukin-1 in type 1 diabetes. Nature Reviews Endocrinology 2010; , 6(3), 158-66.

[148] Patterson, C. C, Dahlquist, G. G, Gyurus, E, Green, A, & Soltesz, G. and EURODIAB Study Group. Incidence t rends for childhood type 1 diabetes in Europe during 1989-2003 and predicted new cases 2005-20: a multicentre prospective registration study. Lancet (2009). , 373(9680), 2027-33.

Chapter 7

Beta Cell Function After Islet Transplantation

Morihito Takita, Nigar Seven, Marlon F. Levy and
Bashoo Naziruddin

Additional information is available at the end of the chapter

http://dx.doi.org/10.5772/ 52952

1. Introduction

1.1. Islet cell transplantation for type 1 diabetes

The transplantation of pancreatic islets of Langerhans is a promising treatment for "brittle" type 1 diabetics, because it is a minimally invasive procedure that replenishes the beta cell mass lost due to autoimmunity. This procedure also provides an opportunity for a "cure" from diabetes based on the achievement of freedom from dependence on exogenous insulin and severe hypoglycemic events. Although islet transplants had been attempted for several decades, they achieved minimum success in terms of post-transplant graft function. The publication of the Edmonton Protocol [1] documenting consistent achievement of insulin independence after islet transplantation, has led to a dramatic increase not only in the number of procedures performed worldwide but also in other related areas in the field of islet transplantation. Breakthroughs have been made in the area of pancreas procurement and preservation with study into ductal preservation, the two layer method, and the type of preservation solution used. Furthermore, there has been much progress in the islet isolation process by bringing standards up to cGMP qualifications, optimization of collagenase enzymes, and using iodixanol for continuous density gradient purification [2]. Some of the hurdles facing further success in this treatment are:

i. lack of suitable donor pancreases;

ii. difficulties in isolating high quality islets on a consistent basis;

iii. improving the engraftment of transplanted islets;

iv. development of an islet-friendly immunosuppression and

v. improving long-term survival of transplanted islets.

1.2. Post-transplant outcome

According to a recent report from the Collaborative Islet Transplant Registry, 677 patients have received either an islet transplant alone (ITA) or islets-after-kidney (IAK) transplants [3]. There has been a remarkable improvement in the post-transplant graft function in recent times. Prior to the publication of Edmonton protocol, the achievement of insulin-independent status by islet transplant recipients was <10%. Patients treated initially under the Edmonton protocol showed remarkable achievement of 82% insulin-independent status at one year post-transplant. However, this result proved to be unsustainable when the five year insulin-independence rates fell to 12.5% at the same center [4]. This data resulted in skepticism on the use of allogeneic islet transplantation as a reliable treatment for long-term success. With the introduction of thymoglobulin at induction phase and the combination of prograf, rapamycin and/or mycophenolate mofetil as maintenance immunosuppressive agents, the islet transplant survival rate has significantly improved to 50% at five year post-transplant [5]. Control of inflammatory reaction during peri-transplant period with the use of TNF-α blockers also played a key role in this improvement. These remarkable results necessitated comparison with whole pancreas transplantation which is considered as an established clinical procedure. Although whole organ treatment achieved high levels of graft survival in the years 1994-1997, the islet survival rate at five years has reached around fifty percent in 2010-2011, comparable to the level of whole pancreas graft success [5]. Moreover, islet cell transplantation seems to confer significantly better glycemic control than maximal medical therapy, and essentially eliminates hypoglycemic unawareness. These results have brought back the enthusiasm in this field.

2. Molecular mechanism of beta cell dysfunction

2.1. Early events after islet transplantation

The liver is the most commonly used site for transplantation of islets. Data supporting the use of this transplant site came from autologous islet transplants in patients with chronic pancreatitis, which showed that islets can function inside the liver for several years. There are several drawbacks associated with the liver as a host site for islets. Major factors affecting islet function include hypoxia, drug toxicity and instant blood-mediated inflammatory reaction (IBMIR). Together, these events may lead to loss of up to 75% of islet transplant mass. IBMIR is primarily a response of innate immune system to isolated islets. Major characteristics of IBMIR include activation of coagulation and complement cascades and infiltration of inflammatory cells. Several approaches are adopted to minimize the deleterious effects of IBMIR which include infusion of low molecular weight dextran sulfate and also inclusion of anti-inflammatory molecules during the infusion of islets. Besides the innate immune response, islets transplanted into liver may experience low oxygen tension. Activation of resident Kupffer cells may pose additional risk to islet survival. In addition, high concentrations of immunosuppressive drugs in the portal vein are likely to exert toxic effect on the transplanted islet mass [6].

2.2. Alloimmunity

The exposure of body to allogeneic tissues via organ/cell transplantation, blood transfusions, pregnancy can cause development of anti-human leukocyte antigen (HLA) antibodies [7]. These *de novo* HLA antibodies have been shown to play a significant role in the early graft loss after solid organ transplantation [8]. Currently, HLA matching between the recipients and donors is not performed before islet cell transplantation. Moreover, to achieve and/or maintain insulin independence and good metabolic control in an islet recipient, multiple islet infusions from multiple donors and high doses of immunosuppressants are generally required. The requirement of multi-donor infusions and reduction or weaning of immunosuppressants due to significant adverse effects could cause patients eventually to develop HLA antibodies against islet graft.

The issue of sensitization of alloantigens after islet cell transplantation has been raised by the Edmonton group in 2007 [9]. 98 islet transplant recipients were screened for HLA antibodies by flow-based methods. Twenty-nine patients (31%) represented *de novo* donor specific antibodies following islet transplantation. Among 14 recipients who discontinued immunosuppression, 10 recipients (71%) were largely sensitized with panel reactive antibody ≥50%. On the other hand, only 11 of 69 (16%) recipients who continued immunosuppression became broadly sensitized posttransplant. This study suggested that development of HLA antibodies after islet transplantation is concerning and withdrawal of immunosuppression completely following failed islet transplantation raises the risk for broad sensitization. Along with the report of Edmonton group, there are several studies that have demonstrated that islet alone transplant recipients develop donor-specific and/or nondonor-specific HLA antibodies, especially following discontinuation of immunosuppression [10-13].

In contrast, in the report of Geneva group it was shown that multiple islet infusions did not act as a risk factor for appearance of anti-HLA antibodies [14]. The group claimed that transplantation of islets in liver might cause less immunogenicity. After combined kidney-islet transplantation and continued immunosuppression even with failed islet graft function, patients had a low risk for sensitization as long as their kidney remained functional.

It has been known that islets express mainly HLA class I antigens on their surfaces. Previous reports demonstrated that patients develop antibodies posttransplant not only against HLA class I antigens, but also against HLA class II antigens [9]. Jackson et al. showed that there would be an induction of HLA class II expression on human islets under inflammatory conditions, which in return may be a possible cause of allosensitization [15]. For this aim, the group conducted an experiment in which they had two groups of isolated human islets; group 1 was control group and cultured at 37°C, whereas group 2 was cultured in the same condition and treated with tumor necrosis factor alpha (TNF-α) and interferon gamma (INF-γ). Presence of HLA class II on islet surface was analyzed by real-time polymerase chain reaction (PCR), immunofluorescence and flow cytometry. Expression of class II transactivator, HLA-DR-α and HLA-DR-β1 increased maximum 9.38, 18.95 and 46.5 fold respectively in group 2 compared to control group after 24 hours of incubation with TNF-α and INF-γ which is shown by real-time PCR analysis. Fluorescent imaging and flow cytometric analysis confirmed the significant increase in the expression of HLA class II expression both on islet α and β cells after cytokine treatment. Inflammatory conditions shortly after islet transplantation up-regulates HLA class II antigens on islet surfaces that trigger alloimmunity. Thus, protocols which provide adequate and efficient control of inflammation after islet transplantation should be considered to improve islet transplant outcome.

Collaborative Islet Transplant Registry reported the sensitization rates against HLA class I antigens pre- and posttransplant in islet alone recipients in 2011 [16]. Data is collected from 303 islet alone recipients between January 1999 and December 2008. Panel reactive antibody (PRA) pretransplant and PRA at 6 months and yearly posttransplant correlated to measures of islet graft failure. Pretransplant PRA showed not to be a predictor of islet graft failure; whereas there was 3.6 fold increased hazard ratio for graft failure when the recipient developed PRA≥20% post-transplant. Each additional islet infusion increased the cumulative number of mismatched HLA alleles from a median of 3 to 9; respectively for one infusion and for 3 infusions. Significantly higher rate of PRA ≥ 20% was observed in recipients who had complete graft loss with discontinued immunosuppression compared to recipients who had functioning grafts with continuing immunosuppression. Development of *de novo* HLA class I antibodies is less pronounced in recipients with exposure to repeat HLA class I mismatched than increased class I mismatch. Reducing the number of islet donors used for each patient and repeating HLA I mismatches with consequent islet transplantation without presence of donor specific anti-HLA antibodies are vital factors to decrease the risk of allosensitization.

Currently, there is no clearly defined monitoring tool for alloimmunity in islet cell transplantation, but researchers have proposed many experimental tools to assess alloreactivity in islet transplanted patients. Alloantibodies, soluble CD30 level, cytotoxic lymphocyte gene expression and microparticles in peripheral blood are the markers which were shown to detect allogeneic rejection after islet transplantation. Monitoring panel reactive antibody in immunosuppressed recipients had little clinical value to assess islet graft survival [16, 17].

Team	Approach	Outcome	References
Edmonton group	Alloantibodies	Pretransplant HLA antibodies reduce graft survival after islet transplantation.	[9]
CITR report	Alloantibodies	Monitoring PRA in immunosuppressed patients had little clinical value for islet graft survival.	[16]
Minnesota group	Soluble CD30	No correlation between sCD30 levels and graft function at 1 year was found. A greater reduction in sCD30 levels posttransplant was associated with full graft function.	[18]
Miami group	Cytotoxic lymphocyte (CL) gene expression	Increased CL gene levels could predict islet allograft loss.	[19]
GRAGIL group	Microparticles	MPs and C-peptide showed opposite pattern. MPs levels in peripheral blood increase with acute rejection of islet allograft.	[20]

Table 1. Immunologic tools to assess alloimmunity after islet cell transplantation

Soluble CD30 (sCD30) is a cell membrane protein of tumor necrosis factor receptor family. sCD30 is released into blood with the activation of CD30 + T cells, leading to speculation that it may act as a marker for immune system activation [21]. Although it has been shown to be predictive for acute rejection in lung, kidney, and heart transplantation [22-24], there are not many reports about the role of sCD30 in the prediction of early graft loss following islet transplantation. In the study of Hire et al., 19 allograft islet recipients treated with three different immunosuppression inductions were evaluated retrospectively for the serum sCD30 levels [18]. Pretransplant, early posttransplant day (day 4–7), one month posttransplant, late posttransplant (day 90–120) sCD30 levels were measured and correlated with islet graft outcomes at 1 year. No correlation between sCD30 levels at any time point and graft function at 1 year was found. However, a greater reduction in SCD30 levels posttransplant was associated with full graft function. Therefore, sCD30 may be of value for immune monitoring of islet allografts.

Cytotoxic lymphocyte (CL) genes granzyme, Fas ligand and perforin may play an active role in the course of acute allograft rejection. University of Miami group studied 13 islet transplant recipients treated with steroid-free immunosuppressive regimen in order to demonstrate whether CL gene expression could be a predictor of allogeneic rejection [19]. All patients attained insulin independence; however, 8 of them restarted insulin therapy. Real-time PCR was used to assess CL gene mRNA levels. The group demonstrated that recipients who restarted insulin therapy had a significant elevation of CL gene mRNA levels and the most reliable measure of ongoing graft loss was granzyme B. Hence, increased blood CL gene levels might be a potential marker to predict islet allograft loss.

Microparticles (MP) are plasma membrane fragments of apoptotic cells in peripheral blood. The quantity of microparticles is correlated with the degree of cell death, so they are considered to be indicators of apoptosis. Kessler et al. demonstrated the elevation of microparticles in peripheral blood at the time of acute rejection following intraportal islet transplantation with a case report [25]. Loss of islet graft function without the presence of GAD65, IA2 or anti-HLA antibodies brought up the diagnosis of acute cellular rejection. With a successful steroid bolus therapy, MPs level declined and the patient regained islet function. In 2011, Toti et al. [20] demonstrated from three islet transplant recipients that in the case of rejection, C-peptide and MPs levels exhibited opposite pattern and a decline in C-peptide was related with increased insulin needs. This data suggested an increment in MPs level might indicate allogeneic rejection. Thus, MPs level in peripheral blood might be a useful tool to monitor allogeneic rejection after islet transplantation.

2.3. Autoimmune recurrence

Type 1 diabetes is an autoimmune disease in which pancreatic beta cells are destroyed through a T-cell mediated mechanism in genetically susceptible individuals [26]. Autoantibodies against pancreatic islets comprise anti-glutamate decarboxylase 65 (GAD65), islet cell autoantibody (ICA), anti-insulin autoantibody (IAA), anti-tyrosine phosphatase autoantibody (IA-2) and against zinc transporter ZnT8. Antibodies present in serum against these pancreatic islet antigens are commonly used to predict and or diagnose the disease in clinical practice. For successful islet cell replacement, it is crucial to prevent recurrent destruction of beta cells through existing autoimmune destruction. The graft failure due to recurrent autoimmunity in a pancreas segment transplanted between identical twins was proven with the demonstration of insulitis in the transplanted tissue [27]. Islet specific T cells seem to have a basic role in the process of autoimmune destruction of beta cells [28].

To investigate T-cell allo- and autoreactivities in peripheral blood following islet transplantation, Roep et al. examined 7 islet allograft recipients [29]. They showed that three patients who got thymoglobulin for induction immunosuppression and retained full islet function for more than 1 year exhibited minor autoreactivites but no alloreactivities. Three patients who did not get thymoglobulin had rapid decline (<3 weeks) in islet function and showed alloreactivities; but one out of these three patients had rapid increase in autoreactivity to several islet autoantigens prior to alloreactivity. One recipient who did not receive thymoglobulin exhibited hyperautoreacivity with no detectable alloreaactivity and developed delayed loss of islet graft function consequently (<33 weeks); which indicated that autoimmune recurrence might be the cause of chronic islet graft dysfunction. In this study, because of the excellent outcomes in thymoglobulin group, the authors evaluated allo- and autoimmunity again in a bigger sample sized group in 2008 [30]. 21 islet recipients under thymoglobulin induction and tacrolimus plus mycophenolate mofetil maintenance immunosuppressive regimen were studied. Immunity against allo- and autoantigens were checked at pretransplant and at 1 year posttransplant. The analyses showed that existence of cellular autoimmunity pretransplant and posttransplant was related with delayed insulin independence and lower levels of circulating C-peptide during the first year posttransplant. Seven out of eight patients with no previous T-cell autoreactivity achieved insulin independence; whereas none of the four patients with autoantibodies against GAD and IA-2 before transplantation became insulin independent. Cellular alloreactivity and autoantibody levels did not show significant involvement with the outcome. Based on these findings, the authors commented that thymoglobulin may cope sufficiently with alloimmunity, but insufficient to control islet autoreactivity in an early period. The issue of autoimmunity remains unaddressed and needs further investigation.

Team	Approach	Outcome	References
Roep *et al.*	Autoantibodies	Autoandibodies increased due to autoimmune activity, but did not indicate loss of graft function.	[29]
Roep *et al.*	T-cell autoreactivity in peripheral blood	Pre- and posttransplant cellular autoimmunity were associated with delayed insulin independence. Autoantibody levels did not affect islet allograft outcome.	[30]
Matsumoto *et al.*	GAD65 specific global immune assay	Broad repertoire of islet antigen-specific T cells secreting various cytokines were related with chronic graft failure.	[31]

Table 2. Immunologic tools to assess autoimmunity after islet cell transplantation

Autoimmunity recurrence might be assessed by monitoring islet specific autoantibodies and T-cell autoreactivity. But the association between autoantibodies and insulin independence and islet graft outcome are variable; increase in autoantibody levels were shown due to autoimmune activity but did not indicate loss of islet graft function [29, 32]. Assays that measure anti-islet cellular autoimmunity before and after islet transplantation demonstrated that pre-and posttransplant cellular autoimmunity were related with delayed insulin independence and lower levels of circulating C-peptide during the first year posttransplant [30]. Nonetheless, in this study islet allograft outcome did not seem to be affected by autoantibody levels or cellular alloreactivity.

Matsumoto et al. have reported on a global immune assay specific for GAD65 (EpiMax) in order to analyze the property of autoreactive T-cell responses [31]. Five type 1 diabetic patients were studied 1 year after allogeneic islet transplantation. All patients achieved insulin independence at 1 year. Three out of five patients maintained long-term insulin independence and EpiMax affirmed minimum T-cell responses in these patients. In contrast, the two patients who developed chronic graft failure and lost insulin independence showed broad repertoire of GAD65 specific T-cells secreting various types of cytokines, including IL-5, IL-13, IL-17, TNF- alpha, and IFN-gamma. In addition to those observations, IFN-γ and IL-13 expressing CD4+ T cells and IFN-γ expressing CD8+ T cells were encountered in the other two failed patients. These findings suggested that broad repertoire of islet antigen-specific T cells which secrete variable types of cytokines were related with chronic graft failure, preventing islet recipients from maintaining long-term insulin independence.

Immunosuppression

Following transplantation of islets, administration of immunosuppression is essential to maintain graft function. However, most of the immunosuppressive drugs also have adverse effects on beta cell function. Careful selection of immunosuppressive regimen is critical for prolonged function of transplanted islets.

2.3.1. Early period of islet cell transplantation

Corticosteroid was a widely used agent as maintenance immunosuppression in the pioneering days of islet cell transplantation in 1990's (Table 3). During this decade, majority of islet cell transplants were after or performed simultaneously with kidney transplantation. Corticosteroid has antiinflammatory as well as immunosuppressive effects by direct or indirect actions on various leukocytes, including T lymphocytes, monocytes and macrophages, through glucocorticoid receptor [33, 34]. However, steroid therapy leads to β cell dysfunction and insulin resistance. [35, 36] Deterioration of insulin secretion from β cell by steroid treatment has been reported, caused by enhanced α-adrenergic receptor signaling [37], β cell apoptosis [38] and activated K^+ channel [39]. Insulin resistance in liver, adipose tissue and skeletal muscle by long-term steroid administration are well known clinically and in basic studies [40-42]. Thus, steroid use for the purpose of maintenance immunosuppression has been averted in the recent decade of islet transplantation (Table 3).

The calcineurin inhibitors (CNIs) have been major players in maintenance immunosuppression of islet cell transplantation. Cyclosporine A and tacrolimus are currently available CNIs in clinic. They inhibit calcineurin, a serine-threonine phosphatase, which is responsible for dephosphorylation of nuclear factor for activated T cells (NF-AT), which in turn results in inactivation of the transcription of cytokine genes. However, CNIs might have β cell toxicity since calcineurin is expressed in β cell and regulates β cell growth as well as function [43, 44].

Azathioprine is a purine analog, serving as a blocker of de novo pathway in purine synthesis in actively proliferative cells such as T cells and B cells [45]. Currently this drug is used for immunosuppression in allogeneic transplantation and autoimmune disease like rheumatoid arthritis as well as therapy in hematologic malignancies [46]. Azathioprine may also prevent the onset of diabetes [47, 48] and no major β cell toxicity of azathioprine has been reported.

2.3.2. Edmonton protocol

Remarkable success in islet transplant survival was achieved by the University of Alberta group using steroid-free immunosuppression regimen that included daclizumab, tacrolimus and sirolimus, resulting in that all 7 recipients achieving insulin independence [1]. The benefit of Edmonton protocol is to eliminate the risk of steroid-induced β cell toxicity as well as insulin resistance and increasing the dose of transplanted islets. However, the protocol uses tacrolimus that has the effect of β cell deterioration.

Publication year	Pts no.	Induction therapy	Maintenance therapy			Transplant type	Donor no.*	Major outcomes	Refs
			Steroid	CNIs	Other				
1990	9			✓Tac		Islet after liver transplant	M/S	5 pts achieved II	[49]
1991	3		✓Pred	✓CsA	✓Aza	ITA	M/S	Rejected 2 weeks after ITA	[50]
	3	✓mALG	✓Pred	✓CsA	✓Aza	IAK	S	Partial function**	
	3	✓mALG	✓Pred	✓CsA	✓Aza	IAK	M	II for 7, 14 and 121 days	
1991	4	✓ATG (3 pts)	✓Pred	✓CsA	✓Aza	IAK	M/S	1 pt achieved II	[51]
	2	✓ATG	✓Pred	✓CsA	✓Aza	SIK	M/S		
1992	10			✓Tac		Simultaneous Islet-Liver transplant	S	6 pts achieved II	[52]

Publication year	Pts no.	Induction therapy	Maintenance therapy			Transplant type	Donor no.*	Major outcomes	Refs
	4		✓Pred	✓Tac		Simultaneous Islet-Liver transplant	S	Partial function**	
	7		✓Pred	✓Tac		SIK	M	Partial function**	
1993	2	✓mALG ✓15-DSG	✓Pred	✓CsA	✓Aza	SIK	S	1 pt achieved II	[53]
1997	6		✓mPred	✓Tac		Simultaneous Islet-Liver-Bone marrow transplant	S	3 pts achieved II	[54]
1997	8	✓OKT3	✓mPred	✓CsA	✓Aza	IAK (7 pts) or SIK (1 pt)	M/S	2 pts achieved II	[55]
1997	20	✓ATG	✓Pred	✓CsA	✓Aza	IAK (7 pts) or SIK (13 pt)	M/S	7 pts achieved II	[56]
1997	3	✓ATG	✓Pred	✓CsA	✓MMF	SIK (2 pts) or IAK (1 pt)	M/S	Partial function**	[57]
1998	7	✓ATG (3pts)	✓Pred	✓CsA	✓Aza	IAK	M	2 pts achieved II	[58]
1999	12	✓ATG	✓Pred	✓CsA	✓Aza	IAK (12 pts) or SIK (12pts)	M/S	Partial function**	[59]

Table 3. Immunosuppression protocols in clinical islet transplants published in 1990's. *M: Multiple donor transplants, S: Single donor transplant. ** Not achieved II, but positive C-peptide or decreased insulin requirement was confirmed. Abbreviations; 15-DSG: 15-deoxyspergualin, ATG: antithymocyte globulin, Aza: azathioprine, CNIs: Calcineurin inhibitors, CsA: Cyclosporine A, IAK: Islet after kidney transplantation, II: Insulin Independence, ITA: Islet transplantation alone, mALG: Minnesota antilymphoblast globulin, MMF: mycophenolic mofetil, mPred: methylprednisolone, Pred: Prednisone, SIK: Simultaneous islet kidney transplantation, Tac: Tacrolimus.

Publication year	Pts no.	Induction therapy	Maintenance therapy			Transplant type	Donor no.*	Major outcomes	Refs
			Steroid	CNIs	Other				
2000	13	✓ATG or ✓Bas	✓Pred	✓CsA	✓Aza or ✓MMF	SIK, IAK or Islet after lung transplant	M/S	2 pts achieved II	[60]
2000	7	✓Dac		✓Tac	✓Sir	ITA	M	100% II	[1]
2001	2	✓ATG or ✓Bas	✓Pred	✓CsA	✓MMF	SIK (5 pts) or IAK (2 pts)	M/S	Partial function**	[61]

Publication year	Pts no.	Induction therapy	Maintenance therapy			Transplant type	Donor no.*	Major outcomes	Refs
2001	10	✓Bas	✓Pred	✓CsA	✓MMF	IAK	M/S	2 pts achieved II	[62]
2003	6	✓Dac		✓Tac	✓Sir	ITA	M/S	3 pts achieved II	[63]
2004	6	✓OKT3γ1		✓Tac	✓Sir	ITA	S	4 pts achieved II	[64]
2004	13	✓Dac		✓Tac	✓Sir	ITA (9 pts) or IAK (4 pts)	M	11 pts achieved II	[65]
2004	10	✓Dac		✓Tac	✓Sir	ITA	M/S	5 pts achieved II	[66]
2004	6	✓Dac		✓Tac	✓Sir	SIK	M	5 pts achieved II	[67]
2005	8	✓ATG ✓Dac ✓Eta		✓Tac	✓MMF ✓Sir	ITA	S	100% II after single infusion	[68]
2005	16	✓Dac ✓Inf (8pts)		✓Tac	✓Sir	ITA	M/S	14 pts achieved II	[69]
2005	22	✓Dac/ ✓Bas		✓Tac/ ✓CsA	✓Sir/ ✓Eve	IAK or ITA	M/S	15 pts achieved II	[70]
2005	65	✓Dac		✓Tac	✓Sir	ITA	M/S	44 pts achieved II	[4]
2005	10	✓ATG or ✓Bas		✓Tac	✓Sir or ✓MMF	ITA	M/S	100% II	[71]
2006	8	✓Dac		✓Tac	✓Sir	IAK	M/S	100% II	[72]
2006	6	✓Dac		✓Tac	✓Sir	ITA	M	3 pts achieved II	[73]
2006	36	✓Dac		✓Tac	✓Sir	ITA	M/S	16 pts achieved II	[74]
2007	11	✓Dac		✓Tac	✓Sir or ✓MMF plus ✓Exe		M/S	8 pts achieved II	[75]
2007	10	✓Dac		✓Tac	✓Sir	ITA	M/S	6 pts achieved II	[76]
2007	19	✓Dac		✓Tac	✓Sir or ✓MMF	ITA	M/S	16 pts achieved II	[77]

Publication year	Pts no.	Induction therapy	Maintenance therapy			Transplant type	Donor no.*	Major outcomes	Refs
2008	5	✓ATG		✓Tac	✓Sir	ITA	M	3 pts achieved II	[78]
	5	✓ATG			✓Sir	ITA	M	Partial function**	
2008	13	✓Dac		✓Tac	✓Sir	SIK	M/S	7 pts achieved II	[79]
2008	7	✓Dac ✓Inf ✓Eta	✓ Pred (2 pts) or mPred (1 pt)	✓Tac	✓Sir ✓MMF (2 pts)	IAK	M/S	6 pts achieved II	[80]
2008	6	✓ATG ✓Eta		✓CyA	✓Eve →MMF	ITA	M/S	5 pts achieved II	[81]
2008	4	✓Dac		✓Tac	✓Sir	ITA	M	100% II	[82]
	6	✓Dac ✓Eta		✓Tac	✓Sir ✓Exe	ITA	M/S	100% II	
2008	3	✓Ale		✓Tac	✓Sir ✓MPA	ITA	M/S	2 pts achieved II	[83]
2008	6	✓Dac ✓Inf		✓Tac	✓Sir	Islet transplant with Bone marrow	S	3 pts achieved II	[84]
2009	14	✓Dac		✓Tac	✓Sir	ITA	M	100% II	[85]
2009	15	✓Dac or ✓Bas		✓Tac	✓Sir	IAK	M/S	100 pts achieved II	[86]
2010	8	✓ATG			✓Sir ✓MMF ✓Efa	ITA	M/S	100% II	[87]
2010	8	✓Dac		✓Tac	✓Sir	ITA	M/S	100% II	[88]
	4	✓Dac		✓Tac	✓Sir ✓Efa	ITA	S	100% II after single infusion	
2010	5	✓ATG ✓Bela			✓Sir or ✓MMF	ITA	M/S	100% II after single infusion	[89]
	5	✓ATG ✓Efa			✓Sir or ✓MMF	ITA	M/S	100% II after single infusion	
2011	3	✓ATG ✓Eta ✓Ana		✓Tac	✓MMF	ITA	M/S	100% II after single infusion	[90]
	3	✓Dac		✓Tac	✓Sir	ITA	M	100% II	

Publication year	Pts no.	Induction therapy	Maintenance therapy	Transplant type	Donor no.*	Major outcomes	Refs
2011	4			ITA**	M/S	Partial function***	[91]

Table 4. Immunosuppression protocols in clinical islet transplants published after 2000. *M: Multiple donor transplants, S: Single donor transplant. **Microencapsulated islets transplanted. *** Not achieved II, but positive C-peptide or decreased insulin requirement was confirmed. Abbreviations; Ale: Alemtuzumab, ATG: antithymocyte globulin, Aza: azathioprine, Ana: anakinra, Bas: basiliximab, Bela: belatacept, CNIs: Calcineurin inhibitors, CsA: Cyclosporine A, Dac: daclizumab, Efa: efalizumab, Eta: etanercept, Eve: everolimus, Exe: exenatide, IAK: islet after kidney transplantation, II: insulin independence, Inf: infliximab, ITA: islet transplantation alone, mALG: Minnesota antilymphoblast globulin, MMF: mycophenolic mofetil, MPA: mycophenolic acid, mPred: methylprednisolone, Pred: prednisone, SIK: simultaneous islet kidney transplantation, Sir: sirolimus, Tac: tacrolimus

Sirolimus is an inhibitor of mammalian target of rapamycin (mTOR), which plays an important role in cell cycle from late G1 to S phase in T cells [92]. The effect of sirolimus in β cell function is still unclear; impaired β cell proliferation and islet graft function by sirolimus has been reported [93-95] while Melzi et al found no significant adverse effect of sirolimus in islet engraftment [96]. Gao et al reported sirolimus and daclizumab did not show any individual or synergistic negative effects on islet proliferation [97]. However, insulin independence in Edmonton protocol was not sustained for a long-term resulting in 12.5% at 5 year after islet transplant [4].

2.3.3. *Newer immunosuppression protocols*

Recent clinical trials implementing monoclonal antibodies such as basiliximab (anti-IL-2 receptor)[70], efalizumab (anti-LFA-1)[89], alemtuzumab (anti-CD52)[83] have shown high rate of insulin independence after transplant. These monoclonal antibodies are produced as molecular targeting agents and considered as less likely to have direct effects on β cell function.

Currently major islet transplant centers are increasingly adopting stronger induction immunosuppression comprised of T cell depletion using anti-thymocyte globulin, alemtuzumab or OKT3γ1 (anti-CD3) plus anti-TNF-α treatment. This has resulted in significantly improved long-term maintenance of insulin independence [3, 5].

In maintenance immunosuppression, tacrolimus is still a key medication; although, there is controversy on the use of tacrolimus and its effect to islet graft function as described above (See § 2.5.1). Mycophenolate mofetil (MMF) is also used for maintenance immunosuppression, inhibiting proliferation of T and B cells and promoting apoptosis of activated T cells [98, 99]. Gallo et al recently showed that MMF was able to reduce survival of β cells, impair glucose-stimulated insulin secretion and β cell proliferation [100]. Posselt et al reported excellent islet transplant outcome using CNI-free immunosuppression that included belatacept [89], which is a fusion protein with Fc fragment of a human IgG linked to cytotoxic T lymphocyte-associated antigen 4 (CTLA-4) that allows costimulation blockade of CD80 and CD86 on antigen presenting cells [101]. Overall islet investigators have continued to make efforts to find effective immunosuppression with less effect on β cell function while enhancing β cell function such as exenatide which is a glucagon-like peptide-1 (GLP-1) analog [75].

2.4. Islet encapsulation

The islet encapsulation aims to eliminate or reduce the dose of immunosuppression, which is a major obstacle in current islet transplantation, by isolating islets from blood flow and avoiding direct interaction with antibodies and immune cells such as lymphocytes and macrophages. However, few clinical trials using encapsulation technique have been reported [91, 102]. The University of Peruga group demonstrated the efficacy of microencapsulated human islets with sodium alginate in 4 type 1 diabetic patients, who were able to reduce HbA1c level and the amounts of exogenous insulin injection [91]. Elliot RB et al. showed a case report on xenotransplantation using alginate-encapsulated porcine islets, also allowing reduction of insulin dose [102]. In both reports, islet recipients did not use any immunosuppressants although insulin independence was not achieved, suggesting the advantage and limitation of current encapsulation strategy (Figure 1).

There are several methods of islet encapsulation; macrocapsular devices, microencapsulation and surface modification. A macrocapsular device that is composed of polytetrafluoroethylene membrane enabled delayed onset of diabetes in mice model [103]. Microencapsulation of islets has been prepared using various materials such as alginate, agarose and collagen [104-106]. An issue of microencapsulation is the enlargement of the size of islet mass; microencapsulation of an islet can increase the size by as much as 3 to 5 folds of the original islet. Alternatively, surface modification of islets is a strategy to reduce the tissue volume. Polyethylene glycol (PEG) is a hydrogen polymer and can be used for conformal coating to encapsulate islets in the process of polymerization [107]. PEGylation, i.e. PEG conjugation at the islet surface, is the another way of islet encapsulation without significant increase in tissue size [108]. Recently, PEGylation attached with biologically active agents of heparin, activated protein C, urokinase or thrombomodulin has been developed to prevent the local coagulation immediately after islet infusion [109-112]. These techniques were recently developed and the sustainability of PEGylation needs to be proven.

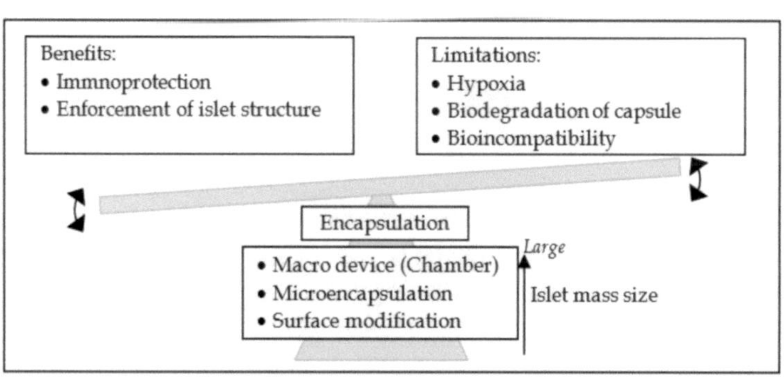

Figure 1. Benefits and current limitations of islet encapsulation.

3. Clinical assessment of beta cell function

Monitoring graft function is a major concern in clinical management of islet recipients since islet graft dysfunction in both acute phase after transplant and chronic phase is an obstacle to its widespread use as a standard care for type 1 diabetes. Furthermore, isolated islets are transplanted via the portal vein into the liver, making it difficult to employ biopsy examination of engrafted islets. Hence, several methodologies to predict islet graft function indirectly have been proposed. In this section, indices currently available for clinical assessment of islet graft function are discussed (Table 5).

3.1. Blood tests and clinical indices

3.1.1. Glucose tolerance/stimulation test

Glucose tolerance test (GTT) is a basic assessment method to diagnose diabetes although glucose stimulation; in itself has risk of artificial hyperglycemia for type 1 diabetic patients. Baidal et al reported that acute insulin/C-peptide release, mixed meal stimulation index, time-to-peak C-peptide, 90min glucose level and area under the curve of glucose values could predict islet dysfunction [113]. Arginine stimulation test is also useful for the evaluation of islet graft function. Glucose-potentiation slope and the maximal response in arginine stimulation test were significantly associated with β cell secretory capacity in a report from University of Pennsylvania group [114].

3.1.2. HYPO score and LI

Hypoglycemic (HYPO) score and lability index (LI) are calculated based on patients' journals of self-monitoring blood glucose (SMBG) for a month, providing a link to graft function through the quality of glycemic control [115]. These assessment tools are beneficial since a major endpoint of clinical allogeneic islet transplantation is to prevent hypoglycemic events; however, HYPO and LI calculations require a number of glucose measurements and hence are only calculated on a monthly or yearly basis using a complex scoring system.

3.1.3. SUITO index

A simple evaluation method using fasting blood glucose and C-peptide levels has been proposed, called secretory unit of islet transplant objects (SUITO) index [116]. The SUITO index was originally developed using the concept of the homeostasis model assessment for insulin secretion (HOMA-β) model, where healthy person has 100 of SUITO index. The calculation uses serum C-peptide levels instead of insulin levels, since islet recipient may be administering exogenous insulin during graft dysfunction and overlapped measurement of endogenous and exogenous insulin amounts are avoided [117]. SUITO index can provide reference value for insulin independence and elimination of hypoglycemia [118]. In addition, SUITO index allows extensive link to quality of life in islet recipients [119].

*3.1.4. C-peptide/glucose ratio and C-peptide/glucose*creatinine ratio*

C-peptide per glucose ratio (CP/G) is also a simple technique to predict islet graft function using blood glucose and C-peptide, similar to the SUITO index [120]. To correct islet graft function in patients with renal dysfunction, C-peptide/glucose*creatinine ratio has also been proposed. University of Miami group showed that CP/G correlated with 90min glucose level and β score [120].

3.1.5. β score

This scoring system uses data on fasting blood glucose, HbA1c, stimulated C-peptide, and absence of insulin or oral diabetic medication, that cover multiple aspect of glycemic control in islet recipients [121]. Correlation between β score and 90 min glucose level after mixed meal tolerance test has also been reported.

3.1.6. TEF

Transplant estimated function (TEF) is calculated by a formula using daily exogenous insulin requirements and HbA1c, that are routinely measured at clinic, eliminating glucose stimulation test when compared to β score [122]. TEF correlated well with β score and insulin response to arginine stimulation test.

3.1.7. TFIM model

Transplanted functional islet mass (TFIM) model is a recently proposed index that is aimed to guide the decision to use a specific islet preparation [123]. TFIM model is composed of transplanted islet volume, increment of insulin secretion, cold ischemia time and exocrine tissue volume transplanted, and can predict islet graft function.

3.2. Clinical image study

Functional mass of transplanted islets can be observed by the combination of the radioisotope-labeled grafts using 18F-fluorodeoxyglucose ([^{18}F]FDG) and positron emission tomography with computed tomography (PET/CT) [124, 125]. Although this technique is only applicable to capture early phase of transplantation up to 60 min after transplant, islet graft loss as well as transplanted islet distribution in the liver can be observed. Nano-iron particle also visualizes engrafted islet mass using magnetic resonance imaging (MRI) and allows longer follow-up when compared to PET/CT technique [126, 127].

Method	Variables required	Advantage	Disadvantage	Reference
GTT	A series of glucose or C-peptide values during glucose stimulation	Widely available method in clinic	The risk of hyperglycemia Repeated blood collection	[113, 114]
HYPO score and LI	Detailed self-recorded journal of glucose levels and hypoglycemic episodes	Direct evaluation of hypoglycemia that is a major outcome in islet transplantation	Number of records for monthly basis are required Complex calculation for LI	[115]
SUITO index	Fasting serum C-peptide and glucose level	Simple calculation Easy prediction of graft function corresponding to insulin independence.	Limited application to other species	[118, 119]
CP/G	Fasting serum C-peptide and glucose level	Simple calculation	Limited information on extended outcomes of hypoglycemia	[120]
β score	Fasting glucose, HbA1c, Daily insulin dose, Stimulated C-peptide	To capture multiple aspects of glycemic control	Composite scoring system requiring 4 variables including the results from glucose stimulation test	[121]
TEF	A series of records on HbA1c and daily insulin amounts	To eliminate glucose stimulation test compared to β score Calculation using variables that can be collected in standard diabetes care	Adjustment of coefficients by individual patient	[122, 128]
TFIM Model	Volume of transplanted islets, increment of insulin secretion, cold ischemia time and volume of transplanted exocrine tissue	To follow graft function using isolation results	Validated using data on islet after kidney transplantation	[123]
Radiologic imaging technique; PET/CT	Radioisotope-labeled islets PET/CT machine	To allow evaluation of islet graft mass and the distribution in the liver	The measurement only applicable for early phase of transplantation due to half-time of radioisotope Labeling procedure required	[124, 125]
Radiologic imaging technique; MRI	Iron-nanoparticle labeled islets MRI machine	To allow longitudinal follow up of islet mass	Labeling procedure required Iron overload	[126, 127]

Table 5. Clinical assessment of β cell function

3.3. Autologous Islet Transplantation

Patients with refractory chronic pancreatitis undergo total or partial pancreatectomy to alleviate pain and also autologous islet transplantation to retain pancreatic endocrine function after surgery. Islets isolated from pancreas are infused intraportally into the liver. Assessment of beta cell function in such autologous islet transplant patients typically follows the methods described for allogeneic islet transplantation. For example, the SUITO index can be applicable to autologous islet transplantation and was founded as an excellent predictor of insulin independence [129]. However, no immune response against infused islets is expected in these patients. Post-transplant function of autologous islets has been shown to be much better than in allogeneic combination; β cell mass more than 10,000 IEQ/kg of islet yield is considered for a factor of insulin independence in allogeneic transplants while islet yield over 5,000 IEQ/kg is the successful factor in autologous transplantation [130]. After achievement of insulin independent status, patients receiving autologous islets have better long term survival of graft. Most patients also achieve significant relief from pain and improve their quality of life.

4. Conclusion

Islet transplantation has been shown to be a very promising treatment that could result in freedom from requirement of exogenous insulin in type 1 diabetic patients. One of the major advantages of islet transplantation is the minimally invasive nature of the procedure when compared to whole organ pancreas transplantation. Despite its wide spread use at several major transplant centers, the volume of patients receiving islet transplants remain low when compared to the number of "brittle" type 1 diabetic patients eligible for this procedure. Recently impressive gains have been made in the improvement of post-transplant islet function. This is primarily due to the use of T-cell depleting immunosuppression during induction phase after transplant followed by use of tacrolimus, rapamycin and or mycophenolic mofetil during the maintenance phase. In addition several advances made in donor selection, pancreas procurement, enzymatic digestion, islet purification and islet culture seem to have contributed to this success. Recent completion of a large scale phase III clinical trial sponsored by the NIH has given hope that soon this procedure may be approved for clinical use. In light of these advances, there is optimism that the remaining hurdles could be overcome to improve the long term function of the transplanted islets.

Acknowledgements

This work was supported by grants from the National Institute of Diabetes and Digestive and Kidney Diseases (1R21DK090513-01 to M.F.L.), the Juvenile Diabetes Research Foundation (#5-2010-668 to B.N. and #3-2011-447 to M.T.) and by the Baylor Health Care System Foundation.

Author details

Morihito Takita[1], Nigar Seven[1], Marlon F. Levy[2] and Bashoo Naziruddin[2*]

*Address all correspondence to: BashooN@Baylorhealth.edu

1 Baylor Research Institute, Islet Cell Laboratory, Dallas, USA

2 Baylor Simmons Transplant Institute, Dallas, USA

References

[1] Shapiro, A. M., Lakey, J. R., Ryan, E. A., Korbutt, G. S., Toth, E., Warnock, G. L., et al. (2000). Islet transplantation in seven patients with type 1 diabetes mellitus using a glucocorticoid-free immunosuppressive regimen. *N Engl J Med*, 343(4), 230-8.

[2] Matsumoto, S. (2010). Islet cell transplantation for Type 1 diabetes. *J Diabetes*, 2(1), 16-22.

[3] Barton, F. B., Rickels, M. R., Alejandro, R., Hering, B. J., Wease, S., Naziruddin, B., et al. (2012). Improvement in outcomes of clinical islet transplantation: 1999-2010. *Diabetes Care*, 35(7), 1436-45.

[4] Ryan, E. A., Paty, B. W., Senior, P. A., Bigam, D., Alfadhli, E., Kneteman, N. M., et al. (2005). Five-year follow-up after clinical islet transplantation. *Diabetes*, 54(7), 2060-9.

[5] Bellin, MD, Barton, F. B., Heitman, A., Harmon, J. V., Kandaswamy, R., Balamurugan, A. N., et al. (2012). Potent induction immunotherapy promotes long-term insulin independence after islet transplantation in type 1 diabetes. *Am J Transplant*, 12(6), 1576-83.

[6] Carlsson, P. O. (2011). Influence of microenvironment on engraftment of transplanted β-cells. *Ups J Med Sci*, 116(1), 1-7.

[7] Terasaki, P. I., & Cai, J. (2005). Humoral theory of transplantation: further evidence. *Curr Opin Immunol*, 17(5), 541-5.

[8] Terasaki, P. I. (2003). Humoral theory of transplantation. *Am J Transplant*, 3(6), 665-73.

[9] Campbell, P. M., Senior, P. A., Salam, A., Labranche, K., Bigam, D. L., Kneteman, N. M., et al. (2007). High risk of sensitization after failed islet transplantation. *Am J Transplant*, 7(10), 2311-7.

[10] Rickels, M. R., Kamoun, M., Kearns, J., Markmann, J. F., & Naji, A. (2007). Evidence for allograft rejection in an islet transplant recipient and effect on beta-cell secretory capacity. *J Clin Endocrinol Metab*, 92(7), 2410-4.

[11] Campbell, P. M., Salam, A., Ryan, E. A., Senior, P., Paty, B. W., Bigam, D., et al. (2007). Pretransplant HLA antibodies are associated with reduced graft survival after clinical islet transplantation. *Am J Transplant*, 7(5), 1242-8.

[12] Mohanakumar, T., Narayanan, K., Desai, N., Ramachandran, S., Shenoy, S., Jendrisak, M., et al. (2006). A significant role for histocompatibility in human islet transplantation. *Transplantation*, 82(2), 180-7.

[13] Kessler, L., Parissiadis, A., Bayle, F., Moreau, F., Pinget, M., Froelich, N., et al. (2009). Evidence for humoral rejection of a pancreatic islet graft and rescue with rituximab and IV immunoglobulin therapy. *Am J Transplant*, 9(8), 1961-6.

[14] Ferrari-Lacraz, S., Berney, T., Morel, P., Marangon, N., Hadaya, K., Demuylder-Mischler, S., et al. (2008). Low risk of anti-human leukocyte antigen antibody sensitization after combined kidney and islet transplantation. *Transplantation*, 86(2), 357-9.

[15] Jackson, A. M., Connolly, J. E., Matsumoto, S., Noguchi, H., Onaca, N., Levy, M. F., et al. (2009). Evidence for Induced Expression of HLA Class II on Human Islets: Possible Mechanism for HLA Sensitization in Transplant Recipients. *Transplantation*, 87(4), 500-6.

[16] Naziruddin, B., Wease, S., Stablein, D., Barton, F. B., Berney, T., Rickels, M. R., et al. (2012). HLA Class I Sensitization in Islet Transplant Recipients- Report from the Collaborative Islet Transplant Registry. *Cell Transplant*, 21(5), 901-908.

[17] Cardani, R., Pileggi, A., Ricordi, C., Gomez, C., Baidal, D. A., Ponte, G. G., et al. (2007). Allosensitization of islet allograft recipients. *Transplantation*, 84(11), 1413-27.

[18] Hire, K., Hering, B., & Bansal-Pakala, P. (2010). Relative reductions in soluble CD30 levels post-transplant predict acute graft function in islet allograft recipients receiving three different immunosuppression protocols. *Transpl Immunol*, 23(4), 209-14.

[19] Han, D., Xu, X., Baidal, D., Leith, J., Ricordi, C., Alejandro, R., et al. (2004). Assessment of cytotoxic lymphocyte gene expression in the peripheral blood of human islet allograft recipients: elevation precedes clinical evidence of rejection. *Diabetes*, 53(9), 2281-90.

[20] Toti, F., Bayle, F., Berney, T., Egelhofer, H., Richard, MJ, Greget, M., et al. (2011). Studies of circulating microparticle release in peripheral blood after pancreatic islet transplantation. *Transplant Proc*, 43(9), 3241-5.

[21] Del Prete, G., De Carli, M., D'Elios, MM, Daniel, K. C., Almerigogna, F., Alderson, M., et al. (1995). CD30-mediated signaling promotes the development of human T helper type 2-like T cells. *J Exp Med*, 182(6), 1655-61.

[22] Platt, R. E., Wu, K. S., Poole, K., Newstead, C. G., & Clark, B. (2009). Soluble CD30 as a prognostic factor for outcome following renal transplantation. *J Clin Pathol*, 62(7), 662-3.

[23] Shah, A. S., Leffell, M. S., Lucas, D., & Zachary, A. A. (2009). Elevated pretransplantation soluble CD30 is associated with decreased early allograft function after human lung transplantation. *Hum Immunol*, 70(2), 101-3.

[24] Spiridon, C., Hunt, J., Mack, M., Rosenthal, J., Anderson, A., Eichhorn, E., et al. (2006). Evaluation of soluble CD30 as an immunologic marker in heart transplant recipients. *Transplant Proc*, 38(10), 3689-91.

[25] Kessler, L., Toti, F., Egelhofer, H., Richard, MJ, Greget, M. N. K., Moreau, F., et al. (2011). Acute cellular rejection of a pancreatic islet graft and rescue by steroid therapy: study of microparticles release in peripheral blood. In , 151.

[26] Kolb, H., Kolb-Bachofen, V., & Roep, B. O. (1995). Autoimmune versus inflammatory type I diabetes: a controversy? *Immunol Today*, 16(4), 170-2.

[27] Sutherland, D. E., Goetz, F. C., & Sibley, R. K. (1989). Recurrence of disease in pancreas transplants. *Diabetes*, 38, 1, 85-7.

[28] Roep, B. O. (2003). The role of T-cells in the pathogenesis of Type 1 diabetes: from cause to cure. *Diabetologia*, 46(3), 305-21.

[29] Roep, B. O., Stobbe, I., Duinkerken, G., van Rood, J. J., Lernmark, A., Keymeulen, B., et al. (1999). Auto- and alloimmune reactivity to human islet allografts transplanted into type 1 diabetic patients. *Diabetes*, 48(3), 484-90.

[30] Huurman, V. A., Hilbrands, R., Pinkse, G. G., Gillard, P., Duinkerken, G., van de Linde, P., et al. (2008). Cellular islet autoimmunity associates with clinical outcome of islet cell transplantation. *PLoS One*, 3(6), e2435.

[31] Matsumoto, S., Chujo, D., Shimoda, M., Takita, M., Sugimoto, K., Itoh, T., et al. (2011). Analysis of long-term insulin independence cases after allogeneic islet transplantation. *Am J Transplant*, 11(2), 175-176.

[32] Braghi, S., Bonifacio, E., Secchi, A., Di Carlo, V., Pozza, G., & Bosi, E. (2000). Modulation of humoral islet autoimmunity by pancreas allotransplantation influences allograft outcome in patients with type 1 diabetes. *Diabetes*, 49(2), 218-24.

[33] Ashwell, J. D., Lu, F. W., & Vacchio, M. S. (2000). Glucocorticoids in T cell development and function*. *Annu Rev Immunol*, 18, 309-45.

[34] Mc Ewen, B. S., Biron, C. A., Brunson, K. W., Bulloch, K., Chambers, W. H., Dhabhar, F. S., et al. (1997). The role of adrenocorticoids as modulators of immune function in health and disease: neural, endocrine and immune interactions. *Brain Res Brain Res Rev*, 23(1-2), 79-133.

[35] Daneman, D. (2006). Type 1 diabetes. *Lancet*, 367(9513), 847-58.

[36] Association, A. D. (2012). Diagnosis and classification of diabetes mellitus. *Diabetes Care*, 35(1), S64-71.

[37] Davani, B., Portwood, N., Bryzgalova, G., Reimer, M. K., Heiden, T., Ostenson, C. G., et al. (2004). Aged transgenic mice with increased glucocorticoid sensitivity in pancreatic beta-cells develop diabetes. *Diabetes*, 53(1), S51-9.

[38] Ranta, F., Avram, D., Berchtold, S., Düfer, M., Drews, G., Lang, F., et al. (2006). Dexamethasone induces cell death in insulin-secreting cells, an effect reversed by exendin-4. *Diabetes*, 55(5), 1380-90.

[39] Ullrich, S., Berchtold, S., Ranta, F., Seebohm, G., Henke, G., Lupescu, A., et al. (2005). Serum- and glucocorticoid-inducible kinase 1 (SGK1) mediates glucocorticoid-induced inhibition of insulin secretion. *Diabetes*, 54(4), 1090-9.

[40] Vegiopoulos, A., & Herzig, S. (2007). Glucocorticoids, metabolism and metabolic diseases. Mol Cell Endocrinol; , 275(1-2), 43-61.

[41] Walker, B. R. (2007). Glucocorticoids and cardiovascular disease. *Eur J Endocrinol*, 157(5), 545-59.

[42] Schäcke, H., Döcke, W. D., & Asadullah, K. (2002). Mechanisms involved in the side effects of glucocorticoids. *Pharmacol Ther*, 96(1), 23-43.

[43] Heit, J. J., Apelqvist, A. A., Gu, X., Winslow, M. M., Neilson, J. R., Crabtree, G. R., et al. (2006). Calcineurin/NFAT signalling regulates pancreatic beta-cell growth and function. *Nature*, 443(7109), 345-9.

[44] Soleimanpour, S. A., Crutchlow, M. F., Ferrari, A. M., Raum, J. C., Groff, D. N., Rankin, M. M., et al. (2010). Calcineurin signaling regulates human islet {beta}-cell survival. *J Biol Chem*, 285(51), 40050-9.

[45] Elion, G. B. (1993). The George Hitchings and Gertrude Elion Lecture. *The pharmacology of azathioprine. Ann N Y Acad Sci*, 685, 400-7.

[46] Maltzman, J. S., & Koretzky, G. A. (2003). Azathioprine: old drug, new actions. *J Clin Invest*, 111(8), 1122-4.

[47] Calafiore, R., Basta, G., Falorni, A., Pietropaolo, M., Picchio, M. L., Calcinaro, F., et al. (1993). Preventive effects of azathioprine (AZA) on the onset of diabetes mellitus in NOD mice. *J Endocrinol Invest*, 16(11), 869-73.

[48] Harrison, L. C., Colman, P. G., Dean, B., Baxter, R., & Martin, F. I. (1985). Increase in remission rate in newly diagnosed type I diabetic subjects treated with azathioprine. *Diabetes*, 34(12), 1306-8.

[49] Tzakis, A. G., Ricordi, C., Alejandro, R., Zeng, Y., Fung, J. J., Todo, S., et al. (1990). Pancreatic islet transplantation after upper abdominal exenteration and liver replacement. *Lancet*, 336(8712), 402-5.

[50] Scharp, D. W., Lacy, P. E., Santiago, J. V., Mc Cullough, C. S., Weide, L. G., Boyle, P. J., et al. (1991). Results of our first nine intraportal islet allografts in type 1, insulin-dependent diabetic patients. *Transplantation*, 51(1), 76-85.

[51] Socci, C., Falqui, L., Davalli, A. M., Ricordi, C., Braghi, S., Bertuzzi, F., et al. (1991). Fresh human islet transplantation to replace pancreatic endocrine function in type 1 diabetic patients. *Report of six cases. Acta Diabetol*, 28(2), 151-7.

[52] Ricordi, C., Tzakis, A. G., Carroll, P. B., Zeng, Y. J., Rilo, H. L., Alejandro, R., et al. (1992). Human islet isolation and allotransplantation in 22 consecutive cases. *Transplantation*, 53(2), 407-14.

[53] Gores, P. F., Najarian, J. S., Stephanian, E., Lloveras, J. J., Kelley, S. L., & Sutherland, D. E. (1993). Insulin independence in type I diabetes after transplantation of unpurified islets from single donor with 15-deoxyspergualin. *Lancet*, 341(8836), 19-21.

[54] Ricordi, C., Alejandro, R., Angelico, M. C., Fernandez, L. A., Nery, J., Webb, M., et al. (1997). Human islet allografts in patients with type 2 diabetes undergoing liver transplantation. *Transplantation*, 63(3), 473-5.

[55] Alejandro, R., Lehmann, R., Ricordi, C., Kenyon, N. S., Angelico, M. C., Burke, G., et al. (1997). Long-term function (6 years) of islet allografts in type 1 diabetes. *Diabetes*, 46(12), 1983-9.

[56] Secchi, A., Socci, C., Maffi, P., Taglietti, M. V., Falqui, L., Bertuzzi, F., et al. (1997). Islet transplantation in IDDM patients. *Diabetologia*, 40(2), 225-31.

[57] Tibell, A., Brendel, M., Wadström, J., Brandhorst, D., Brandhorst, H., Eckhard, M., et al. (1997). Early experience with a long-distance collaborative human islet transplant programme. *Transplant Proc*, 29(7), 3124-5.

[58] Keymeulen, B., Ling, Z., Gorus, F. K., Delvaux, G., Bouwens, L., Grupping, A., et al. (1998). Implantation of standardized beta-cell grafts in a liver segment of IDDM patients: graft and recipients characteristics in two cases of insulin-independence under maintenance immunosuppression for prior kidney graft. *Diabetologia*, 41(4), 452-9.

[59] Bretzel, R. G., Brandhorst, D., Brandhorst, H., Eckhard, M., Ernst, W., Friemann, S., et al. (1999). Improved survival of intraportal pancreatic islet cell allografts in patients with type-1 diabetes mellitus by refined peritransplant management. *J Mol Med (Berl)*, 77(1), 140-3.

[60] Oberholzer, J., Triponez, F., Mage, R., Andereggen, E., Bühler, L., Crétin, N., et al. (2000). Human islet transplantation: lessons from 13 autologous and 13 allogeneic transplantations. *Transplantation*, 69(6), 1115-23.

[61] Tibell, A., Bolinder, J., Hagström-Toft, E., Tollemar, J., Brendel, M., Eckhard, M., et al. (2001). Experience with human islet transplantation in Sweden. *Transplant Proc*, 33(4), 2535-6.

[62] Benhamou, P. Y., Oberholzer, J., Toso, C., Kessler, L., Penfornis, A., Bayle, F., et al. (2001). Human islet transplantation network for the treatment of Type I diabetes: first data from the Swiss-French GRAGIL consortium (1999-2000). Groupe de Recherche Rhin Rhĵne Alpes Genève pour la transplantation d'Ilots de Langerhans. *Diabetologia*, 44(7), 859-64.

[63] Hirshberg, B., Rother, K. I., Digon, B. J., Lee, J., Gaglia, J. L., Hines, K., et al. (2003). Benefits and risks of solitary islet transplantation for type 1 diabetes using steroid-sparing immunosuppression: the National Institutes of Health experience. *Diabetes Care*, 26(12), 3288-95.

[64] Hering, B. J., Kandaswamy, R., Harmon, J. V., Ansite, JD, Clemmings, S. M., Sakai, T., et al. (2004). Transplantation of cultured islets from two-layer preserved pancreases in type 1 diabetes with anti-CD3 antibody. *Am J Transplant*, 4(3), 390-401.

[65] Frank, A., Deng, S., Huang, X., Velidedeoglu, E., Bae, Y. S., Liu, C., et al. (2004). Transplantation for type I diabetes: comparison of vascularized whole-organ pancreas with isolated pancreatic islets. Ann Surg discussion 640-3., 240(4), 631-40.

[66] Goss, J. A., Goodpastor, S. E., Brunicardi, F. C., Barth, M. H., Soltes, G. D., Garber, A. J., et al. (2004). Development of a human pancreatic islet-transplant program through a collaborative relationship with a remote islet-isolation center. *Transplantation*, 77(3), 462-6.

[67] Lehmann, R., Weber, M., Berthold, P., Züllig, R., Pfammatter, T., Moritz, W., et al. (2004). Successful simultaneous islet-kidney transplantation using a steroid-free immunosuppression: two-year follow-up. *Am J Transplant*, 4(7), 1117-23.

[68] Hering, B. J., Kandaswamy, R., Ansite, Eckman. P. M., Nakano, M., Sawada, T., et al. (2005). Single-donor, marginal-dose islet transplantation in patients with type 1 diabetes. *JAMA*, 293(7), 830-5.

[69] Froud, T., Ricordi, C., Baidal, D. A., Hafiz, M. M., Ponte, G., Cure, P., et al. (2005). Islet transplantation in type 1 diabetes mellitus using cultured islets and steroid-free immunosuppression: Miami experience. *Am J Transplant*, 5(8), 2037-46.

[70] Kempf, M. C., Andres, A., Morel, P., Benhamou, P. Y., Bayle, F., Kessler, L., et al. (2005). Logistics and transplant coordination activity in the GRAGIL Swiss-French multicenter network of islet transplantation. *Transplantation*, 79(9), 1200-5.

[71] Warnock, G. L., Meloche, R. M., Thompson, D., Shapiro, R. J., Fung, M., Ao, Z., et al. (2005). Improved human pancreatic islet isolation for a prospective cohort study of islet transplantation vs best medical therapy in type 1 diabetes mellitus. *Arch Surg*, 140(8), 735-44.

[72] Toso, C., Baertschiger, R., Morel, P., Bosco, D., Armanet, M., Wojtusciszyn, A., et al. (2006). Sequential kidney/islet transplantation: efficacy and safety assessment of a steroid-free immunosuppression protocol. *Am J Transplant*, 6(5 Pt 1), 1049-1058.

[73] O'Connell, P. J., Hawthorne, W. J., Holmes-Walker, D. J., Nankivell, B. J., Gunton, J. E., Patel, A. T., et al. (2006). Clinical islet transplantation in type 1 diabetes mellitus: results of Australia's first trial. *Med J Aust*, 184(5), 221-5.

[74] Shapiro, A. M., Ricordi, C., Hering, B. J., Auchincloss, H., Lindblad, R., Robertson, R. P., et al. (2006). International trial of the Edmonton protocol for islet transplantation. *N Engl J Med*, 355(13), 1318-30.

[75] Ghofaili, K. A., Fung, M., Ao, Z., Meloche, M., Shapiro, R. J., Warnock, G. L., et al. (2007). Effect of exenatide on beta cell function after islet transplantation in type 1 diabetes. *Transplantation*, 83(1), 24-8.

[76] Badet, L., Benhamou, P. Y., Wojtusciszyn, A., Baertschiger, R., Milliat-Guittard, L., Kessler, L., et al. (2007). Expectations and strategies regarding islet transplantation: metabolic data from the GRAGIL 2 trial. *Transplantation*, 84(1), 89-96.

[77] Maffi, P., Bertuzzi, F., De Taddeo, F., Magistretti, P., Nano, R., Fiorina, P., et al. (2007). Kidney function after islet transplant alone in type 1 diabetes: impact of immunosuppressive therapy on progression of diabetic nephropathy. *Diabetes Care*, 30(5), 1150-5.

[78] Gillard, P., Ling, Z., Mathieu, C., Crenier, L., Lannoo, M., Maes, B., et al. (2008). Comparison of sirolimus alone with sirolimus plus tacrolimus in type 1 diabetic recipients of cultured islet cell grafts. *Transplantation*, 85(2), 256-63.

[79] Gerber, P. A., Pavlicek, V., Demartines, N., Zuellig, R., Pfammatter, T., Wüthrich, R., et al. (2008). Simultaneous islet-kidney vs pancreas-kidney transplantation in type 1 diabetes mellitus: a 5 year single centre follow-up. *Diabetologia*, 51(1), 110-9.

[80] Cure, P., Pileggi, A., Froud, T., Messinger, S., Faradji, RN, Baidal, D. A., et al. (2008). Improved metabolic control and quality of life in seven patients with type 1 diabetes following islet after kidney transplantation. *Transplantation*, 85(6), 801-12.

[81] Bellin, M. D., Kandaswamy, R., Parkey, J., Zhang, H. J., Liu, B., Ihm, S. H., et al. (2008). Prolonged insulin independence after islet allotransplants in recipients with type 1 diabetes. *Am J Transplant*, 8(11), 2463-70.

[82] Gangemi, A., Salehi, P., Hatipoglu, B., Martellotto, J., Barbaro, B., Kuechle, J. B., et al. (2008). Islet transplantation for brittle type 1 diabetes: the UIC protocol. *Am J Transplant*, 8(6), 1250-61.

[83] Froud, T., Baidal, D. A., Faradji, R., Cure, P., Mineo, D., Selvaggi, G., et al. (2008). Islet transplantation with alemtuzumab induction and calcineurin-free maintenance immunosuppression results in improved short- and long-term outcomes. *Transplantation*, 86(12), 1695-701.

[84] Mineo, D., Ricordi, C., Xu, X., Pileggi, A., Garcia-Morales, R., Khan, A., et al. (2008). Combined islet and hematopoietic stem cell allotransplantation: a clinical pilot trial to induce chimerism and graft tolerance. *Am J Transplant*, 8(6), 1262-74.

[85] Vantyghem, M. C., Kerr-Conte, J., Arnalsteen, L., Sergent, G., Defrance, F., Gmyr, V., et al. (2009). Primary graft function, metabolic control, and graft survival after islet transplantation. *Diabetes Care*, 32(8), 1473-8.

[86] Borot, S., Niclauss, N., Wojtusciszyn, A., Brault, C., Demuylder-Mischler, S., Müller, Y., et al. (2011). Impact of the number of infusions on 2-year results of islet-after-kidney transplantation in the GRAGIL network. *Transplantation*, 92(9), 1031-8.

[87] Posselt, A. M., Bellin, M. D., Tavakol, M., Szot, G. L., Frassetto, L. A., Masharani, U., et al. (2010). Islet transplantation in type 1 diabetics using an immunosuppressive protocol based on the anti-LFA-1 antibody efalizumab. *Am J Transplant*, 10(8), 1870-80.

[88] Turgeon, N. A., Avila, J. G., Cano, J. A., Hutchinson, J. J., Badell, I. R., Page, A. J., et al. (2010). Experience with a novel efalizumab-based immunosuppressive regimen to facilitate single donor islet cell transplantation. *Am J Transplant*, 10(9), 2082-91.

[89] Posselt, A. M., Szot, G. L., Frassetto, L. A., Masharani, U., Tavakol, M., Amin, R., et al. (2010). Islet transplantation in type 1 diabetic patients using calcineurin inhibitor-free immunosuppressive protocols based on T-cell adhesion or costimulation blockade. *Transplantation*, 90(12), 1595-601.

[90] Matsumoto, S., Takita, M., Chaussabel, D., Noguchi, H., Shimoda, M., Sugimoto, K., et al. (2011). Improving Efficacy of Clinical Islet Transplantation with Iodixanol Based Islet Purification, Thymoglobulin Induction and Blockage of IL-1-beta and TNF-alpha. Cell. *Transplant*, 20(10), 1641-1647.

[91] Basta, G., Montanucci, P., Luca, G., Boselli, C., Noya, G., Barbaro, B., et al. (2011). Long-term metabolic and immunological follow-up of nonimmunosuppressed patients with type 1 diabetes treated with microencapsulated islet allografts: four cases. *Diabetes Care*, 34(11), 2406-9.

[92] Raught, B., Gingras, A. C., & Sonenberg, N. (2001). The target of rapamycin (TOR) proteins. *Proc Natl Acad Sci U S A*, 98(13), 7037-44.

[93] Niclauss, N., Bosco, D., Morel, P., Giovannoni, L., Berney, T., & Parnaud, G. (2011). Rapamycin impairs proliferation of transplanted islet β cells. *Transplantation*, 91(7), 714-22.

[94] Zhang, N., Su, D., Qu, S., Tse, T., Bottino, R., Balamurugan, A. N., et al. (2006). Sirolimus is associated with reduced islet engraftment and impaired beta-cell function. *Diabetes*, 55(9), 2429-36.

[95] Tanemura, M., Ohmura, Y., Deguchi, T., Machida, T., Tsukamoto, R., Wada, H., et al. (2012). Rapamycin causes upregulation of autophagy and impairs islets function both in vitro and in vivo. *Am J Transplant*, 12(1), 102-14.

[96] Melzi, R., Maffi, P., Nano, R., Sordi, V., Mercalli, A., Scavini, M., et al. (2009). Rapamycin does not adversely affect intrahepatic islet engraftment in mice and improves early islet engraftment in humans. *Islets*, 1(1), 42-9.

[97] Gao, R., Ustinov, J., Korsgren, O., & Otonkoski, T. (2007). Effects of immunosuppressive drugs on in vitro neogenesis of human islets: mycophenolate mofetil inhibits the proliferation of ductal cells. *Am J Transplant*, 7(4), 1021-6.

[98] Allison, A. C., & Eugui, E. M. (2005). Mechanisms of action of mycophenolate mofetil in preventing acute and chronic allograft rejection. *Transplantation*, 80(2), S181-90.

[99] Cohn, R. G., Mirkovich, A., Dunlap, B., Burton, P., Chiu, S. H., Eugui, E., et al. (1999). Mycophenolic acid increases apoptosis, lysosomes and lipid droplets in human lymphoid and monocytic cell lines. *Transplantation*, 68(3), 411-8.

[100] Gallo, R., Natale, M., Vendrame, F., Boggi, U., Filipponi, F., Marchetti, P., et al. (2012). In vitro effects of mycophenolic acid on survival, function, and gene expression of pancreatic beta-cells. *Acta Diabetol.*

[101] Vincenti, F., Dritselis, A., & Kirkpatrick, P. (2011). Belatacept. *Nat Rev Drug Discov*, 10(9), 655-6.

[102] Elliott, R. B., Escobar, L., Tan, P. L., Muzina, M., Zwain, S., & Buchanan, C. (2007). Live encapsulated porcine islets from a type 1 diabetic patient 9.5 yr after xenotransplantation. *Xenotransplantation*, 14(2), 157-61.

[103] Lee, S. H., Hao, E., Savinov, A. Y., Geron, I., Strongin, A. Y., & Itkin-Ansari, P. (2009). Human beta-cell precursors mature into functional insulin-producing cells in an immunoisolation device: implications for diabetes cell therapies. *Transplantation*, 87(7), 983-91.

[104] Siebers, U., Horcher, A., Bretzel, R. G., Federlin, K., & Zekorn, T. (1997). Alginate-based microcapsules for immunoprotected islet transplantation. *Ann N Y Acad Sci*, 831, 304-12.

[105] Kobayashi, T., Aomatsu, Y., Iwata, H., Kin, T., Kanehiro, H., Hisanaga, M., et al. (2003). Indefinite islet protection from autoimmune destruction in nonobese diabetic mice by agarose microencapsulation without immunosuppression. *Transplantation*, 75(5), 619-25.

[106] Lee, B. R., Hwang, J. W., Choi, Y. Y., Wong, S. F., Hwang, Y. H., Lee, D. Y., et al. (2012). In situ formation and collagen-alginate composite encapsulation of pancreatic islet spheroids. *Biomaterials*, 33(3), 837-45.

[107] Cruise, G. M., Scharp, D. S., & Hubbell, J. A. (1998). Characterization of permeability and network structure of interfacially photopolymerized poly(ethylene glycol) diacrylate hydrogels. *Biomaterials*, 19(14), 1287-94.

[108] Lee, D. Y., Lee, S., Nam, J. H., & Byun, Y. (2006). Minimization of immunosuppressive therapy after islet transplantation: combined action of heme oxygenase-1 and PEGylation to islet. *Am J Transplant*, 6(8), 1820-8.

[109] Cabric, S., Sanchez, J., Lundgren, T., Foss, A., Felldin, M., Källen, R., et al. (2007). Islet surface heparinization prevents the instant blood-mediated inflammatory reaction in islet transplantation. *Diabetes*, 56(8), 2008-15.

[110] Contreras, J. L., Eckstein, C., Smyth, C. A., Bilbao, G., Vilatoba, M., Ringland, S. E., et al. (2004). Activated protein C preserves functional islet mass after intraportal transplantation: a novel link between endothelial cell activation, thrombosis, inflammation, and islet cell death. *Diabetes*, 53(11), 2804-14.

[111] Stabler, C. L., Sun, X. L., Cui, W., Wilson, J. T., Haller, CA, & Chaikof, E. L. (2007). Surface re-engineering of pancreatic islets with recombinant azido-thrombomodulin. *Bioconjug Chem*, 18(6), 1713-5.

[112] Totani, T., Teramura, Y., & Iwata, H. (2008). Immobilization of urokinase on the islet surface by amphiphilic poly(vinyl alcohol) that carries alkyl side chains. *Biomaterials*, 29(19), 2878-83.

[113] Baidal, D. A., Faradji, R. N., Messinger, S., Froud, T., Monroy, K., Ricordi, C., et al. (2009). Early metabolic markers of islet allograft dysfunction. *Transplantation*, 87(5), 689-97.

[114] Rickels, M. R., Schutta, M. H., Markmann, J. F., Barker, C. F., Naji, A., & Teff, K. L. (2005). {beta}-Cell function following human islet transplantation for type 1 diabetes. *Diabetes*, 54(1), 100-6.

[115] Ryan, E. A., Shandro, T., Green, K., Paty, B. W., Senior, P. A., Bigam, D., et al. (2004). Assessment of the severity of hypoglycemia and glycemic lability in type 1 diabetic subjects undergoing islet transplantation. *Diabetes*, 53(4), 955-62.

[116] Matsumoto, S., Noguchi, H., Hatanaka, N., Shimoda, M., Kobayashi, N., Jackson, A., et al. (2009). SUITO index for evaluation of efficacy of single donor islet transplantation. *Cell Transplant*, 18(5), 557-62.

[117] Yamada, Y., Fukuda, K., Fujimoto, S., Hosokawa, M., Tsukiyama, K., Nagashima, K., et al. (2006). SUIT, secretory units of islets in transplantation: An index for therapeutic management of islet transplanted patients and its application to type 2 diabetes. *Diabetes Res Clin Pract*, 74(3), 222-6.

[118] Takita, M., Matsumoto, S., Qin, H., Noguchi, H., Shimoda, M., Chujo, D., et al. (2011). Secretory Unit of Islet Transplant Objects (SUITO) Index can predict severity of hypoglycemic episodes in clinical islet cell transplantation. *Cell Transplant.*

[119] Takita, M., & Matsumoto, S. (2012). SUITO Index for Evaluation of Clinical Islet Transplantation. *Cell Transplant.*

[120] Faradji, R. N., Monroy, K., Messinger, S., Pileggi, A., Froud, T., Baidal, D. A., et al. (2007). Simple measures to monitor beta-cell mass and assess islet graft dysfunction. Am J Transplant ., 7(2), 303-8.

[121] Ryan, E. A., Paty, B. W., Senior, P. A., Lakey, J. R., Bigam, D., & Shapiro, A. M. (2005). Beta-score: an assessment of beta-cell function after islet transplantation. *Diabetes Care*, 28(2), 343-7.

[122] Caumo, A., Maffi, P., Nano, R., Bertuzzi, F., Luzi, L., Secchi, A., et al. (2008). Transplant estimated function: a simple index to evaluate beta-cell secretion after islet transplantation. *Diabetes Care*, 31(2), 301-5.

[123] Friberg, A. S., Lundgren, T., Malm, H., Felldin, M., Nilsson, B., Jenssen, T., et al. (2012). Transplanted functional islet mass: donor, islet preparation, and recipient fac-

tors influence early graft function in islet-after-kidney patients. *Transplantation*, 93(6), 632-8.

[124] Eriksson, O., Eich, T., Sundin, A., Tibell, A., Tufveson, G., Andersson, H., et al. (2009). Positron emission tomography in clinical islet transplantation. *Am J Transplant*, 9(12), 2816-24.

[125] Eich, T., Eriksson, O., & Lundgren, T. (2007). Transplantation NNfCI. Visualization of early engraftment in clinical islet transplantation by positron-emission tomography. *N Engl J Med*, 356(26), 2754-5.

[126] Saudek, F., Jirák, D., Girman, P., Herynek, V., Dezortová, M., Kríz, J., et al. (2010). Magnetic resonance imaging of pancreatic islets transplanted into the liver in humans. *Transplantation*, 90(12), 1602-6.

[127] Medarova, Z., & Moore, A. (2009). MRI as a tool to monitor islet transplantation. *Nat Rev Endocrinol*, 5(8), 444-52.

[128] Caumo, A., Maffi, P., Nano, R., Luzi, L., Hilbrands, R., Gillard, P., et al. (2011). Comparative evaluation of simple indices of graft function after islet transplantation. *Transplantation*, 92(7), 815-21.

[129] Matsumoto, S., Takita, M., Shimoda, M., Itoh, T., Iwahashi, S., Chujo, D., et al. (2011). Usefulness of the Secretory Unit of Islet Transplant Objects (SUITO) Index for Evaluation of Clinical Autologous Islet Transplantation. *Transplant Proc*, 43(9), 3246-9.

[130] Sutherland, D. E., Gruessner, A. C., Carlson, A. M., Blondet, J. J., Balamurugan, A. N., Reigstad, K. F., et al. (2008). Islet autotransplant outcomes after total pancreatectomy: a contrast to islet allograft outcomes. *Transplantation*, 86(12), 1799-802.

Chapter 8

Endoplasmic Reticulum (ER) Stress in the Pathogenesis of Type 1 Diabetes

Jixin Zhong

Additional information is available at the end of the chapter

http://dx.doi.org/10.5772/52644

1. Introduction

As one of the major health problems in the world, diabetes affects over 346 million people worldwide. In United States alone, according to the statistical fact sheet released 2011 by American Diabetes Association, 25.8 million children and adults accounting for 8.3% of the population are affected by diabetes. Unfortunately, the therapy of diabetes remains unsatisfied despite of extensive studies in the last decades. Diabetes can be categorized into two main types: type 1 and type 2. Type 1 diabetes mellitus, used to known as juvenile diabetes, is typically developed in children and juveniles. Despite the increasing rate of Type 2 diabetes in the United States, type 1 diabetes accounts for over 2/3 of new adolescent diabetes diagnoses. Although most commonly presented in childhood, type 1 diabetes also accounts for 5-10% cases of adult diabetes (1). Recent epidemiologic studies revealed that the incidence for type 1 diabetes in most regions of the world has increased by 2-5% (2).

Unlike type 2 diabetes, which is caused by the loss of insulin sensitivity, type 1 diabetes is caused by insulin deficiency following destruction of insulin-producing pancreatic β cells. Autoimmune-mediated β cell death has been considered as the major cause of β-cell loss in type 1 diabetes. However, the underlying mechanisms are not fully understood. Accumulating evidence suggests an involvement of endoplasmic reticulum (ER) stress in multiple biological processes during the development of type 1 diabetes. Pancreatic β cells exhibit exquisite sensitivity to ER stress due to their high development in order to secrete large amounts of insulin. There is also evidence supporting that ER stress regulates the immune cell functionality and cytokine production that is relevant to autoimmune processes in type 1 diabetes. Furthermore, β cell loss caused by autoimmune attack results in an increased ER burden on the rest pancreatic β cells and induces unfolded protein response (UPR) and ER stress, which further exacerbates β cell death. Here I will summarize the functional involvement of ER stress in the pathogenesis of type 1 diabetes and the potential underlying mechanisms.

2. Pancreatic β cell and blood glucose regulation

2.1. Blood glucose regulation by pancreas

The major cause of type 1 diabetes is loss of insulin-secreting pancreatic β cell and insulin inadequacy (3;4). For a better understanding of the pathogenesis of type 1 diabetes, the regulatory mechanisms of blood glucose by pancreaswill briefly introduced. Blood glucose level is closely regulated in order to provide a homeostatic microenvironment for tissues and organs. According to the American Diabetes Association, a normal fasting blood glucose level is between 70 to 100 mg/dL, and the recommended fasting level is to aim for 70 to 130 mg/dL and less than 180 mg/dL after meals (5). Blood glucose is monitored by the cells in the islets of Langerhans (6). Islets of Langerhans are clusters of pancreatic cells that execute the endocrine function of pancreas. They contain the following 4 types of cells, in order of abundance: β cells, α cells, δ cells, and γ cells. Pancreatic β cells and α cells make up about 70% and 17% of islet cells respectively, and both of them are responsible for the blood glucose regulation by producing insulin (β cells) and glucagon (α cells) (6). Pancreatic δ cells produce somatostatin which has a major inhibitory effect, including on pancreatic juice production. Pancreatic γ cells secrete pancreatic polypeptide that is responsible for reducing appetite.

Insulin and glucagon have opposite functions on glucose regulation. They keep blood glucose level in a normal range by coordinating with each other (Figure 1). After a meal, the digestive system breaks down the carbohydrates to small sugar molecules, mainly glucose. The glucose is then absorbed across the intestinal wall and travel to the circulating bloodstream. Pancreatic β cells sense increased blood glucose level by taking up glucose through GLUT2, a glucose transporter. The metabolism of glucose in β cells leads to the increase of ATP/ADP ratio, which causes the closing of ATP-sensitive potassium channels and further leads to the open of calcium channels on membrane. The resulting increase of intracellular calcium concentration promotes the secretion of insulin into circulation of blood. Circulating insulin then acts on cells in a variety of tissues including liver, muscle, and fat through interacting with insulin receptor on the cell membrane. Insulin signaling induces the translocation of glucose transporter GLUT4 to cell membrane of muscle cells and adipocytes, leading to the uptake of glucose into cells as an energy source. In addition, insulin signaling also stimulates the conversion of glucose into glycogen, a process called glycogenesis, in liver. Therefore, insulin lowers blood glucose level by promoting glycogenesis and glucose uptake by peripheral tissues (7). In contrast, a drop in blood glucose caused by starving or other situations like extreme exercise suppresses the secretion of insulin by β cells and stimulates α cells of pancreas to release glucagon. Glucagon acts on liver and promotes glucose production by the breakdown of glycogen to glucose (called glycogenolysis), resulting in the increase of blood glucose.

http://dx.doi.org/10.5772/52644

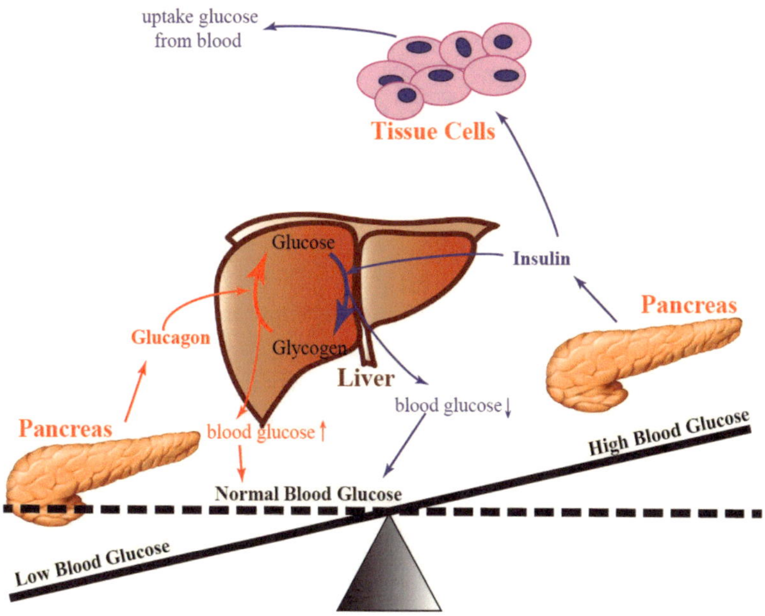

Figure 1. Homeostatic regulation of blood glucose by pancreas. Pancreas is the major organ responsible for maintaining the blood glucose homeostasis. Increase of blood glucose level can be sensed by GLUT2 on β cells, a glucose transporter. The metabolism of glucose in β cells promotes the secretion of insulin into circulation of blood. Circulating insulin then increases the glucose uptake by a variety of tissues including liver, muscle, and fat. In liver, insulin signaling also stimulates the conversion of glucose into glycogen, a process called glycogenesis. Both glycogenesis and glucose uptake by peripheral tissues can lead to a decrease of glucose level in blood stream. In contrast, a drop of blood glucose level suppresses the secretion of insulin by β cells and stimulates α cells to release glucagon. Glucagon acts on liver and promotes glucose production by the breakdown of glycogen to glucose, a process called glycogenolysis, and results in the increase of blood glucose.

2.2. Pancreatic β cells and insulin biosynthesis

Either insulin deficiency or insulin inefficiency can cause diabetes. As the only cell type producing insulin, β cell plays a critical role in the development of diabetes. In type 1 diabetes, autoimmune-mediated destruction of β cell leads to insufficient insulin production and inability of cells to take up glucose. In contrast, type 2 diabetes is caused by loss of insulin sensitivity. In response to insulin resistance, the body secretes more insulin to overcome the impaired insulin action. However, pancreatic β cells fail to secrete sufficient insulin to overcome insulin resistance in some individuals, resulting in type 2 diabetes (8;9). Therefore, dysfunction of β cell exists in both types of diabetes.

Pancreatic β cell is specialized for production of insulin to control blood glucose level. In response to hyperglycemia, insulin is secreted from a readily available pool in β cells. In the meantime, the secretion of insulin activates the biosynthesis of insulin (10). Insulin is first synthesized as preproinsulin with a signal peptide in the ribosomes of the rough endoplasmic reticulum. Preproinsulin is translocated into ER lumen by interaction of signal peptide with signal recognition particle on the ER membrane. Preproinsulin is converted to proinsulin by removing the signal peptide forming three disulfide bonds in the ER. Proinsulin is then translocated into Golgi apparatus and packaged into secretory granules that are close to the cell membrane. In the secretory granules, proinsulin is cleaved into equal amounts of insulin and C-peptide (Figure 2). Insulin is accumulated and stored in the secretory granules. When the β cell is appropriately stimulated, insulin is secreted from the cell by exocytosis (11). As the major site for protein synthesis, ER plays an important role in insulin biosynthesis. To fulfill the requirement for secreting large amount of insulin, the pancreatic β cells are equipped with highly developed ER, leading to the vulnerability of β cell to ER stress (12). In type 1 diabetes, the loss of β cell increases the burden of insulin secretion on the residual β cells. On the on hand, this compensated action is beneficial for the control of blood glucose. On the other hand, it also increases the ER burden of residual β cells, which further exacerbates β cell death.

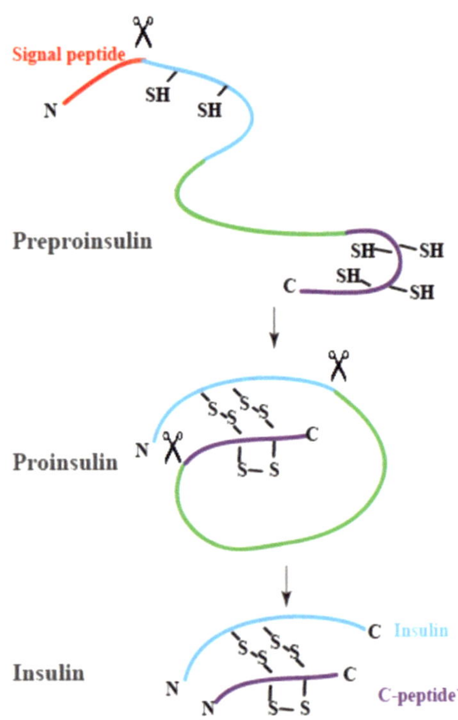

Figure 2. Biosynthesis of insulin in β cell. In the ribosomes of rough endoplasmic reticulum, insulin is first synthesized as a precursor, preproinsulin. Preproinsulin has a signal peptide that directs it to translocate into ER lumen by interacting with signal recognition particle on the ER membrane. In ER lumen, preproinsulin is converted to proinsulin by removing the signal peptide and forming three disulfide bonds. Proinsulin is then translocated into Golgi apparatus and packaged into secretory granules where it is cleaved into equal amounts of insulin and C-peptide. After synthesis, insulin is stored in the secretory granules and secreted from the cell until the β cell is appropriately stimulated.

http://dx.doi.org/10.5772/52644

3. Biological characterization of endoplasmic reticulum (ER) and ER stress

3.1. Endoplasmic reticulum

Endoplasmic Reticulum (ER) is an organelle of eukaryotic cells that is responsible for the facilitation of protein folding and assembly (13-15), manufacture of the membranes(16), biosynthesis of lipid and sterol, storage of intracellular Ca^{2+}, and transport of synthesized proteins in cisternae.It is a membranous network of tubules, vesicles, and cisternae that are interconnected by the cytoskeleton.The ER is well developed in endocrine cells such as β cell in which large amounts of secretory proteins are synthesized.

ER is categorized into two types: rough endoplasmic reticulum (RER) and smooth endoplasmic reticulum (SER). As featured by its name, RER looks bumpy and rough under a microscope due to the ribosomes on the outer surfaces of the cisternae. RER is in charge for protein synthesis. The newly synthesized proteins are folded into 3-dimensional structure in RER and sent to Golgi complex or membrane via small vesicles. In contrast, SER appears to have a smooth surface under the microscope as it does not have ribosomes on its cisternae. SER is responsible for the synthesis of lipids and steroids, regulation of calcium concentration, attachment of receptors on cell membrane proteins, and detoxification of drugs. It is found commonly in places such as in the liver and muscle. It is important for the liver to detoxify poisonous substances. Sarcoplasmic reticulum is a special type of SER. It is found in smooth and striated muscle, and is important for the regulation of calcium levels. It sequesters a large store of calcium and releases them when the muscle cell is stimulated.

3.2. Unfolded protein response and ER stress

ER stress is defined as the cellular responses to the disturbances of normal function of ER. The most common cause of ER stress is protein mis-folding. ER is the place where newly produced proteins fold into 3-dimensional conformation which is essential for their biological function. The sensitive folding environment could be disturbed by a variety of pathological insults like environmental toxins, viral infection, and inflammation. In addition to pathological insults, it can also be induce by many physiological processes such as overloaded protein biosynthesis on ER, For example, in case of type 1 diabetes, increased insulin synthesis in residual β cell exceeds the folding capacity of ER, resulting in the accumulation of unfolded insulin. The accumulation of unfolded or mis-folded proteins in the ER leads a protective pathway to restore ER function, termed as unfolded protein response (UPR).

Protein folding requires a serial of ER-resident protein folding machinery. A special type of proteins called chaperones is used as a quality control mechanism in the ER. As the major mechanisms to promote protein folding, chaperones assist protein folding by interacting with the newly synthesized proteins.In addition,chaperones also help to break down unfolded or incorrectly folded proteins in the ER via a process called ER associated degradation.The monitoring mechanism ensures the correct protein folding in the ER. The unfolded proteins usually have a higher number of hydrophobic surface patches than that of proteins with native conformation (17). Thus, unfolded proteins are prone to aggregate with each other in a crowed environment and directed to degradative pathway (18). Molecular chaperones in the ER preferentially interact with hydrophobic surface patches on unfolded proteins and create a private folding environment by preventing unfolded proteins from interaction and aggregation with other unfolded proteins. In addition, the concentration of Ca^{2+} in ER also impairs protein folding by inhibiting the activity of ER-resident chaperones and foldases (19-22). ER is the major site for Ca^{2+} storage in mammalian cells. The concentration of Ca^{2+} in ER is thousands times higher than that in the cytosol (23). Most chaperones and foldases in ER are vigorous Ca^{2+} binding proteins. Their activity, therefore, is affected by the concentration of Ca^{2+} in ER.

Exhaustion of the protein folding machineries or insufficient energy supply increases the accumulation of unfolded or mis-folded proteins in ER, which is responsible for the activation of UPR. UPR is a protective mechanism by which it monitors and maintains the homeostasis of ER. Various physiological and pathological insults such as increased protein synthesis, failure of posttranslational modifications, nutrient/glucose starvation, hypoxia, and alterations in calcium homeostasis, can result in the accumulation of unfolded or mis-folded proteins in ER which further causes ER stress (24).For example, altered expression of antithrombin III (25;26) or blood coagulation factor VIII (27;28), may result in the exhaustion of protein folding machinery and thus induces UPR. Some physiological processes such as the differentiation of B lymphocytes into plasma cells along with the development of highly specialized secretory capacity can also cause unfolded protein accumulation and activate UPR (29-31). In response to those physiological and pathological insults, cells initiate UPR process to get rid of the unfolded or mis-folded proteins. For instance, UPR can increase the folding capacity by up-regulating ER chaperones and foldases, as well as attenuate the biosynthetic burden through down-regulating the expression of secreted proteins (32-34). In addition, UPR also eliminates unfolded or mis-folded proteins by activating ER associated degradation process (35-37). However, once the stress is beyond the compensatory capacity of UPR, the cells would undergo apoptosis. As such, UPR and ER stress are reported to be implicated in a variety of pathological processes, including diabetes, neurodegenerative diseases, pathogenic infections, atherosclerosis, and ischemia (24;38).

In addition to protein folding, a variety of post-translational modifications including N-linked glycosylation, disulfide bond formation, lipidation, hydroxylation, and oligomerization, occur in ER. Disruption of those post-translational modifications can also result in the accumulation of incorrectly folded proteins and thereby induce UPR or ER stress. For example, glucose deprivation impairs the process for N-linked protein glycosylation and thus leads to ER stress (39).

3.3. ER stress pathways

As a protective mechanism during ER stress, UPR initiates a variety of process to ensure the homeostasis of ER. UPR can be mediated by three major pathways, which are initiated by the three transmembrane signaling proteins located on the ER membrane. Those transmembrane proteins function as a bridge linking cytosol and ER with their C-terminal in the cyto-

http://dx.doi.org/10.5772/52644

sol and N-terminal in the ER lumen. The N-terminal is usually engaged by an ER resident chaperone BiP (Grp78) to avoid aggregation. When unfolded proteins accumulate in ER, chaperons are occupied by unfolded proteins and release those transmembrane signaling proteins. There are three axes of signals that are initiated by the pancreatic endoplasmic reticulum kinase (PERK), the inositol-requiring enzyme 1 (IRE1), and the activating transcription factor 6 (ATF6) respectively. The release of these proteins from BiP triggers UPR and ER stress (Figure 3).

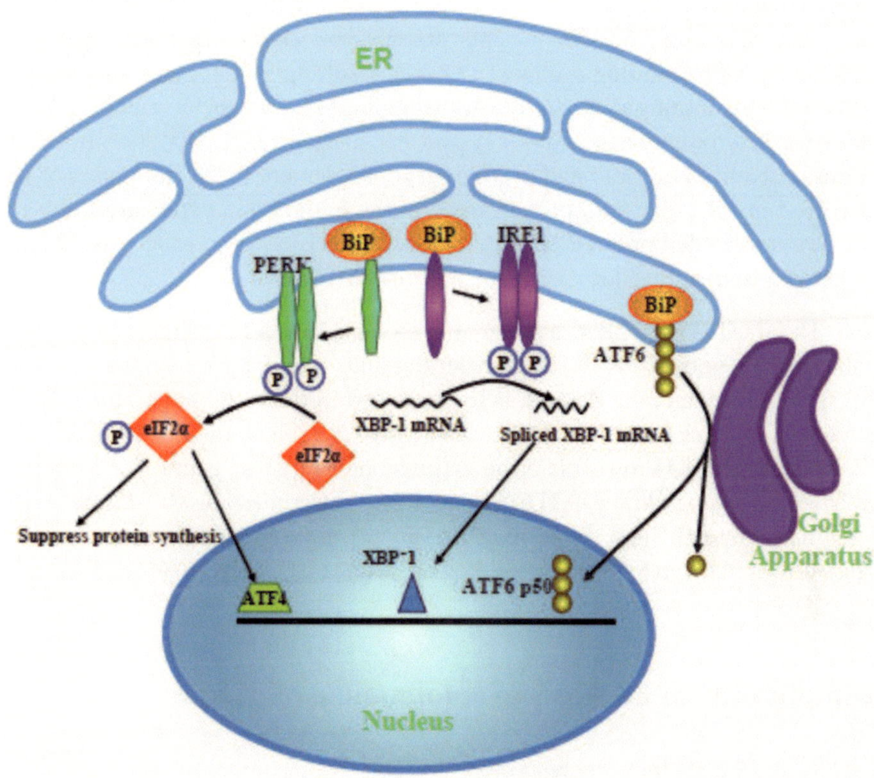

Figure 3. UPR signal pathways. Under normal condition, PERK, IRE1, and ATF6 binding to the ER chaperone BiP to remain inactive state. Upon the accumulation of unfolded proteins, BiP preferentially binds to the unfolded proteins, leading to the release of PERK, IRE1, and ATF6. PERK becomes oligomerized and activated once released from BiP, and subsequently phosphorylates eIF2α. The phosphorylation of eIF2α results in the suppression of the overall transcription of mRNAs and selectively enhanced transcription of genes implicated in UPR such as the ATF4 mRNA. Similar to PERK, IRE1 is dimerized and activated after released from BiP. Activated IRE1 induces XBP-1 by enhancing the splicing of its mRNA. XBP-1 enhances UPR by regulating the transcription of its target genes. The detachment of ATF6 from BiP results in the translocation of ATF6 to the Golgi apparatus and cleavage of ATF6. Cleaved ATF6 then translocates into the nucleus and initiates the transcription of target genes.

PERK/eIF2α/ATF4 axis: PERK is a type I transmembrane Ser/Thr protein kinase uniquely present in ER. In response to ER stress, the binding of unfolded proteins to BiP leads to the release of PERK from BiP. Once released from BiP, PERK becomes oligomerized and autophosphorylated. As a result, PERK inactivates eukaryotic initiation factor 2α (eIF2α) by the phosphorylation of Ser51 to inhibit mRNA translation and protein load on ER (34;40). In addition, phosphorylated eIF2α also promotes the expression of stress-induced genes including the transcription factors ATF4 and CCAAT/enhancer binding protein (C/EBP) homologous protein (CHOP) (41). Deficiency of PERK results in an abnormally elevated protein synthesis in response to the accumulation of unfolded proteins in ER.

IRE1/XBP-1 axis: IRE1 is another axis of signal involved in UPR. There are 2 isoforms of IRE1: IRE1α and IRE1β. IRE1α is expressed in most cells and tissues, while IRE1β is restricted in intestinal epithelial cells (42;43). Once disassociated with BiP, IRE1 becomes activated. Activated IRE1 possesses endoribonuclease activity and cleaves 26 nucleotides from the mRNA encoding X-box binding protein-1 (XBP-1), resulting in the increased production of XBP-1 (44). XBP-1 is a transcriptional factor belonging to basic leucine zipper transcription factorfamily. It heterodimerizes with NF-Y and enhances gene transcription by binding to the ER stress enhancer and unfolded protein response element in the promoters of targeted genes involved in ER expansion, protein maturation, folding and export from the ER, and degradation of mis-folded proteins (44-49). In addition, IRE1α also mediates the degradation of ER-targeted mRNAs, thus decreasing the ER burden (50).

ATF6 axis: The third axis of ER stress signal is mediated by ATF6. Unlike PERK and IRE1 which oligomerize upon UPR, ATF6 translocates into the Golgi apparatus after released from BiP. The transmembrane domain is then cleaved in the Golgi apparatus (51). The 50-kDa cleaved ATF6 is relocated into the nucleus where it binds to the ER stress response element CCAAT(N)9CCACG to regulate the expression of targeted genes. For example, once released from the ER membrane, ATF6 enhances the transcription of XBP-1 mRNA which is further regulated by IRE1 (44). In addition, ATF6 also increases the expression of the two major chaperon systems in the ER: calnexin/calreticulin and BiP/GRP94 (44;52;53).

4. The implication of ER stress in autoimmune responses

4.1. ER stress and innate immune response

The importance of innate immunity was highlighted in the pathophysiology of type 1 diabetes (54-57). Type 1 diabetes was initially considered a T-cell-mediated autoimmune disease (58), in which T-cell was believed as the major immune cell causing β cell destruction while the involvement of innate immune response has been ignored for a long time. However, recent studies suggest a critical role of innate immune responses in the development of type 1 diabetes (54;55). As the first line of defense mechanism, innate immunity is implicated in the initiation as well as the progression of autoimmune responses against pancreatic β cell.

Innate immune response is regulated by elements of the UPR pathway (59). For example, Cyclic-AMP-responsive-element-binding protein H(CREBH), an ER stress-associated transcription factor, regulates the expression of serum amyloid P-component and C-reactive

http://dx.doi.org/10.5772/52644

protein, the two critical factors implicated in innate immune responses. Like ATF6, CREBH is an ER-membrane-bound protein. In response to ER stress, CREBH release an N-terminal fragment and transit to nucleus to regulate the expression of target genes. Innate immune response, in turn, regulates the expression of CREBH through inflammatory cytokines such as IL-1β and IL-6 (60). The development of dendritic cells, the major innate immune cells, is also regulated by ER stress response (61). High levels of mRNA splicing for XBP-1 are found in dendritic cell, and mice deficient in XBP-1 show defective differentiation of dendritic cell. Both conventional ($CD11b^+$ CD11c+
) and plasmacytoid dendritic cells ($B220^+$ CD11c+
) are decreased by >50%. Dendritic cells deficient for XBP-1 are vulnerable to ER stress-induced apoptosis (61). Moreover, the secretion of inflammatory cytokine IL-23 by dendritic cell also involves ER stress response. CHOP, a UPR mediator, can directly bind to the *IL-23* gene and regulate its transcription. ER stress combined with Toll-like receptor (TLR) agonists was found to markedly increase the mRNA of IL-23 p19 subunit and the secretion of IL-23, while knockdown of CHOP suppressed the induction of IL-23 by ER stress and TLR signaling (62).

The association of ER stress with innate immune response is confirmed in many disease models. Richardson and coworkers reported that innate immune response induced by *P. aeruginosa* infection causes ER stress in *C. elegans*, and loss-of-function mutations of XBP-1 lead to larval lethality (63). In consistent with that, polymorphisms of *XBP-1* gene were found to be associated with Crohn's disease and ulcerative colitis in humans (64), the two autoimmune diseases share similar properties with type 1 diabetes. Lack of XBP-1 in intestinal epithelial cells may induce Paneth cell dysfunction which further results in impaired mucosal defense to *Listeria monocytogenes* and increased sensitivity to colitis (64).

In addition to IRE1/XBP-1 axis, PERK/eIF2α/ATF4 axis of UPR is also associated with innate response. TLR signaling, the most important innate signaling pathway, can induce selective suppression of the PERK/eIF2α/ATF-4/CHOP axis of UPR pathway (65). The activation of TLR decreases eIF2α-induced ATF4 translation. For instance, pretreatment of LPS, an agonist for TLR4, attenuated ATF4/CHOP signaling and prevented systemic ER stress-induced apoptosis in macrophages, renal tubule cells, and hepatocytes (65). In contrast, loss of Toll-IL-1R-containing adaptor inducing IFN-β (TRIF), an important adapter for TLR signaling, abrogated the protective effect of LPS on renal dysfunction and hepatosteatosis induced by ER stress, suggesting that TLR signaling suppresses ATF4/CHOP via a TRIF-dependent pathway (65).

4.2. ER stress and adaptive immune response

The presence of β cell specific autoantibodies is a marker for autoimmune diabetes (66). IRE1/XBP1 axis is required for the differentiation of antibody-producing B lymphocytes. IRE1 is necessary for the Ig gene rearrangement, production of B cell receptors, and lymphopoiesis. The expression multiple UPR components including BiP, GRP94, and XBP-1 is upregulated during the differentiation of B cells (67). Mice with a deficiency of IRE1 in hematopoietic cells have a defective differentiation of pro-B cells towards pre-B cells (68). XBP-1, an IRE1 downstream molecule, is also involved in the differentiation of B cell and antibody production by mature B cells. It was found that the engagement of B-cell receptor induces ubiquitin-mediated degradation of BCL-6, a repressor for B-lymphocyte-induced maturation protein 1 (69), while B-lymphocyte-induced maturation protein 1 negatively regulates the expression of B-cell-lineage-specific activator protein (70), a repressor for XBP-1 (71). In line with these results, B lymphocytes deficient in B-lymphocyte-induced maturation protein 1 failed to express XBP-1 in response to LPS stimulation (72). The expression of XBP-1 is rapidly up-regulated when B cells differentiate into plasma cells. Furthermore, XBP-1is able to initiate plasma cell differentiation when introduced into B-lineage cells. XBP-1-deficient lymphoid chimeras have a defective B-cell-dependent immune response due to the absence of immunoglobulin and plasma cells (30). In addition to IRE1/XBP-1 axis, ATF6 axis may also implicated in the differentiation of B cells, as increased ATF6 cleavage is found in differentiating B cells (67). However, PERK axis does not seem to be involved in the B-cell differentiation and maturation (68;73).

Activation of T lymphocyte, another important adaptive immune cell, seems also involves UPR. TCR engagement, the first T cell activation signal, induces the expression of ER chaperons including BiP and GRP94. Inhibition of protein kinase C, a serine/threonine protein kinase downstream of TCR signaling, suppresses the activation of ER stress response induced by T cell activation (74). IRE1/XBP-1 axis regulates the differentiation of effector $CD8^+$ T cell. IRE1/XBP-1 pathway is activated in effector $CD8^+$ T cell during acute infection. IL-2 promotes XBP-1 mRNA transcription, while TCR ligation induces the splicing of XBP-1 mRNA. The differentiation of $CD8^+$ T cell is reduced by suppression of XBP-1 (75). Other than IRE1/XBP-1, CHOP is also involved in the functionality of T cells. A recent report suggests GTPase of the immunity-associated protein 5 (Gimap5) mutation in BioBreeding diabetes-prone rat, a model for type 1 diabetes, leads to ER stress and thus induces spontaneous apoptosis of T cells. Inhibition of CHOP protects $Gimap5^{-/-}$ T cells from ER stress-induced apoptosis (76).

4.3. ER stress regulates cytokine production

Cytokine production is an important inflammatory process in response to insults of pathogens, mutated self-antigens or tissue damage. ER stress is interconnected with the induction of inflammatory cytokines through multiple mechanisms including reactive oxygen species (ROS), NFκB and JNK (Figure 4). ROS are defined as highly reactive small molecules with unpaired electrons. They are important mediators of inflammatory response., Oxidative stress, caused by the accumulation of ROS, was confirmed to be associated with ER stress (77). For example, the disulphide bond formation during the process of protein folding requires oxidizing condition (78). Therefore, increased protein folding load may lead to oxidative stress. The PERK axis of UPR is able to activate antioxidant pathway by promoting ATF4 and nuclear factor-erythroid-derived 2-related factor 2 (NRF2) (79;80). Therefore, deficiency of PERK markedly increases ROS accumulation in response to toxic chemicals (79;81). The IRE1 axis of UPR can activate NFκB, a key regulator in inflammation, by recruiting IκB kinase (82). As a result, loss of IRE1 reduces the activation of NFκB activation and production of TNF-α (82). In addition, the IRE1 axis can also activate JNK, and subsequently induce the expression of inflammatory genes by activating activator protein 1 (AP1) (83). ATF6, the third axis of UPR signaling, can also activate NFκB pathway and induce inflammatory response. Therefore, suppression of ATF6 reduces NFκB activation caused by BiP degradation (84).

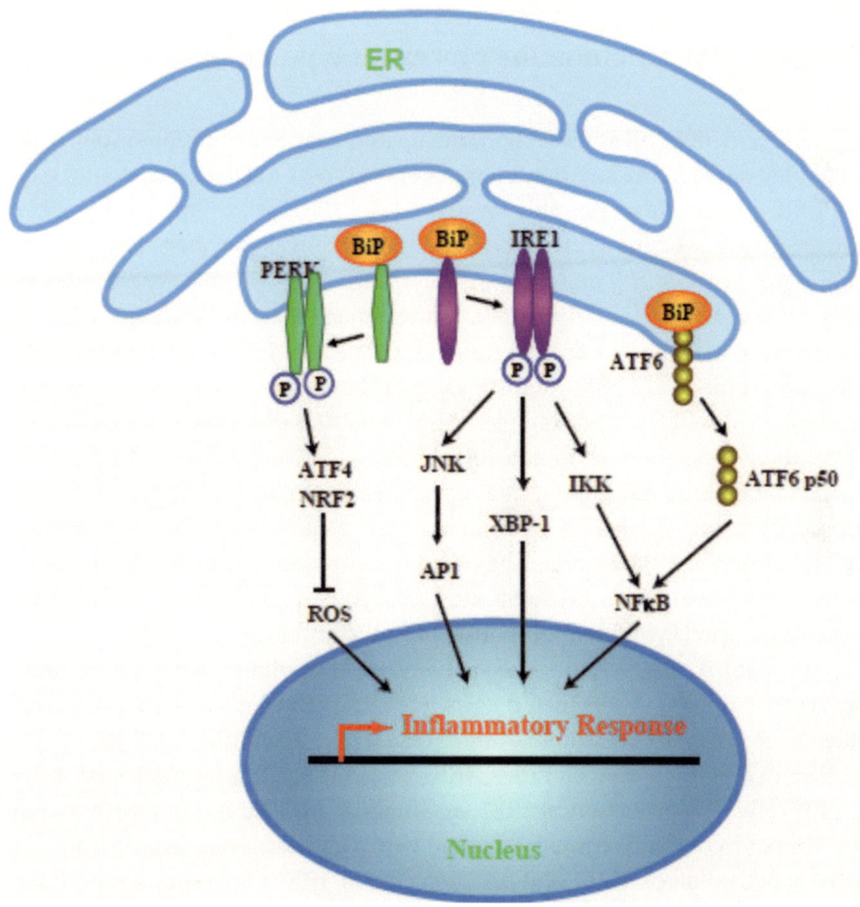

Figure 4. UPR-mediated inflammatory signaling. UPR regulates inflammation through a variety of mechanisms involving ROS, JNK, and NFκB. PERK promotes ATF4 and NRF2, which then suppress ROS production by activating antioxidant pathway. Upon activation, IRE1/TRAF2 complex recruits IKK (IκB Kinase), leading to the phosphorylation of IκBα and subsequent activation of NFκB. IRE1/TRAF2 can also activate JNK, followed by the activation of AP1. XBP-1 induced by IRE1 can also induce the expression of various genes implicated inflammation. Furthermore, cleaved ATF6 can promote inflammation via activating NFκB.

ER stress regulates the expression of cytokines, while cytokines in turn may also induce ER stress via pathways including inducible nitric oxide synthase (iNOS) and JNK. JNK pathway is activated by IL-1β. Suppression of JNK by its inhibitor SP600125 can protectβ cells from IL-1β-induced apoptosis (85). Inflammatory cytokines induce iNOS expression in β cells and produce copious amount of nitric oxygen (86).Nitric oxygen is an important mediator of β-cell death in type 1 diabetes. Excessive nitric oxygencan induce DNA damage, which leads to β cell apoptosis through p53 pathway or necrosis through poly (ADP-ribose) polymerase pathway (87). In addition, nitric oxygencan also deplete ER Ca^{2+} stores by activating Ca^{2+} channels or inhibiting Ca^{2+} pumps (88-90). Depletion of Ca^{2+} then leads to the activation of CHOP and induces ER stress and apoptosis of β cells (91;92).

4.4. ER stress in the autoimmune process of type 1 diabetes

Given the involvement of ER stress in both innate and adaptive immune systems, pathways of ER stress play a role in the autoimmune process of type 1 diabetes. For example, mice deficient in PERK, a molecule responsible for regulating UPR, are extremely susceptible to diabetes. Although the exocrine and endocrine pancreas developed normally, the *null* mice display a progressive loss of β mass and insulin insufficiency postnatally (93) (93). A severe defect of β cell proliferation and differentiation was also found in *PERK null* mice, resulting in low pancreatic β mass and proinsulin trafficking defects (94). Consistent with those observations in mice, some infant-onset diabetic cases in humans are confirmed to be associated with the mutations in PERK. For example, loss of *EIF2AK3* (the gene encodes PERK) develops Wolcott-Rallison syndrome, an autosomal recessive disorder featured by early infancy insulin-dependency and multiple systemic manifestations including growth retardation, hepatic/renal dysfunction, mental retardation, and cardiovascular abnormalities (86;95). Similarly, disruption of UPR by mutating eIF2α, the downstream molecule of PERK signaling, enhances the sensitivity to ER stress-induced apoptosis and results in defective gluconeogenesis. Mice carrying a homozygous Ser51Ala mutation for eIF2α show multiple defects in pancreatic β cells including the smaller core of insulin-secreting β cells and attenuated insulin secretion (41). Altogether, defects in PERK/eIF2α signaling render β cells highly vulnerable to ER stress in both humans and mice (87;96). In addition to PERK/eIF2α signaling, the other two pathways of ER stress, IRE1 and ATF6, are also implicated in the functionality of β cells. The activation of IRE1 signaling is involved in the insulin biosynthesis induced by hyperglycemia. Transient exposure to high glucose enhances IRE1α phosphorylation without activation of XBP-1 and BiP dissociation. IRE1α activation induced by transient exposure to high glucose induces insulin biosynthesis by up-regulating WFS1, a component involved in UPR and maintaining ER homeostasis (10;97). However, chronic exposure of β cells to high glucose may cause activation of IRE1 but with a different downstream signaling, leading to the suppression of insulin biosynthesis (10). The activation of ATF6 induced by ER stress also suppressed the expression of insulin by up-regulating orphan nuclear receptor small heterodimer partner (98).

5. The role of ER stress in β cell destruction

5.1. The involvement of ER stress in β cell destruction

Increasing evidence suggests an important role of ER stress in autoimmune-mediated β cell destruction (99;100). It was noted that β cell loss is the direct causing factor for insufficient insulin secretion in type 1 diabetes patients. Pancreatic β cells have a very well-developed ER to fulfill their biological function for secreting insulin and other glycoproteins, causing the high sensitivity of β cells to ER stress and the subsequent UPR. Severe or long-term ER stress would direct β cells undergoing apoptosis (99). As described earlier, all the three pathways of ER stress are important in the execution of β cell function and involved in the autoimmune responses during the process of type 1 diabetes.

Pro-inflammatory cytokines are believed as the major mediators contributing to ER stress in β cell mediated by autoimmune response. Autoreactive immune cells infiltrated in pancreas produce pro-inflammatory cytokines, the primary causing factor for β cell death in type 1 diabetes(101). Autoreactive macrophages and T-lymphocytes present in the pancreatic islets in the early stage of type 1 diabetes and secrete massive pro-inflammatory cytokines including IL-1β, IFN-γ and TNF-α. Pro-inflammatory cytokines have been confirmed as strong inducers of ER stress in pancreatic β cells. Insult of β cells with IL-1β and IFN-γ was reported to induce the expression of death protein 5, a protein involved in the cytokine-induced ER stress and β cell death (102). Suppression of death protein 5 by siRNA provides protection for β cells against pro-inflammatory cytokine-induced ER stress (102). In addition, stimulation of β cells with IL-1β and IFN-γ can decrease the expression of sarcoendoplasmic reticulum pump Ca^{2+} ATPase 2b, leading to subsequent depletion of Ca^{2+} in the ER (103). It has been well demonstrated that altered ER Ca^{2+} concentration induces the accumulation of unfolded proteins in ER associated with the induction of UPR and ER stress in β cells (104). Reactive oxygen species such as nitric oxygen produced during inflammation are believed to play a critical role in ER stress-induced β cell death. Excessive nitric oxygen production during insulitis induces β cell apoptosis in a CHOP-dependent manner (91).

In addition to cytokine-induced ER stress, defective protein processing and trafficking are also a direct cause of ER stress in β cell. For instance, mis-folding of insulin in β cells directly induces chronic ER stress as evidenced by the observations in Akita mice. The mutation of *Ins2* gene in Akita mouse disrupts a disulfide bond betweenα and β chain of proinsulin, leading to the mis-folding of the mutated insulin. This mutation therefore induces chronic ER stress in β cells and finally causes diabetes in Akita mouse (105). The inefficiency of protein trafficking from ER to Golgi apparatus also causes ER stress in β cells (106).

Hyperglycemia occurs only when β cells fail to compensate the increased demand for insulin. Therefore, β cells are usually "exhausted" in diabetic patients (87). The increased insulin demandrequires the remaining functional β cellsto increase insulin synthesis to compensate the decrease of β mass. The altered insulin synthesis causes ER stress in the β cells of patients with type 1 diabetes. In later case, this compensation is beneficial for control of blood glucose homeostasisin a short term.However, the long term alterations of insulin synthesis in the β cells also induce ER stress which in turn exacerbates β cell dysfunction and promotes disease progression. Collectively, there is convincing evidence that ER stress plays an essential role in β cell destruction during the course of type 1 diabetes.

5.2. Mechanisms underlying ER stress-induced β cell death

The primary purpose of ER stress response is to compensate the damage caused by the disturbances of normal ER function. However, persistence of ER dysfunction would eventually render cells undergoing apoptosis. The mechanisms underlying ER stress induced cell death are not fully elucidated, due to the fact that multiple potential participants involved but little clarity on the dominant death effectors in a particular cellular context. Generally, the process of cell death by ER stress can be illustrated in three phases: adaptation, alarm, and apoptosis (39).

The adaptation response phase is to protect cells from damage induced by the disturbances of ER function and restore the homeostasis of ER. As described earlier, UPR signaling involves three axes of responses: IRE1, PERK, and ATF6. These axes interact between each other and form a feedback regulatory mechanism to control the activity of UPR. The accumulation of unfolded proteins in ER results in the engagement of ER resident chaperon BiP, and as a consequence, IRE1, PERK, and ATF6 are released from BiP. Therefore, over-expression of BiP can prevent cell death induced by oxidative stress, Ca^{2+} disturbances, and hypoxia (107). Upon ER stress, the transcription of BiP is enhanced by ATF6p50, the cleaved form of ATF6 (108). PERK is oligomerized and phosphorylated upon the release from BiP. Activated PERK inactivates eIF2α to reduce mRNA translation and protein load on ER. Therefore, PERK deficiency results in an abnormally elevated protein synthesis in response to ER stress, and renders cells highly sensitive to ER stress-induced apoptosis (109). Consistently, as a downstream molecule of PERK, eIF2α is required for cell survival upon the insult of ER stress. A mutation at the phosphorylation site of eIF2α (Ser51Ala) abolishes the translational suppression in response to ER stress (41). When released from BiP, IRE1 becomes dimerized and activated. Activated IRE1 then induces XBP-1 by promoting the splicing of its mRNA (44). XBP-1 is responsible for the transcription of many adaptation genes implicated in UPR. Unlike PERK and IRE1, ATF6 translocates into the Golgi apparatus once released from BiP. The transmembrane domain of ATF6 is cleaved in the Golgi apparatus and is then relocated into the nucleus, by which it regulates gene expression (51).

During the alarm phase, many signal pathways are activated to alert the system. For instance, the cytoplasmic part of IRE1 can bind to TNF receptor-associated factor 2 (TRAF2), a key adaptor mediating TNF-induced innate immune response. TRAF2 then activates NFκB pathway via activating IKK and activates the signaling for c-Jun N-terminal kinases (JNK) by apoptosis signal-regulating kinase 1 (Ask1). It is reported that dominant negative TRAF2 suppresses the activation of JNK in response to ER stress (110). In addition, TRAF2 is also a critical component for E3 ubiquitin-protein ligase complex (111). E3 ubiquitin-protein ligase complex binds to Ubc13 and mediates the noncanonical ubiquitination of substrates, which is suggested to be required for the activation of JNK (112).

Furthermore, IRE1 can also activate JNK signaling by interacting with c-Jun N-terminal inhibitory kinase (JIK) (113).

Although the purpose of UPR is to maintain the homeostasis of ER, apoptosis could occur when the insult of ER stress exceeds the cellular regulatory capacity. Apoptosis is initiated by the activation of several proteases including caspase-12, caspase-4, caspase-2, and caspase-9. Studies in rodents suggest that caspase-12 is activated by IRE1 and is involved in ER stress-induced apoptosis. Mice deficient for caspase-12 are resistant to ER stress-induced apoptosis, but remain susceptible to apoptosis induced by other stimuli (114). Caspase-12 can also be activated by TRAF2, a downstream molecule of IRE1 (113). In response to ER stress, caspase-7 is translocated from the cytosol to the ER surface, and then activates procaspase-12 (115). Human caspase-4, the closest paralog of rodent caspase-12, can only be activated by ER stress-inducing reagents not by the other apoptotic reagents. Knockdown of caspase-4 by siRNA reduces ER stress-induced apoptosis in neuroblastoma cells, suggesting the involvement of human caspase-4 in ER stress-induced cell death (116). Similarly, caspase-2 and caspase-9 are also activated in the early phase of ER stress. Inhibition of their activation either by inhibitors or siRNA reduces ER stress-induced apoptosis (117). Other than caspase proteins, Ask1 kinase and CHOP are also critical mediators for ER stress-induced cell death. IRE1/TRAF2 complex recruits Ask1 and activates subsequent JNK signaling. The activation of JNK then induces apoptosis by inhibiting anti-apoptotic protein BCL-2 (118) and inducing pro-apoptotic protein Bim (119;120). Deficiency of Ask1 suppresses ER stress-induced JNK activation and protects cells against ER stress-induced apoptosis (121). CHOP, a transcription factor belonging to basic leucine zipper transcription factor family, can be activated by many inducers of UPR including ATF4, ATF6, and XBP-1. Upon activation, CHOP induces cells undergoing apoptosis through suppressing anti-apoptotic protein BCL-2 (122-124).

6. Conclusions and future directions

Although exogenous insulin therapy partly compensates the function of β cells, it cannot regulate blood glucose as accurately as the action of endogenous insulin. As a result, long-term improperly control of blood glucose homeostasis predisposes patients with type 1 diabetes to the development of diverse complications such as diabetic retinopathy (125-127), nephropathy (128;129), neuropathy (130-132), foot ulcers (133-135), and cardiovascular diseases (136-138). Due to the long-term health consequences of diabetes, impact of insulin dependence on life quality, and increasing appearance in both young and old populations, understanding the pathophysiology of diabetes and finding a better way to treat diabetes has become a high priority. Although the underlying mechanisms leading to type 1 diabetes have yet to be fully addressed, accumulating evidence suggests that ER stress plays a critical role in autoimmune-mediated β cell destruction during the course of type 1 diabetes. ER stress in β cells can be triggered by either autoimmune responses against β-cell self-antigens or the increase of compensated insulin synthesis. During the course of type 1 diabetes, autoreactive immune cells secrete copious amount of inflammatory cytokines, leading to excessive production of nitric oxygenand β cell destruction in an ER stress-dependent pathway. ER stress also regulates the functionality of immune cells with implications in autoimmune progression. The inadequate insulin secretion in patients with type 1 diabetes renders the residual β cells for compensated insulin secretion to maintain blood glucose homeostasis. This increase in insulin biosynthesis could overwhelm the folding capacity of ER, and exacerbate β cell dysfunction by inducing ER stress in β cells.

Although ER stress is a critical factor involved in the pathogenesis of type 1 diabetes, it should be kept in mind that the mechanisms underlying autoimmune-mediated β cell destruction in type 1 diabetes are complex, and ER stress is unlikely the exclusive mechanism implicated in disease process. Despite recent significant progress in this area, there are still many questions yet to be addressed. Are there additional factors inducing ER stress in β cells during type 1 diabetes development? Can ER stress be served as a biomarker for β cell destruction and autoimmune progression in the clinic setting? Does blockade of ER stress in immune cells attenuate autoimmune progression and protect β cells? Future studies aimed to dissect these questions would provide a deep insight for type 1 diabetes pathogenesis and would have great potential for developing novel therapeutic strategies against this devastating disorder.

Acknowledgements

This work is supported by a grant from the National Natural Science Foundation of China (81101553/H1604) to JZ. The author declares no competing financial interest.

Abbreviations

AP1, activator protein 1; Ask1, apoptosis signal-regulating kinase 1; ATF6, Activating Transcription Factor 6; C/EBP, CCAAT/enhancer binding protein; CHOP, C/EBP homologous protein; CREBH, Cyclic-AMP-responsive-element-binding protein H; eIF2α, eukaryotic initiation factor 2α; ER, Endoplasmic Reticulum; ER stress, Endoplasmic Reticulum stress; iNOS, inducible nitric oxide synthase; IRE1, inositol-requiring enzyme 1; IRS-1, insulin receptor substrate-1; JIK, c-Jun N-terminal inhibitory kinase; JNK, c-Jun N-terminal kinases; NRF2, nuclear factor-erythroid-derived 2-related factor 2; PERK, pancreatic endoplasmic reticulum kinase; RER, rough endoplasmic reticulum; ROS, reactive oxygen species; SER, smooth endoplasmic reticulum; TLR, Toll-like receptor; TRAF2, TNF receptor-associated factor 2; TRIF, Toll-IL-1R-containing adaptor inducing IFN-β; UPR, unfolded protein response; XBP-1, X box protein-1.

http://dx.doi.org/10.5772/52644

Author details

Jixin Zhong[1,2]

Address all correspondence to: zhongjixin620@163.com

1 Department of Medicine, Affiliated Hospital of Guangdong Medical College, Zhanjiang, Guangdong, China

2 Davis Heart & Lung Research Institute, The Ohio State University College of Medicine, Columbus, Ohio, USA

References

[1] Espino-Paisan L, Urcelay E, Concha EGdl, Santiago JL: Early and Late Onset Type 1 Diabetes: One and the Same or Two Distinct Genetic Entities? In Type 1 Diabetes Complications. Wagner D, Ed. InTech, 2011,

[2] Maahs,DM, West,NA, Lawrence,JM, Mayer-Davis,EJ: Epidemiology of type 1 diabetes. Endocrinol Metab Clin North Am 39:481-497, 2010

[3] Lehuen,A, Diana,J, Zaccone,P, Cooke,A: Immune cell crosstalk in type 1 diabetes. Nat Rev Immunol 10:501-513, 2010

[4] Zhong J, Xu J, Yang P, Liang Y, Wang C-Y: Innate immunity in the recognition of beta-cell antigens in type 1 diabetes. In Type 1 Diabetes - Pathogenesis, Genetics and Immunotherapy. Wagner D, Ed. InTech, 2011,

[5] American Diabetes Association: Standards of medical care in diabetes--2006. Diabetes Care 29 Suppl 1:S4-42, 2006

[6] Tortora GJ, Derrickson BH: Principles of Anatomy and Physiology. John Wiley & Sons Inc., 2008,

[7] Layden,VT, Durai,V, Lowe,WL: G-Protein-Coupled Receptors, Pancreatic Islets, and Diabetes. Nature Education 3:13, 2010

[8] Gerich,JE: The genetic basis of type 2 diabetes mellitus: impaired insulin secretion versus impaired insulin sensitivity. Endocr Rev 19:491-503, 1998

[9] Lillioja,S, Mott,DM, Spraul,M, Ferraro,R, Foley,JE, Ravussin,E, Knowler,WC, Bennett,PH, Bogardus,C: Insulin resistance and insulin secretory dysfunction as precursors of non-insulin-dependent diabetes mellitus. Prospective studies of Pima Indians. N Engl J Med 329:1988-1992, 1993

[10] Lipson,KL, Fonseca,SG, Ishigaki,S, Nguyen,LX, Foss,E, Bortell,R, Rossini,AA, Urano,F: Regulation of insulin biosynthesis in pancreatic beta cells by an endoplasmic reticulum-resident protein kinase IRE1. Cell Metab 4:245-254, 2006

[11] Rhodes CJ: Processing of the insulin molecule. in: D. LeRoith, S.I. Taylor, J.M. Olefsky (Eds.), Diabetes Mellitus, Lippincott Williams & Wilkins. In Diabetes Mellitus: A Fundamental and Clinical Text. 3rd ed. LeRoith D, Taylor SI, Olefsky JM, Eds. Lippincott Williams & Wilkins, 2003,

[12] D'Hertog,W, Maris,M, Ferreira,GB, Verdrengh,E, Lage,K, Hansen,DA, Cardozo,AK, Workman,CT, Moreau,Y, Eizirik,DL, Waelkens,E, Overbergh,L, Mathieu,C: Novel insights into the global proteome responses of insulin-producing INS-1E cells to different degrees of endoplasmic reticulum stress. J Proteome Res 9:5142-5152, 2010

[13] Hubbard,SC, Ivatt,RJ: Synthesis and processing of asparagine-linked oligosaccharides. Annu Rev Biochem 50:555-583, 1981

[14] Kornfeld,R, Kornfeld,S: Assembly of asparagine-linked oligosaccharides. Annu Rev Biochem 54:631-664, 1985

[15] Fewell,SW, Travers,KJ, Weissman,JS, Brodsky,JL: The action of molecular chaperones in the early secretory pathway. Annu Rev Genet 35:149-191, 2001

[16] Paltauf F, Kohlwein S.D., Henry S.A.: Regulation and compartmentalization of lipid synthesis in yeast. In The Molecular and Cellular Biology of the Yeast Saccharomyces. Jones E.W., Broach J.R., Eds. NY, Cold Spring Harbor Laboratory Press, 1992, p. 415-500

[17] Stevens,FJ, Argon,Y: Protein folding in the ER. Semin Cell Dev Biol 10:443-454, 1999

[18] Schroder,M: Endoplasmic reticulum stress responses. Cell Mol Life Sci 65:862-894, 2008

[19] Suzuki,CK, Bonifacino,JS, Lin,AY, Davis,MM, Klausner,RD: Regulating the retention of T-cell receptor alpha chain variants within the endoplasmic reticulum: Ca(2+)-dependent association with BiP. J Cell Biol 114:189-205, 1991

[20] Li,LJ, Li,X, Ferrario,A, Rucker,N, Liu,ES, Wong,S, Gomer,CJ, Lee,AS: Establishment of a Chinese hamster ovary cell line that expresses grp78 antisense transcripts and suppresses A23187 induction of both GRP78 and GRP94. J Cell Physiol 153:575-582, 1992

[21] Corbett,EF, Oikawa,K, Francois,P, Tessier,DC, Kay,C, Bergeron,JJ, Thomas,DY, Krause,KH, Michalak,M: Ca2+ regulation of interactions between endoplasmic reticulum chaperones. J Biol Chem 274:6203-6211, 1999

[22] Zhang,JX, Braakman,I, Matlack,KE, Helenius,A: Quality control in the secretory pathway: the role of calreticulin, calnexin and BiP in the retention of glycoproteins with C-terminal truncations. Mol Biol Cell 8:1943-1954, 1997

[23] Orrenius,S, Zhivotovsky,B, Nicotera,P: Regulation of cell death: the calcium-apoptosis link. Nat Rev Mol Cell Biol 4:552-565, 2003

[24] Lee,AS: The glucose-regulated proteins: stress induction and clinical applications. Trends Biochem Sci 26:504-510, 2001

[25] Schroder,M, Friedl,P: Overexpression of recombinant human antithrombin III in Chinese hamster ovary cells results in malformation and decreased secretion of recombinant protein. Biotechnol Bioeng 53:547-559, 1997

[26] Schroder,M, Schafer,R, Friedl,P: Induction of protein aggregation in an early secretory compartment by elevation of expression level. Biotechnol Bioeng 78:131-140, 2002

[27] Dorner,AJ, Wasley,LC, Kaufman,RJ: Increased synthesis of secreted proteins induces expression of glucose-regulated proteins in butyrate-treated Chinese hamster ovary cells. J Biol Chem 264:20602-20607, 1989

[28] Kaufman,RJ, Wasley,LC, Dorner,AJ: Synthesis, processing, and secretion of recombinant human factor VIII expressed in mammalian cells. J Biol Chem 263:6352-6362, 1988

[29] Schroder,M, Kaufman,RJ: ER stress and the unfolded protein response. Mutat Res 569:29-63, 2005

[30] Reimold,AM, Iwakoshi,NN, Manis,J, Vallabhajosyula,P, Szomolanyi-Tsuda,E, Gravallese,EM, Friend,D, Grusby,MJ, Alt,F, Glimcher,LH: Plasma cell differentiation requires the transcription factor XBP-1. Nature 412:300-307, 2001

[31] Iwakoshi,NN, Lee,AH, Vallabhajosyula,P, Otipoby,KL, Rajewsky,K, Glimcher,LH: Plasma cell differentiation and the unfolded protein response intersect at the transcription factor XBP-1. Nat Immunol 4:321-329, 2003

[32] Martinez,IM, Chrispeels,MJ: Genomic analysis of the unfolded protein response in Arabidopsis shows its connection to important cellular processes. Plant Cell 15:561-576, 2003

[33] Pakula,TM, Laxell,M, Huuskonen,A, Uusitalo,J, Saloheimo,M, Penttila,M: The effects of drugs inhibiting protein secretion in the filamentous fungus Trichoderma reesei. Evidence for down-regulation of genes that encode secreted proteins in the stressed cells. J Biol Chem 278:45011-45020, 2003

[34] Harding,HP, Zhang,Y, Ron,D: Protein translation and folding are coupled by an endoplasmic-reticulum-resident kinase. Nature 397:271-274, 1999

[35] Casagrande,R, Stern,P, Diehn,M, Shamu,C, Osario,M, Zuniga,M, Brown,PO, Ploegh,H: Degradation of proteins from the ER of S. cerevisiae requires an intact unfolded protein response pathway. Mol Cell 5:729-735, 2000

[36] Friedlander,R, Jarosch,E, Urban,J, Volkwein,C, Sommer,T: A regulatory link between ER-associated protein degradation and the unfolded-protein response. Nat Cell Biol 2:379-384, 2000

[37] Travers,KJ, Patil,CK, Wodicka,L, Lockhart,DJ, Weissman,JS, Walter,P: Functional and genomic analyses reveal an essential coordination between the unfolded protein response and ER-associated degradation. Cell 101:249-258, 2000

[38] Kaufman,RJ: Orchestrating the unfolded protein response in health and disease. J Clin Invest 110:1389-1398, 2002

[39] Xu,C, Bailly-Maitre,B, Reed,JC: Endoplasmic reticulum stress: cell life and death decisions. J Clin Invest 115:2656-2664, 2005

[40] Kaufman,RJ, Scheuner,D, Schroder,M, Shen,X, Lee,K, Liu,CY, Arnold,SM: The unfolded protein response in nutrient sensing and differentiation. Nat Rev Mol Cell Biol 3:411-421, 2002

[41] Scheuner,D, Song,B, McEwen,E, Liu,C, Laybutt,R, Gillespie,P, Saunders,T, Bonner-Weir,S, Kaufman,RJ: Translational control is required for the unfolded protein response and in vivo glucose homeostasis. Mol Cell 7:1165-1176, 2001

[42] Tirasophon,W, Welihinda,AA, Kaufman,RJ: A stress response pathway from the endoplasmic reticulum to the nucleus requires a novel bifunctional protein kinase/ endoribonuclease (Ire1p) in mammalian cells. Genes Dev 12:1812-1824, 1998

[43] Wang,XZ, Harding,HP, Zhang,Y, Jolicoeur,EM, Kuroda,M, Ron,D: Cloning of mammalian Ire1 reveals diversity in the ER stress responses. EMBO J 17:5708-5717, 1998

[44] Lee,K, Tirasophon,W, Shen,X, Michalak,M, Prywes,R, Okada,T, Yoshida,H, Mori,K, Kaufman,RJ: IRE1-mediated unconventional mRNA splicing and S2P-mediated ATF6 cleavage merge to regulate XBP1 in signaling the unfolded protein response. Genes Dev 16:452-466, 2002

[45] Yoshida,H, Matsui,T, Yamamoto,A, Okada,T, Mori,K: XBP1 mRNA is induced by ATF6 and spliced by IRE1 in response to ER stress to produce a highly active transcription factor. Cell 107:881-891, 2001

[46] Calfon,M, Zeng,H, Urano,F, Till,JH, Hubbard,SR, Harding,HP, Clark,SG, Ron,D: IRE1 couples endoplasmic reticulum load to secretory capacity by processing the XBP-1 mRNA. Nature 415:92-96, 2002

[47] Lee,AH, Iwakoshi,NN, Glimcher,LH: XBP-1 regulates a subset of endoplasmic reticulum resident chaperone genes in the unfolded protein response. Mol Cell Biol 23:7448-7459, 2003

[48] Yoshida,H, Matsui,T, Hosokawa,N, Kaufman,RJ, Nagata,K, Mori,K: A time-dependent phase shift in the mammalian unfolded protein response. Dev Cell 4:265-271, 2003

[49] Lee,AH, Chu,GC, Iwakoshi,NN, Glimcher,LH: XBP-1 is required for biogenesis of cellular secretory machinery of exocrine glands. EMBO J 24:4368-4380, 2005

[50] Hollien,J, Weissman,JS: Decay of endoplasmic reticulum-localized mRNAs during the unfolded protein response. Science 313:104-107, 2006

[51] Ye,J, Rawson,RB, Komuro,R, Chen,X, Dave,UP, Prywes,R, Brown,MS, Goldstein,JL: ER stress induces cleavage of membrane-bound ATF6 by the same proteases that process SREBPs. Mol Cell 6:1355-1364, 2000

[52] Okada,T, Yoshida,H, Akazawa,R, Negishi,M, Mori,K: Distinct roles of activating transcription factor 6 (ATF6) and double-stranded RNA-activated protein kinase-like endoplasmic reticulum kinase (PERK) in transcription during the mammalian unfolded protein response. Biochem J 366:585-594, 2002

[53] Ni,M, Lee,AS: ER chaperones in mammalian development and human diseases. FEBS Lett 581:3641-3651, 2007

[54] Han,J, Zhong,J, Wei,W, Wang,Y, Huang,Y, Yang,P, Purohit,S, Dong,Z, Wang,MH, She,JX, Gong,F, Stern,DM, Wang,CY: Extracellular high-mobility group box 1 acts as an innate immune mediator to enhance autoimmune progression and diabetes onset in NOD mice. Diabetes 57:2118-2127, 2008

[55] Zhang,S, Zhong,J, Yang,P, Gong,F, Wang,CY: HMGB1, an innate alarmin, in the pathogenesis of type 1 diabetes. Int J Clin Exp Pathol 3:24-38, 2009

[56] Zhong J, Yang P, Wang C: Environmental Triggers and Endogenous Alarmins Linking Innate Immunity to the Pathogenesis of Type 1 Diabetes. In: Type 1 Diabetes Mellitus: Etiology, Diagnosis and Treatment. Nova Science Publishers, Inc., 2011, p. 177-206

[57] Zhong J, Xu J, Yang P, Liang Y, Wang C-Y: Innate immunity in the recognition of ? cell antigens in type 1 diabetes. In Type 1 Diabetes - Pathogenesis, Genetics and Immunotherapy. Wagner D, Ed. InTech, 2011,

[58] Pietropaolo,M, Barinas-Mitchell,E, Kuller,LH: The heterogeneity of diabetes: unraveling a dispute: is systemic inflammation related to islet autoimmunity? Diabetes 56:1189-1197, 2007

[59] Zhao,L, Ackerman,SL: Endoplasmic reticulum stress in health and disease. Curr Opin Cell Biol 18:444-452, 2006

[60] Zhang,K, Shen,X, Wu,J, Sakaki,K, Saunders,T, Rutkowski,DT, Back,SH, Kaufman,RJ: Endoplasmic reticulum stress activates cleavage of CREBH to induce a systemic inflammatory response. Cell 124:587-599, 2006

[61] Iwakoshi,NN, Pypaert,M, Glimcher,LH: The transcription factor XBP-1 is essential for the development and survival of dendritic cells. J Exp Med 204:2267-2275, 2007

[62] Goodall,JC, Wu,C, Zhang,Y, McNeill,L, Ellis,L, Saudek,V, Gaston,JS: Endoplasmic reticulum stress-induced transcription factor, CHOP, is crucial for dendritic cell IL-23 expression. Proc Natl Acad Sci U S A 107:17698-17703, 2010

[63] Richardson,CE, Kooistra,T, Kim,DH: An essential role for XBP-1 in host protection against immune activation in C. elegans. Nature 463:1092-1095, 2010

[64] Kaser,A, Lee,AH, Franke,A, Glickman,JN, Zeissig,S, Tilg,H, Nieuwenhuis,EE, Higgins,DE, Schreiber,S, Glimcher,LH, Blumberg,RS: XBP1 links ER stress to intestinal inflammation and confers genetic risk for human inflammatory bowel disease. Cell 134:743-756, 2008

[65] Woo,CW, Cui,D, Arellano,J, Dorweiler,B, Harding,H, Fitzgerald,KA, Ron,D, Tabas,I: Adaptive suppression of the ATF4-CHOP branch of the unfolded protein response by toll-like receptor signalling. Nat Cell Biol 11:1473-1480, 2009

[66] Baekkeskov,S, Nielsen,JH, Marner,B, Bilde,T, Ludvigsson,J, Lernmark,A: Autoantibodies in newly diagnosed diabetic children immunoprecipitate human pancreatic islet cell proteins. Nature 298:167-169, 1982

[67] Gass,JN, Gifford,NM, Brewer,JW: Activation of an unfolded protein response during differentiation of antibody-secreting B cells. J Biol Chem 277:49047-49054, 2002

[68] Zhang,K, Wong,HN, Song,B, Miller,CN, Scheuner,D, Kaufman,RJ: The unfolded protein response sensor IRE1alpha is required at 2 distinct steps in B cell lymphopoiesis. J Clin Invest 115:268-281, 2005

[69] Niu,H, Ye,BH, la-Favera,R: Antigen receptor signaling induces MAP kinase-mediated phosphorylation and degradation of the BCL-6 transcription factor. Genes Dev 12:1953-1961, 1998

[70] Lin,KI, ngelin-Duclos,C, Kuo,TC, Calame,K: Blimp-1-dependent repression of Pax-5 is required for differentiation of B cells to immunoglobulin M-secreting plasma cells. Mol Cell Biol 22:4771-4780, 2002

[71] Reimold,AM, Ponath,PD, Li,YS, Hardy,RR, David,CS, Strominger,JL, Glimcher,LH: Transcription factor B cell lineage-specific activator protein regulates the gene for human X-box binding protein 1. J Exp Med 183:393-401, 1996

[72] Shaffer,AL, Shapiro-Shelef,M, Iwakoshi,NN, Lee,AH, Qian,SB, Zhao,H, Yu,X, Yang,L, Tan,BK, Rosenwald,A, Hurt,EM, Petroulakis,E, Sonenberg,N, Yewdell,JW, Calame,K, Glimcher,LH, Staudt,LM: XBP1, downstream of Blimp-1, expands the secretory apparatus and other organelles, and increases protein synthesis in plasma cell differentiation. Immunity 21:81-93, 2004

[73] Gass,JN, Jiang,HY, Wek,RC, Brewer,JW: The unfolded protein response of B-lymphocytes: PERK-independent development of antibody-secreting cells. Mol Immunol 45:1035-1043, 2008

[74] Pino,SC, O'Sullivan-Murphy,B, Lidstone,EA, Thornley,TB, Jurczyk,A, Urano,F, Greiner,DL, Mordes,JP, Rossini,AA, Bortell,R: Protein kinase C signaling during T cell activation induces the endoplasmic reticulum stress response. Cell Stress Chaperones 13:421-434, 2008

[75] Kamimura,D, Bevan,MJ: Endoplasmic reticulum stress regulator XBP-1 contributes to effector CD8+ T cell differentiation during acute infection. J Immunol 181:5433-5441, 2008

[76] Pino,SC, O'Sullivan-Murphy,B, Lidstone,EA, Yang,C, Lipson,KL, Jurczyk,A, diIorio,P, Brehm,MA, Mordes,JP, Greiner,DL, Rossini,AA, Bortell,R: CHOP mediates endoplasmic reticulum stress-induced apoptosis in Gimap5-deficient T cells. PLoS One 4:e5468, 2009

[77] Malhotra,JD, Kaufman,RJ: Endoplasmic reticulum stress and oxidative stress: a vicious cycle or a double-edged sword? Antioxid Redox Signal 9:2277-2293, 2007

[78] Tu,BP, Weissman,JS: Oxidative protein folding in eukaryotes: mechanisms and consequences. J Cell Biol 164:341-346, 2004

[79] Harding,HP, Zhang,Y, Zeng,H, Novoa,I, Lu,PD, Calfon,M, Sadri,N, Yun,C, Popko,B, Paules,R, Stojdl,DF, Bell,JC, Hettmann,T, Leiden,JM, Ron,D: An integrated stress response regulates amino acid metabolism and resistance to oxidative stress. Mol Cell 11:619-633, 2003

[80] Cullinan,SB, Zhang,D, Hannink,M, Arvisais,E, Kaufman,RJ, Diehl,JA: Nrf2 is a direct PERK substrate and effector of PERK-dependent cell survival. Mol Cell Biol 23:7198-7209, 2003

[81] Cullinan,SB, Diehl,JA: PERK-dependent activation of Nrf2 contributes to redox homeostasis and cell survival following endoplasmic reticulum stress. J Biol Chem 279:20108-20117, 2004

[82] Hu,P, Han,Z, Couvillon,AD, Kaufman,RJ, Exton,JH: Autocrine tumor necrosis factor alpha links endoplasmic reticulum stress to the membrane death receptor pathway through IRE1alpha-mediated NF-kappaB activation and down-regulation of TRAF2 expression. Mol Cell Biol 26:3071-3084, 2006

[83] Davis,RJ: Signal transduction by the JNK group of MAP kinases. Cell 103:239-252, 2000

[84] Yamazaki,H, Hiramatsu,N, Hayakawa,K, Tagawa,Y, Okamura,M, Ogata,R, Huang,T, Nakajima,S, Yao,J, Paton,AW, Paton,JC, Kitamura,M: Activation of the Akt-NF-kappaB pathway by subtilase cytotoxin through the ATF6 branch of the unfolded protein response. J Immunol 183:1480-1487, 2009

[85] Wang,Q, Zhang,H, Zhao,B, Fei,H: IL-1beta caused pancreatic beta-cells apoptosis is mediated in part by endoplasmic reticulum stress via the induction of endoplasmic reticulum Ca2+ release through the c-Jun N-terminal kinase pathway. Mol Cell Biochem 324:183-190, 2009

[86] Delepine,M, Nicolino,M, Barrett,T, Golamaully,M, Lathrop,GM, Julier,C: EIF2AK3, encoding translation initiation factor 2-alpha kinase 3, is mutated in patients with Wolcott-Rallison syndrome. Nat Genet 25:406-409, 2000

[87] Oyadomari,S, Mori,M: Roles of CHOP/GADD153 in endoplasmic reticulum stress. Cell Death Differ 11:381-389, 2004

[88] Messmer,UK, Brune,B: Nitric oxide-induced apoptosis: p53-dependent and p53-independent signalling pathways. Biochem J 319 (Pt 1):299-305, 1996

[89] Viner,RI, Ferrington,DA, Williams,TD, Bigelow,DJ, Schoneich,C: Protein modification during biological aging: selective tyrosine nitration of the SERCA2a isoform of the sarcoplasmic reticulum Ca2+-ATPase in skeletal muscle. Biochem J 340 (Pt 3): 657-669, 1999

[90] Xu,KY, Huso,DL, Dawson,TM, Bredt,DS, Becker,LC: Nitric oxide synthase in cardiac sarcoplasmic reticulum. Proc Natl Acad Sci U S A 96:657-662, 1999

[91] Oyadomari,S, Takeda,K, Takiguchi,M, Gotoh,T, Matsumoto,M, Wada,I, Akira,S, Araki,E, Mori,M: Nitric oxide-induced apoptosis in pancreatic beta cells is mediated by the endoplasmic reticulum stress pathway. Proc Natl Acad Sci U S A 98:10845-10850, 2001

[92] Xu,L, Eu,JP, Meissner,G, Stamler,JS: Activation of the cardiac calcium release channel (ryanodine receptor) by poly-S-nitrosylation. Science 279:234-237, 1998

[93] Harding,HP, Zeng,H, Zhang,Y, Jungries,R, Chung,P, Plesken,H, Sabatini,DD, Ron,D: Diabetes mellitus and exocrine pancreatic dysfunction in perk-/- mice reveals a role for translational control in secretory cell survival. Mol Cell 7:1153-1163, 2001

[94] Zhang,W, Feng,D, Li,Y, Iida,K, McGrath,B, Cavener,DR: PERK EIF2AK3 control of pancreatic beta cell differentiation and proliferation is required for postnatal glucose homeostasis. Cell Metab 4:491-497, 2006

[95] Araki,E, Oyadomari,S, Mori,M: Endoplasmic reticulum stress and diabetes mellitus. Intern Med 42:7-14, 2003

[96] Mathis,D, Vence,L, Benoist,C: beta-Cell death during progression to diabetes. Nature 414:792-798, 2001

[97] Fonseca,SG, Fukuma,M, Lipson,KL, Nguyen,LX, Allen,JR, Oka,Y, Urano,F: WFS1 is a novel component of the unfolded protein response and maintains homeostasis of the endoplasmic reticulum in pancreatic beta-cells. J Biol Chem 280:39609-39615, 2005

[98] Seo,HY, Kim,YD, Lee,KM, Min,AK, Kim,MK, Kim,HS, Won,KC, Park,JY, Lee,KU, Choi,HS, Park,KG, Lee,IK: Endoplasmic reticulum stress-induced activation of activating transcription factor 6 decreases insulin gene expression via up-regulation of orphan nuclear receptor small heterodimer partner. Endocrinology 149:3832-3841, 2008

[99] Eizirik,DL, Cardozo,AK, Cnop,M: The role for endoplasmic reticulum stress in diabetes mellitus. Endocr Rev 29:42-61, 2008

[100] Laybutt,DR, Preston,AM, Akerfeldt,MC, Kench,JG, Busch,AK, Biankin,AV, Biden,TJ: Endoplasmic reticulum stress contributes to beta cell apoptosis in type 2 diabetes. Diabetologia 50:752-763, 2007

http://dx.doi.org/10.5772/52644

[101] Eizirik,DL, Colli,ML, Ortis,F: The role of inflammation in insulitis and beta-cell loss in type 1 diabetes. Nat Rev Endocrinol 5:219-226, 2009

[102] Gurzov,EN, Ortis,F, Cunha,DA, Gosset,G, Li,M, Cardozo,AK, Eizirik,DL: Signaling by IL-1beta+IFN-gamma and ER stress converge on DP5/Hrk activation: a novel mechanism for pancreatic beta-cell apoptosis. Cell Death Differ 16:1539-1550, 2009

[103] Cardozo,AK, Ortis,F, Storling,J, Feng,YM, Rasschaert,J, Tonnesen,M, Van,EF, Mandrup-Poulsen,T, Herchuelz,A, Eizirik,DL: Cytokines downregulate the sarcoendoplasmic reticulum pump Ca2+ ATPase 2b and deplete endoplasmic reticulum Ca2+, leading to induction of endoplasmic reticulum stress in pancreatic beta-cells. Diabetes 54:452-461, 2005

[104] Rutkowski,DT, Kaufman,RJ: A trip to the ER: coping with stress. Trends Cell Biol 14:20-28, 2004

[105] Ron,D: Proteotoxicity in the endoplasmic reticulum: lessons from the Akita diabetic mouse. J Clin Invest 109:443-445, 2002

[106] Preston,AM, Gurisik,E, Bartley,C, Laybutt,DR, Biden,TJ: Reduced endoplasmic reticulum (ER)-to-Golgi protein trafficking contributes to ER stress in lipotoxic mouse beta cells by promoting protein overload. Diabetologia 52:2369-2373, 2009

[107] Liu,H, Bowes,RC, III, van de,WB, Sillence,C, Nagelkerke,JF, Stevens,JL: Endoplasmic reticulum chaperones GRP78 and calreticulin prevent oxidative stress, Ca2+ disturbances, and cell death in renal epithelial cells. J Biol Chem 272:21751-21759, 1997

[108] Haeri,M, Knox,BE: Endoplasmic Reticulum Stress and Unfolded Protein Response Pathways: Potential for Treating Age-related Retinal Degeneration. J Ophthalmic Vis Res 7:45-59, 2012

[109] Harding,HP, Zhang,Y, Bertolotti,A, Zeng,H, Ron,D: Perk is essential for translational regulation and cell survival during the unfolded protein response. Mol Cell 5:897-904, 2000

[110] Urano,F, Wang,X, Bertolotti,A, Zhang,Y, Chung,P, Harding,HP, Ron,D: Coupling of stress in the ER to activation of JNK protein kinases by transmembrane protein kinase IRE1. Science 287:664-666, 2000

[111] Zheng,C, Kabaleeswaran,V, Wang,Y, Cheng,G, Wu,H: Crystal structures of the TRAF2: cIAP2 and the TRAF1: TRAF2: cIAP2 complexes: affinity, specificity, and regulation. Mol Cell 38:101-113, 2010

[112] Habelhah,H, Takahashi,S, Cho,SG, Kadoya,T, Watanabe,T, Ronai,Z: Ubiquitination and translocation of TRAF2 is required for activation of JNK but not of p38 or NF-kappaB. EMBO J 23:322-332, 2004

[113] Yoneda,T, Imaizumi,K, Oono,K, Yui,D, Gomi,F, Katayama,T, Tohyama,M: Activation of caspase-12, an endoplastic reticulum (ER) resident caspase, through tumor ne-

crosis factor receptor-associated factor 2-dependent mechanism in response to the ER stress. J Biol Chem 276:13935-13940, 2001

[114] Nakagawa,T, Zhu,H, Morishima,N, Li,E, Xu,J, Yankner,BA, Yuan,J: Caspase-12 mediates endoplasmic-reticulum-specific apoptosis and cytotoxicity by amyloid-beta. Nature 403:98-103, 2000

[115] Rao,RV, Hermel,E, Castro-Obregon,S, del,RG, Ellerby,LM, Ellerby,HM, Bredesen,DE: Coupling endoplasmic reticulum stress to the cell death program. Mechanism of caspase activation. J Biol Chem 276:33869-33874, 2001

[116] Hitomi,J, Katayama,T, Eguchi,Y, Kudo,T, Taniguchi,M, Koyama,Y, Manabe,T, Yamagishi,S, Bando,Y, Imaizumi,K, Tsujimoto,Y, Tohyama,M: Involvement of caspase-4 in endoplasmic reticulum stress-induced apoptosis and Abeta-induced cell death. J Cell Biol 165:347-356, 2004

[117] Cheung,HH, Lynn,KN, Liston,P, Korneluk,RG: Involvement of caspase-2 and caspase-9 in endoplasmic reticulum stress-induced apoptosis: a role for the IAPs. Exp Cell Res 312:2347-2357, 2006

[118] Yamamoto,K, Ichijo,H, Korsmeyer,SJ: BCL-2 is phosphorylated and inactivated by an ASK1/Jun N-terminal protein kinase pathway normally activated at G(2)/M. Mol Cell Biol 19:8469-8478, 1999

[119] Putcha,GV, Le,S, Frank,S, Besirli,CG, Clark,K, Chu,B, Alix,S, Youle,RJ, LaMarche,A, Maroney,AC, Johnson,EM, Jr.: JNK-mediated BIM phosphorylation potentiates BAX-dependent apoptosis. Neuron 38:899-914, 2003

[120] Lei,K, Davis,RJ: JNK phosphorylation of Bim-related members of the Bcl2 family induces Bax-dependent apoptosis. Proc Natl Acad Sci U S A 100:2432-2437, 2003

[121] Nishitoh,H, Matsuzawa,A, Tobiume,K, Saegusa,K, Takeda,K, Inoue,K, Hori,S, Kakizuka,A, Ichijo,H: ASK1 is essential for endoplasmic reticulum stress-induced neuronal cell death triggered by expanded polyglutamine repeats. Genes Dev 16:1345-1355, 2002

[122] McCullough,KD, Martindale,JL, Klotz,LO, Aw,TY, Holbrook,NJ: Gadd153 sensitizes cells to endoplasmic reticulum stress by down-regulating Bcl2 and perturbing the cellular redox state. Mol Cell Biol 21:1249-1259, 2001

[123] Matsumoto,M, Minami,M, Takeda,K, Sakao,Y, Akira,S: Ectopic expression of CHOP (GADD153) induces apoptosis in M1 myeloblastic leukemia cells. FEBS Lett 395:143-147, 1996

[124] Zinszner,H, Kuroda,M, Wang,X, Batchvarova,N, Lightfoot,RT, Remotti,H, Stevens,JL, Ron,D: CHOP is implicated in programmed cell death in response to impaired function of the endoplasmic reticulum. Genes Dev 12:982-995, 1998

[125] Bandurska-Stankiewicz,E, Wiatr,D: [Programme preventing vision loss due to diabetes]. Klin Oczna 109:359-362, 2007

[126] Cheung,N, Wong,TY: Diabetic retinopathy and systemic vascular complications. Prog Retin Eye Res 27:161-176, 2008

[127] Studholme,S: Diabetic retinopathy. J Perioper Pract 18:205-210, 2008

[128] Monhart,V: [Diabetes mellitus, hypertension and kidney]. Vnitr Lek 54:499-504, 507, 2008

[129] Navarro-Gonzalez,JF, Mora-Fernandez,C: The role of inflammatory cytokines in diabetic nephropathy. J Am Soc Nephrol 19:433-442, 2008

[130] Boulton,AJ: Diabetic neuropathy: classification, measurement and treatment. Curr Opin Endocrinol Diabetes Obes 14:141-145, 2007

[131] Cornell,RS, Ducic,I: Painful diabetic neuropathy. Clin Podiatr Med Surg 25:347-360, 2008

[132] Otto-Buczkowska,E, Kazibutowska,Z, Soltyk,J, Machnica,L: [Neuropathy and type 1 diabetes mellitus]. Endokrynol Diabetol Chor Przemiany Materii Wieku Rozw 14:109-116, 2008

[133] Gardner,SE, Frantz,RA: Wound bioburden and infection-related complications in diabetic foot ulcers. Biol Res Nurs 10:44-53, 2008

[134] Malgrange,D: [Physiopathology of the diabetic foot]. Rev Med Interne 29 Suppl 2:S231-S237, 2008

[135] Ochoa,O, Torres,FM, Shireman,PK: Chemokines and diabetic wound healing. Vascular 15:350-355, 2007

[136] Anselmino,M, Gohlke,H, Mellbin,L, Ryden,L: Cardiovascular prevention in patients with diabetes and prediabetes. Herz 33:170-177, 2008

[137] Inoguchi,T, Takayanagi,R: [Role of oxidative stress in diabetic vascular complications]. Fukuoka Igaku Zasshi 99:47-55, 2008

[138] Marwick,TH: Diabetic heart disease. Postgrad Med J 84:188-192, 2008

Chapter 9

Biochemical Evaluation of Oxidative Stress in Type 1 Diabetes

Donovan A. McGrowder,
Lennox Anderson-Jackson and
Tazhmoye V. Crawford

Additional information is available at the end of the chapter

http://dx.doi.org/10.5772/52836

1. Introduction

1.1. Type 1 diabetes mellitus

Diabetes mellitus is considered to be one of the most common chronic diseases worldwide, and recognized as one of the leading causes of morbidity and mortality (American Diabetes Association, 2010). It has been reported that the prevalence of diabetes mellitus will increase from 6% to over 10% in the next decade (Rosen et al., 2001). According to the World Health Organization in 2000, a total of 171 million people in all age groups worldwide (2.8% of the global population) have been affected by diabetes mellitus, and the number of persons is expected to increase to 366 million (4.4% of the global population) by 2030 (Wild et al., 2004).

Type 1 diabetes mellitus accounts for 5-10% of all diagnosed cases of diabetes mellitus, and exhibits hyperglycemia as its hallmark. It is caused by pancreatic β-islet cell failure with resulting insulin deficiency mortality and risk factors may be autoimmune, genetic, or environmental (American Diabetes Association, 2004). Type 1 diabetes mellitus is an autoimmune disorder involving immune-mediated recognition of islet β-cells by auto-reactive T cells. This subsequently leads to the liberation of pro-inflammatory cytokines and reactive oxygen species. There is destruction of pancreatic β-cells in the islets of Langerhans and loss of insulin secretion (Delmastro & Piganelli, 2011). The Jun kinase pathway is also activated by the pro-inflammatory cytokines, and there is evidence that oxidative stress is involved in β-cell destruction (Kaneto et al., 2007). The loss of β-cell mass consequential to the activation of pro-apoptotic signaling events is increasingly recognized as a causal and committed stage in the development of type 1 diabetes mellitus (Watson & Loweth, 2009).

Moreover, pancreatic β-cells are sensitive to cytotoxic damage caused by reactive oxygen species as gene expression and activity of antioxidant enzymes such as glutathione peroxidase activity is decreased in these cells (Lenzen et al., 1996).

Increasing evidence in both experimental and clinical studies suggests that oxidative stress plays a central role in the onset of diabetes mellitus as well as in the development of vascular and neurologic complications of the disease (Niedowicz & Daleke, 2005). Studies advancing the role of oxidative stress in vascular endothelial cells proposed that oxidative stress mediate the diversion of glycolytic intermediates into pathological pathways (Rolo & Palmeira, 2006; Turk, 2010). Oxidative stress is increased in diabetes mellitus owing to an increase in the production of oxygen free radicals and a deficiency in antioxidant defense mechanisms. Free radicals are formed disproportionately in diabetes by glucose oxidation, non-enzymatic glycation of proteins, and the subsequent oxidative degradation of glycated proteins (Rodiño-Janeiro et al., 2010). Abnormally high levels of free radicals and the simultaneous decline of antioxidant defense mechanisms can lead to damage of cellular organelles and enzymes, increased lipid peroxidation, and development of insulin resistance (Ceriello, 2006).

This review will explore recent evidence in the literature of the use of biomarkers to assess oxidative stress which is recognized as a significant mediator in the development of macrovascular or cardiovascular complication in type 1 diabetes mellitus, as well as the potential for prevention of complications through the use of antioxidants. There is also a search for other biomarker of oxidative stress which might be clinically useful in patients with diabetes mellitus. Such a biomarker could potentially indicate the severity of disease, identify those at increased risk of complications and monitor response to treatment.

2. Oxidative stress and beta-cell destruction

Impairment in the oxidant/antioxidant equilibrium creates a condition known as oxidative stress. There is a complex interaction between antioxidants and oxidants such as reactive oxygen species, which modulates the generation of oxidative stress. Oxidative stress takes place in a cellular system when the generation of reactive oxygen species increases and overwhelms the body's antioxidant capacity and defenses (Baynes, 1991). If the free radicals are not removed by the cellular antioxidants, they may attack and damage lipids, carbohydrates, proteins and nucleic acids (Baynes & Thorpe, 1999).

Oxidative stress is known to be a component of molecular and cellular tissue damage mechanisms in a wide spectrum of human diseases (Maritim et al., 2003; Isabella et al., 2006). There is growing evidence that have connected oxidative stress to a variety of pathological conditions, including cancer, cardiovascular diseases, chronic inflammatory disease, post-ischaemic organ injury, diabetes mellitus, xenobiotic/drug toxicity, and rheumatoid arthritis (El Faramawy & Rizk, 2011; Samanthi et al., 2011). In recent years, much attention has been focused on the role of oxidative stress. It has been reported that oxidative stress participates in the progression and pathogenesis of secondary diabetic complications. This includes impairment of insulin action and elevation of the complication incidence (Ceriello, 2006). Furthermore, there is evidence for the role of reactive oxygen species and oxidative stress in the development of type 1 diabetic complications including retinopathy, nephropathy, neuropathy, and accelerated coronary artery disease (Phillips et al., 2004; Niedowicz & Daleke, 2005).

It has also been reported that oxidative stress induced by reactive oxygen and nitrogen species is critically involved in the impairment of β-cell function, and thus play a role in the pathology of type 1 diabetes mellitus (West, 2000). Islet β-cells are highly susceptible to oxidative stress because of their reduced levels of endogenous antioxidants (*Azevedo-Martins et al., 2003; Kajikawa et al., 2002).* With decreased antioxidant capacity, β-cells are extremely sensitive towards oxidative stress. Cell metabolism and potassium (adenosine-5′-triphosphate) channels in β-cells are important targets for reactive oxygen species and other oxidants. The alterations of potassium (adenosine-5′-triphosphate) channel activity by the oxidants, is crucial for oxidant-induced dysfunction as genetic ablation of potassium (adenosine-5′-triphosphate) channels attenuates the effects of oxidative stress on β-cell function (Drews, 2010).

Oxidative stress may reduce insulin sensitivity and damage the β-cells within the pancreas. The reactive oxygen species produced by oxidative stress can penetrate through cell membranes and cause damage to the β-cells of pancreas (Chen et al., 2005; Lepore et al., 2004). Reactive oxygen species produced from free fatty acids can cause mitochondrial deoxyribonucleic acid damage and impaired pancreatic β-cell function (Rachek et al., 2006). Mitochondrial and nitrogen oxides (NO_x)-derived reactive oxygen species have been implicated in β-cell destruction and subsequently type 1 diabetes mellitus. Furthermore, increased glucose can cause rapid induction of the Krebs cycle within the β-cell mitochondria, leading to augmented reactive oxygen species production (Newsholme et al., 2007). The superoxide leaked from the mitochondria can contribute to the formation of hydrogen peroxide which may play a role in uncoupling glucose metabolism from insulin secretion (Maechler et al., 1999).

3. Oxidative stress induced by hyperglycaemia in type 1diabetes

3.1. Pathways involved in the production of oxidants

There are multiple sources of reactive oxygen species production in diabetes including those of non-mitochondrial and mitochondrial origins. Reactive oxygen species accelerates four important molecular mechanisms that are involved in oxidative tissue damage induced by hyperglycemia. These four pathways are increased advanced glycation end product, increased hexosamine pathway flux, activation of protein kinase C, and increased polyol pathway flux (also known as the sorbitol-aldose reductase pathway) (Rolo & Palmeira, 2006).

In the polyol pathway, the two enzymes aldose reductase and sorbitol dehydrogenase cause reactive oxygen species production. Glucose is reduced to sorbitol through the use of reduced nicotinamide adenine dinucleotide phosphate, a reaction catalyzed by aldose reductase. This pathway metabolizes 30 - 35% of the glucose present during hyperglycemia. The available reduced nicotinamide adenine dinucleotide phosphate is depleted resulting in the reduction of glutathione regeneration and nitric oxide synthase activity (Ramana et al., 2003). The oxidation of sorbitol to fructose with the concomitant production of reduced nicotinamide adenine dinucleotide is catalyzed by sorbitol dehydrogenase. The reduced nicotinamide adenine dinucleotide phosphate may be used by nicotinamide adenine dinucleotide phosphate oxidases to generate superoxide anion (Moore & Roberts, 1998). Vitamin C supplementation has been found to be effective in reducing sorbitol accumulation in the red blood cells of diabetic patients. In a study conducted by Cunningham et al. (1994) who investigated the effect of two different doses of vitamin C supplements (100 and 600 mg) during a 58 day trial on young adults with type 1 diabetes mellitus, vitamin C supplementation at either dose within 30 days normalized sorbitol levels.

Glucose at high concentrations undergoes non-enzymatic reactions with primary amino groups of proteins to form glycated residues called Amadori products. These early glycation products undergo further complex reactions, such as rearrangement, dehydration, and condensation, to become irreversibly cross-linked, heterogeneous fluorescent derivatives called advanced glycation end products (Thornalley, 2002). The advanced glycation end products binds to a cell surface receptor known as receptor for advanced glycation end product. As a result of interaction of advanced glycation end products, with receptor for advanced end product, there is the induction of the synthesis of reactive oxygen species via a mechanism which involves localization of pro-oxidant molecules at the cell surface (Yan et al., 1994) and the participation of activated nicotinamide adenine dinucleotide phosphate oxidase (Wautier et a., 2001). The reactive aldehydes methylglyoxal and glyoxal are produced from enzymatic and non-enzymatic degradation of glucose, lipid and protein catabolism, and lipid peroxidation. These aldehydes form advanced glycation end products with proteins that are implicated in diabetic complications. Han et al. (2007) assessed plasma methylglyoxal and glyoxal using a novel liquid chromatography-mass spectrophotometry method in 56 young patients (6 - 22 years) with type 1 diabetes mellitus without complications. They found that mean plasma methylglyoxal and glyoxal levels were higher in the diabetic patients compared with their non-diabetic counterparts. They suggest that increased plasma methylglyoxal and glyoxal levels give an indication of future diabetic complications and emphasized the need for aggressive management (Han et al., 2007).

It has been shown that through receptor for advanced glycation end products mediated effects, advanced glycation end product induces reactive oxygen species production possibly through an nicotinamide adenine dinucleotide phosphate oxidase, and the subsequent expression of inflammatory mediators and activation of redox-sensitive transcription factors (Wautier et al., 2001; Schmidt et al., 1996). Furthermore, advanced glycation end products, binding to receptor for advanced glycation end product activate protein kinase C-α-mediated activation of nuclear factor-κB (NFκβ) and nicotinamide adenine dinucleotide phosphate oxidase. This may cause the generation of mitochondrial reactive oxygen species and induce the production of various inflammatory cytokines further aggravating oxidative stress (Simm et al., 1997).

http://dx.doi.org/10.5772/52836

Advanced glycation end product in high concentration in body is toxic and can modify the structure of intracellular proteins especially those involved in gene transcription, and can cause damage to biological membranes and the endothelium. It may diffuse to the extracellular space and directly modify extracellular proteins such as laminin and fibronectin to disturb signaling between the matrix and cells that act via receptor for advanced glycation end products, which is present on many vascular cells (Bierhaus et al. 1998). In addition, advanced glycation end products can modify blood proteins such as albumin, causing them to bind to advanced glycation end product receptors on macrophages/mesangial cells and increase the production of growth factors and proinflammatory cytokines (Brownlee, 2005). Kostolanská et al. (2009) observed significantly higher glycated hemoglobin, serum advanced glycation end products and advanced oxidation protein products concentrations in 81 patients with type 1 diabetes mellitus compared with controls. They suggest that the measurement of glycated hemoglobin, serum advanced glycation end products and advanced oxidation protein products may be useful to predict the risk of development of diabetic complications (Kostolanská et al., 2009).

Antioxidants or antibodies against receptor for advanced glycation end product prevent both oxidative stress and the downstream signaling pathways that can be activated by ligation of receptor for advanced glycation end product. Advanced glycation end product-mediated reaction oxygen species production is implicated in diabetic vascular complications and in blood vessel endothelial activation (Cameron & Cotter, 1999; Mullarkey et al., 1990). The formation and accumulation of advanced glycation end products have been involved in the development and progression of diabetic micro- and macroangiopathy. The advanced glycation end product-receptor for advanced glycation end product interaction produces oxidative stress and subsequently evokes thrombosis and vascular inflammation, thereby playing an important role in diabetic vascular complications (Yamagishi, 2009; Niiya et al., 2006). In a recent study, median levels of malondialdehyde and increased plasma levels of soluble receptor for advanced glycation end product were found in 42 type 1 diabetic patients during the early years after diagnosis (0-10 years). These findings suggest that increased plasma levels of soluble receptor for advanced glycation end product in type 1diabetes may provide protection against cell damage and may be sufficient to eliminate excessive circulating malondialdehyde during early years after disease onset (Reis et al., 2012).

4. Free radicals formed during oxidative stress

4.1. Reactive oxygen species in type 1 diabetes

Reactive oxygen species consist of oxygen free radicals such as superoxide anion ($O_2^{\bullet-}$), hydrogen peroxide (H_2O_2), hydroxyl radical ($^{\bullet}OH$), singlet oxygen, nitric oxide, and peroxynitrite (Chong et al., 2005). Most of these free radicals are produced at low concentrations during normal physiological conditions in the body and are scavenged by endogenous enzymatic and non-enzymatic antioxidant systems that include superoxide dismutase, glutathione peroxidase, catalase, and small molecule substances such as vitamins C and E.

Reactive oxygen species induced tissue injury as well as they are involved in signaling pathways and gene expression (Ha & Lee, 2000). Excess generation of reactive oxygen species such as superoxide anion, hydrogen peroxide, hydroxyl radical and reactive nitrogen species such as nitric oxide oxidize target cellular proteins, nucleic acids, or membrane lipids and damage their cellular structure and function (Brownlee, 2001). There is also evidence that reactive oxygen species also regulate the expression of genes encoding for proteins involved in immune response, inflammation and cell death (Ho & Bray, 1999).

Hydroxyl radicals, hydrogen peroxide, and superoxide anion are byproducts of xanthine oxidase. Xanthine oxidase and xanthine dehydrogenase catalyze the conversion of hypoxanthine to xanthine and then to uric acid, with the former reducing oxygen as an electron acceptor while the latter can reduce either oxygen or nicotinamide adenine dinucleotide (NAD^+) (Fatehi-Hassanabad et al., 2010). Superoxide anion is also produced by nicotinamide adenine dinucleotide phosphate oxidases and cytochrome P450, and is the most commonly occurring oxygen free radical that produces hydrogen peroxide by dismutation. This is achieved via the Haber-Weiss reaction in the presence of ferrous iron by copper (Cu)-superoxide dismutase or manganese (Mn)-superoxide dismutase. Mitochondrial superoxide anion is produced from excess reduced nicotinamide adenine dinucleotide produced in the Krebs cycle (Fubini & Hubbard, 2003). Elevated free or non-esterified fatty acids in type 1 diabetic patients enter the Krebs cycle causing the production of acetyl-CoA to subsequently excess reduced nicotinamide adenine dinucleotide (Steinberg & Baron, 2002). The superoxide anion undergo dismutation to hydrogen peroxide, which if not degraded by catalase or glutathione peroxidase, and in the presence of transition metals, can lead to production of hydroxyl radical, the most active oxygen free radical. Hydroxyl radical alternatively may be formed through an interaction between superoxide anion and nitric oxide (Fubini & Hubbard, 2003; Wolff, 1993).

Superoxide anion can also react with nitric oxide to form the reactive peroxynitrite radicals (Hogg & Kalyanaraman, 1998). Excess production of superoxide anion by the mitochondrial electron transport chain, induced by hyperglycaemia has been reported to have a role in triggering protein kinase C, hexosamine and polyol pathway fluxes, and advanced glycation end product formation pathways which are involved in the pathogenesis of diabetic complications (Nishikawa et al., 2000; Brownlee, 2001). In a study conducted by Hsu et al. (2006), plasma superoxide anion (determined by a chemiluminescent assay) gave photoemission which was considerably higher in 47 type 1 diabetic children than those in controls. The findings confirm the presence of oxidative stress in children with type 1 diabetes mellitus (Hsu et al., 2006).

4.2. Reactive nitrogen species in type 1 diabetes

Nitric oxide is an important regulator of endothelial function and the impairment of its activity is determinant of the endothelial dysfunction (Ignarro, 2002). It is an important vascular target for ROS and is produced by constitutive and inducible nitric oxide synthases. These enzymes oxidize L-arginine to citrulline in the presence of biopterin, reduced nicotinamide adenine dinucleotide phosphate, and oxygen (Alp & Channon, 2004). Constitutive endothelial nitric oxide synthase contains reductase and oxygenase domains that are connected by a calmodulin-binding region and requires cofactor groups such as heme, flavin mononucleotide, flavin adenine dinucleotide, tetrahydrobiopterin, and Ca^{2+}-calmodulin for activation (Gorren & Mayer, 2002; Andrew & Mayer, 1999). If there is none or insufficient L-arginine, the endothelial nitric oxide synthase produce superoxide instead of nitric oxide and this is referred to as the uncoupled state of nitric oxide synthase (Channon, 2004).

Oxidative stress decreases the bioavailability of endothelium-derived nitric oxide in diabetic patients. In a 3-year longitudinal study involving 37 patients with recent-onset (less than 2 years) type 1 diabetes, oxidative stress was evident by elevated malondialdehyde excretion and serum NO_x (nitrate and nitrite) (Hoeldtke et al., 2011). In a latter study, NO_x was also higher in 99 female subjects with uncomplicated type 1 diabetes (duration disease <10 years) compared with 44 sex-matched controls (Pitocco et al., 2009). Mylona Karayanni et al. (2006) examined possible correlation between oxidative stress parameters and adhesion molecules derived from endothelial/platelet activation, P-selectin and tetranectin in a group of juveniles with type 1 diabetes mellitus. Significantly elevated NO_x and lipid hydroperoxide levels, elevated tetranectin and P-selectin plasma levels, and lower glutathione peroxidase activity were found in the diabetic children compared with healthy controls. Based on these findings the authors suggested that decreased anti-oxidative protection from overproduction of lipid hydroperoxide and NO_x overproduction is present in juveniles with type 1 diabetes mellitus. There is also a parallel endothelial/platelet activation which contributes to the vascular complications of type 1 diabetes mellitus (Mylona-Karayanni et al., 2006).

Nitric oxide can react with superoxide to form peroxynitrite which in turn oxidizes tetrahydrobiopterin and causes further uncoupling of nitric oxide formation (Yung et al., 2003). In diabetes mellitus, elevated glucose may cause an increase in the expression of both reduced nicotinamide adenine dinucleotide phosphate and of inducible nitric oxide synthase via the activation of NF-κB, (Spitaler & Graier, 2002). The upregulated inducible nitric oxide synthase will synthesize the superoxide anion instead of nitric oxide, leading to oxidative and nitrosative stress (Llorens & Nava, 2003). The stable protein adduct, nitrotyrosine, is a marker of peroxynitrite (Ischiropoulos, 1998) and nitrogen dioxide (Prutz et al., 1985). Moreover, increased oxidative and nitrosative stress activates poly(ADP-ribose) polymerase-1, which substrate, nicotinamide adenine dinucleotide (NAD^+) as well as slows the rate of glycolysis, electron transport, and adenosine triphosphate formation (Pacher & Szabó, 2006).

The formation of peroxynitrite can further lead to the generation of peroxynitrous acid. The spontaneous decomposition of peroxynitrous acid results in the formation of hydroxyl radicals that can cause endothelial damage (Elliott et al., 1993; Beckman & Koppenol, 1996) thereby reduces the efficacy the endothelium-derived vasodilator system that participates in the general homeostasis of the vasculature (Benz et al., 2002). Overproduction of both nitric oxide and superoxide anion has been reported in response to hyperglycemia (Cosentino et al., 1997; Ceriello et al., 2002), and nitric oxide may work through peroxynitrite to directly alter cellular structure and function (Pfeiffer et al., 2001). Increased nitric oxide levels have been reported in both saliva and plasma of diabetic patients in comparison to healthy subjects (Astaneie et al., 2005).

5. Enzymatics and non-enzymatic antioxidants

5.1. Intracellular enzymes activity in type 1 diabetes

A number of natural antioxidants are present in the body to scavenge oxygen free radicals and prevent oxidative damage to biological membranes. Antioxidant defense mechanisms involve both non-enzymatic and enzymatic strategies. One group of these antioxidants is intracellular enzymes such as manganese superoxide dismutase, catalase, glutathione peroxidase, and glutathione-S-transferases. These enzymes represent a protective mechanism against the damage caused by the oxidative stress and most of these enzymes are polymorphic (Fang et al., 2002; Mates et al., 1999).

Superoxide dismutase is considered a primary enzyme since it is involved in the direct elimination of reactive oxygen synthase (Halliwell, 1994). Isoforms of superoxide dismutase are Cu/Zn-superoxide dismutase which is found in both the cytoplasm and the nucleus, and Mn-superoxide dismutase that is present in the mitochondria. The latter can be released into extracellular space (Reiter et al., 2000). Cu/Zn-superoxide dismutase over-expression inhibits oxidized low density lipoprotein which is can elevate deoxyribonucleic acid binding activity of activator protein-1 and NF-κB (Yung et al., 2006). Superoxide dismutase catalyzes the conversion of superoxide anion radicals produced in the body to hydrogen peroxide. This decreases the possibility of superoxide anion interacting with nitric oxide to form reactive peroxynitrite (Reiter et al., 2000). Low Cu/Zn-superoxide dismutase is a potential early marker of susceptibility to diabetic vascular disease. Suys et al. (2007) found that erythrocyte superoxide dismutase activity and Cu/Zn-superoxide dismutase were higher in type 1 diabetic subjects and was positively associated with flow-mediated dilatation. Based on these findings the authors suggest that higher circulating Cu/Zn-superoxide dismutase could protect type 1 diabetic children and adolescents against endothelial dysfunction (Suys et al., 2007). Furthermore, Reznick and colleagues analyzed both serum and salivary superoxide dismutase activity in 20 patients with type 1 diabetes mellitus. A significant association was found between the level of glycemic control as indicated by the glycated hemoglobin values and an increase in both salivary and serum superoxide dismutase activity (Reznick et al., 2006). On the contrary, in a study which assessed correlations between increase of oxidative stress and the development of microalbuminuria in 87 type 1 diabetic patients (44 with normal urinary protein excretion, and 43 with microalbuminuria), there was a decreased in activity of superoxide dismutase. This was associated with an increased microalbuminuria in type 1 diabetic patients (Artenie et al., 2005).

Selenium-dependent glutathione peroxidase works in conjunction with superoxide dismutase in protecting cell proteins and membranes against oxidative damage. In the literature, glutathione peroxidase response to diabetes has been conflicting. Diabetics have been reported to be associated with increased glutathione peroxidase activity in 90 pregnant women with type 1 diabetes mellitus (Djordjevic et al., 2004) and in young diabetic patients (Ndahimana et al., 1996). On the other hand, decreased glutathione peroxidase activity was reported in the early stages of type 1 diabetes in children and adolescents (Dominguez et al., 1998) or unchanged in type 1 diabetic patients with early retina degenerative lesions (Faure et al., 1995). The low glutathione peroxidase activity could be directly explained by either low glutathione content or enzyme inactivation under sever oxidative stress (Faure et al., 1995). However, some authors found no differences between glutathione peroxidase activity of type 1 diabetic patients and control subjects (Jain et al., 1994; Murakami et al., 1993; Majchrzak et al., 2001).

Catalase, located in peroxisomes, decomposes hydrogen peroxide to water and oxygen (Winterbourn & Metodiewa, 1994). In addition, glutathione peroxidase in the mitochondria and the lysosomes also catalyses the conversion of hydrogen peroxide to water and oxygen (Yung et al., 2006). A significant increase in the catalase activity in lymphocytes was found in 40 children with type 1 diabetes during all phases (at the beginning of diabetes, in remission period and in the later chronic course) compared with the control group. The highest catalase activity occurs in the early course of disease followed by a linear decrease and the lowest activity in chronic course (Zivić, 2008). Conversely Dave and colleagues (2007) reported significant decreased glutathione peroxidase, catalase and glutathione, and significant increase in thiobarbituric acid reactive substances concentration in type 1 diabetic patients with and without nephropathy compared with normal healthy individuals (Dave et al., 2007).

5.2. Non-enzymatic antioxidant levels in type 1 diabetes

In addition to enzymatic antioxidants, the major natural antioxidants, most of which are derived from dietary sources are vitamin A, vitamin C or ascorbic acid, vitamin E and carotenoids. Water-soluble vitamin C and fat-soluble vitamin E together make up the antioxidant system for mammalian cells (Engler et al., 2003). Vitamins A, C, and E are obtained from the diet and function to directly detoxify free radicals. Vitamin C forms the first line of defense against plasma lipid peroxidation is considered the most important antioxidant in plasma (Frei et al., 1990). Vitamin C under certain conditions may foster toxicity by generating prooxidants, and is also engaged in the recycling processes which involved the generation of reduced forms of the vitamins. In the processes of regeneration, α-tocopherol is reconstituted when ascorbic acid recycles the tocopherol radical; dihydroascorbic acid, which is formed, is recycled by glutathione (Weber, 1997).

Vitamin E involves all tocopherol and tocotrienol derivatives that comprise the major lipophilic exogenous antioxidant in tissues (Di Mambro et al., 2003). Vitamin E, a component of the total peroxyl radical-trapping antioxidant system reacts directly with superoxide and peroxyl radicals, and singlet oxygen and in so doing protects membranes from lipid peroxidation (Weber & Bendich, 1997). In a study by Gupta et al. 2011 that evaluated the oxidative stress in 20 type 1 diabetic children, reduced glutathione and vitamin E levels were decreased and malondialdehyde levels were elevated compared with controls. After supplementation with vitamin E (600 mg/daily for three months) there was a significant decrease in malondialdehyde levels and significant increase in glutathione and vitamin E. The findings indicate that vitamin E ameliorates oxidative stress in type 1 diabetes mellitus patients and improves antioxidant defense system. In a latter study high-dose vitamin E supplementation (1200 mg/day) reduces markers of oxidative stress and improves antioxidant defense in young patients with type 1 diabetes mellitus. However vitamin E supplementation did not decreased albumin excretion rate in these patients (Giannini et al., 2007).

α-Tocopherol is very effective in lipid peroxidation inhibition and is the primary *in vivo* chain-breaking, lipid-soluble antioxidant in human serum. A reduction in serum α-tocopherol could be attributed to its consumption while scavenging free radicals in lipoproteins or biomembranes (Frei, 1994). In the Pittsburgh Epidemiology of Diabetes Complications Study cohort, a 10-year prospective study of childhood-onset type 1 diabetes, α-tocopherol or γ-tocopherol did not showed protection against incident coronary artery disease overall. However, high α-tocopherol levels among patients with renal disease and in those using vitamin supplements were associated with lower coronary artery disease risk in type 1 diabetes (Costacou et al., 2006). All the antioxidants work in a synergistic manner with each other and against different types of free radicals. This is shown in the way in which vitamin E suppresses the propagation of lipid peroxidation, and vitamin C working with vitamin E inhibits hydroperoxide formation (Laight et al., 2000).

Glutathione functions as a direct free-radical scavenger, and as a co-substrate for glutathione peroxidase activity (Meister & Anderson, 1983). Glutathione, a tri-peptide present in millimolar concentrations is the most prevalent low-molecular weight peptide antioxidant in cells. Reduced glutathione normally plays the role of a direct intracellular free-radical scavenger through interaction with free radicals and is the substrate of many xenobiotic elimination reactions (Gregus et al., 1996). It is also involved in other cellular functions such as the elimination of hydrogen peroxide, detoxification processes such as protection of the sulfhydryl group of cysteine in proteins, and regeneration of oxidized vitamin E (Lu, 1999). In 30 children with type 1 diabetes at onset, there was a significant reduction in all glutathione forms (total, reduced, oxidized, and protein-bound glutathione). This indicates that there is glutathione depletion upon early onset of type 1 diabetes mellitus (Pastore et al., 2012). In another study, Likidlilid et al. (2007) compared the glutathione level, and glutathione peroxidase activity in 20 type 1 diabetic patients (with fasting glucose > 140 mg/dL) and a normal healthy group. They found that the level of red cell reduced glutathione was significantly lower in type 1 diabetic patients but red cell glutathione peroxidase activity was significantly increased. The decrease of red cell glutathione may be due to its higher rate of consumption, increasing glutathione peroxidase activity or a reduction of pentose phosphate pathway, stimulated by insulin, resulting in lowered glutathione recycle (Likidlilid et al., 2007). In a recent study, reduced glutathione and vitamin E levels were decreased and malondialdehyde levels were higher in 20 type 1 diabetic children compared with healthy controls. After supplementation with vitamin E (600 mg/daily for three months), there was a significant decrease in malondialdehyde levels and significant increase in glutathione and vitamin E levels. This shows that vitamin E ameliorates oxidative stress in type 1 diabetic patients and improves antioxidant defense system (Gupta et al., 2011).

Other nonenzymatic antioxidants include α-lipoic acid, mixed carotenoids, coenzyme Q_{10}, several bioflavonoids, antioxidant minerals (copper, zinc, manganese and selenium), and the cofactors (folic acid, vitamins B_1, B_2, B_6, B_{12}). β-carotene is a lipid soluble and chain-breaking antioxidant that effectively quenches singlet oxygen and inhibits lipid peroxida-

http://dx.doi.org/10.5772/52836

tion. At low physiological oxygen pressures, it exhibits effective radical-trapping antioxidant behaviour (Frei, 1994). Coenzyme Q_{10} has been found to have a very important role in mitochondrial bioenergetics. It is an electron carrier-proton translocator in the respiratory chain and potent antioxidant which works by directly scavenging radicals or indirectly by regenerating vitamin E. In a study by Menke and colleagues (2008), plasma concentrations of coenzyme Q_{10} in 39 children with type 1 diabetes mellitus were higher than in healthy children. The findings suggest that elevated plasma concentration and the intracellular redox capacity of coenzyme Q_{10} in diabetic children may contribute to the body's self-protection during a state of enhanced oxidative stress (Menke et al., 2008). In another study, Salardi and colleagues (2004) determine whether serum hydroperoxides as oxidative markers and vitamin E and coenzyme Q_{10} as indexes of antioxidant capacity could be related to metabolic control in 75 unselected children, adolescents, and young adults with type 1 diabetes. Vitamin E and coenzyme Q_{10} were not significantly different from age-matched control subjects. However, there were significant positive correlations between coenzyme Q_{10} and glycated hemoglobin, and vitamin E and glycated hemoglobin. It was also observed that diabetic patients with poor metabolic control and complications had elevated vitamin E levels and coenzyme Q_{10} levels (Salardi et al., 2004).

Small molecules that have antioxidant capacity such as glutathione and uric acid are synthesized or produced within the body (Engler et al., 2003). A study by Maxwell et al. (1997) found significantly reduced total serum antioxidant status in 28 patients with type 1 diabetes mellitus as attributed by lower uric acid and vitamin C levels. Furthermore, multiple regression analysis showed that uric acid, vitamin E and vitamin C were the main contributors to serum total antioxidant activity.

6. Markers of oxidative stress in type 1 diabetes

6.1. Biomarkers of lipid peroxidation in type 1 diabetes

Oxidative stress and its contribution to low-density lipoprotein oxidation have been implicated in the pathogenesis of vascular diabetic complications. Diabetes produces disturbances of lipid profiles, especially an increased susceptibility to lipid peroxidation, which is responsible for increased incidence of atherosclerosis, a major complication of diabetes mellitus (Siu & To, 2002). Polyunsaturated fatty acids with multiple bonds and lipoproteins in the plasma membrane are very susceptible to attack by reactive oxygen species (Esterbauer & Schaur, 1991). The hydroxyl radicals extract a hydrogen atom from one of the carbon atoms in the polyunsaturated fatty acid and lipoproteins, initiating a free radical chain reaction which leads to lipid peroxidation. This characterized by membrane protein damage through subsequent free radical attacks (Halliwell, 1995). Lipid peroxidation can produce advanced products of oxidation, such as aldehydes, alkanes and isoprostanes (Moore & Roberts, 1998). Elevation of lipid peroxidation negatively affects membrane function causing reduced membrane fluidity and changing the activity of membrane bound enzymes and receptors (Acworth et al., 1997).

In diabetes mellitus, persistence of hyperglycemia was reported to cause increased production of oxidative parameters of lipid peroxidation including malondialdehyde. In a study by Firoozrai and colleagues (2007), malondialdehyde levels were significantly elevated in diabetic patients. The level of malondialdehyde was positively correlated with duration of diabetes and glycated hemoglobin and negatively with ferric reducing ability of plasma (Firoozrai et al., 2007). In a latter study that investigated the effect of glycemic control on oxidative stress and the lipid profile of pediatric type 1 diabetes mellitus patients, total cholesterol, low density lipoprotein-cholesterol, apolipoprotein A, apolipoprotein B, and malondialdehyde levels were significantly elevated compared with controls. In addition, serum malondialdehyde levels and malondialdehyde/low density lipoprotein-cholesterol index were significantly elevated in metabolically poorly controlled in relation to metabolically well-controlled diabetic patients. Based on these findings the authors suggested that type 1 diabetic children, especially those who are metabolically poorly controlled are at high risk of atherosclerosis and vascular complications of diabetes mellitus, and that there is a significant relationship between the lipid profile and oxidative stress (Erciyas et al., 2004).

Isoprostanes are prostaglandin-like compounds formed through peroxidation of arachidonic acid, and have been used extensively as biomarkers of lipid peroxidation as a risk factor for atherosclerosis and other diseases (Roberts & Marrow, 2000). Oxidative stress parameters such as advanced oxidation protein products, total peroxyl radical-trapping antioxidant parameter, and F2-isoprostanes (8-epi-prostaglandin-F2: 8-isoPGF2alpha) were not significantly different in 27 pre-pubertal patients with type 1 diabetes mellitus (with less than 5 years of disease) compared with controls (Gleisner et al., 2006). In another study, Flores and colleagues (2004) evaluated the effect of the normalization of blood glucose levels on urinary F2-isoprostanes at the onset of type 1 diabetes in 14 patients. There was a statistically significant reduction in F2-isoprostanes after insulin therapy (after 16 weeks) which was accompanied by a significant reduction in glycated hemoglobin (Flores et al., 2004).

Lipid hydroperoxides are potentially atherogenic and are degraded by enzymes such as paraoxonase-1 and lipoprotein-associated phospholipase A_2 (Van Lenten et al., 2001; Macphee et al., 2005). Paraoxonase-1 is an enzyme associated with high density lipoprotein surface and the antioxidant effect of the latter is partially related to paraoxonase. This enzyme is able to hydrolyze lipid hydroperoxides and to delay or inhibit the initiation of oxidation of lipoproteins induced by metal ions (Watson et al., 1995). It has been suggested that individuals with low paraoxonase-1 activity may have a greater risk of developing diseases such as diabetes mellitus in which oxidative damage and lipid peroxidation are involved, compared with those with high paraoxonase-1 activity (Durrington et al., 2001; Nourooz-Zadehet al., 1995).

Wegner et al. (2011) reported that 80 type 1 diabetic patients had lower paraoxonase-1 arylesterase activity and higher lipid hydroperoxide levels, and that there was a negative correlation between paraoxonase-1arylesterase activity and lipid hydroperoxide levels. In a latter study, paraoxonase-1 activity was reduced in patients with type 1 diabetes mellitus with retinopathy, confirming that oxidative stress could play a role in pathogenesis of diabetic retinopathy (Nowak et al., 2010). A similar finding of lower high density lipoprotein-paraoxonase-1 activity in 31 type 1 diabetic patients compared with the same number of sex-

and age-matched healthy subjects was reported by Ferretti et al. (2004). These findings confirm a linkage between paraoxonase-1 activity and lipid peroxidation of lipoproteins and suggest that the ability of high density lipoprotein to protect erythrocyte membranes might be related to the paraoxonase-1 activity (Ferretti et al., 2004). The low paraoxonase-1 arylesterase activity suggests insufficient high density lipoprotein capacity to protect against lipid oxidation in patients with type 1 diabetes (Wegner et al., 2011). It is also hypothesized that the lower high density lipoprotein protective action against membrane peroxidation and decrease paraoxonase-1 activity in diabetic patients could contribute to acceleration of arteriosclerosis in patients with type 1 diabetes mellitus (Ferretti et al., 2004). Furthermore, there are several studies linking diabetes and even postprandial hyperglycemia with increased low density lipoprotein oxidative susceptibility (Ceriello, 2000). Decreased insulin in diabetes mellitus increases the activity of fatty acyl coenzyme A oxidase, which intiates β-oxidation of fatty acids, resulting in lipid peroxidation (Horie et al., 2006).

6.2. Biomarkers of protein peroxidation and oxidative damage to DNA in type 1 diabetes

High plasma glucose concentrations can increase the levels of glycation and oxidative damage to cellular and plasma proteins in diabetes mellitus. Glycation of proteins is a complex series of reactions where early-stage reactions leads to the formation of the early glycation adduct, fructosyl-lysine and NH_2-terminal fructosyl-amino acids, and later-stage reactions form advanced glycation end products (Thornalley, 2002). The oxidation of proteins produces nitrotyrosine and protein carbonyl derivatives and nitrotyrosine (Adams et al., 2001). The oxidized or nitrosylated products of free radical attack have reduced biological activity, leading to loss of cell signaling, energy metabolism, transport, and other major cellular functions. These altered oxidized products also are targeted for proteosome degradation, further reducing cellular function. There is also cell death through necrotic or apoptotic mechanisms as a result of the accumulation of cellular injury (Rosen et al., 2001).

Carbonyl group formation is considered an early and stable marker for protein oxidation in the body. Diabetes mellitus is associated with carbonyl stress where there is an increase of reactive carbonyl compounds caused by their enhanced formation and/or decreased degradation or excretion (Miyata et al., 1999.) This leads to the formation of advanced glycation end products such as pentosidin and carboxymethyllysine and advanced oxidation protein products, and damage to a number of biologically important compounds (Miayta et al. 1999; Witko-Sarsat et al., 1996). Telci et al. (2000) examined the influence of oxidative stress on oxidative protein damage in 51 young type 1 diabetic patients clinically free of complications and 48 healthy normolipidaemic age-matched controls. The levels of plasma carbonyl and plasma lipid hydroperoxide were increased in adolescent and young adult type 1 diabetic patients compared with controls.

Modifications in endothelial cell function are proposed to play an important role in atherogenesis. These perturbations include increased permeability to circulating lipoproteins particularly low density lipoprotein, increased retention of these lipoproteins, the loss of endothelial cell-directed vasodilatation, and the increased expression of intercellular cell adhesion molecule-1 and vascular cell adhesion molecule-1 (Ross, 1999). Koitka et al. (2004) reported evidence of endothelial dysfunction in patients with type 1 diabetes. In another study of 45 type 1 diabetic children, there was significantly lower peak brachial artery flow-mediated dilation response and increased carotid artery intima-media thickness. This suggests that altered endothelium function in children with type 1 diabetes may predispose them to the development of early atherosclerosis (Jarvisalo et al., 2004). Furthermore, in a double-blind, placebo-controlled, randomized study of 41 young subjects with type I diabetes mellitus, vitamin E supplementation (1,000 IU for three months) had a positive effect on the endothelial function as evident by improved endothelial vasodilator function in both the conduit and resistance vessels (Skyrme-Jones, 2000).

In addition to lipids and proteins, reactive oxygen species reacts with deoxyribonucleic acid resulting in various products, such as 8-hydroxydeoxyguanosine, that is excrete in urine owing to deoxyribonucleic acid repair processes. Urinary 8-hydroxydeoxyguanosine has been proposed as an indicator of oxidative damage to deoxyribonucleic acid. Goodarzi and colleagues (2010) evaluated the relationship between oxidative damage to deoxyribonucleic acid and protein glycation in 32 patients with type 1 diabetes. There were elevated levels of urinary 8-hydroxydeoxyguanosine, glycated hemoglobin, plasma malondialdehyde, and glycated serum protein in 32 patients with type 1 diabetes. There was a significant correlation between urinary 8-hydroxydeoxyguanosine and glycated hemoglobin. The findings indicate that that deoxyribonucleic acid is associated to glycemic control level (Goodarzi et al., 2010). In a study which investigated whether advanced glycation end product production and oxidative stress are augmented in young patients with type 1 diabetes at early clinical stages of the disease, advanced glycation end products, pentosidine, and 8-hydroxydeoxyguanosine and acrolein-lysine were significantly higher in the patients with type 1 diabetes compared with healthy control subjects (Tsukahara et al., 2003).

6.3. Biomarkers of oxidative stress present in breath

Oxidative stress has been implicated in the major complications of diabetes mellitus, including retinopathy, nephropathy, neuropathy and accelerated coronary artery disease (Ceriello & Morocutti, 2000; Androne et al., 2000; Mackness et al., 2002). There is a clinical need for markers of oxidative stress which could potentially identify diabetic patients at increased risk for these complications. The introduction of breath microassays has enhanced the detection of oxidative stress because reactive oxygen species oxidize polyunsaturated fatty acids in membranes to alkanes such as ethane and pentane. These are excreted in the breath as volatile organic compounds (Kneepkens & Lepage, 1994). Another marker of oxidative stress is the breath methylated alkane contour, comprising a three-dimensional display of C4 to C20 alkanes and monomethylated alkanes in the breath (Phillips et al., 2004). Phillips et al. (2004) reported significantly increased volatile organic compounds and breath methylated alkane contour in the breath of type 1 diabetic patients which was independent of glycemic as they did with blood glucose concentration or with glycation hemoglobin levels.

http://dx.doi.org/10.5772/52836

7. Conclusion

This review presented convincing experimental and clinical evidence that the aetiology of oxidative stress in diabetes mellitus arises from a number of mechanisms that includes excessive reactive oxygen species production from the peroxidation of lipids, auto-oxidation of glucose, glycation of proteins, and glycation of antioxidative enzymes, which limit their capacity to detoxify oxygen radicals. There is also evidence that supports the role of hyperglycemia in producing oxidative stress and, eventually, severe endothelial dysfunction in blood vessels of individuals with type 1 diabetes mellitus. The induction of oxidative stress is a key process in the onset and development of diabetic complications, but the precise mechanisms has not been fully elucidated. A number of biomarkers of oxidative stress have been studied in type 1 diabetic patients such as malondialdehyde, F2-isoprostanes, advanced glycation end product and nitrotyrosine. The introduction of breath microassays has enhanced the detection of oxidative stress.

Type 1 diabetic patients have been found to have decreased amounts and efficiency of antioxidant defenses (both enzymatic and non-enzymatic) due to increased consumption of distinct antioxidant components (e.g. intracellular glutathione) or to primarily low levels of antioxidant substances (flavonoids, carotenoids, vitamin E and C). This review also presents small clinical studies that have demonstrated improvements in a variety of oxidative stress biomarkers in type 1 diabetic patients who have received vitamin A, C or E supplements. However, the findings of key prospective randomized controlled antioxidant clinical trials have failed to demonstrate a significant benefit, in the prevention of cardiovascular events. There is a need for continued investigation of the association between reactive oxygen species, type 1 diabetes mellitus and its complications in order to clarify the molecular mechanisms by which increased oxidative stress accelerates the development of diabetic complications. This will have implication for the prevention and development of therapeutic choices for type 1 diabetic patients.

Author details

Donovan A. McGrowder[1], Lennox Anderson-Jackson[2] and Tazhmoye V. Crawford[3]

1 Department of Pathology, Faculty of Medical Sciences, The University of the West Indies, Mona, Kingston, Jamaica

2 Radiology West, Montego Bay, Jamaica

3 Health Policy Department, Independent Health Policy Consultant, Christiana, Manchester, Jamaica

References

[1] Acworth, I.N., Mccabe, D.R. & Maher, T. (1997). The analysis of free radicals, their reaction products, and antioxidants, in: S.I. Baskin, H. Salem (Eds.), Oxidants, Antioxidants and Free Radicals, Taylor and Francis, Washington, DC, Chapter 2.

[2] Adams, S., Green, P., Claxton, R., Simcox, S., Williams, M.V., Walsh, K. & Leeuwenburgh, C. (2001). Reactive carbonyl formation by oxidative and non-oxidative pathways. Front Biosci Vol. 6, pp. A17-A24.

[3] Alp, N.J. & Channon, K.M. (2004). Regulation of endothelial nitric oxide synthase by tetrahydrobiopterin in vascular disease. Arterioscler Thromb Vasc Biol Vol. 24, pp. 413-420.

[4] American Diabetes Association (2010). Diagnosis and classification of diabetes mellitus. J Diabetes Care Vol 33, pp. S62-S69.

[5] American Diabetes Association (2004). Diagnosis and classification of diabetes mellitus. J Diabetes Care Vol. 27, pp. S5-S10.

[6] Andrew, P.J. & Mayer, B. (1999). Enzymatic function of nitric oxide synthases. Cardiovasc Res Vol. 43, pp. 521-531.

[7] Artenie, A., Artenie, R., Ungureanu, D. & Covic, A. (2004). Correlation between increase of oxidative stress and microalbuminuria in type 1 diabetic patients. Rev Med Chir Soc Med Nat Iasi Vol. 108, pp. 777-781.

[8] Astaneie, F., Afshari, M., Mojtahedi, A., Mostafalou, S., Zamani, M.J., Larijani, B. & Abdollahi, M. (2005).Total antioxidant capacity and levels of epidermal growth factor and nitric oxide in blood and saliva of insulin-dependent diabetic patients. Arch Med Res Vol. 36, pp. 376-381.

[9] Azevedo-Martins, A.K., Lortz, S., Lenzen, S., Curi, R., Eizirik, D.L. & Tiedge, M. Improvement of the mitochondrial antioxidant defense status prevents cytokine-induced nuclear factor-kappaB activation in insulin-producing cells. Diabetes Vol. 52, pp. 93-101.

[10] Baynes, J. & Thorpe, S. (1999). Role of oxidative stress in diabetic complications: a new perspective on an old paradigm. Diabetes Vol. 48, pp. 1-9.

[11] Baynes, J.W. (1991). Role of oxidative stress in development of complications in diabetes. Diabetes Vol. 40, pp. 405-412.

[12] Beckman, J.S. & Koppenol, W.H. (1996). Nitric oxide, superoxide, and peroxynitrite: the good, the bad, and ugly. Am J Physiol Vol. 271, pp. C1424-C1437.

[13] Benz, D., Cadet, P., Mantione, K., Zhu, W. & Stefano, G.B. (2002). Total nitric oxide and health - a free radical and scavenger of free radicals. Med Sci Monit Vol. 8, pp. RA1-RA4.

[14] Bierhaus, A., Hofmann, MA, Ziegler, R. & Nawrothn, P.P. (1998). AGEs and their interaction with AGE-receptors in vascular disease and diabetes mellitus 1. The AGE concept. Cardiovasc Res Vol. 37, pp. 586-600.

[15] Brownlee, M. (2001). Biochemistry and molecular cell biology of diabetic complications. Nature Vol. 414, pp. 813-820.

[16] Brownlee, M. (2005). The pathobiology of diabetic complications: a unifying mechanism. Diabetes. Vol. 54, pp. 1615-1625.

[17] Cameron, N.E. & Cotter, M.A. (1999). Effects of antioxidants on nerve and vascular dysfunction in experimental diabetes. Diabetes Res Clin Pract Vol. 45, pp. 137-146.

[18] Ceriello, A. (2006). Oxidative stress and diabetes-associated complications. Endocr Pract Vol. 12(Suppl 1), pp. 60-62.

[19] Ceriello, A. (2000). The post-prandial state and cardiovascular disease: relevance to diabetes mellitus. Diabetes Metab Res Rev Vol. 16, pp. 125-132.

[20] Ceriello, A., Morocutti, A., Mercuri, F., Quagliaro, L., Moro, M., Damante, G. & Viberti GC. (2000). Defective intracellular antioxidant enzyme production in type 1 diabetic patients with nephropathy. Diabetes Vol. 49, pp. 2170-2177.

[21] Ceriello, A., Quagliaro, L., Catone, B., Pascon, R., Piazzola, M., Bais, B., Marra, G., Tonutti, L., Taboga, C. & Motz, E. (2002). Role of hyperglycemia in nitrotyrosine postprandial generation. Diabetes Care Vol. 25, pp. 1439-1443.

[22] Channon, K.M. (2004). Tetrahydrobiopterin: regulator of endothelial nitric oxide synthase in vascular disease. Trends Cardiovasc Med Vol. 14, pp. 323-327.

[23] Chen, H., Li, X. & Epstein, P.N. (2005). MnSOD and catalase transgenes demonstrate that protection of islets from oxidative stress does not alter cytokine toxicity. Diabetes Vol. 54, pp. 1437-1446.

[24] Chong, Z.Z., Li, F. & Maiese, K. (2005). Oxidative stress in the brain: Novel cellular targets that govern survival during neurodegenerative disease. Prog Neurobiol Vol. 75, pp. 207-246.

[25] Cosentino, F., Hishikawa, K., Katusic, Z.S. & Lüscher, T.F. (1997). High glucose increases nitric oxide synthase expression and superoxide anion generation in human aortic endothelial cells. Circulation Vol. 96, pp. 25-28.

[26] Costacou, T., Zgibor, J.C., Evans, R.W., Tyurina, Y.Y., Kagan, V.E. & Orchard, T.J. (2006). Antioxidants and coronary artery disease among individuals with type 1 diabetes: Findings from the Pittsburgh Epidemiology of Diabetes Complications Study. J Diabetes Complications Vol. 20, pp. 387-394.

[27] Dalle-Donne, I., Ranieri, R., Roberto, C., Daniela, G. & Aldo, M. (2006). Biomarkers of oxidative damage in human disease. Clinical Chemistry Vol. 52, pp. 601-623.

[28] Dave, G.S. & Kalia, K. (2007). Hyperglycemia induced oxidative stress in type-1 and type-2 diabetic patients with and without nephropathy. Cell Mol Biol (Noisy-le-grand). Vol. 53, pp. 68-78.

[29] Delmastro, M.M. & Piganelli J. D. (2011). Oxidative stress and redox modulation potential in type 1 diabetes. Clin Dev Immunol Vol. 1.

[30] Di Mambro, V.M., Azzolini, A.E., Valim, Y.M. & Fonseca, M.J. (2003). Comparison of antioxidant activities of tocopherols alone and in pharmaceutical formulations. Int J Pharm Vol. 262, pp. 93-99.

[31] Djordjevic, A., Spasic, S., Jovanovic-Galovic, A., Djordjevic, R. & Grubor- Lajsic, G. (2004). Oxidative stress in diabetic pregnancy: SOD, CAT and GSH-Px activity and lipid peroxidation products. J Matern Fetal Neonatal Med Vol. 16, pp. 367-372.

[32] Dominguez, C., Ruiz, E., Gussinye, M. & Carrascisa, A. (1998). Oxidative stress at onset and in early stages of type I diabetes in children and adolescents. Diabetes Care Vol. 21, pp. 1736-1742.

[33] Drews, G., Krippeit-Drews, P. & Düfer M. (2010). Oxidative stress and beta-cell dysfunction. Pflugers Arch Vol. 460, pp. 703-718.

[34] Durrington, P.N., Mackness, B. & Mackness, M.I. (2001). Paraoxonase and atherosclerosis. Arterioscler Thromb Vasc Biol Vol. 21, pp.473-480.

[35] El Faramawy, S.M. & Rizk, R.A. (2011). Spectrophotometric studies on antioxidants-doped liposomes. J Am Sci Vol. 7, pp. 363-369.

[36] Elliott, T.G., Cockcroft, J.R., Groop, P.H., Viberti, G.C. & Ritter, J.M. (1993). Inhibition of nitric oxide synthesis in forearm vasculature of insulin- dependent diabetic patients: blunted vasoconstriction in patients with microalbuminuria. Clin Sci Vol. 85, pp. 687-693.

[37] Engler, M.M., Engler, M.B., Malloy, M.J., Chiu, E.Y., Schloetter, M.C., Paul, S.M., Stuehlinger, M., Lin, K.Y., Cooke, J.P., Morrow, J.D., Ridker, P.M., Rifai, N., Miller, E., Witztum, J.L. & Mietus-Snyder, M. (2003). Antioxidant vitamins C and E improve endothelial function in children with hyperlipidemia: Endothelial Assessment of Risk from Lipids in Youth (EARLY) Trial. Circulation Vol. 108, pp. 1059-1010.

[38] Erciyas, F., Taneli, F., Arslan, B. & Uslu, Y. (2004). Glycemic control, oxidative stress, and lipid profile in children with type 1 diabetes mellitus. Arch Med Res Vol. 35, pp. 134-40.

[39] Fang, Y-Z., Yang, S. & Wu, G. (2002). Free radicals, antioxidants and nutrition. Nutrition Vol. 18, pp. 872-879.

[40] Fatehi-Hassanabad, Z., Chan, C.B. & Furman, B.L. (2010). Reactive oxygen species and endothelial function in diabetes. European Journal of Pharmacology Vol. 636, pp. 8-17.

[41] Faure, P., Benhamou, P.Y., Perard, A., Halimi, S. & Roussel, A.M. (1995). Lipid peroxidationin insulin dependent diabetic patients with early retina degenerative lesions: Effects of an oral zinc supplementation. Eur J Clin Nutr Vol. 49, pp. 282-288.

[42] Ferretti, G., Bacchetti, T., Busni, D., Rabini, R.A. & Curatola G. (2004). Protective effect of paraoxonase activity in high-density lipoproteins against erythrocyte membranes peroxidation: a comparison between healthy subjects and type 1 diabetic patients. Clin Endocrinol Metab. Vol. 89, pp. 2957-2962.

[43] Firoozrai, M., Nourbakhsh, M., Razzaghy-Azar, M. (2007). Erythrocyte susceptibility to oxidative stress and antioxidant status in patients with type 1 diabetes. Diabetes Res Clin Pract Vol. 77, pp. 427-432.

[44] Flores, L., Rodela, S., Abian, J., Clària, J. & Esmatjes, E. (2004). F2 isoprostane is already increased at the onset of type 1 diabetes mellitus: effect of glycemic control. Metabolism Vol. 53, pp. 1118-1120.

[45] Frei, B. (1994). Reactive oxygen species and antioxidant vitamins: mechanisms of action. Am Med Vol. 97, pp. 5S-13S.

[46] Frei, B., Stocker, R., England, L. & Ames, B.N. (1990). Ascorbate: the most effective antioxidant in human blood plasma. Adv Exp Med Biol Vol. 264, pp. 155-163.

[47] Fubini, B. & Hubbard, A. (2003). Reactive oxygen species (ROS) and reactive nitrogen species (RNS) generation by silica in inflammation and fibrosis. Free Radic Biol Med. Vol. 34, pp. 1507-1516.

[48] Giannini, C., Lombardo, F., Currò, F., Pomilio, M., Bucciarelli, T., Chiarelli, F. & Mohn, A. (2007). Effects of high-dose vitamin E supplementation on oxidative stress and microalbuminuria in young adult patients with childhood onset type 1 diabetes mellitus. Diabetes Metab Res Rev Vol. 23, pp. 539-546.

[49] Gleisner, A., Martinez, L., Pino, R., Rojas, I.G., Martinez, A., Asenjo, S. & Rudolph, M.I. (2006). Oxidative stress markers in plasma and urine of prepubertal patients with type 1 diabetes mellitus. J Pediatr Endocrinol Metab Vol. 19, pp. 995-1000.

[50] Goodarzi, M.T., Navidi, A.A., Rezaei, M. & Babahmadi-Rezaei, H. (2010). Oxidative damage to DNA and lipids: correlation with protein glycation in patients with type 1 diabetes. J Clin Lab Anal. Vol. 24, pp. 72-76.

[51] Gorren, A.C. & Mayer, B. (2002). Tetrahydrobiopterin in nitric oxide synthesis: a novel biological role for pteridines. Curr Drug Metab Vol. 3, pp. 133-157.

[52] Gregus, Z., Fekete, T., Halaszi, E. & Klaassen, C.D. (1996). Lipoic acid impairs glycine conjugation of benzoic acid and renal excretion of benzoylglycine, Drug Metab Dispos Vol. 24, pp. 682-688.

[53] Gupta, S., Sharma, T.K., Kaushik, G.G. & Shekhawat, V.P. (2011). Vitamin E supplementation may ameliorate oxidative stress in type 1 diabetes mellitus patients. Clin Lab Vol. 57, pp. 379-386.

[54] Ha, H. & Lee, H.B. (2000). Reactive oxygen species as glucose signaling molecules in mesangial cells cultured under high glucose. Kidney Int Vol. Suppl 77, pp. S19-S25.

[55] Halliwell, B. (1994). Free radicals, antioxidants, and human disease: cause or consequence? Lancet Vol. 344, pp. 721-724.

[56] Halliwell, B. (1995). Oxidation of low-density lipoproteins: questions of initiation, propagation, and the effect of antioxidants. J Clin Nutr Vol. 61, pp. 670-677S.

[57] Han, Y., Randell, E., Vasdev, S., Gill, V., Gadag, V., Newhook, L.A., Grant, M. & Hagerty D. (2007). Plasma methylglyoxal and glyoxal are elevated and related to early membrane alteration in young, complication-free patients with Type 1 diabetes. Mol Cell Biochem Vol. 305, pp. 123-131.

[58] Ho, E. & Bray, T.M. (1999). Antioxidants, NFkappaB activation, and diabetogenesis. Proc Soc Exp Biol Med Vol. 222, pp. 205-213.

[59] Hoeldtke, R.D., Bryner, K.D. & VanDyke, K. (2011). Oxidative stress and autonomic nerve function in early type 1 diabetes. Clin Auton Res Vol. 21, pp. 19-28.

[60] Hogg, N. & Kalyanaraman, B. (1998). The use of NO gas in biological systems. Methods Mol Biol Vol. 100, pp. 231-234.

[61] Horie, S., Ishii, H. & Suga, T. (1981). Changes in peroxisomal fatty acid oxidation in diabetic rat

[62] liver. J Biochem (Tokyo) Vol. 90, pp. 1691-1696.

[63] Hsu, W.T., Tsai, L.Y., Lin, S.K., Hsiao, J.K. & Chen, B.H. (2006). Effects of diabetes duration and glycemic control on free radicals in children with type 1 diabetes mellitus. Ann Clin Lab Sci Vol. 36, pp. 174-178.

[64] Ignarro, L.J. (2002). Nitric oxide as a unique signaling molecule in the vascular system: a historical overview. J Physiol Pharmacol Vol. 53, pp. 503-514.

[65] Ischiropoulos, H. (1998). Biological tyrosine nitration: a pathophysiological function of nitric oxide and reactive oxygen species. Arch Biochem Biophys Vol. 356, pp. 1-11.

[66] Jain, S.K. & McVie, R. (1994). Effect of glycemic control race (white vs. black), and duration of diabetes on reduced glutathione content in erythrocytes of diabetic patients. Metabolism Vol. 43, pp. 306-309.

[67] Järvisalo, M.J., Raitakari, M., Toikka, J.O., Putto-Laurila, A., Rontu, R., Laine, S., Lehtimäki, T., Rönnemaa, T., Viikari, J. & Raitakari OT. Endothelial dysfunction and increased arterial intima-media thickness in children with type 1 diabetes. Circulation Vol. 109, pp. 1750-1755.

[68] Kaneto, H., Katakami, N., Kawamori, D., Miyatsuka, T., Sakamoto, K., Matsuoka, T.A., Matsuhisa, M. & Yamasaki, Y. (2007). Involvement of oxidative stress in the pathogenesis of diabetes. Antioxid Redox Signal Vol. 9, pp. 355-366.

[69] Kajikawa, M., Fujimoto, S., Tsuura, Y., Mukai, E., Takeda, T., Hamamoto, Y., Takehiro, M., Fujita. J., Yamada, Y. & Seino Y. (2002). Ouabain suppresses glucose-induced mitochondrial ATP production and insulin release by generating reactive oxygen species in pancreatic islets. Diabetes Vol. 51, pp. 2522-2529.

[70] Kostolanská, J., Jakus, V. & Barák, L. (2009). HbA1c and serum levels of advanced glycation and oxidation protein products in poorly and well controlled children and adolescents with type 1 diabetes mellitus. J Pediatr Endocrinol Metab Vol. 22, pp. 433-442.

[71] Laight, D.W., Carrier, M.J. & Anggard, E.E. (2000). Antioxidants, diabetes and endothelial dysfunction. Cardiovasc Res Vol. 47, pp. 457-464.

[72] Lenzen, S., Drinkgern, J. &Tiedge, M. (1996). Low antioxidant enzyme gene expression in pancreatic islets compared with various other mouse tissues. Free Radio Biol Med Vol. 20, pp. 463-466.

[73] Lepore, D.A., Shinkel, T.A., Fisicaro, N., Mysore, T.B., Johnson, L.E., d'Apice, A.J. & Cowan P.J. (2004). Enhanced expression of glutathione peroxidase protects islet beta cells from hypoxia-reoxygenation. Xenotransplantation Vol. 11, pp. 53-59.

[74] Li, F., Chong, Z.Z. & Maiese, K. (2006). Cell life versus cell longevity: the mysteries surrounding the NAD(+) precursor nicotinamide. Curr Med Chem Vol. 13, pp. 883-895.

[75] Likidlilid, A., Patchanans, N., Poldee, S. & Peerapatdit, T. (2007). Glutathione and glutathione peroxidase in type 1 diabetic patients. J Med Assoc Thai Vol. 90, pp. 1759-1767.

[76] Llorens, S. & Nava, E. (2003). Cardiovascular diseases and the nitric oxide pathway. Curr Vasc Pharmacol Vol. 1, pp. 335-346.

[77] Lu, S.C. (1999). Regulation of hepatic glutathione synthesis: current concepts and controversies, FASEB J Vol. 13, pp. 1169-1183.

[78] Mackness, B., Durrington, P.N., Boulton, A.J., Hine, D. & Mackness, M.I. (2002). Serum paraoxonase activity in patients with type 1 diabetes compared to healthy controls. Eur J Clin Invest Vol. 32, pp. 259-264.

[79] Macphee, C.H., Nelson, J.J. & Zalewski, A. (2005). Lipoprotein-associated phospholipase A2 as a target of therapy. Curr. Opin. Lipidol Vol. 16, pp. 442-446.

[80] Maechler, P., Jornot, L. & Wollheim, C.B. (1999). Hydrogen peroxide alters mitochondrial activation and insulin secretion in pancreatic beta cells. Journal of Biological Chemistry, Vol. 274, pp. 27905-27913.

[81] Majchrzak, A., Zozulińska, D. & Wierusz-Wysocka, B. (2001). Evaluation of selected components in antioxidant systems of blood in patients with diabetes. Pol Merkur Lekarski Vol. 10, pp. 150-152.

[82] Maritim, A.C., Sanders, R.A. & Watkins, J.B. 3rd. (2003). Diabetes, oxidative stress, and antioxidants: a review. J Biochem Mol Toxicol Vol. 17, pp. 24-38.

[83] Mates, J.M., Perez-Gomez, C. & Castro, I.N. (1999). Antioxidant enzymes and human diseases. Clinical Biochemistry Vol. 32, pp. 595-603.

[84] Maxwell, S.R., Thomason, H., Sandler, D., Leguen, C., Baxter, M.A., Thorpe, G.H., Jones, A.F. & Barnett, A.H. (1997). Antioxidant status in patients with uncomplicated insulin-dependent and non-insulin-dependent diabetes mellitus. Eur J Clin Invest Vol. 27, pp. 484-490.

[85] Meister, A. Anderson, M.E. (1983). Glutathionne. Annu Rev Biochem Vol. 52, pp. 711-760.

[86] Menke, T., Niklowitz, P., Wiesel, T. & Andler, W. (2008). Antioxidant level and redox status of coenzyme Q10 in the plasma and blood cells of children with diabetes mellitus type 1. Pediatr Diabetes. Vol. 9, pp. 540-545.

[87] Miyata, T., Van Ypersele S.C., Kurokawa, K. & Baynes, J.W. (1999). Alterations in nonenzymatic biochemistry in uremia: origin and significance of .carbonyl stress. in long-term uremic complications. Kidney Int Vol. 55, pp. 389-399.

[88] Moore, K. & Roberts, L.J. 2nd. (1998). Measurement of lipid peroxidation. Free Radic Res Vol. 28, pp. 659-671.

[89] Mullarkey, C.J., Edelstein, D. & Brownlee, M. (1990). Free radical generation by early glycation products: a mechanism for accelerated atherogenesis in diabetes. Biochem Biophys Res Commun Vol. 173, pp. 932-939.

[90] Murakami, K., Kondo, T., Ohtsuka, Y., Fujiwara, Y., Shimada, M. & Kawakami, Y. (1989). Impairment of glutathione metabolism in erythrocytes from patients with diabetes mellitus. Metabolism Vol. 38, pp. 753-758.

[91] Mylona-Karayanni, C., Gourgiotis, D., Bossios, A. & Kamper, E.F. (2006). Oxidative stress and adhesion molecules in children with type 1 diabetes mellitus: a possible link. Pediatr Diabetes Vol. 7, pp. 51-59.

[92] Ndahimana, J., Dorchy, H. & Vertongen, E.C. (1996). Erythrocyte and plasma antioxidant activity in type I diabetes mellitus. Press Med Vol. 25, pp. 188-192.

[93] Newsholme, P., Haber, E. P., Hirabara, M., Rebelato, E. L., Procopio, J., Morgan, D., Oliveira-Emilio, H.C., Carpinelli, A. & Curi, R. (2007). Diabetes associated cell stress and dysfunction: role of mitochondrial and non-mitochondrial ROS production and activity. Journal of Physiology, Vol. 583, pp. 9-24.

[94] Niedowicz, D. & Daleke, D. (2005). The role of oxidative stress in diabetic complications. Cell Biochem Biophys Vol. 43, pp. 289-330.

[95] Niiya, Y., Abumiya, T., Shichinohe, H., Kuroda, S., Kikuchi, S., Ieko, M., Yamagishi, S.I., Takeuchi, M., Sato, T. & Iwasaki, Y. (2006). Susceptibility of brain microvascular

endothelial cells to advanced glycation end products-induced tissue factor upregulation is associated with intracellular reactive oxygen species. Brain Res Vol. 1108, pp. 179-187.

[96] Nishikawa, T., Edelstein, D., Du, X., Yamagishi, S., Matsumura, T., Kaneda, Y., Yorek, M., Beebe, D., Oates, P., Hammes, H., Giardino, I. & Brownlee, M. (2000). Normalizing mitochondrial superoxide production blocks three pathways of hyperglycemic damage. Nature Vol. 404, pp. 787-790.

[97] Nourooz-Zadeh, J., Tajaddini-Sarmadi, J., McCarthy, S., Betteridge, D.J. & Wolff, S.P. (1995). Elevated levels of authentic plasma hydroperoxides in NIDDM. Diabetes Vol. 44, pp. 1054-1058.

[98] Nowak, M., Wielkoszyński, T., Marek, B., Kos-Kudła, B., Swietochowska, E., Siemińska, L., Karpe, J., Kajdaniuk, D., Głogowska-Szelag, J. & Nowak, K. (2010). Antioxidant potential, paraoxonase 1, ceruloplasmin activity and C-reactive protein concentration in diabetic retinopathy. Clin Exp Med Vol. 10, pp. 185-192.

[99] Pacher, P. & Szabo, C. (2006). Role of peroxynitrite in the pathogenesis of cardiovascular complications of diabetes. Curr Opin Pharmacol Vol. 6, pp. 136-141.

[100] Pastore, A., Ciampalini, P., Tozzi, G., Pecorelli, L., Passarelli, C., Bertini, E. & Piemonte, F. (2012). All glutathione forms are depleted in blood of obese and type 1 diabetic children Diabetes Care Vol. 23, pp. 1182-1186.

[101] Pfeiffer, S., Lass, A., Schmidt, K. & Mayer, B. (2010). Protein tyrosine nitration in mouse peritoneal macrophages activated in vitro and in vivo: evidence against an essential role of peroxynitrite. FASEB J Vol. 15, pp. 2355-2364.

[102] Phillips, M., Cataneo, R.N., Cheema, T. & Greenberg, J. (2004). Increased breath biomarkers of oxidative stress in diabetes mellitus. Clin Chim Acta Vol. 344, pp. 189-194.

[103] Pitocco, D., Zaccardi, F., Di Stasio, E., Romitelli, F., Martini, F., Scaglione, G.L., Speranza, D., Santini, S., Zuppi, C. & Ghirlanda, G. (2009). Role of asymmetric-dimethyl-L-arginine (ADMA) and nitrite/nitrate (NOx) in the pathogenesis of oxidative stress in female subjects with uncomplicated type 1 diabetes mellitus. Diabetes Res Clin Pract Vol. 86, pp. 173-176.

[104] Prutz, W.A., Monig, H., Butler, J. & Land, E.J. (1985). Reactions of nitrogen dioxide in aqueous model systems: oxidation of tyrosine units in peptides and proteins. Arch Biochem Biophys Vol. 243, pp. 125-134.

[105] Rachek, L.I., Thornley, N.P., Grishko, V.I., LeDoux, S.P. & Wilson, G.L. (2006). Protection of INS-1 cells from free fatty acid-induced apoptosis by targeting hOGG1 to mitochondria. Diabetes Vol. 55, pp. 1022-1028.

[106] Ramana, K.V., Chandra, D., Srivastava, S., Bhatnagar, A. & Srivastava, S.K. (2003). Nitric oxide regulates the polyol pathway of glucose metabolism in vascular smooth muscle cells. The FASEB Journal Vol. 17, pp. 417-425.

[107] Reis, J.S., Veloso, C.A., Volpe, C.M., Fernandes, J.S., Borges, E.A., Isoni, C.A., Dos Anjos, P.M. & Nogueira-Machado, J.A. (2012). Soluble RAGE and malondialdehyde in type 1 diabetes patients without chronic complications during the course of the disease. Diab Vasc Dis Res Vol.

[108] Feb 15. [Epub ahead of print].

[109] Reiter, R.J., Tan, D.X., Osuna, C. & Gitto, E. (2000). Actions of melatonin in the reduction of oxidative stress. A review. J Biomed Sci Vol. 7, pp. 444-458.

[110] Reznick, A.Z., Shehadeh, N., Shafir, Y. & Nagler, R.M. (2006). Free radicals related effects and antioxidants in saliva and serum of adolescents with Type 1 diabetes mellitus. Arch Oral Biol Vol. 51, pp. 640-648.

[111] Roberts, L.J. & Morrow, J.D. (2000). Measurement of F_2-isoprostanes an index of oxidative stress in vivo. Free Radic Biol Med Vol. 28, pp. 505-513.

[112] Rodiño-Janeiro, B.K., González-Peteiro, M., Ucieda-Somoza, R., González-Juanatey, J.R. Alvarez, E. (2010). Glycated albumin, a precursor of advanced glycation end-products, up-regulates NADPH oxidase and enhances oxidative stress in human endothelial cells: molecular correlate of diabetic vasculopathy. Diabetes Metab Res Rev Vol. 26, pp. 550-558.

[113] Rolo, A.P. & Palmeira, C.M. (2006). Diabetes and mitochondrial function: role of hyperglycemia and oxidative stress. Toxicol Appl Pharmacol Vol. 212, pp. 167-178.

[114] Rosen, P., Nawroth, P.P., King, G., Moller, W., Tritschler, H.J. & Packer, L. (2001). The role of oxidative stress in the onset and progression of diabetes and its complications: A summary of a Congress Series sponsored by UNESCO MCBN, the American Diabetes Association and the German Diabetes Society. Diabetes Metab Res Rev Vol. 17, pp. 189-912.

[115] Ross, R. (1999). Atherosclerosis-an inflammatory disease. N Engl J Med Vol. 340, pp. 115-126.

[116] Salardi, S., Zucchini, S., Elleri, D., Grossi, G., Bargossi, A.M., Gualandi, S., Santoni, R., Cicognani, A. & Cacciari, E. (2004). High glucose levels induce an increase in membrane antioxidants, in terms of vitamin E and coenzyme Q10, in children and adolescents with type 1 diabetes. Diabetes Care Vol. 27, pp. 630-631.

[117] Samanthi, R.P.M., Rolf, E.A., Jelena, A.J., Maria, A. & Paresh, C.D. (2011). Novel conjugates of 1,3-diacylglycerol and lipoic acid: synthesis, DPPH assay, and RP-LC-MS-APCI analysis. J Lipids Vol. 10, pp. 1-10.

[118] Schmidt, A.M., Hori, O., Cao, R., Yan, S.D., Brett, J., Wautier, J.L., Ogawa, S., Kuwabara, K., Matsumoto, M. & Stern, D. (1996). RAGE: a novel cellular receptor for advanced glycation end products. Diabetes Vol. 45(Suppl 3), pp. S77-S80.

[119] Simm, A., Münch, G., Seif, F., Schenk, O., Heidland, A., Richter, H., Vamvakas, S. & Schinzel R. (1997). Advanced glycation endproducts stimulate the MAP-kinase pathway in tubuluscell line LLC-PK1. FEBS Lett Vol. 410. pp. 481-484.

[120] Siu, A.W. & To, C.H. (2002). Nitric oxide and hydroxyl radical-induced retinal lipid peroxidation in vitro. Clin Exp Optom. Vol. 85, pp. 378-382.

[121] Skyrme-Jones, R.A., O'Brien, R.C., Berry, K.L. & Meredith, I.T. (2000). Vitamin E supplementation improves endothelial function in type I diabetes mellitus: a randomized, placebo-controlled study. J Am Coll Cardiol Vol. 36, pp. 94-102.

[122] Spitaler, M.M. 7 Graier, W.F. (2002). Vascular targets of redox signalling in diabetes mellitus. Diabetologia Vol. 45, pp. 476-494.

[123] Steinberg, H.O. & Baron, A.D. (2002). Vascular function, insulin resistance and fatty acids. Diabetologia Vol. 45, pp. 623-634.

[124] Suys, B., de Beeck, L.O., Rooman, R., Kransfeld, S., Heuten, H., Goovaerts, I., Vrints, C., de Wolf, D., Matthys, D. & Manuel-y-Keenoy, B. (2007). Impact of oxidative stress on the endothelial dysfunction of children and adolescents with type 1 diabetes mellitus: protection by superoxide dismutase? Pediatr Res Vol. 62, pp. 456-461.

[125] Telci, A., Cakatay, U., Salman, S., Satman, I. & Sivas, A. (2000). Oxidative protein damage in early stage Type 1 diabetic patients. Diabetes Res Clin Pract Vol. 50, pp. 213-223.

[126] Thornalley, P.J. (2002). Glycation in diabetic neuropathy: characteristics, consequences, causes, and therapeutic options. Int Rev Neurobiol Vol. 50, pp. 37-57.

[127] Tsukahara, H., Sekine, K., Uchiyama, M., Kawakami, H., Hata, I., Todoroki, Y., Hiraoka, M., Kaji, M., Yorifuji, T, Momoi, T., Yoshihara, K., Beppu, M. & Mayumi, M. (2003). Formation of advanced glycosylation end products and oxidative stress in young patients with type 1 diabetes. Pediatr Res Vol. 54, pp. 419-424.

[128] Turk, Z. (2010). Glycotoxines, carbonyl stress and relevance to diabetes and its complications. Physiol Res Vol. 59, pp. 147-156.

[129] Van Lenten, B. J., Navab, M., Shih, D., Fogelman, A. M. & Lusis, A. J. (2001). The role of high-density lipoproteins in oxidation and inflammation. Trends Cardiovasc Med Vol. 11, pp. 155-161.

[130] Watson, A.D., Berliner, J.A., Hama, S.Y., La Du, B.N., Faull, K.F., Fogelman, A.M. & Navab, M. (1995). Protective effect of high density lipoprotein associated paraoxonase. Inhibition of the biological activity of minimally oxidized low density lipoprotein. J Clin Invest Vol. 6, pp. 2882-2891.

[131] Watson, D. & Loweth, A.C. (2009). Oxidative and nitrosative stress in beta-cell apoptosis: their contribution to beta-cell loss in type 1 diabetes mellitus. Br J Biomed Sci Vol. 66, pp. 208-215.

[132] Wautier, M.P., Chappey, O., Corda, S., Stern, D.M., Schmidt, A.M & Wautier, J.L. (2001). Activation of NADPH oxidase by AGE links oxidant stress to altered gene expression via RAGE. Am J Physiol Vol. 280, pp. E685-E694.

[133] Weber, P., Bendich, A. & Machlin, L.J. (1997). Vitamin E and human health: rationale for determining recommended intake levels. Nutrition Vol. 13, pp. 450-460.

[134] Wegner, M., Pioruńska-Stolzmann, M., Araszkiewicz, A., Zozulińska-Ziołkiewicz, D. & Wierusz-Wysocka, B. (2011). Evaluation of paraoxonase 1 arylesterase activity and lipid peroxide levels in patients with type 1 diabetes. Pol Arch Med Wewn Vol. 121, pp. 448-455.

[135] West, I.C. (2000). Radicals and oxidative stress in diabetes. Diabetic Med Vol. 17, pp. 171-180.

[136] Wild, S., Roglic, G., Green, A., Sicree, R. & King, H. (2004). Global prevalence of diabetes: estimates for the year 2000 and projections for 2030. Diabetes Care Vol. 27, pp. 1047-1053.

[137] Winterbourn, C.C. & Metodiewa, D. (1994). The reaction of superoxide with reduced glutathione. Arch Biochem Biophys Vol. 314, pp. 284-290.

[138] Witko-Sarsat, V., Friedlander, M., Capeillère-Blandin, C., Nguyen-Khoa, T., Nguyen, A.T., Zingraff, J., Jungers, P., Descamps-Latscha, B. (1996). Advanced oxidation protein products as a novel marker of oxidative stress in uraemia. Kidney Int Vol. 49, pp. 1304-1313.

[139] Yamagishi, S. (2009). Advanced glycation end products and receptor-oxidative stress system in diabetic vascular complications. Ther Apher Dial Vol. 13, p. 534-539.

[140] Yan, S.D., Schmidt, A.M., Anderson, G.M., Zhang, J., Brett, J., Zou, Y.S., Pinsky, D. & Stern, D. (1994). Enhanced cellular oxidant stress by the interaction of advanced glycation endproducts with their receptors/ binding proteins. J Biol Chem Vol. 269, pp. 9889-9897.

[141] Yung, L.M., Leung, F.P., Yao, X., Chen, Z.Y. & Huang, Y. (2006). Reactive oxygen species in vascular wall. Cardiovascular and Hematological Disorders Vol. 6, pp. 1-19.

[142] Zivić, S., Vlaski, J., Kocić, G., Pesić, M., Cirić, V. & Durić, Z. (2008). The importance of oxidative stress in pathogenesis of type 1 diabetes-determination of catalase activity in lymphocytes of diabetic patients. Med Pregl Vol. 61, pp. 458-463.

Section 4

Complications

Chapter 10

Diabetic Ketoacidosis

Mustafa Cesur and Irmak Sayin

Additional information is available at the end of the chapter

http://dx.doi.org/10.5772/53199

1. Introduction

A chronic autoimmune destruction of the pancreatic beta cells results in decreasing endogenous insulin secretion and the clinical manifestation of type 1 diabetes mellitus (T1DM). The clinical onset of the disease is often acute in children and adolescents and diabetic ketoacidosis (DKA) is present in 20-74% of the patients [1-7]. DKA is a serious condition that requiring immediate intervention. Even with appropriate intervention, DKA is associated with significant morbidity and possible mortality in diabetic patients in the pediatric age group [8]. Young age and female sex have been associated with an increased frequency of DKA [3,9]. The triad of uncontrolled hyperglycemia, metabolic acidosis and increased total body ketone concentration characterizes DKA [10]. In addition to possible acute complications, it may also influence the later outcome of diabetes [11].

2. Epidemiology

Worldwide, an estimated 65 000 children under 15 years old develop T1DM each year, and the global incidence in children continues to increase at a rate of 3% a year [12,13]. The current incidence in the UK is around 26/100 000 per year [14]. Patterson et al. were aimed to establish 15-year incidence trends for childhood T1DM in European centres with EURODIAB study. 29 311 new cases of T1DM were diagnosed in children before their 15th birthday during a 15-year period between 1989-2003. The overall annual increase was 3.9% and the increases in the age groups 0-4 years, 5-9 years, and 10-14 years were found to be 5.4%, 4.3%, and 2.9% respectively. If present trends continue, prevalent cases younger than 15 years will rise by 70% in 2020 [15].

The incidence of DKA was found to be 5-8% in large community-based studies [16]. Approximately 115 000 patients admitted to the hospital because of DKA in one year in USA

[17]. In a Turkish study conducted among the patients with diabetic adults who admitted to the hospital, the ratio of T1DM was found to be 6.6% and DKA was 38% of the group [18]. There is wide geographic variation in the frequency of DKA at onset of diabetes. The ratio inversely correlates with the regional incidence of T1DM. Frequencies range from 15 to 70% in Europe, Australia, and North America [11,19-25]. The most occurrence ages of DKA are between the 18-44 years (56%), than 45-65 years (24%) continues with only 18% of patients <20 years of age. Two-thirds of DKA patients are considered to have T1DM and 34% to have type 2 diabetes. DKA is the most common cause of death in children and adolescents with T1DM. Half of all deaths in diabetic patients younger than 24 years of age are caused from DKA [26,27]. In adult subjects with DKA, the overall mortality is usually given <1% (13), however mortality rates may increase over 5% in the elders and in patients with concomitant life-threatening illnesses [28,29].

3. Pathogenesis

There are some factors as a reason of acute metabolic complications in diabetic patiens. These factors are insulin deficiency as the initial primary event in progressive beta-cell failure, its failure in a patient with established disease or its ineffectiveness when insulin action is antagonized by physiological stress such as sepsis and in the context of counterregulatory hormone (catecholamines, cortisol, glucagon, and growth hormone) excess. These hormonal changes increase glucose production from glycogenolysis and gluconeogenesis and impair glucose utilization by peripheral tissues, resulting in hyperglycemia, osmotic diuresis, electrolyte loss, dehydration, decreased glomerular filtration (further compounding hyperglycemia) and hyperosmolarity. [26, 30-35].

The combination of insulin deficiency and increased counterregulatory hormones in DKA also leads to the release of free fatty acids into the circulation from adipose tissue (lipolysis). This is augmented by transient insulin resistance due to the hormone imbalance itself as well as the elevated free fatty acid concentrations [8,10,26,28-39]. Uncontrolled hepatic fatty acid oxidation in the liver to ketone bodies (beta-hydroxybutyrate and acetoacetate) results ketonemia and metabolic acidosis [40]. The pathogenesis causing to hyperglycemia and ketoacidosis are schematized in Figure 1 [30].

A number of clinical studies showed that the hyperglycemia in patients with hyperglycemic crises is associated with a severe inflammatory state characterized by an elevation of proinflammatory cytokines tumor necrosis factor alpha (TNF-α) and interleukin-6, and -8 (IL-6,8), C-reactive protein, reactive oxygen species, and lipid peroxidation, as well as cardiovascular risk factors, plasminogen activator inhibitor-1 and free fatty acids in the absence of obvious infection or cardiovascular pathology. Insulin therapy and hydration recover these parameters to near-normal values within 24 hours [41]. Recent studies focused on the role of interleukin-1 beta (IL-1ß), interleukin-12 (IL-12) and interferon-gamma (IFN-γ). As demonstrated *in vitro,* these cytokines can directly influence beta cell function and viability [42]. Karavanaki et al. studied plasma levels of cytokines IL-1β, interleukin-2 (IL-2), IL-6, IL-8, and interleukin-10 (IL-10), TNF-

http://dx.doi.org/10.5772/53199

α and also white blood cell count (WBC), high sensitivity C-reactive protein (hs-CRP), growth hormone (GH) and cortisol in 38 newly diagnosed T1DM children with DKA (mean age 7.68±3.07 years), prior to, during and 120 hours after DKA management, with the aim to monitor their levels at different time-points and in different degrees of DKA severity. Prior to DKA management the levels of IL- 6, IL-8, IL-10,WBC and cortisol were elevated, but all parameters were reduced within 120 hours after DKA management [43].

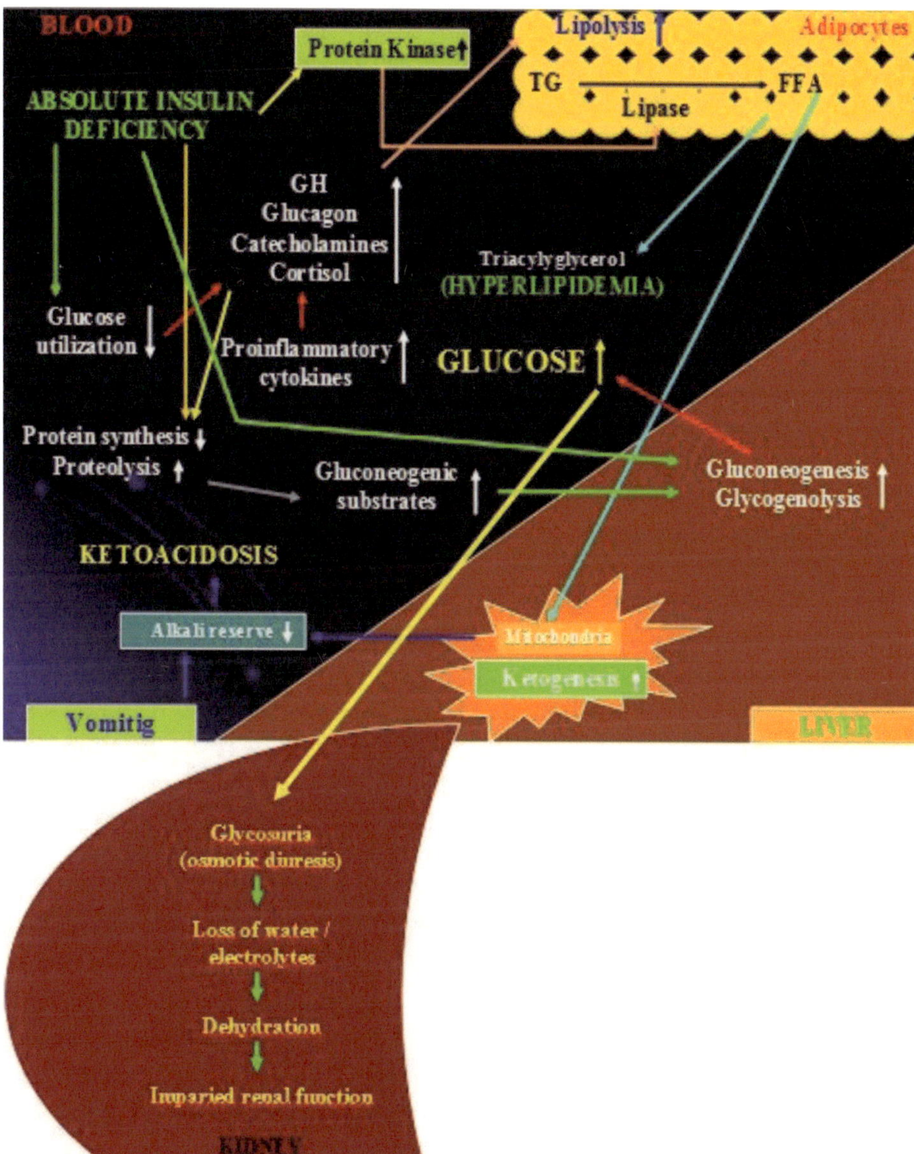

Figure 1. The pathogenesis causing to hyperglycemia and ketoacidosis in DKA (Data adapted from reference [17])

Recent studies have reported that an upregulated production of and interleukin-18 (IL-18) could be an important pathogenic event in the dysregulated production of IFN-γ and other type 1 cytokines thought to predispose T1DM [44-46] and the potential role of IL-18 in the pathophysiology of the chronic complications of diabetes mellitus [7-11]. But the potential role of IL-18 in the acute complications of diabetes mellitus such as DKA is controversial. Dong et al. compared serum IL-18 levels and other cytokines (IL-12 and IFN-γ) in newly diagnosed T1DM with DKA, T1DM without DKA and age/sex-matched healthy controls. Serum IL-18 levels were significantly higher in patients than those in healthy controls. Serum IL-12 and IFN-γ levels were not different between patients and controls. But there was a positive correlation between serum IL-18 and islet cell antibody (ICA) and C-peptide levels, but not between serum IL-18 and HbA1C, insulin and glucose in T1DM. Serum IL-18 levels also correlated positively with serum IL-12 levels. Serum IL-18 levels was significantly higher in patients with DKA than those in patients without DKA while C-peptide levels were markedly lower in patients with DKA. These results point that serum IL-18 levels are elevated and correlated with C-peptide levels and ICA in patients with T1DM, with marked increase in T1DM with DKA. Clinicans should be aware of the risk of DKA in diabetic patients with high serum IL-18 [47]. The procoagulant and inflammatory states may be due to nonspecific phenomena of stress and may partially explain the association of hyperglycemic crises with a hypercoagulable state [48].

4. Precipitating factors

A careful search for precipitating factors should be made, as correction of these contributes to improved outcomes and less frequent recurrences.

The most common precipitating factor in the development of DKA is infection [37,49,50] including viral syndromes, urinary tract infections, pelvic inflammatory disease, pneumonia, mucormycosis, malignant otitis externa (with pseudomonas aeruginosa), periodontal abscess and dental infection [51]. Other precipitating factors include discontinuation of, or inadequate insulin therapy, acute pancreatitis, myocardial infarction, stroke, major trauma and other severe/acute illnesses and drugs [30,32,37]. New-onset T1DM or discontinuation of insulin in T1DM frequently leads to the development of DKA. In young patients with T1DM, psychological problems complicated by eating disorders may be a contributing factor in 20% of recurrent ketoacidosis. In younger patients fear of weight gain and hypoglycemia, stresss of chronic disease may lead to insulin omission.

In the past, before the improvement in technology and sufficient education of patients continuous subcutaneous insulin infusion devices had also been associated with an increased frequency of DKA [52]; nowadays the incidence of DKA appears to have reduced in pump users [53]. Additional prospective studies are needed to document reduction of DKA incidence with the use of continuous subcutaneous insulin infusion devices [54].

Drugs that affect carbohydrate metabolism, such as corticosteroids, thiazides, sympathomimetic agents and pentamidine may precipitate the development of DKA [10]. The association between antipsychotic drugs, especially with atypical antipsychotics and hyperglycemia and even DKA have been reported in some cases [55,56]. Arefi et al. reported the first case of DKA due to nalidixic acid overdosage [57]. It has been available for the treatment of urinary tract infections for many years [58]. There are reports of hyperglycemia, convulsions and glycosuria in overdosage of nalidixic acid [58-61]. Interferon-alpha (IFN-α), a natural protein with anti-viral, anti-proliferative and immunomodulatory effects is routinely administered in chronic hepatitis C (CHC). Classical IFN-α has been correlated with the development of a variety of autoimmune disorders including Hashimoto thyroiditis, immune-mediated thrombocytopenia, hemolytic anemia, psoriasis, rheumatoid arthritis, systemic lupus erythematosus, primary biliary cirrhosis and sarcoidosis. It is unclear whether IFN-α treatment is associated with the development of T1DM. The prevalence of diabetes mellitus development in patients receiving classical IFN-α for CHC is very low ranging from 0.08% to 0.7% [62,63]. Fabris et al. reviewed 9 relative studies; the prevalence of pancreatic auto-antibodies appeared to rise from 3% to 7% prior to and following initiation of IFN-α treatment [64]. Soultati et al. reported a 38 year-old female patient developed simultaneously DKA and hyperthyroidism 5 months following initiation of treatment with pegylated IFN-α and ribavirin for CHC. High titers of glutamic acid decarboxylase, antinuclear and thyroid (thyroid peroxidase and thyroglobulin) antibodies were detected [65]. Until 2005, 35 cases of IFN-α related T1DM had been reported in the medical literature [64,66-69]. DKA was reported in a few classical IFN-α related cases [70-73], in three pegylated IFN-α related cases [65,74,75]. The development of DKA and the permanent insulin dependency may be related with a rapidly developing T helper-1-mediated pathogenic mechanism [72]. Tacrolimus, a reversible calcineurin inhibitor, is known for its diabetogenic potential. The incidence of diabetes is less frequent among the patients of nephrotic syndrome in comparison to organ transplant recipients. DKA is even rarer. Sarkar et al. reported in a 12-year-old girl with steroid resistant nephrotic syndrome, DKA as the first presentation of new onset tacrolimus induced transient T1DM despite a lower dose range and low trough level of the drug is being [76].

Cocaine abuse causes recurrent DKA with several mechanisms, including therapeutic non-compliance, stimulation of adrenal release of epinephrine and norepinephrine and increased release of other counter regulatory hormones [30,77]. Cytomegalovirus infection [78,79], protease inhibitor treatment [80,81] and highly active antiretroviral therapy (via immune restoration) may precipitate DKA in HIV-infected patients [82].

5. Diagnosis

5.1. History and physical examination

The acute DKA episode in T1DM evolution should be done rapidly. The symptoms of poorly controlled diabetes may be present for several days, but the metabolic changes typical of ketoacidosis usually occurs within a short time (typically 24 h). Occasionally, the entire symptomatic presentation may evolve or develop more acutely and the patient may present with DKA with no prior clues or symptoms. For DKA, the typical clinical findings includes a history of polyuria, polydipsia, weight loss, vomiting, dehydration, weakness and mental status change. Physical examination may include poor skin turgor, Kussmaul respirations, tachycardia and hypotension. Mental status can vary from full alertness to profound lethargy or coma [10,37]. The symptoms and physical signs of DKA are listed in Table 1.

MANIFESTATIONS OF DIABETIC KETOACIDOSIS	
Symptoms	Physical findings
Nausea / vomiting	Tachycardia
Thirst / polyuria	Dry mucous membranes / reduced skin turgor
Abdominal pain	Dehydration / hypotension
Shortness of breath	Tachypnea / Kussmaul respirations
	Abdominal tenderness
	Lethargy / obtundation / cerebral edema / possibly coma

Table 1. The symptoms and physical signs of DKA

Although infection is a common precipitating factor for DKA, patients can be normothermic or even hypothermic. Severe hypothermia, if present, is a poor prognostic sign and could be fatal. The major complications of hypothermia are acute renal failure, aspiration pneumonia, rhabdomyolysis, acute respiratory distresss syndrome and acute pancreatitis [83]. The mechanism of hypothermia complicated by DKA is unclear, but the inability of glucose to endocytose due to insulin deficit which leads to a lack of substrate for cellular heat production has been proposed [84]. A characteristic elevated J point on the electrocardiogram (ECG) (Osborn wave) may be observed when markedly hypothermia occurs [85-87]. The thermoregulatory system could be impaired in diabetic patients with autonomic neuropathy and reduced muscle mass or adipose tissue related with malnutrition. Thus, become prone to hypothermia under certain conditions [88,89].

Nausea, vomiting, diffuse abdominal pain are frequent in patients with DKA (50%) [90]. Abdominal pain on presentation could be a result of the DKA or an indication of a precipitating cause of DKA, particularly in younger patients or in the absence of severe metabolic acidosis [91,92]. Further evaluation is necessary if this complaint does not resolve with successfull treatment, because this may indicate other underlying complications.

5.2. Laboratory findings

The initial laboratory evaluation should include determination of plasma glucose, blood urea nitrogen, creatinine, electrolytes (with calculated anion gap), osmolality, serum and urinary ketones and urinalysis, as well as initial arterial blood gases and a complete blood count [93]. If laboratory measurement of serum potassium is delayed an ECG should be performed for baseline evaluation of potassium status [94,95]. An increased

http://dx.doi.org/10.5772/53199

WBC count is response to stress is characteristic of DKA and is not indicative of infection. If there is evidence of infection, chest X-ray and urine, sputum, throat or blood cultures should also be obtained [93].

The severity of DKA is classified as mild, moderate, or severe based on the severity of metabolic acidosis (blood pH, bicarbonate, and ketones) and the presence of altered mental status as shown in Table 2.

	DKA		
	Mild (plasma glucose >250 mg/dl)	Moderate (plasma glucose >250 mg/dl)	Severe (plasma glucose >250 mg/dl)
Arterial pH	7.25–7.30	7.00 to <7.24	<7.00
Serum bicarbonate (mEq/l)	15–18	10 to <15	<10
Urine ketone *	Positive	Positive	Positive
Serum ketone *	Positive	Positive	Positive
Effective serum osmolality †	Variable	Variable	Variable
Anion gap ‡	>10	>12	>12
Mental status	Alert	Alert/drowsy	Stupor/coma

*Nitroprusside reaction method.
†Effective serum osmolality: 2[measured Na+ (mEq/l)] + glucose (mg/dl)/18.
‡Anion gap: (Na+) − [(Cl− + HCO3− (mEq/l)].

Table 2. Classification of DKA

One of the major laboratory findings in DKA is the elevation of total blood ketone concentration. Assessment of increased ketonemia is usually performed by the nitroprusside reaction which provides a semiquantitative estimation of acetoacetate and acetone levels. The nitroprusside test (both in urine and in serum) is highly sensitive, but it does not recognize the main metabolic product in ketoacidosis; beta-hydroxybutyrate. In conclusion this assay is insufficient to determine the severity of ketoacidosis [10,31]. Measurement of serum ß- hydroxybutyrate may be an alternative to determine ketoacidosis [96). Ketoacids cause an increased anion gap metabolic acidosis. The anion gap is calculated by subtracting the sum of chloride(Cl) and bicarbonate (HCO3) concentration from the sodium (Na) concentration:

[Na - (Cl +HCO3)]. A normal anion gap is between 7 and 9 mEq/l and an anion gap 10–12 mEq/l indicates the presence of increased anion gap metabolic acidosis [10].

In clinical trials mixed acid–base disorders have been showed in DKA [97,98], but it is very rare the presentation of DKA with alkalaemia. The first case has been reported in 1970, defined as 'diabetic ketoalkalosis' [99] and it was followed by other case reports. The factors related with alkalemia in DKA were; recurrent vomiting which causes hydrogen and chloride ion loss (autonomic neuropathy such as delayed gastric emptying might have been related to recurrent vomiting), alkali ingestion and contraction alkalosis due to dehydration and/or diuretic use [100]. Treatment of diabetic ketoalkalosis does not differ from that of pure DKA.

Hyperglycemia is a key diagnostic criterion of DKA; but plasma glucose level varies in a wide range on admission. Recent studies have reported from normal or near normal [101] to elevated [31,3] hepatic glucose production rates. This factor possibly contributes to the wide range of plasma glucose levels in DKA that are independent of the severity of ketoacidosis [96]. In contrast to this 10% of the DKA patients presents with so-called 'true euglycemic DKA' [blood glucose <200 mg/dl (11.1 mmol/l)] [102]. Due to nausea or vomiting caused by a precipitating illness or by worsening ketoacidosis itself, a decrease in caloric intake occurs. If patients continue to take sufficient amounts of insulin in this situation may maintain euglycemia. But ketone body formation cannot be stopped, so they present as DKA accompanied with only mild elevations of blood glucose or normoglycemia [103-105]. Euglycemic DKA can be associated with other conditions such as; near total glycogen depletion [106,107], accelerated lipolysis [108] and free fatty acid production [109], less effectiveness of insulin suppressing lipolysis and ketogenesis during fasting and when there is sufficient circulating fluid volume to maintain glucose excretion [110]. In women with diabetes, pregnancy is also a condition that is associated with euglycemic ketoacidosis [111,112] as pregnancy is considered to be a state of accelerated starvation [113] with increased lipolysis and ketone body production in the presence of increased insulin insensitivity [114].

At presentation leukocytosis with cell counts in the 10,000 –15,000 mm^3 range is commonly seen in DKA and may not be indicative of an infection. But leukocytosis with cell counts 25,000 mm^3 may indicate infection and require further evaluation [115]. In ketoacidosis, leukocytosis may be correlated to elevated levels of cortisol and norepinephrine which is attributed to stress [116].

On admission serum sodium is usually low because of the osmotic flux of water from the intracellular to the extracellular space as a result of hyperglycemia. An increased or even normal serum sodium concentration in the presence of hyperglycemia indicates severe degree of free water loss. To assess the severity of sodium and water deficit, serum sodium may be corrected by adding 1.6 mg/dl to the measured serum sodium for each 100 mg/dl of glucose above 100 mg/dl [10,31]. In the calculation of effective osmolality, [sodium ion (mEq/l) x 2 + glucose (mg/dl)/18], the urea concentration is not taken into account because it is freely permeable and its accumulation does not induce major changes in intracellular volume or osmotic gradient across the cell membrane [10].

http://dx.doi.org/10.5772/53199

Serum potassium concentration may be increased because of an extracellular shift of potassium caused by insulin deficiency, hypertonicity and acidemia [117]. However, patients have severe total-body potassium deficiency. Treatment could be lowers serum potassium concentration and trigger cardiac arrhythmia. So patients with low normal or low serum potassium concentration should be monitored closely. If necessary appropriate potassium replacement should be done [93].

Insulin mainly affects glucose metabolism, but also protein and lipid metabolism. In the literature there are many cases of DKA presented with severe hyperlipidemia [118,119]. In patients with newly diagnosed T1DM presenting with DKA there is an absolute insulin deficiency that causes increased lipolysis and free fatty acid accumulation to the liver, decreased in utilization and excretion which results with hyperlipidemia. Severe hypertriglyceridemia can complicate DKA by the development of pancreatitis. As it is related with increased morbidity and mortality, clinicians must be aware of this complication. Children under the age of 5 years presenting with DKA have a higher rate of mortality. Therefore, these should be monitored for hyperlipidemia and if there is clinical evidence, for pancreatitis [120-123]. Pseudonormoglycemia [124] and pseudohyponatremia [125] may occur in DKA in the presence of severe chylomicronemia.

On the admission in patients with DKA, serum phosphate level is usually elevated because of an extracellular shift of phosphate caused by insulin deficiency, hypertonicity and increased catabolism. Thus, serum concentration does not reflect an actual body deficit [31,126,127]. Typical total body deficits of water and electrolytes in DKA are seen in Table 3.

Typical deficits	
Total water (L)	6
Water (ml/kg)*	100
Na^+ (mEq/kg)	7-10
Cl^- (mEq/kg)	3-5
K^+ (mEq/kg)	3-5
PO_4 (mmol/kg)	5-7
Mg^{++} (mEq/kg)	1-2
Ca^{++} (mEq/kg)	1-2

Table 3. Typical total body deficits of water and electrolytes in DKA (*Per kg of body weight)

Increased amylase and lipase has been reported in 16-25 % of patients with DKA. The mechanism of elevated enzymes in DKA remains unclear. Amylase elevations could be related with subtle injury to pancreatic acinar cells which causes release of this enzyme to the circulation, release of salivary gland amylase or suboptimal excretion in the urine [128]. There is little correlation between the presence, degree or isoenzyme type of hyperamylasemia and the presence of gastrointestinal symptoms (nausea, vomiting, and abdominal pain) or pancreatic imaging studies [129]. Increase in lipase may be related with release of nonpancreatic lipolytic enzymes into the circulation due to malignant tumors, to acute cholecystitis or esophagitis. Other possible mechanism are; renal insufficiency, delayed blood withdrawal, hypertriglyceridemia or subclinical pancreatitis [130]. Pancreatic enzyme levels reach a peak 12-24 hours after initiation of treatment for DKA [131]. Hyperlipasemia is less reliable for diagnosing acute pancreatitis, but elevated lipase is more spesific.

5.3. Differential diagnosis

Other causes of metabolic acidosis and ketosis must be differentiated from DKA. Differantial diagnosis of DKA can be seen in Table 4.

	DKA	Starvation or high fat intake	Lactic acidosis	Uremic acidosis	Alcholic ketosis	Methanol or ethylenglycol intoxication	Salicylate intoxication
Ph	↓	N	↓	Mild ↓	↓↑	↓	↓↑
Plasma glucose	↑	N	N	N	↓ or N	N	N or ↓
Total plasma ketones	↑↑	Slight ↑	N	N	Slight to moderate ↑	N	N
Anion gap	↑	Slight ↑	↑	Slight ↑	↑	↑	↑
Osmolality	↑	N	N	↑	N	↑↑	N
Uric acid	↑	Mild ↑	N	N	↑	N	N
Glycosuria	++	-	-	-	-	-	-

*Acetest and Ketostix measure acetoacetic acid only, thus misleading low values may be obtained because the majority of 'ketone bodies' are ß-hydroxybutyrate.
*(Data adapted from reference 10)

Table 4. Differantial diagnosis of DKA

Acute renal failure can be seen in ~5-7% of all adult hospitalizations [132,133]. It shares the common feature of an increased anion gap metabolic acidosis but can be easily differentiated from DKA by the absence of hyperglycemia or ketonemia. On the other hand, severe DKA can lead to prerenal azotemia and secondary acute kidney injury [134,135].

Severe uremic acidosis, characterized by an extremely high blood urea nitrogen, often >200 mg/dL (71.4 mmol/L) and creatinine >10 mg/dL (884 umol/L) causes acidosis via retention of anionic solutes in the patient with chronic kidney disease. The pH and anion gap can be found usually mild abnormal, however blood sugar is typically normal. Severe uremia typically occurs when creatinine clearance falls to <10 mL/min (0.1669 ml/s) in irreversible renal disease [136].

Lactic acidosis occasionally contributes to metabolic acidosis in patients hospitalized for either uncomplicated diabetes or DKA [137]. The main reason of lactic acidosis is tissue hypoxia [138]. It occurs in the setting of decreased tissue oxygen delivery which triggers non-oxidative metabolism of glucose to lactic acid. When co-existent with DKA, the anion gap typically exceeds that attributable to lactate alone. If lactic acidosis, with a serum lactate ≥5 mmol/L (45 mg/dL), occurs accompanied with DKA or hyperosmolar hyperglycemic state, severe volume depletion affects cardiac output negatively and also pre-existent cardiovascular disease increases this risk. Underlying liver disease with reduced lactate clearance and sepsis may also contribute more frequent/severe lactic acidosis in hyperglycemic emergencies. For main therapy it should be performed to optimise tissue perfusion and to treat underlying conditions [17,136].

When there is insufficient carbohydrate availability, starvation ketosis may occur by result of physiologically appropriate lipolysis and ketogenesis to provide fuel substrates. Blood glucose and arterial pH are found to be usually in normal level and the anion gap is at most mildly elevated. Although ketonuria may be apparent in urine analysis, modest ketonemia is typical in blood examination [17,136].

Chronical alcohol abuse may be the reason of alcoholic ketosis for ethanol is the predominant caloric source for days or weeks. Ketosis happens in sudden decrease of alcohol and caloric intake. Patients are usually present in normoglycemic or hypoglycemic state on submission, although some have rarely mild hyperglycemia [136].

Toxic ingestions sometimes need to be differentiated and history of the patients with laboratory studies may help for the differantial diagnosis. Salicylate, methanol and ethylene glycol each produce an increased anion gap metabolic acidosis without hyperglycemia or ketosis. Methanol and ethylene glycol will also cause a serum osmolal gap [17,136]. Measurement of suspicious drug/toxin concentrations with high index of suspicion, usually confirms the diagnosis of acute intoxication [139-142].

If there are some gastrointestinal or renal losses for any reason, non-anion gap metabolic acidosis may occur. It is characterized by a low serum bicarbonate concentration with subsequent chloride retention. Diarrhea and renal tubular acidosis are frequent causes of this condition. Carbonic anhydrase inhibitor therapy, rapid dilution of plasma bicarbonate by infused saline may be considered as the other varying reasons [143,144]. DKA can be easily differentiated from this condition by the presence of an increased anion gap and hyperglycemia. In complicated diabetics, especially in diabetic nephropathy, if there is hypoalbunemia, it can affect the apparent anion gap, since albumin is negatively charged protein contibuting 50-60% to the normal anion gap. If albumin is below the normal value of 4 g/dL (40 g/L), the calculated anion gap should be corrected by adding 2.5 for every 10 g/L (1 g/dL) to determine whether excessive abnormal anions are present [145-147].

6. Treatment

Successful treatment of DKA requires correction of dehydration, hyperglycemia and electrolyte imbalances, identification of comorbid precipitating events and above all, frequent patient monitoring. Protocols for the management of patients with DKA is summarized in Fig. 2 [10].

6.1. Fluid therapy

The most important initial therapeutic intervention is fluid replacement followed by insulin administration. DKA is a volume depletion state with water deficit, varying widely but averaging 6 L [51]. Initial fluid therapy is directed toward expansion of the intravascular, interstitial and intracellular volume (all of which are reduced in hyperglycemic crises), to establish tissue perfusion for insulin to reach cells [148] and restoration of renal perfusion. The goal of fluid resuscitation is to replace half of the estimated water deficit over the first 12-24 hours and adding for the ongoing losses (eg: vomiting) [51]. Replacement fluids may decrease the blood glucose by up to 23% because of increased renal perfusion and loss of glucose in urine [149] Hyperglycemia can reduce serum sodium by causing an osmotically driven shift of water from intracellular to extracellular compartments. In the previous estimated models; each 5.5 mmol/L (100 mg/dL) increase in glucose above normal resulted in a decrease of 1.6 mmol/L (1.6 mEq/L) in measured serum sodium [150], Hillier et al. suggested that 2.4 mmol/L (2.4 mEq/L) per 5.5 mmol/L (100 mg/dL) glucose increase is more accurate [151].

The initial fluid of choice is isotonic saline, generally given for the first 4 hours of therapy (Table 4). Subsequent choice for fluid replacement depends on hemodynamics, the state of hydration, serum electrolyte levels and urinary output. Fluid resuscitation should be individualized according to the patient's degree of dehydration, mental status and underlying diseases such as congestive heart failure or renal failure [51]. Glucose, an osmotic diuretic, may produce a high urine output even in severely dehydrated patients. The threshold for glycosuria in healthy adults occurs at plasma glucose concentration of approximately 180 mg/dL (9.99 mmol/L), though adults with long-standing diabetic nephropathy may have considerably higher thresholds. As a result, urine output should not be considered a reliable predictor of volume status in hyperglycemic states [152].

http://dx.doi.org/10.5772/53199

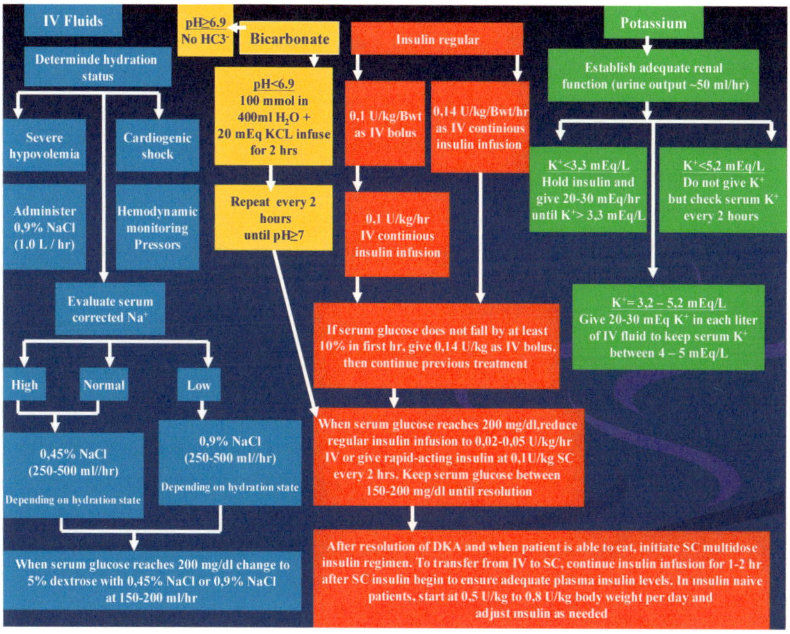

Figure 2. Protocols for the management of patients with DKA (Data adapted from reference 10)

Hours	Volume
1st hour	1,000 – 2,000 mL
2nd hour	1,000 mL
3rd-5th hours	500 – 1,000 mL/hour
6th-12th hours	250 – 500 mL/hour

Table 5. Suggested average initial replacement rate of fluid in DKA (after hemodynamic resuscitation with normal saline when indicated)

Many guidelines recommend initial fluid resuscitation with colloid in hypotensive patients. However, the hypotension results from a loss of electrolyte solution and it is more physiological to replace with crystalloid. A recent Cochrane review did not support the use of colloid in preference to crystalloid fluid [153]. In the absence of cardiac compromise, isotonic saline (0.9% NaCl) is infused at a rate of 15–20 ml kg/body wt/h or 1–1.5 L during the first hour. In general, 0.45% NaCl infused at 250–500 ml/hour is appropriate if the corrected serum sodium is normal or elevated; 0.9% NaCl at a similar rate is appropriate if corrected serum sodium is low (Fig. 2). That total fluid administered should not exceed 4 $L/m^2/24$ hour for fear of causing cerebral edema is most often the mainstay of therapy in many pediatric critical care unit protocols [154,155]. Successful treatment with fluid replacement can be evaluate by hemodynamic monitoring (improvement in blood pressure), measurement of fluid input/output, laboratory values and clinical improvement. In patients with renal or cardiac failure, monitoring of serum osmolality and frequent assessment of cardiac, renal and mental status must be performed during fluid resuscitation to avoid iatrogenic fluid overload [10,37,148]. During treatment of DKA, hyperglycemia is corrected faster than ketoacidosis. The mean duration of treatment until blood glucose is <250 mg/dl and ketoacidosis (pH>7.30; bicarbonate >18 mmol/l) is corrected is 6 and 12 hours [36,156]. Once the plasma glucose falls to <200-250 mg/dL (11.1-13.88 mmol/L), 5% dextrose should be added to replacement fluids to allow continued insulin administration until ketonemia is controlled while at the same time avoiding hypoglycemia [93,135]. In hypotensive patients, aggressive fluid resuscitation with isotonic saline should be continued until blood pressure normalized [51].

6.2. Insulin therapy

Insulin lowers the serum glucose concentration (by decreasing gluconeogenesis and glycogenolysis, increasing tissue glucose uptake) and arrests ketone production (by reducing lipolysis and glucagon secretion). The most important point in the treatment of DKA involves insulin administration. There was major concern about; physiologic or low dose insulin therapy was superior to pharmacologic dose regimen and the administration of regular insulin via continuous intravenous infusion or by frequent subcutaneous or intramuscular injections [10,157-160]. Several randomized controlled studies have shown that physiologic or low dose insulin therapy was superior to pharmacologic dose regimen and low-dose insulin therapy is effective regardless of the route of administration in DKA [118,159,160]. In clinical practice most patients are treated with low dose, intravenous regular insulin until resolution of DKA [30]. The administration of continuous intravenous infusion of regular insulin is preferred because of its short half-life and easy titration and the delayed onset of action and prolonged half-life [107,127,160].

Previous treatment algorithms have recommended the administration of an initial intravenous bolus of regular insulin (0.1 unit/kg) followed by the infusion of 0.1 unit/kg/h [10,17], but a recent prospective randomized study showed that a bolus dose is not required if patients are given hourly insulin infusion at 0.14 unit/kg body weight [161]. Low-dose insulin infusion protocols decrease plasma glucose concentration at a rate of 50–75 mg/d/ h. If plasma glucose does not decrease by 50–75 mg in the first hour, the insulin infusion should be increased every hour until a steady glucose decline is achieved. When the plasma glucose reaches 200 mg/dl in DKA, the insulin infusion rate may decrease to 0.02–0.05 units/kg/h, at the same time dextrose should be added to the intravenous fluids for avoiding hypoglycemia. The rate of insulin administration or the concentration of dextrose may need to be adjusted to maintain glucose values between 150 and 200 mg/dl until DKA resolved [90]. Resolution of ketoacidosis includes these criteria; a blood glucose <200 mg/dl and two of the following criteria: a serum bicarbonate level >15 mEq/l, a venous pH >7.3, and a calculated anion gap in normal range. Once hyperglycemia is corrected, 12-24 hours of intravenous insulin treatment is sufficient to clear ketones from the circulation [51].

Subcutaneous rapid-acting insulin analogs (lispro and aspart) offer an efficacious and cost-effective alternative to continuous intravenous infusions in the treatment of DKA [162-164].

Umpierrez et al. used subcutaneous rapid-acting insulin (insulin lispro or aspart) 0.2 units/kg initially followed by 0.1 unit/kg every hour or an initial dose of 0.3 units/kg followed by 0.2 units/kg every 2 hours, until blood glucose is ≤ 250 mg/dL; the insulin dose is then decreased by half (to 0.05 or 0.1 unit/kg, respectively) every 1-2 hours until resolution [162,163]. There were no differences in length of hospital stay, total amount of insulin needed for resolution of hyperglycemia or ketoacidosis. Patients treated with insulin analogs were managed in the open medical wards which reduced cost of hospitalization by 30% [162-164]. This approach is not widely used for many reasons, including titration difficulties with longer half-life preparations, requirement for hourly nursing interventions and lack of staff experience compared to that with standard insulin infusions. However, until these studies are confirmed outside the research arena, patients with severe DKA, hypotension, anasarca or associated severe critical illness should be managed with intravenous regular insulin in the intensive care unit [93].

In patients younger than 4 years of age there is a prolonged time lag for plasma glucose levels to reach 12 to 14 mmol/L, because young children and adolescents who have high growth velocity and higher levels of the human growth hormone, a diabetogenic hormone. In addition to this, patients with fever or infections and higher metabolic requirements may need 15% to 20% more insulin than the usual dose [165].

In rare cases of patients with allergy to human insulin presenting with hyperglycemic crisis, desensitization to human insulin may be performed before treatment with human insulin. A recent case report documented the successful treatment of a woman with allergy to human insulin and its analogs with continuous subcutaneous infusion of human insulin [166].

6.3. Potassium

Despite a total body potassium deficit resulting from the glycosuric osmotic diuresis, mild-to-moderate hyperkalemia is common in patients with hyperglycemic crises upon initial presentation because of proteolysis, acidosis, and insulin deficiency [10,167]. Insulin therapy, correction of acidosis and volume expansion decrease serum potassium concentration [10].

Occasionally patients with DKA may present with significant hypokalemia, in which case insulin therapy should be delayed until potassium concentration is corrected to >3.5 mequiv./l to avoid arrhythmias and respiratory muscle weakness [168,169]. To prevent hypokalemia, potassium replacement is initiated after serum levels fall below the upper level of normal for the particular laboratory (5.0-5.2 mEq/l) in patients without renal impairment. The treatment goal is to maintain serum potassium levels within the normal range of 4–5 mEq/l. Generally, 20–30 mEq potassium in each liter of infusion fluid is sufficient to maintain serum potassium concentration within the normal range but additional doses may be necessary [10,30].

The rare patient with severe hyperkalemia (>6.0 mEq/l) on admission with concomitant electrocardiographic changes may benefit from bicarbonate therapy [170].

6.4. Bicarbonate therapy

The hepatic metabolism of free fatty acids generates ketoanions, such as beta-hydroxybutyrate and acetoacetate [171,172]. Impaired tissue perfusion due to volume contraction and the adrenergic response to the often severe underlying precipitating illness result in lactate production [173]. Acute kidney injury leads to accumulation of other unmeasured anions, such as sulphate, urate and phosphate [174]. All these, together with hyperchloremia which predominates during the recovery phase of DKA [175], contribute to the development of acidemia, which often is severe [176,177].

Metabolic acidemia can impair myocardial contractility, reduce cardiac output, affect oxyhemoglobin dissociation and tissue oxygen delivery, inhibit intracellular enzymes, such as phosphofructokinase, alter cellular metabolism, and result in vital organ dysfunction [178-181]. In the past, therapy in DKA has placed importance on the rapid reversal of acidemia. But based on currently available evidence, several deleterious effects of bicarbonate therapy have been reported, such as increased risk of hypokalemia, decreased tissue oxygen uptake, cerebral edema and development of paradoxical central nervous system acidosis [182]. The use of bicarbonate in DKA remains a controversial subject.

Since severe acidosis may be associated with adverse effects, patients with pH <6.9 or when pH is <7.1 and hemodynamic instability or hyperkalemic electrocardiographic changes are present [93,135], bicarbonate should be given. A choice is to give 100 mmol sodium bicarbonate (two ampules) in 400 ml sterile water with 20 mEq KCI at a rate of 200 ml/h for 2 hours. If the pH is stil <7.0 after infusion, we recommend repeating infusion every 2 hours until pH reaches >7.0 [17,93]. Potassium replacement should be considered before administering bicarbonate or KCL should be added in the bicarbonate solution at 40 mmol (40 mEq) KCl/L to avoid precipitous hypokalemia [93,135].

6.5. Phosphate

In patients with DKA there is about 1 mmol/kg body weight phosphate depletion. At presentation serum phosphate levels are usually normal or elevated. But with insulin therapy these levels rapidly decrease [90,132]. Randomized studies showed that phosphate replacement have no any additional benefit on the clinical outcome [126,183] and in contrast, phosphate replacement may trigger hypocalcemia and hypomagnesemia [183,184]. Hypophosphatemia can cause hemolysis, refractory acidosis, reduced cardiac output, respiratory muscle weakness, rhabdomyolysis, central nervous system depression, seizures, coma or acute renal failure. Careful phosphate replacement should be planned to the patients with these findings and severe hypophosphatemia (serum phosphate <1 mg/dL) [10,90,132]. In severe deficiency, the amount, added to intravenous replacement fluids can be 20–30 mEq/l potassium phosphate. Secure replacement rate that can correct hypophosphatemia is 4.5 mmol/h (1.5 ml/h of K2 PO4) [185]. In less severe deficiencies 80-110 mmol (2.5-3.5 g) daily in 2-3 divided doses oral phosphate can be given [93,135,186].

http://dx.doi.org/10.5772/53199

6.6. Transition to subcutaneous insulin

When DKA has resolved, patients who are appropriate for oral intake can be started on a multiple dose insulin regimen with a long acting insulin (e.g. glargine or detemir) to cover basal insulin requirements and short/rapid acting insulin (lispro, aspart or glulisine) given before meals to control plasma glucose. To ensure adequate plasma insulin levels and to avoid hyperglycemia and ketonemia intravenous insulin infusion should be continued for 1–2 hours after the subcutaneous insulin is given. Patients who are inappropriate for oral intake the treatment should be continued with an infusion of intravenous fluids and insulin [10,17,49,93,187]. A multiple-dose subcutaneous combination regimen is preferred, as it is related with less hypoglycemia and provides a better physiologic pattern of control than other regimens. In insulin-naïve patients, a multidose insulin regimen should be started at a dose of 0.5-0.8 units/kg body weight per day. Patients with known diabetes, whose blood glucose monitoring are in the normal ranges before DKA, may start with dose of insulin they are receiving [160].

In the past human insulin (NPH and regular) were usually given in two or three doses per day. With the development of new analogue insulins, basal-bolus regimens with basal (glargine and detemir) and rapid-acting (lispro, aspart, or glulisine) insulin treatments became a major concern in the treatment of DKA. A prospective randomized trial compared with a split mixed regimen of NPH plus regular insulin twice daily treatment and a basal-bolus regimen, including glargine once daily and glulisine before meals following the resolution of DKA. Glycemic control were similar between the two groups but the study showed that treatment with basal-bolus insulin regimen was associated with a lower rate of hypoglycemic events (15%) than the rate in those treated with NPH and regular insulin (41%). This trial showed that analogue insulins may offer a more physiologic effect [156].

6.7. Somatostatin therapy in the management of resistant diabetic ketoacidosis

As a inhibiting hormone for counterregulatory hormones, somatostatin may be used in the treatment of DKA. Somatostatin analogues have been successfully used in the treatment of diabetes associated autonomic neuropathy and they have also been shown to decrease the requirements for insulin [188,189]. Continuous subcutaneous octreotide infusion suppresses counterregulatory hormones, increases insulin-mediated glucose metabolism by enhancing glucose storage and reduces energy expenditure [189]. There are limiting data in the literature about somatostatin use in DKA. Diem et al. were assessed preventive effects of octreotide on diabetic ketogenesis during insulin withdrawal. Octreotide led to a marked suppression of beta-hydroxybutyrate, acetoacetate and glucagon levels and an associated diminution of bicarbonate consumption and the fall in pH [190]. Anthony et al. reported a case of DKA with glucagonoma who was unresponsive to conventional therapy and treated with octreotide [191]. In conclusion, for patients who do not respond to conventional DKA treatment, somatostatin could be added to therapy. More data and further randomized controlled clinical trials should be made with the use of somatostatin in treatment of DKA.

6.8. Monitoring

Successful management and early intervention for complications require close monitoring. Timeline in DKA management are listed in Figure-3 [165]. The clinicians should be made a flow chart to obtain all relevant incidents regarding the patient's condition and clinical outcome [192].

Time	Evaluation	Laboratory	Intervention
0-1 st hour	GCS on admission, check pupils, monitor vitals (HR, BP, temperature and pulse oximetry)	CBC, electrolytes (Na, Cl, K, HCO3, PO4, Mg), BUN, Cr, ß- hydroxybutyrate, urine ketones, venous pH, blood glucose, lactic acid level, ECG	Calculate total fluid deficit; start careful fluid ressuciation; plasma volume expanders, goal to achieve normal blood pressure; check urine output (may need catheter)
2 nd hour	Check BP and ensure urine output; check GCS every hour for first 8 hours	Check lactic acid in second hour and follow up on labs	Start insulin (with prior check on K levels) and replace fluids; may need bicarbonate; GCS<8 or CE: intubate and ventilate, nasogastric tube for suction
	High fever	Suspect infection; check WBC (>15000mm3), CRP (high) and urine (WBCs and for nitrates, leukoesterases)	Send appropriate cultures (blood and urine), chest radiograph, use antibiotics with broad spectrum
3-8 th hour	GCS as above; check for ongoing losses	Venous blood pH every 2 hours; electrolytes; and ß- hydroxybutyrate every 4 hours; may check urine ketones	While continuing insulin; reasses adequecy of fluids and ascertain complete rehydration
	Continued abdominal pain	Serum amylase and lipase levels; ultrasound abdomen and abdominal X-ray	May need to manage acute abdominal pain (pancreatitis)
			May need to switch dextrose if serum glucose level is ≤250 mg/dL; continue to check response to ongoing hydration
9-24 th hour	Check GCS every 2 hours	Can change to labs every 8/12 hours at end of 24 hours	Complete rehydration at 48-hour period;transition to pump or subcutaneous insulin
24-48 hours	Check GCS every 2 hours if hypernatremia was initially present	Check for pH, electrolytes, and ß- hydroxybutyrate as above and stop if pH, ß- hydroxybutyrate and HCO3 are normal	

Figure 3. Timeline in DKA management. GCS:Glascow Coma Scale, CBC:Complete Blood Counting, ECG:Electrocardiogram, HR:Heart Rate, BP:Blood Pressure, BUN:Blood Urea Nitrogen, Cr: Creatinine, WBC:White Blood Cell, CRP:C-reactive protein, CE:Cerebral edema (adapted from reference 165)

http://dx.doi.org/10.5772/53199

Recommendations for laboratory monitoring include; hourly vital signs and neurologic checks; hourly blood glucose levels for the first 4-6 hours and then to continue with 2 hour intervals in the following period; venous blood gases every 2 hours for 6 hours, then every 4 hours, Na, K and ionized calcium every 2 hours for 6 hours then every 4 hours; magnesium and phosphorus every 4 hours; blood urea nitrogen and creatinine levels (every 4 hours) should also be monitored until stable; basic metabolic profile at admission and then every morning. Fluid intake and urinary output should be monitored [193-195]. These are the minimum requirements and should be revised for special situations. For example, patients with initially low potassium, more frequent (hourly) K measurements should be made with ECG monitoring [194,195] or if patient's neurological status is unstable and has a high risk of cerebral edema, more frequent neurologic and vital sign checks (20-30 minutes) should be made [192].

Serum bicarbonate and anion gap are good markers of therapeutic response. Close monitoring of arterial blood gases and serum or urine ketones should not be used as predictor of clinical improvement. Despite of successfull treatment by arresting ketogenesis, ketone levels may be considered unchanged or high, as beta-hydroxybutyrate converts to acetoacetate and conventional (nitroprusside) testing detects only acetoacetate and acetone [135]. For avoid this problem laboratory measurement or the use of a bedside fingerstick sample monitor for beta-hydroxybutyrate can be made. It is reasonable to reduce laboratory monitoring frequency when acidosis resolves, the anion gap falls to near normal limits while response to glycemic therapy becomes noticeable [135]. In the presence of persistent acidosis, despite of successfull treatment; sepsis, concomitant illness or inadequate insulin dosing should be kept in mind and further evaluation and intervention should be made [135,193].

7. Complications of diabetic ketoacidosis or it's treatment

Most of the diabetes-related morbidity and mortality in T1DM can be attributed to complications of DKA.

7.1. Hypoglycemia

Decrease in the plasma glucose concentration rate should be kept in the range of 50–75 mg/dl/hour. As ketoacidosis is corrected, a rapid decline in plasma glucose levels can be occur and this may cause the blood glucose drop to hypoglycemia levels. Hypoglycemia leads to the release of counter-regulatory hormones and this results with rebound ketosis which can lengthen the duration of treatment. In addition to this, severe hypoglycemia can cause cardiac arrhythmias, seizure or loss of consciousness, brain injury including coma or death. The insulin infusion rate should be checked every hour until a steady glucose decline is achieved and once the plasma glucose falls to <200-250 mg/dL (11.1-13.88 mmol/L), dextrose should be added to replacement fluids to allow continued insulin administration and avoid hypoglycemia [93].

7.2. Rhabdomyolysis and renal failure

Acute renal failure (ARF) is an uncommon complication of DKA and rarely requires renal replacement therapy and it may be severe and potentially life threatening [196,197]. The etiology of ARF associated with DKA is multifactorial. The most commonly cited causes are hypovolemia, hypotension and rhabdomyolysis [196]. Prolonged profound ketoacidosis and insulin infusions can lead to severe hypophosphatemia, mainly as a result of intracelluar phosphate shifting [198-201]. Hypophosphatemia can be resulted with rhabdomyolysis. Other risk factors for rhabdomyolysis are severe hyperglycemia and high osmolality. But the pathogenic mechanism leading to rhabdomyolysis in DKA remains unclear. There are few reported cases in literature which had rhabdomyolysis in DKA. There may be no symptoms or the condition can present with a mild increase of creatine kinase or rarely significant acute renal failure necessitating hemodialysis [202-205].

7.3. Peripheral venous thrombosis

In DKA treatment, patients may require central vascular access for intensive fluid replacement. However, this route of vascular access causes many complications [206] like venous thromboembolism (VTE) [207]. Children with thrombophilia, malignancy, congenital cardiac disease, acute infection, trauma and surgery have a high risk for complications of central venous catheter (CVC) related VTE [206]. In the medical literature there have been few reported cases CVC related VTE in DKA children without known risk factors. [208-210]. Thus, DKA and its treatment may promote a prothrombotic state and activation of vascular endothelium, predisposing to thrombosis. Whilst, DKA has not been identified as an isolated risk factor for CVC-related VTE in adults [211]. Where essential for, intensive fluid replacement in DKA, these lines should be removed as soon as possible, particularly as CVC-related VTE appears to occur within the first 24-48 hours after insertion [210].

7.4. Pancreatitis

Acute pancreatitis is a well known complication of DKA in adults [212] but is unusual in childhood. In children with DKA, abdominal pain and vomiting are common. In addition to this, patients with DKA also have elevated serum pancreatic enzyme (amylase/lipase) concentrations without clinical signs or symptoms and without radiographic evidence of pancreatitis [213,214]. Although hypertriglyceridemia is a known cause of acute pancreatitis and elevated triglyceride concentrations are frequent during DKA, an association between elevated triglyceride concentrations in DKA and pancreatic enzyme elevation or pancreatitis have not be showned in the previous studies [213,215]. The mechanism responsible for pancreatic enzyme elevation in DKA has thus remained unclear. Physicians should be aware of this phenomenon so that patients with DKA who have abdominal pain and elevated pancreatic enzymes are not erroneously diagnosed with acute pancreatitis unless in the presence of persistent abdominal pain, which does not resolve with a successful treatment.

http://dx.doi.org/10.5772/53199

7.5. Mucormycosis

Mucormycosis is an acute, rapidly progressing, and often fatal facultative fungal infection occurs in patients with diabetes who have poor glycemic control and DKA, which have been well established as predisposing factors for fungal growth. Mucormycosis can be classfied; cutaneous, rhino-cerebral, pulmonary, gastrointestinal, central nervous system and disseminated [216]. The rhino-cerebral forms develops in patients with diabetes, particularly with the complication such as DKA. The most common symptoms are; facial pain, headache, fever, and mental obtundation [217]. In the Figure 4 there is a patient of us, firstly diagnosed T1DM with DKA infected by mucormycozis [218].

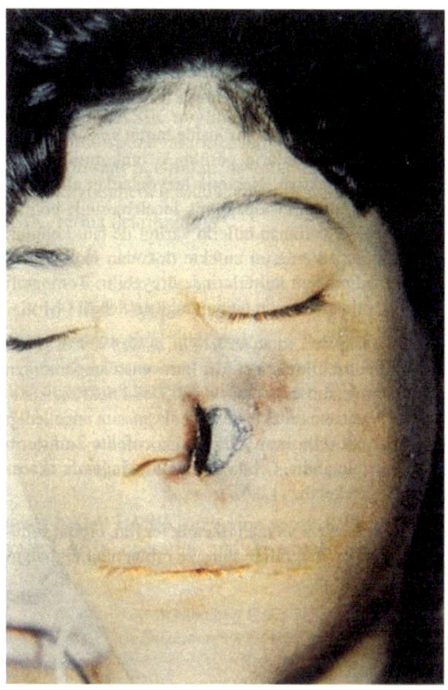

Figure 4. A 15 years old male patient firstly diagnosed T1DM with DKA infected by rhino-orbita-cerebral mucormycozis (Picture from the reference [218])

7.6. Pulmonary oedema

Pulmonary oedema is a rare, iatrogenic complication of DKA. Usually occurs within a few hours of initiation of treatment related with rapid infusion of crystalloids over a short period of time. Elderly patients and those with impaired cardiac/renal function are at high risk and monitoring of central venous pressure should be considered [219].

7.7. Pneumomediastinum

Spontaneous pneumomediastinum is a rare pulmonary complication of DKA [220]. Kussmaul breathing and repeated vomiting increases the intra-alveolar pressure; that leads to alveolar rupture; then, the air penetrates peribronchial and perivascular spaces and reach the mediastinum. Extension into neck and subcutaneous tissue could be seen. The most common sypmtoms include chest pain and dyspnoea. Treatment is mostly supportive; management of nausea/vomiting along with correction of acidosis to break Kussmaul breathing is should be considered. Patients should be carefully monitored in intensive care settings [221-223].

7.8. Cerebral edema

Symptomatic cerebral edema (CE) is rare in adults treated for DKA, although asymptomatic CE may be occur [224] and may be present before treatment [225]. In contrast to this, CE occurs in ~0.3–1.0% of DKA episodes in children [224,226) and is associated with a mortality rate of 20–40% [226] and accounts for 57–87% of all DKA deaths [224,226]. Because of possible delay in diagnosis and more susceptibility to metabolic and vascular changes, children <5 years of age have higher risk for the development of CE. The recognized risk factors for development of CE are acidosis, hypocapnia and elevated serum urea nitrogen (indicator of severity of ketoacidosis and dehydration) [227]. The etiology of CE is unknown; many mechanisms have been proposed including cerebral hypoperfusion with subsequent re-perfusion [228,229], the generation of various inflammatory mediators [230], increased cerebral blood flow, disruption of cell membrane ion transport and a rapid shift in extracellular and intracellular fluids resulting in changes in osmolality. Thus the etiology of DKA-related CE is multifactorial and results of an interplay of complex pathophysiological processes involving the brain [231-235]. The time of onset is not the same in all affected individuals; two-thirds of patients develops signs and symptoms in the first 6-7 hours and the rest from 10-24 hours after start of the treatment with the early-onset individuals tending to be younger [182,236,237].

Muir et al. suggested a model for early detection. The system allowed 92% sensitivity and 96% specificity for the recognition of CE early enough for intervention. One diagnostic criterion, two major criteria or one major plus two minor criteria is suitable to establish CE [236]. Diagnostic criteria, major criteria and minor criteria are shown in Table 6.

Diagnostic criteria	Major criteria	Minor criteria
1. Abnormal motor or verbal response to pain 2.Decorticate or decerebrate posture 3.Cranial nerve palsy (especially III, IV, VI) 4.Abnormal neurogenic respiratory pattern (eg: grunting, tachypnea, Cheyne-Stokes, apneustic)	1.Altered mentation and fluctuating level of consciousness 2.Sustained heart rate deceleration (decline more than 20 per minute) not attributable to improved intravascular volume or sleep state 3. Age inappropriate incontinence	1.Vomiting following initial treatment and its cessation, if present at admission 2. Headache (recurrent and more severe than on admission) 3.Lethargy or not easily aroused from sleep 4. Diastolic blood pressure greater than 90 mmHg 5. Age <5 years

Table 6. Diagnostic criteria, major criteria and minor criteria for Cerebral Edema

http://dx.doi.org/10.5772/53199

To prevent the development CE the following should be made; avoiding excessive hydration and rapid reduction of plasma osmolarity, a gradual decline in serum glucose and maintenance of serum glucose between 250–300 mg/dl until the patient's mental status is improved [238].

First of all the rate of fluid administration should be decreased and head of the bed lifted up [236]. Administration of IV mannitol in a dosage of 1.0 g/kg over 20 minutes when repeated as necessary in 1-2 hours shows an improvement in clinical outcome [224,227,228,239]. Patients who do not respond adequately to mannitol of a dose of 1 g/kg, 5-10 mL/kg 3% saline infusion is an alternative treatment [240].

7.9. Intracerebral complications other than CE

Neurologic collapse during DKA can cause other intracerebral complications, with or without associated edema, but defined not idiopathic CE [227]. These include; subarachnoid hemorrhage, basilar artery thrombosis [224], cerebral venous thrombosis [241,242], meningoencephalitis [243] and disseminated intravascular coagulation [244,245].

8. Preventıon

DKA can be prevented by access to a 24-hours telephone helpline for emergency advice and treatment, sufficient patient education and easier access to medical care. Especially patients should be educated about a clinical condition which increases the risk of developing DKA and the changes in the treatment at this situations.

These are includes the following;

1. Patients should be educated about what are the precipitating factors of DKA.
2. Early contact with a 24-hours telephone helpline or the health care provider should be obtained in an acute illness.
3. The importance of insulin during an acute illness should be emphasized.
4. Patients should be advised never to discontinue insulin before contact with health care provider.
5. Patients should be informed about blood glucose goals, the use of additional dose short or rapid acting insulin and the medications available to suppress a fever and treat an infection.
6. In the case of nause and vomiting an easily digestible liquid diet containing carbohydrates and salt should be initiated.
7. Family members should be educated about sick day management and record keeping including assessing and documenting temperature, blood glucose, and urine/blood ketone testing, insulin administration, oral intake and weight [93].

Home measurement of blood glucose-ketone levels may allow early recognition of hyperglycemia and ketosis. Adjusment of insulin therapy based on these findings may prevent hospitalization for DKA [246].

9. Conclusıon

DKA is a life-threatening condition which is the most common cause of death in children and adolescents with T1DM and a mortality rate <1% in adult subjects. DKA is a preventable complication of T1DM. Education about the precipitating factors of DKA and rapid access to health care providers contributes to better outcomes and fewer recurrences. DKA can be controlled in a period of 12-36 hours with an appropriate treatment. Thus, complications can be prevented and reduction in mortality rates can be achieved.

Author details

Mustafa Cesur[1] and Irmak Sayin[2]

1 Ankara Guven Hospital, Department of Endocrinology and Metabolic Disease, Turkey

2 Ufuk University, Medical Faculty, Department of Internal Medicine, Turkey

References

[1] Struwe FE. Zur Friuherkennung des Diabetes mellitus bei Kindern und Jugendlichen. Mschr Kinderheilk 1973:121:477-9.

[2] Kiiar M-L. Clinical course of diabetes in children. Academic dissertation. Oulu: Acta Universitas Ouluensis, series D, Medica No 100, 1983.

[3] Drash A. Clinical care of the diabetic child. Chicago: Year Book Medical Publishers, 1987.

[4] Daneman D, Knip M, Kaar M-L, Sochett E. Comparison of children with type I (insulin-dependent) diabetes in Northern Finland and Southern Ontario: differences at disease onset. Diabetes Res 1990;14:123-6.

[5] Couper JJ, Hudson I, Werther GA, et al. Factors predicting residual beta-cell function in the first year after diagnosis of childhood type 1 diabetes. Diabetes Res Clin Pract 199 1;11: 9-16.

[6] Elamin A, Omer MIA, Tuvemo T. Islet-cell antibodies and endogenous insulin secretion in Sudanese diabetic children. Diabetes Res Clin Pract 1992;16:91-6.

[7] Pinkney JH, Bingley PJ, Sawtell PA, et al. Presentation andb progress of childhood diabetes mellitus: a prospective population-based study. Diabetologia 1994;37:70-4.

[8] White NH. Diabetic ketoacidosis in children. Endocrinol Metab Clin North Am. 2000 Dec;29(4):657-82.

[9] Usher-Smith JA, Thompson MJ, Sharp SJ, Walter FM. Factors associated with the presence of diabetic ketoacidosis at diagnosis of diabetes in children and young adults: a systematic review. BMJ. 2011 Jul 7;343:d4092. doi: 10.1136/bmj.d4092.

[10] Kitabchi AE, Umpierrez GE, Murphy MB, Barrett EJ, Kreisberg RA, Malone JI, Wall BM. Management of hyperglycemic crises in patients with diabetes. Diabetes Care 2001;24: 131– 153.

[11] Komulainen J, Lounamaa R, Knip M, Kaprio EA, Akerblom HK. Ketoacidosis at the diagnosis of type 1 (insulin dependent) diabetes mellitus is related to poor residual beta cell function. Childhood Diabetes in Finland Study Group. Arch Dis Child. 1996 Nov;75(5):410-5.

[12] DIAMOND Project Group. Incidence and trends of childhood type 1 diabetes world-wide 1990-1999. Diabet Med 2006;23:857-66.

[13] EURODIAB ACE Study Group. Variation and trends in incidence of childhood diabetes in Europe. Lancet 2000;355:873-6.).

[14] Ali K, Harnden A, Edge J. Type 1 diabetes in children. BMJ 2011;342:d294.

[15] Patterson CC, Dahlquist GG, Gyürüs E, Green A, Soltész G; EURODIAB Study Group. Incidence trends for childhood type 1 diabetes in Europe during 1989-2003 and predicted new cases 2005-20: a multicentre prospective registration study. Lancet. 2009 Jun 13;373(9680):2027-33.

[16] Chiasson JL, Aris-Jilwan N, Belanger R, Bertrand S, Beauregard H, Ekoe JM, Fournier H, Havrankova J. Diagnosis and treatment of diabetic ketoacidosis and the hyperglycemic hyperosmolar state. CMAJ. 2003; 168:859-66.

[17] Kitabchi AE, Nyenwe EA. Hyperglycemic crises in diabetes mellitus: diabetic ketoacidosis and hyperglycemic hyperosmolar state. Endocrinol Metab Clin North Am. 2006; 35:725-51.

[18] Gurlek A, Erbas T, Sayinalp S, Gedik O. Frequency of insulin-dependent diabetes mellitus in Turkish adult-onset diabetic population. Acta Diabetol. 1996; 33:216-9.

[19] Lévy-Marchal C, Papoz L, de Beaufort C, Doutreix J, Froment V, Voirin J, Czernichow P. Clinical and laboratory features of type 1 diabetic children at the time of diagnosis. Diabet Med. 1992 Apr;9(3):279-84.

[20] Lévy-Marchal C, Patterson CC, Green A; EURODIAB ACE Study Group. Europe and Diabetes. Geographical variation of presentation at diagnosis of type I diabetes in children: the EURODIAB study. European and Dibetes. Diabetologia. 2001 Oct;44 Suppl. 3:B75-80.

[21] Oyarzabal Irigoyen M, García Cuartero B, Barrio Castellanos R, Torres Lacruz M, Gómez Gila AL, González Casado I, Hermoso López F, Luzuriaga Tomás C, Rica Etxebarrial I, López García MJ, Rodríguez Rigual M. Ketoacidosis at onset of type 1 diabetes mellitus in pediatric age in Spain and review of the literature. Pediatr Endocrinol Rev. 2012 Mar;9(3):669-71.

[22] Hanas R, Lindgren F, Lindblad B. Diabetic ketoacidosis and cerebral oedema in Sweden--a 2-year paediatric population study. Diabet Med. 2007 Oct;24(10):1080-5.

[23] Rewers A, Chase HP, Mackenzie T, Walravens P, Roback M, Rewers M, Hamman RF, Klingensmith G. Predictors of acute complications in children with type 1 diabetes. JAMA. 2002 May 15;287(19):2511-8.

[24] Roche EF, Menon A, Gill D, Hoey H. Roche EF, Menon A, Gill D, Hoey H. Pediatr Diabetes. 2005 Jun;6(2):75-8.

[25] Bui TP, Werther GA, Cameron FJ. Trends in diabetic ketoacidosis in childhood and adolescence: a 15-yr experience. Pediatr Diabetes. 2002 Jun;3(2):82-8.

[26] Wolfsdorf J, Glaser N, Sperling MA. Diabetic ketoacidosis in infants, children, and adolescents: a consensus statement from the American Diabetes Association. Diabetes Care 2006; 29: 1150– 2259.

[27] White NH. Diabetic ketoacidosis in children. Endocrinol Metab Clin North Am 2000; 29: 657– 682.

[28] Graves EJ, Gillium BS. the National Center for Health Statistics Detailed diagnoses and procedures: National Hospital Discharge Survey, 1995. Vital Health Stat 131997; (130): 1– 146.

[29] Malone ML, Gennis V, Goodwin JS. Characteristics of diabetic ketoacidosis in older versus younger adults. J Am Geriatr Soc 1992; 40: 1100– 110.

[30] Kitabchi AE, Umpierrez GE, Murphy MB, Kreisberg RA. Hyperglycemic crises in adult patients with diabetes: a consensus statement from the American Diabetes Association. Diabetes Care. 2006 Dec;29(12):2739-48.

[31] Kitabchi AE, Fisher JN, Murphy MB, Rumbak MJ. Diabetic ketoacidosis and the hyperglycemic hyperosmolar nonketotic state. In Joslin's Diabetes Mellitus 13th ed Kahn CR, Weir GC, editors. Eds. Philadelphia, Lea & Febiger, 1994, p. 738– 770.

[32] DeFronzo RA, Matzuda M, Barret E. Diabetic ketoacidosis: a combined metabolic-nephrologic approach to therapy. Diabetes Rev 1994; 2: 209– 238.

[33] Luzi L, Barrett EJ, Groop LC, Ferrannini E, DeFronzo RA. Metabolic effects of low-dose insulin therapy on glucose metabolism in diabetic ketoacidosis. Diabetes 1988; 37: 1470– 1477.

[34] van de Werve G, Jeanrenaud B. Liver glycogen metabolism: an overview. Diabetes Metab Rev 1987; 3: 47– 78.

[35] Felig P, Sherwin RS, Soman V, Wahren J, Hendler R, Sacca L, Eigler N, Goldberg D, Walesky M. Hormonal interactions in the regulation of blood glucose. Recent Prog Horm Res 1979; 35: 501– 532.

[36] Umpierrez GE, Kelly JP, Navarrete JE,Casals MM, Kitabchi AE. Hyperglycemic crises in urban blacks. Arch Intern Med 1997;157:669–675.

[37] Ennis ED, Stahl EJVB, Kreisberg RA. The hyperosmolar hyperglycemic syndrome. Diabetes Rev 1994;2:115–126.

[38] Lorber D. Nonketotic hypertonicity in diabetes mellitus. Med Clin North Am 1995;79:39–52.

[39] Barrett EJ, DeFronzo RA, Bevilacqua S, Ferrammi E. Insulin resistance in diabetic ketoacidosis. Diabetes 1982;31:923–928.

[40] Miles JM, Haymond MW, Nissen S, Gerich JE. Effects of free fatty acid availability, glucagon excess and insulin deficiency on ketone body production in postabsorptive man. J Clin Invest 1983; 71:1554–1561.

[41] Stentz FB, Umpierrez GE, Cuervo R, Kitabchi AE. Proinflammatory cytokines, markers of cardiovascular risks, oxidative stresss, and lipid peroxidation in patients with hyperglycemic crises. Diabetes 2004; 53:2079–2086.

[42] Holstad M, Sandler S. A transcriptional inhibitor of TNF-alpha prevents diabetes induced by multipe lowdose streptozotocin injections in mice. J Autoimmun 2001; 16: 441-447.

[43] Karavanaki K, Karanika E, Georga S, Bartzeliotou A, Tsouvalas M, Konstantopoulos I, Fotinou A, Papassotiriou I, Karayianni C. Cytokine response to diabetic ketoacidosis (DKA) in children with type 1 diabetes T1DM). Endocr J. 2011;58(12):1045-53.

[44] Nicoletti F, Conget I, Di Marco R, Speciale AM, Morinigo R, Bendtzen K, et al. Serum levels of the interferon-gamma-inducing cytokine interleukin-18 are increased in individuals at high risk of developing Type 1 diabetes. Diabetologia 2001; 44: 309-311.

[45] Mironczuk K, Okruszko, Wawrusiewicz-Kurylonek AN, Kretowski A, Kinalska I, Gorska M. Interleukin 18 and sICAM-1 serum levels in families with type 1 diabetes mellitus. Rocz Akad Med Bialymst 2005; 50: 151-154.

[46] Mahmoud RA, el-Ezz SA, Hegazy AS. Increased serum levels of interleukin-18 in patients with diabetes nephropathy. Ital J Biochem 2004; 53: 73-81.

[47] Dong G, Liang L, Fu J, Zou C. Serum interleukin-18 levels are raised in diabetic ketoacidosis in Chinese children with type 1 diabetes mellitus. Indian Pediatr. 2007 Oct; 44(10):732-6.

[48] Buyukasik Y, Ileri NS, Haznedaroglu IC, Karaahmetoglu S, Muftuoglu O, Kirazli S, Dundar S. Enhanced subclinical coagulationbactivation during diabetic ketoacidosis. Diabetes Care 1998;21:868–870.

[49] National Center for Health Statistics. National hospital discharge and ambulatory surgery data. http://www.cdc.gov/nchs/ about/major/hdasd/nhds.htm. (Accessed 24 January 2009).

[50] Weinert LS, Scheffel RS, Severo MD, Cioffi AP, Teló GH, Boschi A, Schaan BD. Precipitating factors of diabetic ketoacidosis at a public hospital in a middle-income country. Diabetes Res Clin Pract. 2012 Apr;96(1):29-34.

[51] Chaithongdi N, Subauste JS, Koch CA, Geraci SA. Diagnosis and management of hyperglycemic emergencies. Hormones (Athens). 2011 Oct-Dec;10(4):250-60.

[52] Peden NR, Broatan JT, McKenry JB. Diabetic ketoacidosis during long-term treatment with continuous subcutaneous insulin infusion. Diabetes Care 1984;7:1–5.

[53] Cesur M, Cesur A. Double diabetes: possible but unpublished complication of insulin pump therapy. J Diabetes Complications. 2008; 22:147-9.

[54] Weissberg-Benchell J, Antisdel-Lomaglio J, Seshadri R. Insulin pump therapy: a meta-analysis. Diabetes Care 2003;26: 1079–1087.

[55] Avella J, Wetli CV, Wilson JC, Katz M, Hahn T. Fatal olanzapine-induced hyerglycemic ketoacidosis. AmJ Forensic Med Pathol 2004;25:172–175.

[56] Campanella LM, Lartey R, Shih R. Sever hyperglycemic hyperosmolar nonketotic coma in a nondiabetic patient receiving aripiprazole. Am Emerg Med 2009;53: 264–266.

[57] Arefi M, Tabrizchi N. Nalidixic acid and diabetic ketoacidosis. Indian J Endocrinol Metab. 2012 Mar;16 Suppl 1:S124-6.

[58] Goodman LS, Gilman A. The Pharmacological Basis of Therapeutics: A Textbook of Pharmacology, Toxicology, and Therapeutics for Physicians and Medical Students. Am J Med Sci. 1941;202:1179.

[59] Eizadi-Mood N. Nalidixic acid overdose and metabolic acidosis. CJEM. 2006;8:78.

[60] Leslie PJ, Cregeen RJ, Proudfoot AT. Lactic acidosis, hyperglycaemia and convulsions following nalidixic acid overdosage. Hum Toxicol. 1984;3:239–43.

[61] Islam MA, Sreedharan T. convulsions, hyperglycemia, and glycosuria from overdose of nalidixic acid. JAMA. 1965;192:1100–1.

[62] Okanoue T, Sakamoto S, Itoh Y, Minami M, Yasui K, Sakamoto M, Nishioji K, Katagishi T, Nakagawa Y, Tada H, Sawa Y, Mizuno M, Kagawa K, Kashima K. Side effects of high-dose interferon therapy for chronic hepatitis C. J Hepatol 1996; 25: 283-291.

[63] Fattovich G, Giustina G, Favarato S, Ruol A. A survey of adverse events in 11,241 patients with chronic viral hepatitis treated with alfa interferon. J Hepatol 1996; 24: 38-47.

[64] Fabris P, Floreani A, Tositti G, Vergani D, De Lalla F, Betterle C. Type 1 diabetes mellitus in patients with chronic hepatitis C before and after interferon therapy. Aliment Pharmacol Ther 2003; 18: 549-558.

[65] Soultati AS, Dourakis SP, Alexopoulou A, Deutsch M, Archimandritis AJ. Simultaneous development of diabetic ketoacidosis and Hashitoxicosis in a patient treated with pegylated interferon-alpha for chronic hepatitis C. World J Gastroenterol. 2007 Feb 28;13(8):1292-4.

[66] Sasso FC, Carbonara O, Di Micco P, Coppola L, Torella R, Niglio A. A case of autoimmune polyglandular syndrome developed after interferon-alpha therapy. Br J Clin Pharmacol 2003; 56: 238-239.

[67] Christensen UB, Krogsgaard K. Onset of type 1 diabetes mellitus during combination therapy of chronic hepatitis C with interferon-alpha and ribavirin. Ugeskr Laeger 2004; 166: 1024-1025.

[68] Schories M, Peters T, Rasenack J, Reincke M. Autoantibodies against islet cell antigens and type 1 diabetes after treatment with interferon-alpha. Dtsch Med Wochenschr 2004; 129: 1120-1124.

[69] Radhakrishnan S, Upadhyay A, Mohan N, Dhar A, Walia HK, Zubaidi G. Late development of diabetes mellitus after interferon-alfa and ribavirin therapy for chronic hepatitis C: a case report. Med Princ Pract 2005; 14: 281-283.

[70] Bosi E, Minelli R, Bazzigaluppi E, Salvi M. Fulminant autoimmune Type 1 diabetes during interferon-alpha therapy: a case of Th1-mediated disease? Diabet Med 2001; 18: 329-332.

[71] Bhatti A, McGarrity TJ, Gabbay R. Diabetic ketoacidosis induced by alpha interferon and ribavirin treatment in a patient with hepatitis C. Am J Gastroenterol 2001; 96: 604-605.

[72] Recasens M, Aguilera E, Ampurdanes S, Sanchez Tapias JM, Simo O, Casamitjana R, Conget I. Abrupt onset of diabetes during interferon-alpha therapy in patients with chronic hepatitis C. Diabet Med 2001; 18: 764-767.

[73] Mofredj A, Howaizi M, Grasset D, Licht H, Loison S, Devergie B, Demontis R, Cadranel JF. Diabetes mellitus during interferon therapy for chronic viral hepatitis. Dig Dis Sci 2002; 47: 1649-1654.

[74] Jabr FI, Ordinario MM. Sudden onset of diabetic ketoacidosis during pegylated interferon alfa therapy. Am J Med 2003; 115: 158-159.

[75] Cozzolongo R, Betterle C, Fabris P, Paola Albergoni M, Lanzilotta E, Manghisi OG. Onset of type 1 diabetes mellitus during peginterferon alpha-2b plus ribavirin treatment for chronic hepatitis C. Eur J Gastroenterol Hepatol 2006; 18: 689-692.

[76] Sarkar S, Mondal R, Nandi M, Das AK. Tacrolimus Induced Diabetic Ketoacidosis in Nephrotic Syndrome.Indian J Pediatr. 2012 Jun 2.

[77] Warner AE, Greene GS, Buchsbaum MS, et al, Diabetic ketoacidosis associated with cocaine use. Arch Intern Med 1998; 158: 1799-1802.

[78] Evans EM, Nye F, Beeching NJ, et al, 'Disappearing diabetes' – resolution of apparent type 1 diabetes in a patient with AIDS and cytomegalovirus (CMV) infection. Diabet Med 2005; 22: 218-220.

[79] Izumi K, Diabetic ketoacidosis with cytomegalovirus-associated colitis. Intern Med 2009; 48 (5): 343-346.

[80] Besson C, Jubault V, Viard JP, et al, Ketoacidosis associated with protease inhibitor therapy. AIDS 1998;12: 1399-1400.

[81] Kan VL, Nylen ES, Diabetic ketoacidosis in an HIV patient: A new mechanism of HIV protease-inhibitor-induced glucose intolerance. AIDS 1999;13: 1987-1989.

[82] Takarabe D, Rokukawa Y, Takahashi Y, et al, Autoimmune diabetes in HIV-infected patients on highly active antiretroviral therapy. J Clin Endocrinolol Metab 2010; 95: 4056-4060.

[83] Me´garbane B, Axler O, Chary I, Pompier R, Brivet FG. Hypothermia with indoor occurrence is associated with a worse outcome. Intensive Care Med 2000;26:1843–9.

[84] Matz R. Hypothermia in diabetic acidosis. Hormones 1972;3:36–41.

[85] Goldberger ZD. Severe hypothermia with Osborn waves in diabetic ketoacidosis. Respir Care 2008;53:500–2.

[86] Sheikh AM, Hurst JW. Osborn waves in the electrocardiogram, hypothermia not due to exposure, and death due to diabetic ketoacidosis. Clin Cardiol 2003;26:555–60.

[87] Ozawa Y, Maruyama H, Nakano S, Saruta T. An unconscious diabetic patient. Postgrad Med J 1998;74:549–50.

[88] Stansberry KB, Shapiro SA, Hill MA, McNitt PM, Meyer MD, Vinik AI. Impaired peripheral vasomotion in diabetes. Diabetes Care 1996;19:715–21.

[89] Yokoyama M, Noto Y, Kida H. Hypothermia with acute renal failure in a patient suffering from diabetic nephropathy and malnutrition. Diabetes Metab 2000;26:145–7.

[90] Nsien EE, Steinberg WM, Borum M, Ratner R. Marked hyperlipasemia in diabetic ketoacidosis. A report of three cases. J Clin Gastroenterol. 1992; Sep;15(2):117-21.

[91] Umpierrez G, Freire AX. Abdominal pain in patients with hyperglycemic crises. J Crit Care 2002;17:63–67.

[92] Campbell IW, Duncan LJ, Innes JA, Mac-Cuish AC, Munro JF. Abdominal pain in diabetic metabolic decompensation: clinical significance. JAMA 1975;233:166–168.

[93] Kitabchi AE, Umpierrez GE, Miles JM, Fisher JN. Hyperglycemic crises in adult patients with diabetes. Diabetes Care 2009;Jul;32(7):1335-43.

[94] Malone JI, Brodsky SJ. The value of electrocardiogram monitoring in diabetic ketoacidosis. Diabetes Care 1980; Jul-Aug;3(4):543-7.

[95] Soler NG, Bennett MA, Fitzgerald MG, Malins JM. Electrocardiogram as a guide to potassium replacement in diabetic ketoacidosis. Diabetes 1974;Jul;23(7):610-5.

[96] Sheikh-Ali M, Karon BS, Basu A, Kudva YC, Muller LA, Xu J, Schwenk WF, Miles JM. Can serum ß-hydroxybutyrate be used to diagnose diabetic ketoacidosis? Diabetes Care 2008;31:643–647.

[97] M.S. Elisaf, A.A. Tsatsoulis, K.P. Katopodis, K.C. Siamonpoulos, Acid–base and electrolyte disturbances in patients with diabetic ketoacidosis. Diabetes Res. Clin. Prac. 1996;34: 23–27.

[98] K. Tanahashi, K. Yasuda, M. Hayashi, K. Hashimoto, C. Sugiyama, H. Asakawa, et al., Acid–base disturbances in Japanese patients with ketoacidosis, J. Japan. Diab. Soc. 2006;49:259–265.

[99] G.M. Roggin, D. Moses, M. Kautcher, W. Wishner, C. Shuman, Ketosis and metabolic alkalosis in a patient with diabetes, JAMA 1970; Jan 12;211(2):296-8.

[100] Watanabe Y, Noda K, Akazawa K, Fukuyama J. Two cases of type 1 diabetic women with diabetic ketoacidosis presenting as alkalaemia. Diabetes Res Clin Pract. 2009 Feb;83(2):e54-7.

[101] Miles JM, Gerich JE. Glucose and ketone body kinetics in diabetic ketoacidosis. Clin Endocrinol Metab 1983;12:303–319.

[102] Joseph F, Anderson L, Goenka N, Vora J. Starvation-induced true diabetic euglycemic ketoacidosis in severe depression. J Gen Intern Med. 2009 Jan;24(1):129-31.

[103] Munro JF, Campbell IW, McCuish AC, Duncan LJ. Euglycaemic diabetic ketoacidosis. Br Med J. 1973;2:578–80.

[104] Burge MR, Garcia N, Qualls CR, Schade DS. Differential effects of fasting and dehydration in the pathogenesis of diabetic ketoacidosis. Metabolism. 2001;50:171–7.

[105] Foster DW, McGarry JD. The metabolic derangements and treatment of diabetic ketoacidosis. N Engl J Med. 1983;309:159–69.

[106] Burge MR, Hardy KJ, Schade DS. Short-term fasting is a mechanism for the development of euglycemic ketoacidosis during periods of insulin deficiency. J Clin Endocrinol Metab. 1993;76:1192–8.

[107] Rothman DL, Magnusson I, Katz LD, Shulman RG, Shulman GI. Quantitation of hepatic glycogenolysis and gluconeogenesis in fasting humans with 13C NMR. Science. 1991;254:573–6.

[108] Wolfe RR, Peters EJ, Klein S, Holland OB, Rosenblatt J, Gary H Jr. Effect of short-term fasting on lipolytic responsiveness in normal and obese human subjects. Am J Physiol. 1987;252:E189–96.

[109] Jensen MD, Haymond MW, Gerich JE, Cryer PE, Miles JM. Lipolysis during fasting. Decreased suppression by insulin and increased stimulation by epinephrine. J Clin Invest. 1987;79:207–13.

[110] Owen OE, Licht JH, Sapir DG. Renal function and effects of partial rehydration during diabetic ketoacidosis. Diabetes. 1981;30:510–8.

[111] Clark JD, McConnell A, Hartog M. Normoglycaemic ketoacidosis in a woman with gestational diabetes. Diabet Med. 1991;8:388–9.

[112] Franke B, Carr D, Hatem MH. A case of euglycaemic diabetic ketoacidosis in pregnancy. Diabet Med. 2001;18:858–9.

[113] Metzger BE, Ravnikar V, Vileisis RA, Freinkel N. "Accelerated starvation" and the skipped breakfast in late normal pregnancy. Lancet.1982;1:588–92.

[114] Brumfield CG, Huddleston JF. The management of diabetic ketoacidosis in pregnancy. Clin Obstet Gynecol. 1984;27:50–9.

[115] Slovis CM, Mork VG, Slovis RJ, Bain RP. Diabetic ketoacidosis and infection: leukocyte count and differential as early predictors of serious infection. Am J Emerg Med 1987;5:1–5.

[116] Razavi L, Kitabchi AE, Stentz FB, Wan JY, Larijani BA, Tehrani M, Gozashti M, Midfar K, Taheri E. Proinflammatory cytokines in response to insulin-induced hypoglycemic stresss in healthy subjects. Metab Clin Exp 2009;58:443–448.

[117] Adrogue HJ, Wilson H, Boyd AE 3rd, Suki WN, Eknoyan G. Plasma acid-base patterns in diabetic ketoacidosis. N Engl J Med 1982;307:1603–1610.

[118] Potter JL, Stone RT. Massive hyperlipidemia in diabetic ketoacidosis. The clinical importance of laboratory recognition. Clin Pediatr (Phila). 1975;14:412-413.

[119] Nyamugunduru G, Roper H. A difficult case. Childhood onset insulin dependent diabetes presenting with severe hyperlipidaemia. BMJ. 1997;314(7073):62-65.

[120] Hsu JH, Wu JR, Chao MC, Dai ZK, Chiou SS, Chen BH. Severe hyperlipidaemic pancreatitis associated with diabetes. Acta Paediatr. 2006;95:378-379.

[121] Koul PB, Sussmane JB. Metabolic hyperglycemic emergencies with acute pancreatitis in a child with known insulin-dependent diabetes mellitus. Eur J Emerg Med. 2005 ; 12:309-311.

[122] Shenoy SD, Cody D, Rickett AB, Swift PG. Acute pancreatitis and its association with diabetes mellitus in children. J Pediatr Endocrinol Metab. 2004;17:1667-1670.

[123] Nair S, Pitchumoni CS. Diabetic ketoacidosis, hyperlipidemia, and acute pancreatitis: the enigmatic triangle. Am J Gastroenterol. 1997;92:1560-1561.

[124] Rumbak MJ, Hughes TA, Kitabchi AE. Pseudonormoglycemia in diabetic ketoacidosis with elevated triglycerides. Am J Emerg Med 1991;9:61–63.

[125] Kaminska ES, Pourmotabbed G. Spurious laboratory values in diabetic ketoacidosis and hyperlipidemia. Am J Emerg Med 1993;11:77–80.

[126] Fisher JN, Kitabchi AE. A randomized study of phosphate therapy in the treatment of diabetic ketoacidosis. J Clin Endocrinol Metab 1983;57:177–180.

[127] Fisher JN, Shahshahani MN, Kitabchi AE. Diabetic ketoacidosis: low-dose insulin therapy by various routes. N Engl J Med 1977;297:238–241.

[128] Warshaw AL, Feller ER, Lee KH. On the cause of raised serum-amylase in diabetic ketoacidosis. Lancet. 1977 Apr 30;1(8018):929-31.

[129] Yadav D, Nair S, Norkus EP, Pitchumoni CS. Nonspecific hyperamylasemia and hyperlipasemia in diabetic ketoacidosis: incidence and correlation with biochemical abnormalities. Am J Gastroenterol 2000;95:3123–3128.

[130] Frank B, Gottlieb K. Amylase normal, lipase elevated: is it pancreatitis? A case series and review of the literature. Am J Gastroenterol. 1999 Feb;94(2):463-9.

[131] Quiros JA, Marcin JP, Kuppermann N, Nasrollahzadeh F, Rewers A, DiCarlo J, Neely EK, Glaser N. Elevated serum amylase and lipase in pediatric diabetic ketoacidosis. Pediatr Crit Care Med. 2008 Jul;9(4):418-22.

[132] Argarawal M, Swartz R,Acute renal failure. Am Fam Physician 2000 Apr 1;61(7): 2077-88.

[133] Lewington A, Kanagasundaram S, Renal Association Clinical Practice Guidelines on acute kidney injury.Nephron Clin Pract. 2011;118 Suppl 1:c349-90.

[134] Chaithongdi N, Subauste JS, Koch CA, Geraci SA. Diagnosis and management of hyperglycemic emergencies. Hormones (Athens). 2011 Oct-Dec;10(4):250-60.

[135] Eisenbarth GS, Polonsky KS, Buse JB 2008 Acute diabetic emergencies: Diabetic ketoacidosis. In: Kronenberg HM, Melmed S, Polonsky KS et al (eds). Williams Textbook of Endocrinology, 11th edn, Saunders Elsevier, Pennsylvania; pp, 1407-1416.

[136] Vanholder R, De Smet R, Glorieux G, et al, Review on uremic toxins: classification, concentration, and interindividual variability. Kidney Int 2003;63: 1934-1943.

[137] Watkins PJ, Smith JS, Fitzgerald MG, et al, Lactic acidosis in diabetes. Br Med J 1969;1: 744-747.

[138] Cesur M, Cekmen N, Cetinbas RR, Badalov P, Erdemli O. A clinical case of development of lactic acid acidosis in a diabetic patient taking metformin. Anesteziol Reanimatol. 2006; 2:65-7.

[139] Samlan SR, Jordan MT, Chan SB, et at, Tinitus as a measure of salicylate toxicity in the overdose setting. West J Emerg Med 2008;9: 146-149.

[140] Chyka PA, Erdman AR, Christianson G, et al, Salicylate poisoning: an evidence-based consensus guideline for out-of-hospital management. Clin Toxicol 2007; 45: 95-131.

[141] Mégarbane B, Borron SW, Baud FJ, Current recommendations for treatment of severe toxic alcohol poisonings. Intensive Care Med 2005;31: 189-195.

[142] Brent J, Fomepizole for the treatment of pediatric ethylene and diethylene glycol, butoxyethanol, and methanol poisonings. Clin Toxicol 2010;48: 401-406.

[143] Eisenhut M, Causes and effects of hyperchloremic acidosis. Crit Care 2006;10: 413.

[144] Walmsley RN, White GH, Normal "anion gap" (hyperchloremic) acidosis. Clin Chem 1985;31: 309-313.

[145] Charles JC, Heilman RL, Metabolic acidosis. Hosp Physician 2005;41: 37-42.

[146] Walmsley RN, White GH, Normal "Anion Gap" (Hyperchloremic) Acidosis. Clin Chem 1985;31: 309-313.

[147] Emmett M, Narins R, Clinical use of the anion gap. Medicine (Baltimore) 1997;56: 38-54.

[148] Hillman K. Fluid resuscitation in diabetic emergencies: a reappraisal. Intensive Care Med 1987;13:4–8.

[149] Halperin M, Maccari C, Kamel K. Strategies to diminish the danger of cerebral edema in pediatric diabetes. Pediatr Diabetes. 2006;7:191-195.

[150] Katz MA, Hyperglycemia induced hyponatremia – calculation of expected serum sodium depression. N Engl J Med 1973;289: 843-844.

[151] Hillier TA, Abbott RD, Barrett EJ, Hyponatraemia: evaluating the correction factor for hyperglycemia. Am J Med 1999; 106: 399-403.

[152] Cowart SL, Stachura ME. Glucosuria. In: Walker HK, Hall WD, Hurst JW (eds). Clinical Methods: The History, Physical, and Laboratory Examinations, 3rd edn, Butterworths, Boston; 1990;pp, 653-657.

[153] Perel P, Roberts I. Colloids versus crystalloids for fluid resuscitation in critically ill patients. Cochrane Database Syst Rev 2007; 3:CD000567.

[154] Bigham M, Kaplan J. Endocrine emergencies. Pediatr Crit Care Mag. 2007:1114.

[155] Duck SC, Waytt DT. Factors associated with brain herniation in the treatment of diabetic keto acidosis. J Pediatr. 1988;113:10-14.

[156] Umpierrez GE, Jones S, Smiley D, Mulligan P, Keyler T, Temponi A, Semakula C, Umpierrez D, Peng L, Cero′n M, Robalino G. Insulin analogs versus human insulin in the treatment of patients with diabetic ketoacidosis: a randomized controlled trial. Diabetes Care. 2009 Jul;32(7):1164-9.

[157] Alberti KG, Hockaday TDR, Turner RC. Small doses of intramuscular insulin in the treatment of diabetic 'coma.' Lancet 1973;5:515–522

[158] Al Hanshi S, Shann F. Insulin infused at 0.05 versus 0.1 units/kg/hr in children admitted to intensive care with diabetic ketoacidosis. Pediatr Crit Care Med. 2011 Mar; 12(2):137-40.

[159] Kitabchi AE, Ayyagari V, Guerra SMO. Medical House Staff. The efficacy of low dose versus conventional therapy of Insulin for treatment of diabetic ketoacidosis. Ann Intern Med 1976;84:633–8.

[160] Kitabchi AE, Umpierrez GE, Fisher JN, Murphy MB, Stentz FB. Thirty years of personal experience in hyperglycemic crises: diabetic ketoacidosis and hyperglycemic hyperosmolar state. J Clin Endocrinol Metab. 2008 May;93(5):1541-52.

[161] Kitabchi AE, Murphy MB, Spencer J, Matteri R, Karas J. Is a priming dose of insulin necessary in a low-dose insulin protocol for the treatment of diabetic ketoacidosis? Diabetes Care. 2008 Nov;31(11):2081-5.

[162] Umpierrez GE, Latif K, Stoever J, et al, Efficacy of subcutaneous insulin lispro versus continuous intravenous regular insulin for the treatment of patients with diabetic ketoacidosis. Am J Med 2004;117: 291-296.

[163] Umpierrez GE, Cuervo R, Karabell A, et al, Treatment of diabetic ketoacidosis with subcutaneous insulin aspart. Diabetes Care 2004;27: 1873-1878.

[164] Della Manna T, Steinmetz L, Campos PR, et al, Subcutaneous use of a fast-acting insulin analog: An alternative treatment for pediatric patients with diabetic ketoacidosis. Diabetes Care 2005;28: 1856-1861.

[165] Koul PB. Diabetic ketoacidosis: a current appraisal of pathophysiology and management. Clin Pediatr (Phila). 2009 Mar;48(2):135-44.

[166] Zhang L, Zhang M, Liu YY, Hu M, Zhou X, Luo Y. Successful treatment with continuous subcutaneous insulin infusion for allergy to human insulin and its analogs. Diabetes Res Clin Pract. 2011 Oct;94(1):e1-2.

[167] Peterson LN, Levi M. Disorder of potassium and metabolism. In: Schrier RW (ed). Renal and electrolyte disordes, 6th edn, Lippincott Williams & Wilkins, Philadelphia; 2002; pp, 171-215.

[168] Beigelman PM. Potassium in severe diabetic ketoacidosis. Am J Med 1973;54:419–20 [Editorial].

[169] Abramson E, Arky R. Diabetic acidosis with initialmhypokalemia: therapeutic implications. JAMA 1966;196:401–3.

[170] Nyenwe EA, Kitabchi AE. Evidence-based management of hyperglycemic emergencies in diabetes mellitus. Diabetes Res Clin Pract. 2011 Dec;94(3):340-51.

[171] McGarry J, Wright PH, Foster DW: Hormonal control of ketogenesis. Rapid activation of hepatic ketogenic capacity in fed rats by anti-insulin serum and glucagon. J Clin Invest 1975, 55:1202-1209.

[172] McGarry JD, Foster DW: Regulation of hepatic fatty acid oxidation and ketone body production. Annu Rev Biochem 1980; 49:395-420.

[173] Zimmet PZ, Taft P, Ennis GC, Sheath J, Acid production in diabetic acidosis; a more rational approach to alkali replacement. British Medical Journal 1970; 3:610-612.

[174] Calzavacca P, Lacari E, Bellomo R. In: Stewart's Textbook of Acid-Base. Ebers P, Kellum J Lulu.com, editor. 2009. Renal failure; pp. 394–395. Clinical applications of quantitative acid-base medicine.

[175] Oh MS, Carroll HJ, Goldstein DA, Fein IA. Hyperchloremic acidosis during the recovery phase of diabetic ketosis. Annals of Internal Medicine 1978; 89:925-927.

[176] Adrogue HJ, Wilson H, Boyd AE, Suki WN, Eknoyan G. Plasma acid-base patterns in diabetic ketoacidosis. N Engl J Med 1982; 307:1603-1610.

[177] Foster DW, McGarry JD. The metabolic derangements and treatment of diabetic ketoacidosis. N Engl J Med 1983; 309:159-169.

[178] Mitchell JH, Wildenthal K, Johnson RL Jr. The effects of acid-base disturbances on cardiovascular and pulmonary function. Kidney Int 1972;1:375-389.

[179] Kono N, Kuwajima M, Tarui S. Alteration of glycolytic intermediary metabolism in erythrocytes during diabetic ketoacidosis and its recovery phase. Diabetes 1981; 30:346-353.

[180] [180 Adrogue HJ, Madias NE. Management of life-threatening acid-base disorders. First of two parts. N Engl J Med 1998; 338:26-34.

[181] Kraut JA, Kurtz I. Use of base in the treatment of severe acidemic states. American Journal of Kidney Diseases 2001; 38:703-727.

[182] Glaser N, Barnett P, McCaslin I, Nelson D,Trainor J, Louie J, Kaufman F, Quayle K, Roback M, Malley R, Kuppermann N, the Pediatric Emergency Medicine Collaborative Research Committee of the American Academy of Pediatrics. Risk factors for cerebral edema in children with diabetic ketoacidosis. N Engl J Med 2001;344:264–269.

[183] Winter RJ, Harris CJ, Phillips LS, Green OC. Diabetic Ketoacidosis: induction of hypocalcemia and hypomagnesemia by phosphate therapy. Am J Med 1979;67:897–900.

[184] Kreisberg RA. Phosphorus deficiency and hypophosphatemia. Hosp Pract 1977;12: 121–128.

[185] Miller DW, Slovis CM. Hypophosphatemia in the emergency department therapeutics. Am J Emerg Med 2000;18:457–461.

[186] Geerse DA, Bindels AJ, Kuiper MA, et al, Treatment of hypophosphatemia in the intensive care unit: a review. Crit Care 2010;14: R147.

[187] Tattersall RB. The history of diabetes mellitus. In: Holt RIG, Cockram CS, Flyvberg A, Goldstein BJ, editors. Textbook of diabetes. 4th ed., West Sussex, UK: Wiley-Blackwell; 2010. p. 3–23.

[188] Ogbonnaya KI, Arem R. Diabetic diarrhea. Pathophysiology, diagnosis, and management. Arch Intern Med. 1990 Feb;150(2):262-7.

[189] Bruttomesso D, Fongher C, Silvestri B, Barberio S, Marescotti MC, Iori E, Valerio A, Crazzolara D, Pianta A, Tiengo A, Del Prato S. Combination of continuous subcutaneous infusion of insulin and octreotide in Type 1 diabetic patients. Diabetes Res Clin Pract. 2001 Feb;51(2):97-105.

[190] Diem P, Robertson RP. Preventive effects of octreotide (SMS 201-995) on diabetic ketogenesis during insulin withdrawal. Br J Clin Pharmacol. 1991 Nov;32(5):563-7.

[191] Anthony LB, Sharp SC, May ME. Case report: diabetic ketoacidosis in a patient with glucagonoma. Am J Med Sci. 1995 Jun;309(6):326-7.

[192] Rosenbloom AL, Hanas R. Diabetic ketoacidosis (DKA): treatment guidelines. Clin Pediatr. 1996;35:261-266.

[193] Ennis ED, Kreisberg RA. Diabetic ketoacidosis and the hyperglycemic hyperosmolar syndrome. In: LeRoith D, Taylor SI, Olefsky JM (eds) Diabetes Mellitus: A Fundamental and Clinical Text 3rd edn, Lippincott Williams & Wilkins, Philadelphia 2003; pp, 627-641.

[194] Malone JI, Brodsky SJ. The value of electrocardiogram monitoring in diabetic ketoacidosis. Diabetes Care. 1980;3:543-547.

[195] Soler NG, Bennett MA, Fitzgerald MG, Malins JM. Electrocardiogram as a guide to potassium replacement in diabetic ketoacidosis. Diabetes 1974 Jul;23(7):610-5.

[196] Murdoch IA, Pryor D, Haycock GB, Cameron SJ. Acute renal failure complicating diabetic ketoacidosis. Acta Paediatr 1993 May;82(5):498-500.

[197] Kawata H, Inui D, Ohto J, Miki T, Suzue A, Fukuta Y, Nishimura M. The use of continuous hemodiafiltration in a patient with diabetic ketoacidosis. J Anesth. 2006;20(2):129-31.

[198] Riley MS, Schade DS, Eaton RP. Effects of insulin infusion on plasma phosphate in diabetic patients. Metabolism 1979 Mar;28(3):191-4.

[199] Kebler R, McDonald FD, Cadnapaphornchai P. Dynamic changes in serum phosphorus levels in diabetic ketoacidosis. Am J Med 1985 Nov;79(5):571-6.

[200] Becker DJ, Brown DR, Steranka BH, Drash AL. Phosphate replacement during treatment of diabetic ketosis. Effects on calcium and phosphorus homeostasis. Am J Dis Child. 1983 Mar;137(3):241-6.

[201] Liu PY, Jeng CY. Severe hypophosphatemia in a patient with diabetic ketoacidosis and acute respiratory failure. J Chin Med Assoc. 2004 Jul;67(7):355-9.

[202] Joffe HV, Abrahamson MJ. Case study: tea colored urine in a patient with diabetic ketoacidosis. Clin Diabetes 2004;22:197Y198.

[203] Casteels K, Beckers D, Wouters C, Van Geet C. Rhabdomyolysis in diabetic ketoacidosis. Pediatr Diabetes 2003 Mar;4(1):29-31.

[204] Singhal PC, Abramovici M, Venkatesan J. Rhabdomyolysis in the hyperosmolal state. Am J Med 1990 Jan;88(1):9-12.

[205] Al-Matrafi J, Vethamuthu J, Feber J. Severe acute renal failure in a patient with diabetic ketoacidosis. Saudi J Kidney Dis Transpl 2009 Sep;20(5):831-4.

[206] Massicotte M, Dix D, Monagle P, Adams M, Andrew M. Central venous catheter related thrombosis in children: analysis of the Canadian Registry of Venous Thromboembolic Complications. J Pediatr 1998;133: 770-776.

[207] Beck C, Dubois J, Grigon A, Lacroix J, David M. Incidence and risk factors of catheter-related deep vein thrombosis in a pediatric intensive care unit: a prospective study. J Pediatr 1998; 133: 237-241.

[208] Gutierrez JA, Bagatelle R, Samson MP, Theodorou AA, Berg RA. Femoral central venous catheter associated deep venous thrombosis in children with diabetic ketoacidosis. Crit Care Med 2003; 31: 80-83.

[209] Worly JM, Fortenberry JD, Hansen I, Chambliss CR, Stockwell J. Deep Venous Thrombosis in Children with Diabetic Ketoacidosis and Femoral Central Venous Catheters. Pediatrics 2004;113: e57-60.

[210] Woolley SL. Femoral venous thrombosis in a 5-week old with diabetic ketoacidosis and a femoral venous catheter. Indian Pediatr 2007 Oct;44(10):779-81.

[211] Carr ME. Diabetes mellitus: A hypercoaguable state. J Diabetes Complications 2001; 15: 44-54.

[212] Rosenbloom AL. Hyperglycemic hyperosmolar state: an emerging pediatric problem. J Pediatr. 2010;156:180-184.

[213] Haddad NG, Croffie JM, Eugster EA: Pancreatic enzyme elevations in children with diabetic ketoacidosis. J Pediatr 2004; 145:122–124.

[214] Moller-Petersen J, Andersen PT, Hjorne N, et al: Hyperamylasemia, specific pancreatic enzymes, and hypoxanthine during recovery from diabetic ketoacidosis. Clin Chem 1985;31:2001–2004.

[215] Gianfrate L, Ferraris L: Acute pancreatitis, hyperlipidemia, and diabetic ketoacidosis: Who comes first? Am J Gastroenterol 1998; 93:1393–1394.

[216] Martin-Moro JG, Calleja JM, Garcia MB, Carretero JL, Rodriguez JG. Rhinoorbitocerebral mucormycosis: a case report and literature review. Med Oral Patol Oral Cir Bucal 2008; 13: E792-5.

[217] Mandell GL, Dolin R. Principles and Practice of Infectious Disease. 6th ed. Philadelphia: Churchil Livingstone, 2005.

[218] Tomac S, Cakal E, Karaahmetoglu S, Cesur M, Muftuoglu O. A Rhino-orbita-brain mucormycozis in a newly diagnosed diabetic ketoacidozis case. Turk Oftalmoloji Gazetesi 2002; 32:362-64.

[219] Dixon AN, Jude EB, Banerjee AK, Bain SC. Simultaneous pulmonary and cerebral oedema and multiple CNS infarctions as complications of diabetic ketoacidosis: a case report. Diabet Med 2006; 23: 571–573.

[220] LinksLevsky JM, Feuer BH, Di Vito J., Jr Pneumomediastinum in a patient with diabetic ketoacidosis. J Emerg Med 2004; 26: 233–5.

[221] LinksDrolet S, Gagné JP, Langis P. Spontaneous pneumorrhachis associated with pneumomediastinum in a patient with diabetic ketoacidosis: an exceptional manifestation of a benign disease. Can J Surg 2007; 50: 225–6.

[222] O'Sullivan AJ, Casey JH. Spontaneous pneumomediastinum and diabetic ketoacidosis. Med J Aust. 1997 Mar 3;166(5):245-6.

[223] Banday W, Tahir M, Jallu S, Augustine F. Spontaneous pneumomediastinum: rare complication of diabetic ketoacidosis. BMJ Case Rep. 2009;2009. pii: bcr10.2008.1091.

[224] Rosenbloom AL. Intracerebral crises during treatment of diabetic ketoacidosis. Diabetes Care 1990; 13: 22–33.

[225] Hoffman WH, Steinhart CM, el Gammal T, Steele S, Cuadrado AR, Morse PK. Cranial CT in children and adolescents with diabetic ketoacidosis. Am J Neuroradiol 1988; 9: 733–739.

[226] Marcin JP, Glaser N, Barnett P, McCaslin I, Nelson D, Trainor J, Louie J, Kaufman F, Quayle K, Roback M, Malley R, Kuppermann N. Factors associated with adverse outcomes in children with diabetic ketoacidosis-related cerebral edema. J Pediatr 2002;141:793–797.

[227] Wolfsdorf J, Craig ME, Daneman D, et al. Diabetic ketoacidosis in children and adolescents with diabetes. Pediatr Diabetes 2009;10(Suppl. 12): 118-133.

[228] Glaser N, Barnett P, McCaslin I, Nelson D, Trainor J, Louie J et al. Pediatric Emergency Medicine Collaborative Research Committee of the American Academy of Pediatrics. Risk factors for cerebral edema in children with diabetic ketoacidosis. The Pediatric Emergency Medicine Collaborative Research Committee of the American Academy of Pediatrics. N Engl J Med 2001; 344: 264–269.

[229] Yuen N, Anderson SE, Glaser N, Tancredi DJ, O'Donnell ME. Cerebral blood flow and cerebral edema in rats with diabetic ketoacidosis. Diabetes 2008; 57: 2588–94.

[230] Abbott NJ. Inflammatory mediators and modulation of blood-brain barrier permeability. Cell Mol Neurobiol 2000;20:131–147.

[231] Dietrich, WD. Inflammatory factors regulating the blood–brain barrier. In: Feuerstein, GZ., editor. Inflammatory cells and mediators in CNS disease. Amsterdam: Harwood Academic; 1999. p. 137-155.

[232] Jenkinson M, Bannister P, Brady M, et al. Improved optimization for the robust and accurate linear registration and motion correction of brain images. Neruoimage 2002;17:825–841.

[233] Smith S. Fast Robust Automated Brain Extraction. Human Brain Mapping 2002;17:143–155.

[234] Demsar F, Roberts TP, Schwickert HC, et al. A MRI spatial mapping technique for microvascular permeability and tissue blood volume based on macromolecular contrast agent distribution. Magn Reson Med 1997;37:236–242.

[235] Ivanusa T, Katarina B, Medic J, et al. Dynamic contrast enhanced MRI of mouse fibrosarcoma using small-molecular and novel macromolecular contrast agents. Physica Medica 2007;23:85–90.

[236] Muir AB, Quisling RG, Yang MCK, Rosenbloom AL. Cerebral edema in childhood diabetic ketoacidosis. Natural history, radiographic findings, and early identification. Diabetes Care. 2004;27:1541-1546.

[237] Marcin JP, Glaser N, Barnett P, et al. Factors associated with adverse outcomes in children with diabetic ketoacidosis-related cerebral edema. J Pediatr. 2002;141:793-797.

[238] Pappius HM. Fundamental aspects of brain edema. In: Vinkin PJ, Bruyn GW, eds. Handbook of Clinical Neurology. Volume 16. Part 1. Tumors of the Brain and Skull. Amsterdam: North Holland Publishing Co.; 1974:167-185.

[239] Bello FA, Sotos JF. Cerebral oedema in diabetic ketoacidosis in children. Lancet. 1990;336;64.

[240] Rosenbloom AL. The management of diabetic ketoacidosis in children. Diabetes Ther. 2010 Dec;1(2):103-20.

[241] Roberts MD, Slover RH, Chase HP. Diabetic ketoacidosis with intracerebral complications. Pediatr Diabetes. 2001;2:109-114.

[242] Rosenbloom AL. Fatal cerebral infarctions in diabetic ketoacidosis in a child with previously unknown heterozygosity for factor V Leiden deficiency. J Pediatr. 2004;145:561-562.

[243] Yoon J-W, Austin M, Onodera T, Notkins AL. Virus-induced diabetes mellitus. N Engl J Med. 1979;300:1173-1179.

[244] Cooper RM. Turner RA, Hutaff L, Prichard R. Diabetic keto-acidosis complicated by disseminated intravascular coagulation. South Med J. 1973;66:653-657.

[245] Bonfanti R, Bognetti E, Meschi F, Medaglini S, D'Angelo A, Chiumello G. Disseminated intravascular coagulation and severe peripheral neuropathy complicating ketoacidosis in a newly diagnosed diabetic child. Acta Diabetol. 1994;31:173-174.

[246] Laffel LM, Wentzell K, Loughlin C, Tovar A, Moltz K, Brink S. Sick day management using blood 3-hydroxybutyrate (3-OHB) compared with urine ketone monitoring reduces hospital visits in young people with T1DM: a randomized clinical trial. Diabet Med 2006 Mar;23(3):278-84.

Chapter 11

Diabetic Ketoacidosis: Clinical Practice Guidelines

Shereen Abdelghaffar

Additional information is available at the end of the chapter

http://dx.doi.org/10.5772/53020

1. Introduction

Diabetic ketoacidosis (DKA), the most common endocrinal emergency remains a life-threatening condition despite improvements in diabetes care [1]. The mortality and morbidity rates remain high worldwide, especially in developing countries and among non-hospitalized patients [2,3], which highlight the importance of early diagnosis and implementation of effective preventive and management strategies. The adage "The child is not a miniature adult" is most appropriate when considering DKA. The fundamental pathophysiology of DKA is the same in children as in adults; however, the child differs from the adult in a number of characteristics which raise some important considerations in management [2].

The purpose of this chapter is to briefly review the pathophysiology of DKA and discuss recommended treatment protocols and current standards of care pertaining to children, adolescents and adults with type 1 or 2 diabetes presenting with DKA. The information provided is based on evidence from published studies and internationally accepted guidelines whenever possible and, when not, supported by expert opinion or consensus [1-5]. Current concepts of cerebral edema, recommendations and strategies for the prediction and prevention of DKA and hence its complications are finally presented.

The considerations and recommendations included are in agreement with those endorsed by the American Diabetes Association (ADA), Lawson Wilkins Pediatric Endocrine Society (LWPES), European Society for Pediatric Endocrinology (ESPE), and the International Society for Pediatric and Adolescent Diabetes (ISPAD) [2-5]. Thus, this book chapter will provide easy and practical information to guide healthcare professional who manage DKA in all age groups.

2. Definition of Diabetic Ketoacidosis (DKA)

The biochemical criteria for DKA include the following triad [4]:

- Hyperglycemia (blood glucose >11 mmol/L [200 mg/dL])
- Venous pH <7.3 and/or bicarbonate <15 mmol/L
- Ketonemia and ketonuria

3. Pathophysiology of DKA

Diabetic ketoacidosis (DKA) results from absolute or relative deficiency of circulating insulin and the combined effects of increased levels of the counterregulatory hormones: catecholamines, glucagon, cortisol and growth hormone [5].

Absolute insulin deficiency occurs in the following conditions:

- undiagnosed type 1 diabetes mellitus (T1DM); DKA is reported be the first presentation in about 25% of cases especially in those less than 5 years old [2].
- patients on treatment who miss their insulin doses, especially the long-acting component of a basal-bolus regimen. It is estimated that 75% of DKA episodes are associated with insulin omission or treatment error [6].
- patients who use insulin pump if insulin delivery fails [7].

Relative insulin deficiency, on the other hand, occurs when the concentrations of counterregulatory hormones increase in response to stress in conditions such as:

- sepsis,
- trauma, or
- gastrointestinal illness with diarrhea and vomiting.

The combination of low serum insulin and high counterregulatory hormone concentrations results in an accelerated catabolic state with increased glucose production by the liver and kidney (via glycogenolysis and gluconeogenesis), impaired peripheral glucose utilization resulting in hyperglycemia and hyperosmolality, and increased lipolysis and ketogenesis, causing ketonemia and metabolic acidosis [4].

Hyperglycemia and hyperketonemia cause osmotic diuresis, dehydration, and electrolyte loss. This stimulates stress hormone production, which induces insulin resistance and leads to a vicious circle, worsening the hyperglycemia and hyperketonemia. Fatal dehydration and metabolic acidosis will ensue if management is not initiated. Poor tissue perfusion or sepsis may lead to lactic acidosis which can aggravate the ketoacidosis [5].

http://dx.doi.org/10.5772/53020

At presentation, the magnitude of specific deficits of fluid and electrolytes in an individual patient varies depending upon the extent to which the patient was able to maintain intake of fluid and electrolytes, and the content of food and fluids consumed before coming to medical attention and the duration and severity of illness [8].

4. Epidemiology of DKA

There is wide geographic variation in the frequency of DKA at onset of diabetes; rates inversely correlate with the regional incidence of type 1 diabetes. Frequencies range from 15 to 70% in different regions of the world [9 -14].

4.1. Frequency of DKA

At disease onset

DKA at diagnosis of type 1 diabetes occurs more commonly in [15,16]:

- children younger than four years of age
- children with absent first-degree relative with T1DM and
- families of a lower socioeconomic class

Type 2 diabetes mellitus (T2DM), associated with increased rates and severity of obesity, may account for as much as one half of newly diagnosed diabetes in those aged 10 to 21 years, depending on the socioeconomic and ethnic composition of the population [2]. Acute decompensation with DKA has been recognized to occur at the time of diagnosis in as many as 25% of children with type 2Diabetes Mellitus (T2DM0 [17].

In children with established diabetes (recurrent DKA)[4]

The risk of DKA in established T1DM is 1–10% per patient per year

Risk is increased in the following conditions [18]:

- poor metabolic control or previous episodes of DKA
- peripubertal and adolescent girls
- psychiatric disorders, including those with eating disorders
- difficult or unstable family circumstances
- omission of insulin
- limited access to medical services
- insulin pump therapy

4.2. Diagnosis of DKA

Although DKA is defined by the biochemical triad of ketonemia, hyperglycemia and acidemia, several exceptions do exist which may provide a diagnostic dilemma for the physician in the emergency room. Examples of such are:

- **"Euglycemic ketoacidosis"**: Partially treated children and children who have consumed little or no carbohydrate may present rarely with mildly increased blood glucose concentrations [19].
- **Absent or mild metabolic acidosis, ketonemia and ketonuria**: This may occur in the Hyperglycemic Hyperosmolar State (HHS) or if the patient experiences severe vomiting which may lead to alkalosis which can mask the present acidosis.
- Hyperglycemic hyperosmolar state (HHS), also referred to as hyperosmolar nonketotic coma, may occur in young patients withT2DM, but rarely in T1DM subjects. The criteria for HHS include [20-22]:
  - plasma glucose concentration >33.3 mmol/L (600 mg/dL)
  - arterial pH >7.30
  - serum bicarbonate >15 mmol/L
  - small ketonuria, absent to mild ketonemia
  - effective serum osmolality >320 mOsm/kg
  - stupor or coma

It is important to recognize that overlap between the characteristic features of HHS and DKA may occur. Some patients with HHS, especially when there is very severe dehydration, have mild or moderate acidosis. Conversely, some children with T1DM may have features of HHS (severe hyperglycemia) if high carbohydrate containing beverages have been used to quench thirst and replace urinary losses prior to diagnosis [22].

- Other diagnostic difficulties may be faced in the very young age such as the following [2]:
  - Polyuria, polydipsia and weight loss which are characteristic features of diabetes are difficult to demonstrate in the very young.
  - up to 70% of the young have DKA as a first presentation, hence, at presentation, duration of DKA is usually longer, dehydration and acidosis are more severe, as young children have relatively higher basal metabolic rate, and a relatively large surface area relative to body mass.
- Measurement of blood ß-hydroxybutyrate (ß -OHB) concentration, may not be available in all labs, besides, urine Ketone testing can be misleading due the following reasons [2,4]:
  - The used method does not detect the major ketone body B-hydroxybutyrate. (sodium nitroprusside only measures acetoacetate and acetone). Serum ß-OHB concentrations,

may be increased to levels consistent with DKA when a urine ketone test is negative or shows only trace or small ketonuria

- The readings are qualitative depending on color comparisons
- High doses of Vitamin C may cause false-negative results, while some drugs may, on the other hand, give false-positive results.

5. Management of DKA

5.1. Goals of therapy

Management of DKA should be mainly directed to correction of acidosis. Immediate aims of management include [1,4]:

- Expansion of the intravascular volume
- Correction of deficit in fluids, electrolyte & acid base status
- Initiation of Insulin therapy
- Assessment and monitoring of therapy

5.2. Place of management

The child with DKA should receive care in a unit that has:

- Experienced nursing staff trained in DKA management
- Written guidelines for DKA management
- Access to laboratories that can provide frequent and timely measurements of biochemical variables
- A specialist/consultant pediatrician experienced in the management of DKA should supervise inpatient management [4].

Children with severe DKA or those at high risk for cerebral edema should be treated in an intensive care unit (pediatric, if available) or in a unit that has equivalent resources and supervision, such as a children's ward specializing in diabetes care [4].

In a child with established diabetes, whose parents have been trained in sick day management, and who presents with mild DKA, can be managed in an outpatient health care facility (e.g., emergency ward), provided an experienced diabetes team supervises the care [15].

Emergency Assessment [23]

- Clinically evaluate the patient to confirm the diagnosis and determine its cause. Carefully look for evidence of infection.
- Assess level of consciousness

- Weigh the patient.
- Assess clinical severity of dehydration. Signs of dehydration include dry mucus membranes, sunken eyes, absent tears, weak pulses, and cool extremities. The three most useful individual signs for assessing dehydration in young children and predicting at least 5% dehydration and acidosis are:
  - prolonged capillary refill time (normal capillary refill is < 1.5-2 seconds)
  - abnormal skin turgor ('tenting' or inelastic skin)
  - hyperpnea
- .≥10% dehydration is suggested by the presence of weak or impalpable peripheral pulses, hypotension, and oliguria.

Biochemical assessment [1,4]

- Obtain a blood sample for laboratory measurement of serum or plasma glucose, electrolytes, bicarbonate, blood urea nitrogen, creatinine, osmolality, venous (or arterial in critically ill patient) pH, partial pressure of Carbon dioxide(pCO2), calcium, phosphorus, and magnesium concentrations (if possible), Glycosylated Hemoglobin (HbA1c), hemoglobin and hematocrit or complete blood count.
  - Increased serum urea nitrogen and hematocrit may be useful markers of the severity of extracellular fluid (ECF) contraction.
  - It has to be noted that an elevated white blood cell count in response to stress is characteristic of DKA and is not necessarily indicative of infection [24].
  - Metabolic acidosis being an important landmark of DKA is also helpful to grade the severity of the condition and hence the prognosis by assessing its degree as follows [15]:
- Mild DKA: venous pH <7.3 or bicarbonate <15 mmol/L
- Moderate DKA: pH <7.2, bicarbonate <10 mmol/L
- Severe DKA: pH <7.1, bicarbonate <5 mmol/L
- Perform a urinalysis for ketones.
- Measurement of blood ß-OHB concentration, if available, is useful to confirm ketoacidosis and may be used to monitor the response to treatment [25].
- Obtain appropriate specimens for culture (blood, urine, throat), if there is evidence of infection.
- If laboratory measurement of serum potassium is delayed, perform an electrocardiogram (ECG) for baseline evaluation of potassium status.

Supportive measures [1]:

- Secure the airway and empty the stomach by continuous nasogastric suction to prevent pulmonary aspiration, in case there is deterioration in conscious level.

http://dx.doi.org/10.5772/53020

- A peripheral intravenous (IV) catheter should be placed for convenient and painless repetitive blood sampling. An arterial catheter may be necessary in some critically ill patients managed in an intensive care unit.
- Perform continuous electrocardiographic monitoring to assess T-waves for evidence of hyper- or hypokalemia
- Give oxygen to patients with severe circulatory impairment or shock
- Give antibiotics to febrile patients after obtaining appropriate cultures of body fluids
- Catheterize the bladder if the child is unconscious or unable to void on demand (e.g., infants and very ill young children)

6. Further clinical and biochemical monitoring

Meticulous monitoring of the patient's clinical and biochemical response to treatment is mandatory for timely adjustments in treatment as indicated by the patient's clinical or laboratory data. Documentation on a flow chart of hour-by-hour clinical observations, IV and oral medications, fluids, and laboratory results is very helpful.

Monitoring should include the following [4]:

- Hourly (or more frequently as indicated) vital signs (heart rate, respiratory rate, blood pressure)
- Hourly (or more frequently as indicated) neurological observations for warning signs and symptoms of cerebral edema. The latter include:
  - Headache
  - recurrence of vomiting
  - change in neurological status (restlessness, irritability, increased drowsiness, incontinence) or specific neurologic signs (e.g., cranial nerve palsies, abnormal pupillary responses)
  - inappropriate slowing of heart rate
  - rising blood pressure
  - decreased oxygen saturation
- Amount of administered insulin
- Hourly (or more frequently as indicated) accurate fluid input (including all oral fluid) and output.
- Capillary blood glucose should be measured hourly (but must be cross-checked against laboratory venous glucose, as capillary methods may be inaccurate in the presence of poor peripheral circulation and acidosis).

6.1. Laboratory tests

- Serum electrolytes, glucose, blood urea nitrogen, hematocrit and blood gases should be repeated 2-hourly for the first 12 hours, or more frequently, as clinically indicated, in more severe cases.
- Urine ketones until cleared or blood ß-OHB concentrations, if available, every 2 hours
- If the laboratory cannot provide timely results, a portable biochemical analyzer that measures plasma glucose, serum electrolytes and blood ketones on fingerstick blood samples at the bedside is a useful adjunct to laboratory-based determinations [2].
- **Additional calculations that may be informative**:
  - **Anion gap = serum sodium(Na) – {serum chloride (Cl) + serum bicarbonate (HCO3)} : normal is 12 ± 2 (mmol/L).** In DKA, the anion gap is typically 20–30 mmol/L; an anion gap >35 mmol/L suggests concomitant lactic acidosis.
  - **Corrected sodium = measured Na + 2([plasma glucose -5.6]/5.6) (mmol/L)** The measured serum sodium concentration is an unreliable index of the degree of ECF contraction as glucose, largely restricted to the extracellular space, causes osmotic movement of water into the extracellular space thereby causing dilutional hyponatremia.
  - Therefore, it is important to calculate the corrected sodium (using the above formula) and monitor its changes throughout the course of therapy. As the plasma glucose concentration decreases after administering fluid and insulin, the measured serum sodium concentration should increase (positive sodium load), but it is important to appreciate that this does not indicate a worsening of the hypertonic state. A failure of measured serum sodium levels to rise or a further decline in serum sodium levels with therapy is thought to be a potentially ominous sign of impending cerebral edema
  - **Effective osmolality (mOsm/kg)= 2x(Na + K) + glucose (mmol/L)** The effective osmolality (formula above) is frequently in the range of 300–350 mOsm/Kg.

6.2. Fluids and electrolytes

The objectives of fluid and electrolyte replacement therapy are [1]:

- Restoration of circulating volume
- Replacement of sodium and the ECF and intracellular fluid deficit of water
- Improved glomerular filtration with enhanced clearance of glucose and ketones from the blood
- Reduction of risk of cerebral edema

6.3. Fluids

- Establish two I.V. lines: one for fluids and electrolytes and the other for insulin infusion

http://dx.doi.org/10.5772/53020

- Shock with hemodynamic compromise is rare in pediatric DKA. If the patient is shocked, administer shock therapy: 10 ml/Kg 0.9% normal saline (or Ringer's lactate or acetate) through a large bore cannula, over 0.5 hr. Re-assess the patient and repeat up to a maximum of 30 ml/kg if necessary, with reassessment after each bolus.

- The volume and rate of administration depends on circulatory status and, where it is clinically indicated.

- **Calculate the Fluid Requirements**

1. Deficit Fluid Requirements :

   Patients with DKA have a deficit in extracellular fluid (ECF) volume that usually is in the range 5–10%. Clinical estimates of the volume deficit are subjective and inaccurate, therefore, in moderate DKA use 5–7%and in severe DKA 7–10% dehydration [4].

   - Assess the degree of dehydration and calculate the deficit (% dehydration x body weight) considering the age of the patient as shown in Table 1.

Degree of Dehydration	**Infants & children <8 years**		**Children "/>8 years**	
	Degree	Fluids	Degree	Fluids
Mild	5%	50 ml/kg	3%	30 ml/kg
Moderate	8%	80 ml/kg	5%	50 ml/kg
Severe	10%	100 ml/kg	8%	80 ml/kg

Table 1. Calculation of deficit fluid requirements in children presenting with DKA (1)

2. Maintenance Fluid Requirements:

Age (years)	**Amount of fluids**
0-2	80 ml/kg/24hr
3-5	70 ml/kg/24hr
6—9	60 ml/kg/24hr
10-14	50 ml/kg/24hr
Adult ("/>15)	35 ml/kg/24hr

Table 2. Calculation of maintenance fluid requirements (1)

3. Total working fluid = deficit + maintenance (calculated for 48 hours)

- Type of fluids

- If blood glucose is over 300 mg/dl, start with isotonic saline, then when blood glucose goes down to 250 mg/dl, add glucose 5% to isotonic saline in a 1:1 ratio if acidosis is corrected. If acidosis is not corrected, add glucose 10% to isotonic saline in 1:1 ratio.

- In case of hyperosmolarity (> 340 mosm/kg), or if corrected Na is 155 mEq/l or more, use half normal saline (0.45%) instead of normal saline (0.9%), to prevent cerebral edema but only after correction of shock and severe dehydration. It is advisable to use it after 6 hours from initiation of fluid therapy.

Principles of Water and Salt Replacement and Reduction of Risk of Cerebral Edema

There is no convincing evidence of an association between the rate of fluid or sodium administration used in the treatment of DKA and the development of cerebral edema [26]. No treatment strategy can be definitively recommended as being superior to based on evidence. The principles described below were endorsed by a panel of expert physicians representing the Lawson Wilkins Pediatric Endocrine Society (LWPES), the European Society for Paediatric Endocrinology (ESPE), and the International Society for Pediatric and Adolescent Diabetes (ISPAD) [4,5].

- Water and salt deficits must be replaced
- IV or oral fluids that may have been given in another facility before assessment should be factored into calculation of deficit and repair
- In addition to clinical assessment of dehydration, calculation of effective osmolality may be valuable to guide fluid and electrolyte therapy.
- Urinary losses should not routinely be added to the calculation of replacement fluid, but may be necessary in rare circumstances.
- The use of large amounts of 0.9% saline has been associated with the development of hyperchloremic metabolic acidosis [27].

6.4. Insulin therapy

Regardless of the type of diabetes, the child who presents with severe fasting hyperglycemia, metabolic derangements, and ketonemia will require insulin therapy to reverse the metabolic abnormalities [2]

DKA is caused by a decrease in effective circulating insulin associated with increases in counter-regulatory hormones {glucagon, catecholamines, growth hormone (GH), cortisol}. Although rehydration alone causes some decrease in blood glucose concentration, insulin therapy is essential to normalize blood glucose and suppress lipolysis and ketogenesis [1].

Extensive evidence indicates that *'low dose'* IV insulin administration should be the standard of care [4].

- Start insulin infusion 1–2 hours after starting fluid replacement therapy; i.e. after the patient has received initial volume expansion [28].

http://dx.doi.org/10.5772/53020

Correction of insulin deficiency

  - Dose: 0.1 unit/kg/hour (for example, one method is to dilute 50 units regular [soluble] insulin in 50 mL normal saline, 1 unit = 1 mL)

  - Route of administration IV

  - An IV bolus is unnecessary, may increase the risk of cerebral edema, and should not be used at the start of therapy

- The dose of insulin should usually remain at 0.1unit/kg/hour at least until resolution of DKA (pH >7.30, bicarbonate >15 mmol/L and/or closure of the anion gap), which invariably takes longer than normalization of blood glucose concentrations.

- If the patient demonstrates marked sensitivity to insulin (e.g., some young children with DKA, patients with HHS, and some older children with established diabetes), the dose may be decreased to 0.05 unit/kg/hour, or less, provided that metabolic acidosis continues to resolve.

- To prevent an unduly rapid decrease in plasma glucose concentration and hypoglycemia, 5% glucose should be added to the IV fluid (e.g., 5% glucose in 0.45% saline) when the plasma glucose falls to approximately 250–300 mg/dL, or sooner if the rate of fall is precipitous.

  - It may be necessary to use 10% or even 12.5% dextrose to prevent hypoglycemia while continuing to infuse insulin to correct the metabolic acidosis. The fall of blood glucose should not exceed 100 mg per hour. If blood glucose drops more than 100 mg/hr, reduce insulin infusion to 0.05 U/kg/hr. Aim to keep blood glucose at about 11 mmol/L (200 mg/dL) until resolution of DKA

- If biochemical parameters of DKA (pH, anion gap) do not improve, reassess the patient, review insulin therapy, and consider other possible causes of impaired response to insulin; e.g., infection, errors in insulin preparation.

- In circumstances where continuous IV administration is not possible, hourly or 2-hourly subcutaneous (SC) or intramuscular (IM) administration of a short- or rapid-acting insulin analog (insulin lispro or insulin aspart) is safe and may be as effective as IV regular insulin infusion, but should not be used in subjects whose peripheral circulation is impaired.

6.5. Potassium replacement

Pathophysiology of potassium depletion in DKA [4]

Children with DKA suffer total body potassium deficits of the order of 3 to 6 mmol/kg. The major loss of potassium is from the intracellular pool.

Intracellular potassium is depleted because of the following factors:

- increased plasma osmolality drags water and potassium out of cells

- glycogenolysis and proteolysis secondary to insulin deficiency cause potassium efflux from cells
- Potassium is lost from the body from vomiting and as a consequence of osmotic diuresis.
- Volume depletion causes secondary hyperaldosteronism, which promotes urinary potassium excretion.

- Despite potassium depletion, at presentation, serum potassium levels may be normal, increased or decreased. Renal dysfunction, by enhancing hyperglycemia and reducing potassium excretion, contributes to hyperkalemia. Administration of insulin and the correction of acidosis will drive potassium back into the cells, decreasing serum levels. The serum potassium concentration may decrease abruptly, predisposing the patient to cardiac arrhythmias.

Guidelines of Potassium supplementation [1]

- Replacement therapy is required regardless of the serum potassium concentration
- If the patient is hypokalemic, start potassium replacement at the time of initial volume expansion and before starting insulin therapy. Otherwise, start replacing potassium after initial volume expansion and concurrent with starting insulin therapy.
- If the patient is hyperkalemic, postpone potassium replacement until the patient voids urine
- If immediate serum potassium measurements are unavailable, an ECG may help to determine whether the child has hyper- or hypokalemia. Flattening of the T wave, widening of the QT interval, and the appearance of U waves indicate hypokalemia. Tall, peaked, symmetrical, T waves and shortening of the QT interval are signs of hyperkalemia.
- The starting potassium concentration in the infusate should be 40 mmol/L or 20 mmol potassium/L in the patient receiving fluid at a rate >10 mL/kg/h. Subsequent potassium replacement therapy should be based on serum potassium measurements.
- Potassium replacement should continue throughout IV fluid therapy. The maximum recommended rate of intravenous potassium replacement is usually 0.5 mmol/kg/hr
- If hypokalemia persists despite a maximum rate of potassium replacement, reduce the rate of insulin infusion

6.6. Phosphate

Phosphate is lost as a result of osmotic diuresis in DKA. Plasma phosphate levels fall after starting treatment by insulin, which promotes entry of phosphate into cells.

Prospective studies have not shown clinical benefit from phosphate replacement. Severe hypophosphatemia in conjunction with unexplained weakness should be treated. Administration of phosphate may induce hypocalcemia. Potassium phosphate salts may be safely used as an alternative to or combined with potassium chloride or acetate, provided that careful monitoring of serum calcium is performed to avoid hypocalcemia [2]

6.7. Acidosis

Severe metabolic acidosis is hazardous leading to decreased myocardial performance, decreased response of respiratory center, peripheral and cerebral vasodilatation and life threatening hyperkalemia. Nevertheless, it can be reversible by fluid and insulin replacement; insulin stops further ketoacid production and allows ketoacids to be metabolized, which generates bicarbonate. Treatment of hypovolemia improves tissue perfusion and renal function, thereby increasing the excretion of organic acids[1].

Controlled trials have shown no clinical benefit from bicarbonate administration. Moreover, bicarbonate therapy may be more hazardous than acidosis itself. It can cause paradoxical CNS acidosis and promotes intracellular acidosis and cerebral edema. Moreover, rapid correction of acidosis with bicarbonate causes hypokalemia, while sodium overload can result in increasing osmolality. Late alkalemia can lead to shift of oxygen dissociation curve to the left, with impaired O2 delivery to the tissues & increased anaerobic glycolysis[4].

Nevertheless, there may be selected patients who may benefit from cautious alkali therapy[1]. These include: patients with severe acidemia (arterial pH <6.9) in whom decreased cardiac contractility and peripheral vasodilatation can further impair tissue perfusion, and patients with life-threatening hyperkalemia

- Bicarbonate administration is not recommended unless the acidosis is profound and likely to affect adversely the action of adrenaline/epinephrine during resuscitation.
- If bicarbonate is considered necessary, cautiously give 1–2 mmol/kg over 60 minutes.

6.8. Introduction of oral fluids and transition to SC insulin injections

- Oral fluids should be introduced only when the clinical condition has become stable, however mild acidosis/ketosis may still be present.
- When oral fluid is tolerated, IV fluid should be reduced and change to SC insulin is planned.
- To prevent rebound hyperglycemia the first SC injection should be given 15–30 minutes (with rapid acting insulin) or 1–2 hours (with regular insulin) before stopping the insulin infusion to allow sufficient time for the insulin to be absorbed. With intermediate- or long-acting insulin, the overlap should be longer and the IV insulin gradually lowered. For example, for patients on a basal-bolus insulin regimen, the first dose of basal insulin may be administered in the evening and the insulin infusion is stopped the next morning.
- After transitioning to SC insulin, frequent blood glucose monitoring is required to avoid marked hyperglycemia and hypoglycemia [2].

7. Morbidity and mortality from DKA

The mortality rate from DKA in children is 0.15% to 0.30% [11,12]. Cerebral edema accounts for 60% to 90% of all DKA deaths [13,14]. Ten % to 25% of survivors of cerebral edema have significant residual morbidity [29]

Other rare causes of morbidity and mortality include:

- Hypokalemia
- Hyperkalemia
- Severe hypophosphatemia
- Hypoglycemia
- Other central nervous system complications (disseminated intravascular coagulation, dural sinus thrombosis, basilar artery thrombosis)
- Peripheral venous thrombosis
- Sepsis
- Rhinocerebral or pulmonary mucormycosis
- Aspiration pneumonia
- Pulmonary edema
- Adult respiratory distress syndrome (ARDS)
- Pneumothorax, pneumomediastinum and subcutaneous emphysema
- Rhabdomyolysis
- Acute renal failure
- Acute pancreatitis [30]

7.1. Cerebral edema

Cerebral edema is responsible for the majority of deaths related to DKA in children, and significant neurologic morbidity persists in many of the survivors. The incidence of cerebral edema in national population studies is 0.5–0.9% and the mortality rate is 21–24%.The pathogenesis of both its initiation and progression is unclear and incompletely understood, although a number of mechanisms have been proposed. These include cerebral ischemia and hypoxia, fluid shifts caused by inequalities in osmolarity between the extravascular and intravascular intracranial compartments, increased cerebral blood flow, and altered membrane ion transport. Demographic factors that have been associated with an increased risk of cerebral edema include [13,14,29]:

http://dx.doi.org/10.5772/53020

Epidemiological factors

- Newly diagnosed cases
- Young age: < 5 years old
- Longer duration of symptoms
- Prolonged illness
- Extended history of poor metabolic control

Features at presentation

- Severe acidosis (initial pH < 7.1)
- Greater hypocapnia after adjusting for degree of acidosis
- High Blood urea nitrogen
- Severe dehydration
- Abnormal mental status

Therapeutic interventions

- Rapid rehydration (> 50cc/ kg in first 4 hrs)
- Bicarbonate therapy for correction of acidosis
- Insulin administration in the first hour of therapy

Changes in biochemical values during treatment

- Severe Hypernatremia
- Persistent hyponatremia
- An attenuated rise in measured serum sodium concentrations during therapy
- Non closure of the anion gap

Warning signs and symptoms of cerebral edema include:

- Headache & slowing of heart rate
- Change in neurological status (restlessness, irritability, increased drowsiness, incontinence)
- Specific neurological signs (e.g., cranial nerve palsies)
- Rising blood pressure
- Decreased oxygen saturation

Clinically significant cerebral edema usually develops 4–12 hours after treatment has started, but can occur before treatment has begun or, rarely, may develop as late as 24–48 hours after the start of treatment. Symptoms and signs are variable. A method of clinical diagnosis based on bedside evaluation of neurological state is shown below [23]:

7.2. Diagnostic criteria

- Abnormal motor or verbal response to pain
- Decorticate or decerebrate posture
- Cranial nerve palsy (especially III, IV, and VI)
- Abnormal neurogenic respiratory pattern (e.g., grunting, tachypnea, Cheyne-Stokes respiration, apneusis)

7.2.1. Major criteria

- Altered mentation/fluctuating level of consciousness
- Sustained heart rate deceleration (decrease more than 20 beats per minute) not attributable to improved intravascular volume or sleep state
- Age-inappropriate incontinence

7.2.2. Minor criteria

- Vomiting
- Headache
- Lethargy or not easily arousable
- Diastolic blood pressure >90 mm Hg
- Age <5 years

One diagnostic criterion, two major criteria, or one major and two minor criteria have a sensitivity of 92% and a false positive rate of only 4%.

A chart with the reference ranges for blood pressure and heart rate, which vary depending on height, weight, and gender, should be readily available, either in the patient's chart or at the bedside.

8. Treatment of cerebral edema [1,2,4]

- Start as early as you suspect the condition, do not delay treatment until radiographic evidence
- Transfer to the ICU (if not already there)
- Restrict IV fluids to 2/3 maintenance and replace deficit over 72 hr rather than 24 hr

- Give mannitol 0.5-1 g/kg IV (2.5 ml/kg of 20% solution) over 20 minutes and repeat after 6 hours, if there is no initial response in 30 minutes to 2 hours
- Hypertonic saline (3%), 5-10 mL/kg over 30 minutes, may be an alternative to mannitol or a second line of therapy if there is no initial response to mannitol
- Elevate the head of the bed
- Intubation may be necessary for the patient with impending respiratory failure, but aggressive hyperventilation (to a pCO2 <2.9 kPa [22 mm Hg]) has been associated with poor outcome and is not recommended.
- After treatment for cerebral edema has been started, a cranial CT scan should be obtained to rule out other possible intracerebral causes of neurologic deterioration (10% of cases), especially thrombosis or hemorrhage, which may benefit from specific therapy.

9. Prevention of recurrent DKA

Home measurement of blood ß –OHB concentrations, when compared to urine ketone testing, decreases diabetes-related hospital visits (both emergency department visits and hospitalizations) by the early identification and treatment of ketosis. Blood ß -OHB measurements may be especially valuable to prevent DKA in patients who use a pump because interrupted insulin delivery rapidly leads to ketosis. There may be dissociation between urine ketone (sodium nitroprusside only measures acetoacetate and acetone) and serum ß -OHB concentrations, which may be increased to levels consistent with DKA when a urine ketone test is negative or shows only trace or small ketonuria [4].

A psychiatric social worker or clinical psychologist should be consulted to identify the psychosocial reason(s) contributing to development of DKA. Insulin omission can be prevented by schemes that provide education, psychosocial evaluation and treatment combined with adult supervision of insulin administration. Diabetes education of the child and his/her family is the cornerstone to prevent DKA occurrence and recurrence.

10. Conclusion

10.1. Future thoughts and recommendations

1. DKA is the first presentation of ~25% of young diabetics. Cerebral edema is a major risk causing mortality and morbidity.
2. The child is not a miniature adult. Children and adolescents with DKA should be managed in centers experienced in treatment and monitoring of DKA.

3. Successful management of DKA requires meticulous monitoring of the patient's clinical and biochemical response to treatment so that timely adjustments in treatment can be made when indicated by the patient's clinical or laboratory data

4. Fluid administration should rehydrate evenly over 48 hours at a rate rarely in excess of 1.5–2 times the usual daily maintenance requirement.

5. Begin insulin infusion with 0.1 U/kg/h. 1–2 hours after starting fluid replacement therapy. Increase the amount of glucose administered if blood glucose is falling too rapidly or acidosis is not resolving.

6. Even with normal or high levels of serum potassium at presentation, there is always a total body deficit of potassium. Begin with 40 mmol potassium/L in the infusate or 20 mmol potassium/L in the patient receiving fluid at a rate >10 mL/kg/h.

7. There is no evidence that bicarbonate is either necessary or safe in DKA. It is used cautiously in severe acidemia (arterial pH <6.9) and in life-threatening hyperkalemia

8. Despite much effort to identify the cause of cerebral edema, its pathogenesis is incompletely understood. Further research is needed in this area.

9. In case of profound neurological symptoms, Mannitol should be given immediately.

10. All cases of recurrent DKA are preventable

Author details

Shereen Abdelghaffar

Pediatric Endocrinology and Diabetes, Cairo University, Egypt

References

[1] Savage MW, Dhatariya KK, Kilvert A. Rayman G,Rees JAE, Courtney CH, Hilton L, Dyer PH, Hamersley. Diabetes UK Position Statements and Care Recommendations. Joint British Diabetes Societies Guidelines for the management of DKA. Diabet. Med. 2011; 28:508-15

[2] American Diabetes Association. Diabetic Ketoacidosis in infants, children and adolescents. A Consensus statement. Diabetes Care, 2006, May;29(5):1150-59

[3] Wolfsdorf J, Craig ME, Daneman D, Dunger D, Edge J, Lee W, Rosenbloom A, Sperling M, and Hanas R.ISPAD Clinical Practice Consensus Guidelines 2009 Compendium. Diabetic ketoacidosis in children and adolescents with diabetes. Pediatric Diabetes 2009: 10(Suppl. 12): 118–13

[4] Dunger DB, Sperling MA, Acerini CL, et al, for the European Society for Paediatric Endocrinology; Lawson Wilkins Pediatric Endocrine Society. European Society for Paediatric Endocrinology/Lawson Wilkins Pediatric Endocrine Society consensus statement on diabetic ketoacidosis in children and adolescents. Pediatrics 2004;113:e133-40

[5] Kitabchi AE, Umpierrez GE, Murphy MB, Kreisberg RA. Hyperglycemic crises in adult patients with diabetes: a consensus statement from the American Diabetes Association. Diabetes Care 2006 Dec: 29(12):2739–48.

[6] Keenan HT, Foster CM, Bratton SL. Social factors associated with prolonged hospitalization among diabetic children. Pediatrics 2002;109:40-4.

[7] Hanas R, Lindgren F, Lindblad B. A 2-yr national population study of pediatric ketoacidosis in Sweden: predisposing conditions and insulin pump use. Pediatr Diabetes 2009 Feb: 10(1): 33–7.

[8] Mc Donnell CM, Pedreira CC, Vadamalayan B, Cameron FJ, Werther GA. Diabetic ketoacidosis, hyperosmolarity and hypernatremia: are high carbohydrate drinks worsening initial presentation? Pediatr Diabetes 2005 Jun: 6(2): 90–4.

[9] The Writing Group for the SEARCH for Diabetes in Youth Study Group. Incidence of Diabetes in Youth in the United States. JAMA. 2007;297:2716-24

[10] NHS Information Centre. National Diabetes Audit 2008-2009. Available at http://www.ic.nhs.uk/webfiles/Services/NCASP/Diabetes/200910%20annual%20report%20documents/National_Diabetes_Audit_Executive_Summary_2009_2010.pdf. Last accessed 7 August 2012.

[11] Edge JA, Ford-Adams ME, Dunger DB. Causes of death in children with insulin dependent diabetes 1990-1996. Arch Dis Child 1999;81:318-23

[12] Curtis JR, To T, Muirhead S, Cummings E, Daneman D. Recenttrends in hospitalization for diabetic ketoacidosis in Ontario children. Diabetes Care 2002;25:1591-6.

[13] Edge J, Hawkins MM, Winter DL, Dunger DB. The risk and outcome of cerebral oedema developing during diabetic ketoacidosis. Arch Dis Child 2001;85:16-22.

[14] Glaser N, Barnett P, McCaslin I, et al, for the Pediatric Emergency Medicine Collaborative Research Committee of the American Academy of Pediatrics. Risk factors for cerebral edema in children with diabetic ketoacidosis. The Pediatric Emergency Medicine Collaborative Research Committee of the American Academy of Pediatrics. N Engl J Med 2001;344:264-9.

[15] Chase HP, Garg SK, Jelley DH. Diabetic ketoacidosis in children and the role of outpatient management. Pediatr Rev 1990;11:297-304.

[16] Pinkey JH, Bingley PJ, Sawtell PA, Dunger DB, Gale EA. Presentation and progress of childhood diabetes mellitus: A prospective population-based study. The Bart's-Oxford Study Group. Diabetologia 1994;37:70-4.

[17] Hathout EH, Thomas W, El-Shahawy M, Nahab F, Mace JW. Diabetic autoimmune markers in children and adolescents with type 2 diabetes. Pediatrics 2001;107:e102.

[18] Rewers A, Chase HP, Mackenzie T, Walravens P, Roback M, Rewers M, et al. Predictors of acute complications in children with type 1 diabetes. JAMA 2002 May 15: 287(19): 2511–8.

[19] Burge MR, Hardy KJ, Schade DS. Short-term fasting is a mechanism for the development of euglycemic ketoacidosis during periods of insulin deficiency. J Clin Endocrinol Metab 1993 May: 76(5):1192–8.

[20] Morales AE, Rosenbloom AL. Death caused by hyperglycemic hyperosmolar state at the onset of type 2 diabetes. J Pediatr 2004 Feb: 144(2): 270–3.

[21] Kershaw MJ, Newton T, Barrett TG, Berry K, Kirk J. Childhood diabetes presenting with hyperosmolar dehydration but without ketoacidosis: a report of three cases. Diabet Med 2005 May: 22(5):645–7.

[22] Canarie MF, Bogue CW, Banasiak KJ, Weinzimer SA, Tamborlane WV. Decompensated hyperglycemic hyperosmolarity without significant ketoacidosis in the adolescent and young adult population. J Pediatr Endocrinol Metab 2007 Oct: 20(10): 1115–24.

[23] Steiner MJ, Dewalt DA, Byerley JS. Is this child dehydrated? JAMA 2004 Jun 9: 291(22): 2746–54.

[24] Rewers A, Klingensmith G, Davis C, Petitti DB, Pihoker C, Rodriguez B, et al. Presence of diabetic ketoacidosis at diagnosis of diabetes mellitus in youth: the Search for Diabetes in Youth Study. Pediatrics 2008 May: 121(5): e1258–66.

[25] Ham MR, Okada P, White PC. Bedside ketone determination in diabetic children with hyperglycemia and ketosis in the acute care setting. Pediatr Diabetes 2004 Mar: 5(1): 39–43.

[26] Brown TB. Cerebral oedema in childhood diabetic ketoacidosis: is treatment a factor? Emerg Med J 2004 Mar: 21(2): 141–4.

[27] Oh MS, Carroll HJ, Uribarri J. Mechanism of normochloremic and hyperchloremic acidosis in diabetic ketoacidosis. Nephron 1990: 54(1): 1–6.

[28] Edge J, Jakes R, Roy Y, Hawkins M, Winter D, Ford-Adams ME, Murphy NP, Bergomi A, Widmer B, Dunger DB. The UK case-control study of cerebral oedema complicating diabetic ketoacidosis in children. Diabetologia 2006: 49: 2002–9.

[29] Lawrence S. Diagnosis and treatment of diabetic ketoacidosis in children and adolescents. Paediatr Child Health January 200510 (1): 21-24

[30] Haddad NG, Croffie JM, Eugster EA. Pancreatic enzyme elevations in children with diabetic ketoacidosis. J Pediatr 2004 Jul: 145(1): 122–4.

Chapter 12

Distinctive Characteristics and Specific Management of Diabetic Ketoacidosis in Patients with Acute Myocardial Infarction, Stroke and Renal Failure

Aleksandar Jovanovic, Snezana Markovic-Jovanovic,
Vladan Peric and Radojica Stolic

Additional information is available at the end of the chapter

http://dx.doi.org/10.5772/ 52390

1. Introduction

Diabetic ketoacidosis (DKA) is considered a predominantly acute type 1 diabetic complication, although it may occur in type 2 diabetes as well, particularly in patients who already have a decreased insulin secretion capacity. Stress –induced burst in catecholamine and ACTH secretion in acute myocardial infarction (AMI) promotes release of free fatty acids and their hepatic and muscular tissue utilization. The impairment in insulin-mediated intracellular glucose influx owing to the absent or insufficient pancreatic insulin secretion is the prerequisite for the occurrence of diabetic ketoacidosis.

The results of the analysis of acid – base disturbances from our previous study [26] performed in the intensive-care unit in diabetics and non-diabetics suffering acute myocardial infarction are shown in Fig. 1.

Cardiovascular accidents have a marked place among the possible causes of diabetic ketoacidosis. Cardiovascular morbidity influences the severity and duration of diabetic ketoacidosis and limits the first and most important step in its treatment- the fluid resuscitation. The resulting hyperosmolarity of body fluids precipitates a pro-thrombotic state, thus aggravating prognosis in patients with myocardial infarction. The clinical features of hyperglycemic/hyperosmolar state and diabetic ketoacidosis may overlap and are observed simultaneously (overlap cases) [44].

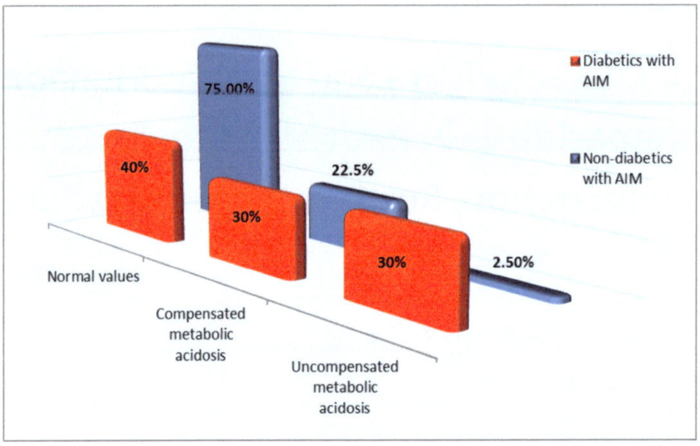

Figure 1. Acid-base disturbances in diabetics and non-diabetics suffering acute myocardial infarction: Almost one-third of diabetic patients with acute myocardial infarction had un-compensated metabolic acidosis defined as pH< 35, HCO3- < 22mmol/L. Although acidosis was mild in most of the cases at least third of these patients had criteria for true diabetic ketoacidosis (pH<30, HCO3- <15mmol/L). Additional 30% had a compensated metabolic acidosis with normal pH and mild to moderately decreased bicarbonate level. The pH was normalized at a price of the increased respiratory effort to lower the PaCO2 which may lead to respiratory muscle fatigue.

Additional risk factors for development of hyperosmolarity include the presence of congestive heart failure, impaired thirst, limited access to water (especially in patients with dementia or who are bed bound), older age, and poor kidney function. Table 1 depicts the significant correlations of pH values and certain clinical and biochemical parameters in diabetics suffering AMI.

	Spearman's correlation coefficients ρ
	pH
Blood glucose	-0.71
Blood ketones	-0.72
Anion gap	-0.77
Noradrenaline	-0.54
Heart failure	-0.41
Rhythm / Conduction disturbances	-0.5
SaO2	0.68
CK	-0.62
Serum lactate	-0.54

Table 1. Significant (p<0.05 and less) correlations between serum pH and clinical and biochemical parameters in diabetics suffering AMIAs expected, serum pH correlated with glycemic control, but also with clinical and biochemical parameters that were related to tissue hypo-perfusion (incidence of heart failure and rhythm/conduction disturbances, haemoglobin oxygen saturation, serum lactate) and to infarct size and stress-hormone release (e.g. serum creatinine – kinase and plasma noradrenaline values)

Hyperosmolar state and circulatory impairment with decreased oxygen tissue delivery may stimulate lactate production. Although true lactic acidosis occurs rarely, the increased lactate load may further contribute to the degree of acidosis. In our study, bicarbonate levels was lower ($p<0.05$) and base deficit were significantly ($p<0.01$) higher in patients with diabetes mellitus and acute myocardial infarction comparing to patients with acute myocardial infarction only. Serum lactate was moderately high (Fig.2), but true lactic acidosis defined as serum lactate > 5 mmol/l was registered only in one case with lethal outcome. Moreover, it seems that rise in the serum lactate level between diabetics and non-diabetics with AMI was not accounted for the differences in oxygen delivery, since hemoglobin saturation was much the same in both groups. Therefore, it seems that DKA itself caused further tissue hypo-perfusion and contributed to serum lactate rise. These findings are compatible with the results of the recent study performed by Cox et al. [14]

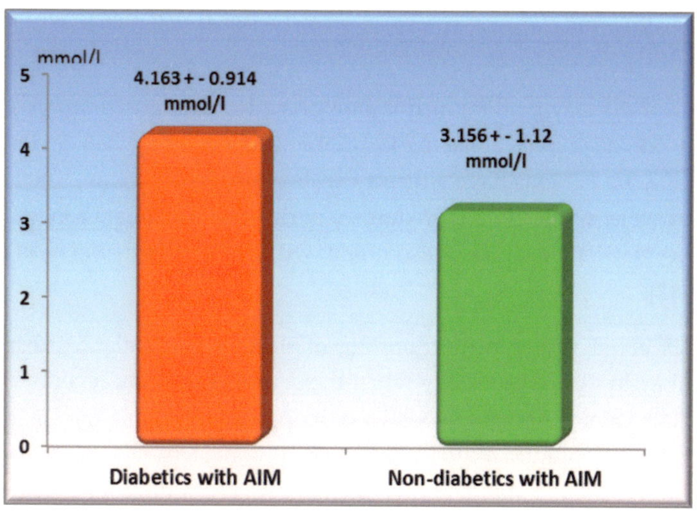

Figure 2. Serum lactate in diabetics and non-diabetics suffering AMIThe lactate level in diabetic / AMI patients was higher (4.143 +- 0.914 vs. 3.156 +- 1.12 mmol/L, $p<0.01$) comparing to patients with acute myocardial infarction only

Finally, the intensive care unit mortality reached 15% among DM/AMI patients comparing to 5% in patients with AMI only.

The excess in-hospital mortality of diabetic patients results primarily from an increased incidence of congestive heart failure, severe coronary artery disease, decreased vasodilatory reserve of epicardial artery resistance, abnormal metabolism of myocardial substrate, diffuse nature of the atherosclerotic disease and hyper-coagulable state. Autonomic neuropathy predisposes patients to ventricular arrhythmia [5]. Also, inhibition of myocardial protective mechanisms against ischaemia / reperfusion injury may contribute to the increased mortality rate [46, 58]. The similar mechanisms are operative in developing cerebrovascular injury in diabetics [18].

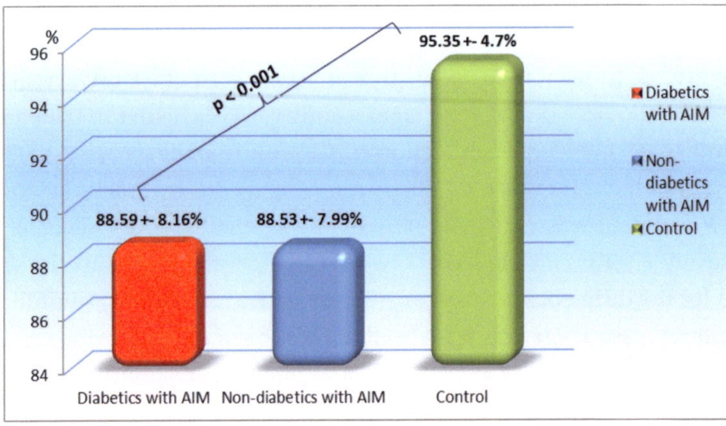

Figure 3. Haemoglobin saturation (SaO2) in diabetics and non-diabetics suffering AMI and in control groupAlthough SaO2 was significantly depressed in all patients suffering AMI comparing to control group subjects, there was no significant difference between diabetics and non-diabetics with AMI.

Diabetic acidosis itself may be the precipitating event for the occurrence of serious arrhythmia, pulmonary edema or even acute myocardial infraction [22]. When acidosis is severe, i.e. pH is less than 7.2 the H+ ions have a direct cardiac depressant action. They cause negative inotropy, bradycardia, reduced cardiac output, peripheral vasodilatation and severe shock. Sometimes, a bio-marker elevation is also noted, without further evidence of a true myocardial infarction [42].

Potassium deficit is one of the most important of electrolyte imbalances seen in DKA, as it can lead to fatal arrhythmia, especially when the serum potassium level is < 3 mmol/L. On the other hand iatrogenic or spontaneously occurring hyperkalemia may lead to ventricular tachycardia or fibrillation, intra-ventricular conduction defects, sine wave, slow ventricular escape rhythm or ventricular stand. Hyperkalemia can also induce a current of injury called 'dialyzable current of injury', which can cause ST-segment elevation and thus be mistaken for acute infarction. [7, 6)].

Pseudo-infarction presents a unique danger for the clinician treating these critically ill patients. While the mechanism of these and other temporary electrocardiographic changes in diabetic ketoacidosis remains unclear, appreciation of their transient nature is essential if misdiagnosis of myocardial infarction and possible inappropriate delay in intravenous fluid administration are to be avoided [21]. However a true myocardial necrosis was also reported with the DKA as the precipitating factor [50], which further complicates the management and the outcome of these patients.

A pulmonary edema in the absence of left ventricular failure has also been reported in DKA and may be a variant of adult respiratory distress syndrome (ARDS). The aetiology may be pulmonary vascular microangiopathy seen in diabetics. Vigorous fluid therapy can precipitate this condition.

http://dx.doi.org/10.5772/52390

Since volume repletion must be done cautiously and gradually, its therapeutic reach in diabetic ketoacidosis is limited. Intravenous insulin remains the keystone in treatment of diabetics with AMI, yet their recovery from ketoacidosis may be prolonged.

Potassium levels must be monitored continuously and corrected as need occurs. If the potassium level is less than 3.3 mEq per L (3.3 mmol per L), potassium replacement should be given immediately and insulin should be started only after the potassium level is above 3.3 mEq per L. Phosphate replacement is needed occasionally.

Bicarbonate therapy is not recommended unless pH falls to critically low levels (<7.0). Even then, positive effects of bicarbonate therapy remain questionable.

Phosphate replacement is done only if the patient's serum phosphate level is below normal. Excessive replacement can lead to hypocalcemia.

A serum deficit of about 1 mmol per L of magnesium usually exists. Severe magnesium deficiency may lead to cardiac dysrhythmias. Magnesium level should be monitored, especially in patients who receive diuretics and low levels should be corrected in order to avoid this and other complications of hypomagnesaemia.

In summary, acute myocardial infarction may precipitate diabetic ketoacidosis. Heart failure following infarction reduces patients' capacity for volume resuscitation, so clinical features of hyperglycemic hyperosmolar state and diabetic ketoacidosis may overlap and are observed simultaneously. Additional risk factors for development of hyperosmolarity include the presence of congestive heart failure, impaired thirst, limited access to water, older age, and poor kidney function.

When acidosis is severe, i.e. pH is less than 7.2, the H+ ions have a direct cardiac depressant action. Another consequence of tissue hypoperfusion resulting both from impaired myocardial output and increased osmolality as well as counter-regulatory hormone metabolic effects is increased lactate production. Increased lactate production may aggravate existing acidosis.

Diabetic acidosis itself may be the precipitating event for the occurrence of a true myocardial necrosis. Also, the ECG changes in hyperkalemia in DKA can mimic acute anteroseptal myocardial infarction. Moreover, a bio-marker elevation was also noted, without further evidence of a true myocardial infarction. Knowing that "silent" myocardial infarction occurs with higher incidence among diabetics, the differential diagnosis between myocardial necrosis and hypokalemic disturbances may be difficult.

Since volume repletion must be done cautiously and gradually, its therapeutic reach in diabetic ketoacidosis is limited. Intravenous insulin remains the keystone in treatment of diabetics with AMI, yet their recovery from ketoacidosis may be prolonged. Potassium levels must be monitored continuously and corrected as need occurs. Phosphate replacement is needed occasionally. Bicarbonate therapy is not recommended unless pH falls to critically low levels (<7.0).

2. Diabetic ketoacidosis and cerebrovascular accidents

Although cerebrovascular accidents represent a significant and well-known precipitating factor for DKA, the literature data on precise mechanisms, distinctive features or management guidelines for patients are quite few or missing. The prevalence of stroke as the precipitating factor for DKA was 0% in some studies [40] to as much as 7% in others [24]. Considering the data from the recent study in USA, most of the DKA patients (e.g. 80%) were in the age 18-65 years, with only 18% younger than 18; even 24% of all patients with DKA were in the age 45-65 years [32] Based on these data, it seems that the prevalence of DKA in patients with stroke may be underestimated and its importance under-appreciated in many cases.

Cerebrovascular accidents lead to increased release of counter-regulatory hormones (catecholamines, cortisol) which lead to hyperglycemia. Hyperglycemia develops as a result of three processes: increased gluconeogenesis, accelerated glycogenolysis, and impaired glucose utilization by peripheral tissues. Also these hormones increase the release of free fatty acids from peripheral tissues and their utilization as the energy source in hepatic and muscle mitochondria (beta-oxidation) with the increased ketone production as the direct consequence. This sequence is identical to the one seen in acute myocardial infarction [32], [19].

There is a significant overlapping of the symptoms in stroke and DKA (table 2). One can assume that an interference of symptoms of the two conditions during the clinical examination may be confusing and their interpretation difficult particularly in elder and less communicative patients.

DKA	STROKE	COMMENTS
Excessive thirst or drinking lots of fluid	Inability to swallow	
Frequent urination	**Incontinence**	Frequent urination and incontinence may be difficult to differentiate in a somnolent/ comatose patient
General weakness	**General weakness**, a feeling of weakness in one arm / leg	
Nausea and vomiting	**Nausea and vomiting**	
Loss of appetite	**Loss of appetite**	Loss of appetite in DKA results from predominantly catabolic pattern of metabolism, nausea and confusion
Confusion, somnolence, stupor, comma	**Confusion, somnolence, stupor, comma**	Mental status changes can be seen with mild-to-moderate DKA; more severe deterioration in mental status is typical with moderate-to-severe DKA.

DKA	STROKE	COMMENTS
Abdominal pain	Headache	
Shortness of breath,**increased rate of breathing** -Kusmaul's type	**Increased or decreased breathing frequency**, abnormal breathing patterns, Cheyne-Stokes type	Breathing patterns may be similar and interchangeably assigned to either of the diseases stroke the clinical examination
A generally ill appearance	**A generally ill appearance**	
Dry skin	**Skin may be dry**, or moisture	A dehydration may occur in case of not having access to water or fluids, or intensive use of osmotic diuretics
Dry mouth,	**Often dry mouth**	
Increased heart rate,	**Increased heart rate**	
Low blood pressure	Mainly high blood pressure, sometimes low	
A distinctive fruity odor on the breath, fruity-scented breath	Different kinds of breath odor not uncommon	Fruity scented breath may be hardly recognizable. Moreover, the odor appearing after ingestion of various sweet and fruits may imitate the characteristic odor of DKA
High blood sugar level	High sugar level in diabetics	Due to the effect of counter-regulatory hormones
High ketone level in serum and urine	Moderately high ketone level in urine in diabetics, alcohol abuse, starvation	
Low (<7.3) plasma pH	Plasma pH usually normal	
Low serum (<15 mmol/l) bicarbonate	Serum bicarbonate usually normal	
Increased (>/12) anion gap	Anion gap usually >/12	

Table 2. Symptoms and signs in diabetic ketoacidosis and stroke: the overlapping features

Blood glucose levels are high in the majority of diabetic patients suffering stroke. Moreover, pH, bicarbonate and anion gap are not routinely monitored in all diabetic patients suffering stroke, at least not in secondary level health institutions worldwide. In conclusion, some of the DKA cases in patients with stroke may easily be overlooked.

Furthermore, there is striking lack of literature data concerning management of adult diabetic patients with stroke. Although there are clear concerns about the volume overload, intensive use of osmotic and Henley's loop diuretics and the need for careful volume and monitoring in patients suffering cerebrovascular accident and DKA no clear guidelines were produced for intensive care units and intensive care neurologic units.

Some of the management guidelines may be defined here:

1. It is important that patients with stroke complicated by DKA avoid dehydration since both DKA and stroke correlate with the pro-thrombotic state and dehydration potentates a tendency toward intravascular thromboembolism. Since the use of osmotic and sometimes also other kinds of diuretics is inevitable in patients with stroke a careful hydration is recommended in order to avoid further thrombotic complications.

2. Fluid resuscitation must be performed carefully, in small aliquots, and with constant monitoring of blood pressure, hematocrit and plasma sodium; novel minimal invasive procedures [39] should have advantages over central venous catheter since CVP itself was reported to be a risk factor for cerebrovascular thromboembolism [33]. Excessive use of diuretics may precipitate pro-thrombotic state.

3. Infused insulin is the principle therapeutic tool for fighting DKA in patients with cerebrovascular accidents. Since fluid resuscitation must be restricted, DKA itself is expected to have more prolonged clinical course. This may be of importance, since DKA itself may be a precipitating factor for stroke (see later)

4. Serum potassium must be carefully monitored in all cardiovascular patients with DKA (see earlier). Hyper or hypokalemia should be promptly corrected; thus said, insulin-induced intracellular shift of potassium must be taken in account when evaluating potassium levels or performing potassium substitution

5. Bicarbonate therapy is not recommended except in extreme acidosis.

Not only does stroke precipitate DKA, but the vice-versa is also true [20]: diabetic ketoacidosis itself was reported as a risk factor for the occurrence of stroke in children and youth. The risk of acute ischemic or hemorrhagic stroke during the acute DKA episode is perhaps under-appreciated.

Systemic inflammation is present in DKA, with resultant vascular endothelial perturbation that may result in coagulopathy and increased hemorrhagic risk. Hyperglycemia and acidosis may contribute to oxidative injury [25], as well as ischemic injury [34]. Thrombotic risk during DKA is also elevated by abnormalities in coagulation factors, platelet activation, blood volume and flow, and vascular reactivity.

Recent data demonstrate that DKA is associated with reduced cerebral blood flow and with brain cell swelling [23]. These data suggest that cerebral injury resulting from DKA may be similar to hypoxic/ischemic brain injury. A cerebral hypo-perfusion occurs in untreated DKA. [23] In analogy with ischemia/reperfusion injury, DKA could be associated with metabolic abnormalities similar to those of hypoxic/ischemic brain injury and that these abnormalities would worsen during initial DKA treatment as normal cerebral perfusion is reestablished [15, 4].

Although a small percentage of children have clinically apparent cerebral injury at presentation of DKA prior to treatment, neurological decline during DKA treatment is more common [16]. During initial DKA treatment with insulin and intravenous saline, key aspects of the cerebral metabolic state worsen. After initiation of DKA therapy, abnormalities in Protein C, Protein S, plasma homo-cysteine, and von Willebrand Factor (vWF) were demonstrated [11, 9]. While protein C levels normalize with treatment, free protein S, the active anticoagulant of protein S, is reduced and does not return to baseline with treatment.

Arterial ischemic stroke [47], cerebral venous thrombosis [29], and hemorrhagic stroke [36] were noted in children following DKA. DKA-associated cerebral edema may also predispose to ischemic injury and hemorrhage, though cases of stroke without concomitant cerebral edema have been identified [49]. As stroke itself may cause cerebral edema, it becomes difficult to ascertain whether cerebral edema in DKA is the cause or an effect of acute cerebral infarction. A sub-arachnoid or intra-ventricular hemorrhage may occur without cerebral edema as was demonstrated using on CT scanning. Clinically, a transcranial Doppler ultrasound in children with DKA demonstrated significant vascular dysregulation with vasodilation, decreased cerebral blood flow velocity, and loss of normal cerebral blood flow regulation that only normalized after treatment. Another group of researchers found normal to increased cerebral blood flow with impaired cerebral auto-regulation during episodes of DKA not associated with overt CE in 6 children [20].

Treatment with bumetanide, [27] an inhibitor of Na-K-2Cl Co-transport, resulted in improvements in metabolic measures during untreated DKA and amelioration of the declines in metabolic measures during initial DKA treatment.

It is clear that at least some of these mechanisms may be operative in adult DKA. Abnormalities in coagulation during DKA or its treatment have been also noted in adults. Indeed, an endothelial injury, platelet activation, relative hypo-fibrinolysis, and activation of the coagulation system [20] even in the absence of clinical signs of thrombosis were all demonstrated in patients with DKA. However, the up-regulation was not to a degree expected for the increase in coagulation activity (thrombin-antithrombin III complex and prothrombin fragment 1 + 2 levels) at DKA presentation.

In summary, cerebrovascular accidents represent a significant and well-known precipitating factor for DKA. It seems that the prevalence of DKA in patients with stroke may be underestimated and its importance under-appreciated in many cases.

It is important that patients with stroke complicated by DKA avoid dehydration since both DKA and stroke correlate with the pro-thrombotic state and dehydration potentates a tendency toward intravascular thromboembolism. Unfortunately, like in acute myocardial infarction, the volume replenishment capacity in patients with stroke is often limited. Intravenous insulin and monitoring and correction of possible electrolyte imbalances are the mainstay of the treatment.

Not only does stroke precipitate DKA, but the vice-versa is also true: diabetic ketoacidosis itself was reported to be a risk factor for the occurrence of stroke in children and youth. A cerebral hypo-perfusion occurs in untreated DKA and may lead to cerebral injury. Arterial ischemic stroke, cerebral venous thrombosis and hemorrhagic stroke were noted following DKA episodes.

Treatment with bumetanide, an inhibitor of Na-K-2Cl co-transport, resulted in improvements in metabolic measures during untreated DKA and prevented cerebral metabolic aggravation during initial DKA treatment.

3. Diabetic ketoacidosis and renal failure

Renal failure occurs with increased frequency in patients with diabetes. Fortunately, the coincidence of type 1 diabetes with DKA and acute renal failure is uncommon. Volume overload and hyperkalemia may complicate the condition. It has been reported that DKA in patients with acute renal failure may be sometimes associated with respiratory distress syndrome [17].

3.1. Diabetic ketoacidosis and acute renal failure

Although acute renal failure (ARF) rarely develops in patients with diabetic ketoacidosis (DKA), these serious complications can be life threatening in critically ill patients [43]. The estimated mortality with combined DKA and ARF still reaches around 50%. ARF pre-renal failure may occur as a result of the severe fluid depletion associated with diabetic ketoacidosis; underlying diabetic nephropathy as well as hypotension, sepsis, renal artery occlusion, serious urinary infections complicated by papillary necrosis and exposure to nephrotoxic agents. Of the latter, a certain antibiotics and radio-contrast agents, but also angiotensin converting enzyme inhibitors were mentioned. [51]. The increased incidence of cardiovascular disease may also lead to renal impairment.

The long-lasting ketoacidosis in combination with infused insulin can lead to severe hypophosphatemia. Patients with uncontrolled diabetes may already be predisposed to hypophosphatemia due to osmotic dieresis and often decreased muscle mass; however, the majority of the imbalance results from phosphate shift from extracellular to intracellular space[30]. In the presence of metabolic acidosis, proximal tubular reabsorption of phosphate is inhibited and their urinary excretion is initially increased, thereby critically reducing the overall level of the extracellular phosphate [10].

Hypophosphatemia, in turn, further contributes to the deepening of the metabolic acidosis. Acidosis cannot be compensated by renal production of ammonia, because later in the course of diabetic ketoacidosis, with a reduction in the total amount of phosphate in the body, a reduction in urinary excretion of phosphate ensues. Prolonged metabolic acidosis accompanied by hypophosphatemia may be the cause of transient rhabdomyolysis. Acidosis and rhabdomyolysis lead to renal injury. In addition, prolonged hypophosphataemia can lead to cardiomyopathy due to decreased concentration of intracellular adenosine - triphosphate and 2.3diphosphoglycerate (DPG). [35]. It is, therefore important to detect changes in serum phosphate levels of order in early to prevent these complications.

Acute hypophosphatemia may be associated with respiratory problems, confusion, irritability, seizures, ataxia or coma, metabolic acidosis due to reduced phosphate reabsorption.

However, even the severe symptoms may be hardly recognizable for they can mimic those of the underlying disease – e.g. DKA itself. Hipophosphatemia may be the cause of rhabdomyolysis, which (though not often) can lead to occurrence of cardiomyopathy and acute renal failure.

Even after initiation of phosphate replacement, serum phosphate levels are often difficult to normalize, and a severe metabolic acidosis can last despite insulin-induced normalization of blood glucose.

In cases of severe acidosis, phosphate replacement is of paramount importance [31]. However, after initial-phase phosphate replacement, the re-institution of acid-base balance phosphate re-shifts from intra- to extracellular space; this can lead to the hyperphosphataemia later in the course of treatment [13]. Therefore, serum phosphate levels should be monitored continuously. With the occurrence of acute renal failure, indications for haemodialysis include oliguria, persistent metabolic acidosis resistant to standard therapy, fluid overload and hypertension. Early initiation of haemodialysis is not only effective against the direct consequences of acute renal failure - uremia and hypervolemia – but also contribute to rapid correction of metabolic acidosis and hypophosphatemia [28]. Indeed, the existing hypophosphataemia is easily corrected once a normal acid-base balance is established by haemodialysis. Prompt institution of dialysis is important as the diabetic patient may tolerate uraemia less well. Uncontrolled ketosis may worsen hyperkaliemia and metabolic acidosis. Insulin requirements may be increased due to insulin resistance, or decreased due to impaired clearance of circulating insulin [38, 56].

The vast majority of patients require intermittent haemodialysis. Patients with cardiac dysfunction or autonomic neuropathy tend to develop hypotension during treatment. Also, anticoagulation with heparin may increase the risk of hemorrhage from proliferative retinopathy, therefore prostacyclin may be a safer alternative [52]. Peritoneal dialysis may be complicated by peritonitis and chest infections. Also, haemodialysis allows greater fluid removal and remove restrictions for administration of drugs and nutrition [56].

3.2. Diabetic ketoacidosis and chronic renal failure

Despite the strong prevalence of compromised immune status, constant state of protein malnutrition, frequent vascular accessing with a predisposition to significant infections, increased incidence of cardiovascular diseases, the occurrence of DKA in patients with chronic renal failure is quite rare. [41, 3]. Kidneys play a major role in insulin breakdown [38]; advanced chronic renal failure is associated with both insulin resistance and decreased insulin degradation. The latter may lead to a marked decrease in insulin requirement. Therefore, many patients see an improvement in glycemic control when they progress to haemodialysis. Furthermore, in hyperglycemic dialysis-dependent patients volume contraction due to osmotic diuresis is not encountered. Since glycosuria and osmotic diuresis account for most of the fluid and electrolyte losses seen in DKA, anuric patients may be somewhat protected from dehydration. However they may still be prone to development of hyperkalemia and metabolic acidosis [37]. In persistent and long-lasting DKA, a substantial volume loss can still occur due to a prolonged decrease in oral intake or increased insensible water losses related to tachypnea and fever.

The uremic environment can affect methods used to assess glycemic control. Changes in dietary intake and exercise (ie, reduced intake due to anorexia prior to starting dialysis) can also affect the response to administered insulin). Renal inability to reabsorb/regenerate bicarbonate and excrete hydrogen ions may lead to metabolic acidosis even in the absence of DKA; in addition, patients often suffer from anorexia, nausea, vomiting, infections, and even acute coronary events predisposing them to catabolic pattern of metabolism. In patients treated with peritoneal dialysis, glucose contained in peritoneal dialysate will tend to increase the need for hypoglycemic therapy.

Therefore, the treatment of oliguric patient certainly differs from the wide accepted DKA treatment guidelines. [8]. First of all, end-stage-renal-disease patients with DKA may be less likely volume depleted; in most cases the extracellular volume is expanded from its baseline secondary to hyperglycemia. The volume expansion may cause dyspnea, nausea, vomiting, seizures and coma [54]. In oliguric patient, fluid hydration in amounts usually administered in the DKA treatment may precipitate severe pulmonary edema. Therefore, the need for fluid resuscitation in these patients must be justified clinically or by laboratory testing and potential volume resuscitation should be performed carefully, using central venous access for continuous monitoring. [2]. When volume overload is apparent, immediate haemodialysis is the therapy of choice.

Metabolic control can be difficult to achieve. Insulin is normally metabolized by kidneys and in chronic renal failure insulin degradation is much slower. Furthermore, insulin is not excreted either by haemodialysis or peritoneal dialysis. Hyperinsulinemia resulting from aggressive glucose – lowering therapies may easily lead to severe and prolonged hypoglycemia. One cannot readily predict insulin requirements in this setting and careful individualized therapy is essential.

As already emphasized, kidneys in end-stage renal disease are not able to contribute to the overall acid-base balance. Therefore, DKA in these patients may be both profound and prolonged. In addition, pulmonary dysfunction related to volume overload and sometimes underlying pulmonary infections can impair respiratory compensation to metabolic acidosis. Bicarbonate administration is rarely of value in DKA [55] and the associated volume, sodium and osmotic overload may be particularly problematic for anuric patients. In this situation, significant metabolic acidosis will only be correctable by haemodialysis [53].

Total body concentration of potassium is unchanged, and patients with DKA and end stage renal failure frequently have a high serum potassium level. Lack of insulin causes translocation of intracellular potassium to the extracellular compartment. Hyperglycemia causes hypertonicity of extracellular fluids, which also leads to shift of potassium from the cells to the extracellular compartment. The important potassium – lowering effect of osmotic diuresis is missing. DKA aggravates hyperkalemia in more than 50% of cases [48]. Even when testing reveals hypokalemia, total body potassium stores may be high, and these patients are unable to excrete a potassium load. Consequently, hypokalemia must be documented and

http://dx.doi.org/10.5772/ 52390

acidosis corrected before potassium supplementation is initiated. All dialysis patients presenting with significant symptoms should undergo immediate cardiac monitoring. If there is clinical suspicion or electrocardiographic evidence of hyperkalemia, they should receive immediate potassium lowering therapies, including emergent haemodialysis. [8].

In a study performed in USA in 2001 [1] the occurrence of diabetic ketoacidosis after renal transplantation was followed. A female sex, recipients of cadaver kidneys, patients age 33–44 (vs. >55), more recent year of transplant, and patients receiving tacrolimus vs. cyclosporine had significantly higher risk of diabetic ketoacidosis. However, the rate of diabetic ketoacidosis decreased more over time in tacrolimus users. Diabetic ketoacidosis was independently associated with increased mortality.

In summary, acute renal failure rarely develops in patients with diabetic ketoacidosis, but it can be life-threatening. Insulin requirements may be increased due to insulin resistance, or decreased due to impaired clearance of circulating insulin.

Patients with uncontrolled diabetes may already be predisposed to hypophosphatemia. In the presence of metabolic acidosis, proximal tubular reabsorption of phosphate is inhibited, and the overall level of the extracellular phosphate is further reduced. In cases of severe acidosis, phosphate replacement is of paramount importance.

Indications for haemodialysis in patients with acute renal failure and DKA include oliguria, persistent metabolic acidosis resistant to standard therapy, fluid overload and hypertension. Early initiation of haemodialysis is not only effective against uremia and hypervolemia but also contribute to rapid correction of metabolic acidosis and hypophosphatemia.

The occurrence of DKA in patients with advanced chronic renal failure is quite rare. Chronic renal failure is associated both with insulin resistance and decreased insulin degradation. The latter may lead to a marked decrease in insulin requirement. In patients treated with peritoneal dialysis, glucose contained in peritoneal dialysate will tend to increase the need for hypoglycemic therapy.

In oliguric patients, fluid hydration in amounts usually administered in DKA treatment may precipitate severe pulmonary edema. Sodium and osmotic overload may be particularly problematic for anuric patients. Pulmonary dysfunction due to frequent pulmonary infections can impair ventilatory compensation to metabolic acidosis. Bicarbonate administration is rarely of value in DKA. In this situation, significant metabolic acidosis will only be correctable by haemodialysis.

Most DKA patients on both peritoneal and haemodialysis are hyperkalemic and the potassium replacement in DKA is usually not necessary.

4. Conclusion

Diabetic ketoacidosis is serious metabolic complication in diabetic patients with acute myocardial infarction, stroke and renal insufficiency. Conversely, severe diabetic ketoacidosis is an important risk factor for acute myocardial infarction, stroke and acute renal failure. The presence of DKA makes patients' management difficult and aggravates the outcome.

Acidosis in these patients is usually deeper, prolonged and resistant to therapy. In all of the three conditions a fluid resuscitation in quantities commonly used in the treatment of DKA can not be performed. In addition, in many cases there is more or less marked insulin resistance. In chronic renal insufficiency, on the contrary, intensive insulin therapy usual for the treatment of ketoacidosis may carry a risk of hyperinsulinemia and prolonged hypoglycemia. Electrolyte imbalance, especially potassium deficiency or excess can have serious consequences, especially in patients with myocardial infarction, and special care should be given to electrolyte monitoring.

Finally, we believe that more attention should be paid to the possible acid-base disorders in diabetic patients suffering cerebrovascular insults. Clinical assesment in these cases is not sufficient because the significant overlapping of the signs and symptoms, therefore DKA symptoms may be attributed to cerebrovascular pathology. The conclusions based on blood glucose levels would not be appropriate, since glycemia tends to be high in distressed patients. Acid-base status should be determined routinely, along with glycemia and HbA1c in all diabetics affected by stroke in order to prevent misdiagnosis.

Author details

Aleksandar Jovanovic*, Snezana Markovic-Jovanovic, Vladan Peric and Radojica Stolic

*Address all correspondence to: aleksandar2403@yahoo.com

Medical Faculty, University of Pristina/K. Mitrovica, Serbia

References

[1] Abbott, K. C., Bernet, V. J., Agodoa, L. Y., & Yuan, C. M. (2003). Diabetic ketoacidosis and hyperglycemic hyperosmolar syndrome after renal transplantation in the United States. *BMC Endocr Disord*, 3, 10.

[2] Al-Khafaji, A., & Webb, A. R. . (2012). Fluid resuscitation. *Oxford journals CEACCP*, 12, 127-131.

[3] Alpert, M. A. (1996). Cardiovascular factors influencing survival in dialysis patients. *Adv Perit Dial*, 12, 110-9.

[4] Alvarez-Sabin, J., Morrison, R., Ribo, M., Arenillas, J., Montaner, J., Huertas, R., Santamarina, E., & Rubiera, M. (2004). Impact of admission hyperglycemia on stroke outcome after thrombolysis: risk stratification in relation to time to reperfusion. *Stroke*, 35, 2493-2498.

[5] Aronson, D., Rayfield, E. J., & Chesebro, J. H. (1997). Mechanisms Determining Course and Outcome of Diabetic Patients Who Have Had Acute Myocardial Infarction. *Ann Intern Med*, 126, 296-306.

[6] Batra, A. S., Acherman, R. J., Wong, P., & Silka, M. J. (2002). Acute myocardial infarction in a 12-year-old as a complication of hyperosmolar diabetic ketoacidosis. *Pediatr Crit Care Med*, 3(2), 194-196.

[7] Bellazzini, M. A., & Meyer, T. (2010). Pseudo-myocardial infarction in diabetic ketoacidosis with hyperkalemia. *J Emerg Med*, 39(4), e139-41.

[8] Blicker, J., Herd, A. M., & Talbot, J. (2004). Diabetic ketoacidosis in the dialysis-dependent patient: two case reports and recommendations for treatment. *CJEM*, 6(4), 281-284.

[9] Burzynski, J. (2005). DKA and thrombosis. *CMAJ*, 173(2), 132.

[10] Busch, A., Waldegger, S., Herzer, T., et al. (1994). Electrophysiological analysis of Na +/Pi cotransport mediated by a transporter cloned from rat kidney and expressed in Xenopus oocytes. *Proc Natl Acad Sci U S A*, 91(17), 8205-8.

[11] Carl, G. F., Hoffman, W. H., Passmore, G. G., et al. (2003). Diabetic ketoacidosis promotes a prothrombotic state. *Endocrine Research*, 29.

[12] Carroll, P., & Matz, R. (1982). Adult respiratory distress syndrome complicating severely uncontrolled diabetes mellitus: report of nine cases and a review of the literature. *Diabetes Care*, 5, 574-580.

[13] Casteels, K., Beckers, D., Wouters, C., & Van Geet, C. (2003). Rhabdomyolysis in diabetic ketoacidosis. *Pediatr Diabetes*, 4(1), 29-31.

[14] Cox, K., Cocchi, M. N., Salciccioli, JD, Carney, E., Howell, M., & Donnino, M. W. (2012). Prevalence and significance of lactic acidosis in diabetic ketoacidosis. *J Crit Care*, 27(2), 132-7.

[15] Dempsey, R., Baskaya, M., Combs, D., Donaldson, D., & Rao, A. (1996). Effect of hyperglycemia on reperfusion-associated recovery of intracellular pH and high energy phosphates after transient cerebral ischemia in gerbils. *Neurol Res*, 18, 546-552.

[16] Edge, J., Hawkins, M., Winter, D., & Dunger, D. (2001). The risk and outcome of cerebral oedema developing during diabetic ketoacidosis. *Arch Dis Child*, 85, 16-22.

[17] Ennis, E. D., & Kreisberg, R. A. (2004). Diabetic Ketoacidosis and the Hyperglycemic Hyperosmolar Syndrome. *LeRoith D, Taylor SI, Olefsky JM (eds): Diabetes mellitus: a fundamental and clinical text.-3rd ed. Lippincott Williams & Wilkins.*

[18] Ergul, A., Li, W., Elgebaly, M. M., Bruno, A., & Fagan, S. C. (2009). Hyperglycemia, diabetes and stroke: focus on the cerebrovasculature. *Vascul Pharmacol*, 51, 44-9.

[19] Felig, P., Sherwin, R. S., Soman, V., Wahren, J., Hendler, R., Sacca, L., Eigler, N., Goldberg, D., & Walesky, M. (1979). Hormonal interactions in the regulation of blood glucose. *Recent ProgHorm Res*, 35, 501-532.

[20] Foster, J. R., Morrison, G., & Fraser, D. D. (2011). Diabetic Ketoacidosis-Associated Stroke in Children and Youth. *Stroke Res Treat*, Article ID 219706, 12.

[21] Fuller, P. J., Colman, P. G., Harper, R. W., & Stockigt, J. R. (1982). Transient anterior electrocardiographic changes simulating acute anterior myocardial infarction in diabetic ketoacidosis. *Diabetes Care*, 5(2), 118-21.

[22] Gandhi, M. J., Tilak, T., & Suvarna, S. (1995). Cardiovascular Complications in Diabetic Ketoacidosis Int. J. Diab. Dev. Countries , 15

[23] Glaser, N., Gorges, S., Marcin, J., Buonocore, M., Di Carlo, J., Neely, E., Barnes, P., Bottomly, J., & Kuppermann, N. (2010). Mechanism of cerebral edema in children with diabetic ketoacidosis. *Diabetes*, March, 59(3), 702-709.

[24] Husain, S. S., Javed, M. R., & Ahmad, Ali. S. (2011). Diabetic Ketoacidosis: The Precipitating Entites in Patients With Type 2 Diabetes Mellitus. *Professional Med J*, 18(1), 80-82.

[25] Jain, S. K., Mc Vie, R., & Bocchini, R. A. Jr. (2006). Hyperketonemia (ketosis), oxidative stress and type 1 diabetes. *Pathophysiology*, 13(3), 163-170.

[26] Jovanovic, A., Peric, V., Sovtic, S., Novakovic, T., & Markovic-Jovanovic, S. (2006). Hyperlactatidemia caused by acute myocardial infarction in patients with type2 diabetes mellitus. *ECE, Glasgow, UK, European Society of Endocrinology and British Endocrine Societies.*

[27] Kahle, K., Barnett, S., Sassower, K., & Saley, K. (2009). Decreased seizure activity in a human neonate treated with bumetanide, an inhibitor of the Na+-K+-2Cl- cotransporter NKCC1. *J Child Neurol*, 24, 572-576.

[28] Kawata, H., Inui, D., Ohto, J., et al. (2006). The use of continuous hemodiafiltration in a patient with diabetic ketoacidosis. *J Anesth*, 20(2), 129-31.

[29] Keane, S., Gallagher, A., Ackroyd, S., Mc Shane, MA, & Edge, J. A. (2002). Cerebral venous thrombosis during diabetic ketoacidosis. *Archives of Disease in Childhood*, 86(3), 204-206.

[30] Kebler, R., et al., Mc Donald, F. D., & Cadnapaphornchai, P. (1985). Dynamic changes in serum phosphorus levels in diabetic ketoacidosis. *Am J Med*, 79(5), 571-6.

[31] Kitabchi, A. E., Umpierrez, G. E., Murphy, M. B., et al. (2004). Hyperglycemic crises in diabetes. *Diabetes Care*, 27(1), S94-102.

[32] Kitabchi, A. E., Umpierrez, G. E., Murphy, M. B., & Kreisberg, R. A. (2006). Hyperglycemic crises in adult patients with diabetes. *Diabetes Care*, 29, 2739-2748.

[33] Kusminski, R. E. (2007). Complications of Central Venous Catetherisation. *J Am Coll Surg*, 204(4).

[34] Lin, J. J., Lin, K. L., Wang, H. S., Wong, A. M. C., & Hsia, S. H. (2008). Occult infarct with acute hemorrhagic stroke in juvenile diabetic ketoacidosis. *Brain and Development*, 30(1), 91-93.

[35] Liu, P. Y., & Jeng, C. Y. (2004). Severe hypophosphatemia in a patient with diabetic ketoacidosis and acute respiratory failure. *J Chin Med Assoc*, 67(7), 355-9.

[36] Mahmud, H., Ramsay, D. A., Levin, S. D., Singh, R. N., Kotylak, T., & Fraser, D. D. (2007). Coma with diffuse white matter hemorrhages in juvenile diabetic ketoacidosis. *Pediatrics*, 120(6), e1540-e1546.

[37] Mak, R. H. (2000). Impact of end-stage renal disease and dialysis on glycemic control. *Semin Dial*, 13(1), 4-8.

[38] Mak, R. H. K., & De Fronzo, R. A. (1992). Glucose and insulin metabolism in uraemia. *Nephron*, 61, 377-82.

[39] Marik, P. E., Xavier, Monnet. X., & Jean-Louis, Teboul. J. L. (2011). Hemodynamic parameters to guide fluid therapy. *Annals of Intensive Care*, 1, 1.

[40] Mbugua, P. K., Otieno, C. F., Kayima, J. K., Amayo, A. A., & Mc Ligeyo, S. O. . (2005). Diabetic ketoacidosis: clinical presentation and precipitating factors at Kenyatta National Hospital, Nairobi. *East African Medical Journal*, 82(12), S191-S196.

[41] Minnaganti, V. R., & Cunha, B. A. (2001). Infections associated with uremia and dialysis. *Infect Dis North Am*, 15(2), 385-406.

[42] Moller, N., Foss, A. C., Gravholt, C. H., Mortensen, U. M., Poulsen, S. H., & Mogensen, CE. (2005). Myocardial injury with biomarker elevation in diabetic ketoacidosis. *J Diabetes Complications*, 19(6), 361-3.

[43] Murdoch, I. A., Pryor, D., Haycock, G. B., & Cameron, S. J. (1993). Acute renal failure complicating diabetic ketoacidosis. *Acta Paediatr*, 82(5), 498-500.

[44] Nugent, B. W. (2005). Hyperosmolar hyperglycemic state. *Emerg Med Clin North Am*, 23(3), 629-48.

[45] Okuda, Y., Adrogue, H. J., Field, J. B., et al. (1996). Counterproductive effects of sodium bicarbonate in diabetic ketoacidosis. *J ClinEndocrinolMetab*, 81, 314-320.

[46] Otter, W., Kleybrink, S., Doering, W., et al. (2004). Hospital outcome of acute myocardial infarction in patients with and without diabetes mellitus. *Diabet Med*, 21, 183-187.

[47] Roe, F., Crawford, T. O., Huff, K. R., Costin, G., Kaufman, F. R., & Nelson, M. D. (1996). Brain infarction in children with diabetic ketoacidosis. *Journal of Diabetes and its Complications*, 10(2), 100-108.

[48] Rohrscheib, M., Tzamaloukas, A. H., Todd, S., et al. (1980). Serum Potassium Concentration in Hyperglycemia of Chronic Dialysis Popp D, Achtenberg JF, Cryer PE:

Hyperkalemia and hyperglycemic increments in plasma potassium in diabetes mellitys. *Arch Intern Med*, 140, 1617-20.

[49] Scibilia, J., Finegold, D., Dorman, J., Becker, D., & Drash, A. (1986). Why do children with diabetes die? *Acta Endocrinologica. Supplementum*, 279, 326-333.

[50] Tretjak, M., Verovnik, F., Vujkovac, B., et al. (2003). Severe Diabetic Ketoacidosis Associated With Acute Myocardial Necrosis. *Diabetes Care*, 26(10), 2959-60.

[51] Tumbridge, W. M. G. (1981). Factors contributing to the deaths of diabetics under fifty years of age. *Lancet*, 2, 569-72.

[52] Turney, J. H., Williams, L. C., Fewell, M. R., Parson, V., & Weston, MJ. (1980). Platelet protection and heparin sparing with prostacyclin during regular dialysis therapy. *Lancet*, 2, 219-22.

[53] Tzamaloukas, A. H., & Avasthi, P. S. (1988). Acid-base disorders in hyperglycemia of insulin-dependent diabetic patients on chronic dialysis. *J Diabet Complications*, 2(2), 75-8.

[54] Tzamaloukas, A. H., Rohrscheib, M., Ing, T. S., Siamopoulos, K. C., Elisaf, M. F., & Spalding, C. T. (2004). Serum tonicity, extracellular volume and clinical manifestations in symptomatic dialysis- associated hyperglycemia treated only with insulin. *Int J Artif Organs*, 27(9), 751-8.

[55] Viallon, A., Zeni, F., Lafond, P., Tardy, B., Page, Y., & Bertrand, J. C. (1999). Does bicarbonate therapy improve the management of severe diabetic ketoacidosis? *Criti Care Med*, 27, 2690-3.

[56] Woodrow, G., Brownjohn, A. M., & Turney, J. H. (1994). Acute renal failure in patients with type 1 diabetes mellitus. *Postgrad Med J*, 70, 192-94.

[57] Woodrow, G., Brownjohn, A. M., & Turney, J. H. (1994). Acute renal failure in patients with type 1 diabetes mellitus. *Postgrad Med J*, 70, 192-194.

[58] Yin, X., Zheng, Y., Zhai, X., et al. (2012). Diabetic Inhibition of Preconditioning- and Postconditioning-Mediated Myocardial Protection against Ischemia/Reperfusion Injury. *Exp Diabetes Res*, 198048.

Chapter 13

Diabetic Neuropathy

Baqiyyah Conway and Amanda Peltier

Additional information is available at the end of the chapter

http://dx.doi.org/10.5772/55372

1. Introduction

Diabetic neuropathy is a common microvascular complication of diabetes mellitus. Diabetic neuropathy is a major risk factor for non-traumatic amputations and is thought to play a role in the pathogenesis of other late complications of diabetes. The two major forms of diabetic neuropathy include generalized neuropathy and autonomic neuropathy. Genreralized neuropathy, affecting motor and sensory peripheral nerves can be subdivided further into polyneuropathies which affect multiple nerves and focal neuropathies. The most common form of generalized neuropathy is distal symmetrical polyneuropathy. Autonomic neuropathy affects peripheral autonomic nerves. These autonomic nerves innervate most organ systems of the body and the skin. Both distal symmetric polyneuropathy and autonomic neuropathy cause substantial morbidity and are associated with a high risk of mortality. The hypothesized mechanisms of diabetic neuropathy include ischemic effects caused by vascular abnormalities, disruption of neuronal metabolism, axonal transport mechanisms and repair capabilities, glycation of peripheral nervous system connective tissue, and glycation of Schwann cells or extracellular matrix. In this chapter, we discuss the diagnostic criteria, pathophysiology, epidemiology, and treatment of peripheral and autonomic neuropathy in type 1 diabetes.

2. Classification

Table 1 gives a detailed classification of the neuropathies observed in diabetes.

Generalized Neuropathy	Focal Neuropathies	Autonomic Neuropathies
Typical: Distal symmetric polyneuropathy (DSP)	*Compression:*	Cardiovascular autonomic neuropathy
Atypical Neuropathy:	Median -carpal tunnel	Gastrointestinal autonomic neuropathy
Insulin Neuritis/Treatment Neuropathy	Ulnar -cubital tunnel	Genitourinary autonomic neuropathy
Inflammatory Neuropathy	Fibular -fibular head	Hypoglycemia unawareness and associated autonomic failure
Chronic inflammatory demyelinating polyneuropathy	Tibial -tarsal tunnel	Sudomotor autonomic neuropathy
Mononeuritis multiplex	Lateral femoral cutaneous -inguinal ligament	
Diabetic amyotrophy	*Ischemic:*	
	Thoracic radiculopathies	
	Cranial nerve palsy (III, VI, VII)	
Dyck et al. 2011 [1] and Vinik et al 2003 [2]		

Table 1. Classification of Diabetic Neuropathy

3. Diabetic distal symmetric polyneuropathy in type 1 diabetes mellitus

3.1. Overview

Distal Symmetric Polyneuropathy (DSP) is the most common type of neuropathy affecting patients with type 1 diabetes. Polyneuropathy is the greatest risk factor for non-traumatic amputations and confers a higher mortality risk [3, 4]. The incidence of DSP increases with duration of diabetes and with degree of hyperglycemia [5]. In type 1 diabetes, typically the incidence of DSP is linked to other microvascular complications of nephropathy and retinopathy [6]. Unlike type 2 diabetes, polyneuropathy is rarely if ever present in the first five years of diagnosis. Metabolic memory in which improved metabolic control, even for a finite period, confers improved outcomes in the future is a phenomenon which was discovered with the Diabetes Complications and Control Treatment Trial, and may be an important factor to consider in the treatment of type 1 diabetic patients [7].

3.2. Diagnostic criteria

The case definition of typical DSP or diabetic sensorimotor polyneuropathy from the American Academy of Neurology, American Association of Neuromuscular and Electrodiagnostic

Medicine, and the American Association of Physical Medicine and Rehabilitation is, "a combination of neuropathic symptoms, multiple signs, and abnormal electrodiagnostic studies" [8]. However, this does not distinguish typical DSP from atypical diabetic neuropathies [1]. A more precise definition for typical DSP proposed by neuromuscular experts at the 2011 Neurodiab Meeting suggested a tiered approach of possible, probable, confirmed and subclinical DSP. Possible DSP includes symptoms or signs of DSP such as decreased distal sensation or depressed ankle reflexes. Probable clinical DSP includes a combination of symptoms and signs of DSP. Confirmed DSP includes symptoms, signs, and abnormal nerve conduction study consistent with DSP (i.e. symmetric). Subclinical DSP would include patients with abnormal nerve conduction studies but no signs or symptoms of neuropathy [1]. Debate is ongoing as to whether abnormal skin biopsy with decreased epidermal nerve fiber density should be considered with nerve conduction study as a confirmatory test.

3.3. Epidemiology

The prevalence of DSP in type 1 diabetes mellitus has been postulated to be over 50% by 25 years of diagnosis [9, 10]. These data depend on measures used for quantification. Nerve conduction studies are typically more sensitive than monofilament tests and often show decreased conduction velocity in sensory and motor nerves prior to the development of signs or symptoms of sensory loss with monofilament and vibration testing [11]. More tests used, and more sensitive measures will increase prevalence statistics.

Risk factors for DSP incidence and severity in addition to duration of diabetes and age are hyperglycemia, systolic blood pressure, smoking, cholesterol, and height. The Diabetes Control and Complications Trial confirmed hyperglycemia as a significant risk factor for DSP in type 1 diabetes[1]. Interestingly, hyperglycemia alone has not been proven in prospective cohort studies of type 2 diabetes to delay progression in this population [12] which raises the question of whether hyperglycemia is the sole cause of DSP in type 2 diabetes.

Typical progression of DSP in type 1 is very slow, with incremental sensory loss over years and decades. The Diabetes Control and Complications Trial/Epidemiology of Diabetes Interventions and Complications study data show minimal changes in conduction velocity and amplitudes over 5 year periods, which can reassure patients [13, 14]. Progression typically affects both large, myelinated fibers conveying tactile sensitivity, vibration and joint position sense, and small, unmyelinated fibers conveying temperature and pain sensation. Motor involvement is typically subclinical until later in the disease course. While slowed conduction velocities, particularly in the fibular nerve, are common early signs of DSP, weakness typically occurs later, first affecting the toes and then more proximal muscles.

Inflammatory neuropathies such as mononeuritis multiplex and diabetic amyotrophy affecting the plexus are less common in type 1 diabetes than type 2 [15]. Chronic inflammatory demyelinating polyneuropathy is also more common in type 2, but has not been shown to

1 *The DCCT was a groundbreaking study of patients with type 1 diabetes in the United States; a large, multicenter study designed to test whether improved glycemic control delayed the onset or progression of diabetic complications. The follow up epidemiologic study, EDIC (Epidemiology of Diabetes Interventions and Complications) continued to follow the same patients enrolled in DCCT, which is still ongoing.

affect diabetic patients at an increased rate than the general population [16]. Acute painful neuropathy associated with weight loss and abrupt improvement in glycemic control occurs in both type 1 and type 2 patients. This type of neuropathy, formerly known as "insulin neuritis" typically has significant resolution within a year of onset [17].

Sensory symptoms include numbness, or alteration of sensation often described by patients as "wearing multiple socks" or "walking on wood". Neuropathic pain when present can vary between sharp shooting pains, stabbing, or dull and aching. Muscle cramps in feet and legs are common complaints. Hand symptoms can occur when DSP progresses to include the hands in a length dependent process, but more commonly occur because of coexisting compression neuropathies in the hands [18, 19].

Coexisting polyneuropathy from other causes also occurs in type 1 diabetes patients and can account for as many as 10% of DSP cases [9]. The most common include alcoholic neuropathy, B12 deficiency and monoclonal gammopathies. Atypical presentations such as severe distal or proximal weakness, spasticity, faster progression over weeks to months should be signals that a coexistent polyneuropathy may be present and needs evaluation.

3.4. Pathophysiology

The polyol pathway was put forth as a possible cause of diabetic neuropathy over 30 years ago when aldose reductase inhibitors were first studied [20]. Since then, the pathophysiology of DSP in type 1 diabetes is still not completely known but several major pathways have been the focus of most studies. 1) increased flux through the polyol pathway; 2) advanced glycation end-products affecting proteins and lipids [21, 22]; 3) increased oxidative stress with impaired mitochondrial function [23, 24], 4) protein kinase C inhibition [25, 26] and 5) loss of nerve growth factors [27, 28]. Additional mechanisms that have been raised include inflammation, loss of nitric oxide, and hypoxia from microvascular damage [29]. Additional metabolic factors such as hypertriglyceridemia may be more pertinent to type 2 diabetes, although this also occurs in type 1 patients [30, 31]. Loss of ATP and AMP production through mitochondrial dysfunction may be a "final common pathway" for these mechanisms to cause neuronal injury [32].

The role of Schwann cells in DSP is still not completely understood. Schwann cells, not neurons produce aldose reductase [33] and are also the source of nerve growth factors such as nerve growth factor (NGF) and brain-derived neurotrophic factor [34, 35]. Schwann cells in culture tend to be more resistant to hyperglycemia than neurons. However, the most recent evidence suggests unmyelinated fibers to be more sensitive to hyperglycemia than myelinated fibers [36]. These may have important implications for biomarkers in treatment studies.

3.5. Assessment

The assessment of DSP in type 1 diabetes significantly affects the sensitivity and specificity cited. The simplest assessments used are loss of ankle deep tendon reflexes and detection of pressure from a 10g monofilament. Monofilament sensitivity alone ranges from 20% to 64% [37, 38] and likely improves if multiple sites on the foot are tested (8 sites recommended). Nerve

http://dx.doi.org/10.5772/55372

conduction studies measuring sensory and motor nerve action potential amplitude, latency, and conduction velocity are typically used for most studies [14]. The most common nerves assessed are sural sensory and fibular motor nerves. These were shown by Dyck et al to be involved earliest [39]. The earliest finding is conduction velocity slowing in the fibular and sural nerves.

Additional measures used include quantitative sensory testing, which can be performed with multiple devices to measure vibration and thermal thresholds [40, 41]. This can be more sensitive than nerve conduction studies but is subjective and not well suited for diagnostic purposes [42]. Quantitative sensory testing is highly reproducible and has been used in several clinical neuropathy studies [43, 44]. Sural nerve biopsy is rarely performed for diagnosis due to its invasiveness (and cannot be repeated) and is usually used to evaluate for other forms of neuropathy such as chronic inflammatory demyelinating polyneuropathy, vasculitis, or inherited neuropathies. Skin biopsy with measurement of intraepidermal nerve fiber density has become more common, especially when combined with chemical axotomy with capsaicin to measure nerve regeneration [36]. Newer noninvasive methods used include confocal microscopy of corneal C fibers [45] or of Meissner corpuscles (mechanoreceptors) in the finger [46, 47].

3.6. Management

Management of DSP is largely supportive. The main therapeutic aim is to achieve normoglycemia or HgA1c less than 7 [13]. This can be accomplished with frequent self-monitoring and using insulin pumps for continuous subcutaneous insulin infusion or multiple daily injections. Both the EURODIAB and the Diabetes Control and Complications Trial confirmed therapeutic efficacy in delaying progression of DSP with lower glycemic levels [5, 13]. For treatment of insulin neuritis, management is largely supportive and usually requires relaxing hyperglycemia control somewhat. Inflammatory neuropathies may respond to pulsed IV steroids and intravenous immunoglobulins but class A evidence is still lacking [48, 49]. Diabetic chronic inflammatory demyelinating polyneuropathy is managed similarly to idiopathic chronic inflammatory demyelinating polyneuropathy [50].

Foot care is critical once DSP occurs. Patients should be instructed to inspect their feet every night for new ulcerations, blisters or cuts. Wearing shoes at all times will also decrease the chance of potential injury. Feeling bathwater with hands or more proximal leg is also helpful to avoid burns from insensate feet. As neuropathy occurs, the foot structure will change due to muscle atrophy and due to fractures from insensate feet (Charcot foot). Orthotic inserts may be helpful in preventing further ulceration and stabilizing the feet [51].

Falls are an important complication in DSP and need to be screened for at clinic visits. Evaluation by a physical therapist can be helpful in identifying whether a cane, four-point canes, walkers, wheelchairs should be singular. Home evaluations to improve lighting, minimize obstructions and irregular floors like loose rugs are also important. Adding grab bars in bath areas and minimizing steps can be helpful changes to homes.

3.7. Treatment of neuropathic pain

A significant number of patients with DSP (16-60%) have symptoms of neuropathic pain [52, 53]. One UK study suggested that painful symptoms were more prevalent in type 2 than type 1 diabetes [53]. Typical pain symptoms are delayed compared to signs of neuropathy in type 1 diabetes [54, 55]. The etiology of neuropathic pain in DSP has been thought to be due to abnormalities in C-fiber nerve endings causing aberrant signaling through protein kinase C [26], increased transient receptor potential vanilloid 1 expression [56], dysregulation of ion channels [57], abnormal nerve growth factor levels [58] and possibly dysregulation of descending pain pathways [59].

Typical pain symptoms described include "burning", "stabbing", "needle-like", "shooting", "electric" etc. Patients often complain of allodynia, e.g. normal sensations become painful such as the touch of bedcovers to the feet, as well as hyperalgesia (painful sensations such as pinprick are unbearably painful). Pain is typically worse at night, and with activities such as walking and standing. Mononeuropathies such as carpal tunnel syndrome can also cause nocturnal paresthesias. Pain symptoms are typically not completely relieved with medications. Pain can be moderate to severe with an average of 5.8/10 on a pain scale [60].

Medications used for neuropathic pain include traditional pain medications such as opioids and tramadol, antiepileptic agents and antidepressants (Table 2) [61]. Typically patients require large doses of opiates for pain relief, and long acting opiates are preferred to provide sustained relief. Sedation, constipation, pharmacologic tolerance and addiction issues are significant barriers and usually prohibit opiates as first line pain treatment in neuropathic pain. Mexiletine, a sodium channel blocker and anti-arrhythmic agent has also been shown to have some analgesic effects [62].

Alpha2-delta inhibitors gabapentin and pregabalin are the most commonly used anti-epileptic medications. These medications act at the dorsal horn of the spinal cord to inhibit voltage gated calcium channels [63, 64]. The advantage of gabapentin and pregabalin is their renal excretion and lack of interaction with other medications. Main side effects include drowsiness, dizziness, peripheral edema, weight gain, and myoclonic jerks at higher doses. Gabapentin is typically initiated at 300 mg up to three times a day and can be escalated up to 4800 mg in divided doses. Its short half-life requires three to four times a day dosing for optimal pain relief. Pregabalin has a longer half-life and is typically dosed twice a day although some patients benefit from dosing three times a day. Pregabalin is usually started at 75 mg twice a day and titrated up to 300 mg twice a day. Consultation with a nephrologist in dialysis dependent patients is needed due to renal excretion, but does not preclude use in these patients. Typically nephrologists will administer one dose after dialysis. Other anticonvulsants used for neuropathic pain include carbamazepine, oxcarbazepine, valproic acid, lamotrigine, lacosamide, and phenytoin.

Antidepressants acting on norepinephrine such as tricyclic antidepressants and the selective serotonin and norepinephrine reuptake inhibitor duloxetine are also helpful in treating neuropathic pain [65, 66]. Duloxetine is well tolerated, with few side effects. Caution should be used in patients with renal insufficiency as elevations of systolic blood pressure have been observed. Nausea can occur initially, but can be avoided with initiation at lower doses such as 20 -30 mg and slow titration up to 60 mg. Effectiveness of 120 mg was not statistically different from 60 mg in clinical studies, although some patients report improved benefit at higher doses [65]. Tricyclic antidepressants also have a benefit in patients reporting difficulty initiating sleep due to pain due to their sedating effects. Dosages of 25-100 mg amitriptyline 2 hours before bedtime are typically used. At higher doses and in elderly patients, an ECG should be obtained because of possible effects of tricyclics on QT prolongation and heart block. Side effects include drowsiness, urinary hesitancy, constipation, orthostatic hypotension and erectile dysfunction.

Topical creams are not typically efficacious for painful DSP. Capsaicin cream/patch has shown efficacy [67], but is typically not well tolerated due to the significant initial pain with application. Gloves need to be worn and avoidance of the eyes is necessary. Occasionally 1% lidocaine patches can be helpful in patients with focal mononeuropathies such as meralgia paresthetica (compression of the lateral femoral cutaneous nerve). Topical compounded creams containing gabapentin, amitriptyline, and ketamine have been used but there are no published reports on efficacy in placebo controlled studies.

Anti-Epileptic Medications	Anti-Depressants	Other
Gabapentin	Tricyclic antidepressants (amitriptyline, nortriptyline, imipramine)	Opiates
Pregabalin*	Duloxetine*	Tramadol
Carbamazepine		Mexiletine
Lamotrigine		Capsaicin Cream/Patch
		Alpha lipoic acid

*FDA approved indication for diabetic neuropathic pain.

Table 2. Pharmacologic Treatments of Neuropathic Pain

4. Focal neuropathies

4.1. Overview and epidemiology

Other types of neuropathy which can occur include mononeuropathies, typically at compression points such as median mononeuropathy at the wrist, e.g. carpal tunnel syndrome, ulnar neuropathy at the elbow, and peroneal neuropathy at the knee. In the Rochester Diabetes Trial, these occurred at about the same frequency or higher in type 1 vs. type 2 patients [9]. Cranial neuropathies and truncal radiculopathy occur at an increased rate in diabetic patients, but prevalence data for type 1 and type 2 patients is not available. Pain is a common presenting symptom in ischemic ocular motor palsies and thoracic radiculopathies in diabetes [68, 69]. The Veterans Affairs study of type II patients showed decreased prevalence of cranial mononeuropathies with stricter glucose control but data is lacking for type 1 patients [70]. It is not uncommon for mononeuropathies to occur prior to the development of DSP or identification of diabetes, particularly in type 2 patients [71, 72]. This has not been described in type 1 patients.

Median mononeuropathy at the wrist, e.g. carpal tunnel syndrome is the most common mononeuropathy in diabetes and occurs three to four times as commonly in diabetics compared to healthy controls, and is more common in diabetics with DSP than without [72-74]. Median mononeuropathy has been reported as early as 11 years old [75]. Risk factors for development of carpal tunnel syndrome include obesity and lipid-lowering medications [74].

4.2. Pathophysiology

The pathophysiology of mononeuropathies in diabetes is not well understood. They are generally divided into compression-site mononeuropathies, occurring at typical compression points such as the transverse ligament in the wrist (median), cubital tunnel (ulnar nerve), across the knee (fibular nerve), the inguinal ligament (lateral femoral cutaneous nerve/meralgia paresthetica) and tarsal tunnel (tibial nerve). Cranial nerve mononeuropathies and thoracic radiculopathies, diabetic amyotrophies are thought to have an ischemic etiology, either due to microvascular disease (such as cranial nerve involvement) or inflammation (diabetic amyotrophy). Some patients (described in type 2 diabetes) have a rapid development of multiple mononeuropathies which is indistinguishable from a vasculitic mononeuritis multiplex in presentation and can be associated with inflammation on biopsy [76].

The greater prevalence of compression mononeuropathies in diabetes (20-30% of Type 1 and 2 patients) [9, 77] has been observed for decades, but the pathophysiology is not well known. Experimental compression neuropathies trigger Schwann cell proliferation, apoptosis causing local demyelination then remyelination. This occurs prior to the development of axonal degeneration [78]. The median nerve when visualized with ultrasonography is larger in patients with compression compared to healthy controls which may be due to remyelination [79]. It has been presumed that hyperglycemia injured nerves are more vulnerable to compression than normal nerves. Another possibility is lack of symptoms in the diabetic may make compression mononeuropathies worse because of delayed recognition [77]. Other possible etiologies include greater edema within the nerve and diabetic cheiroarthropathy (thickening/ fibrosis of the flexor synovium from excessive connective tissue) [80, 81].

4.3. Assessment

Identification of mononeuropathies may be based on signs and symptoms localizable to a specific nerve in a diabetic patient (e.g. ptosis, diploplia in a Cranial nerve III/oculomotor nerve palsy). This is typically the case for cranial nerve palsies, optic neuropathies, thoracic radiculopathies, or lateral femoral cutaneous nerve palsy where the distribution of deficit is pathognemonic. If the symptoms and signs are specific to one cranial nerve in a previously diagnosed diabetic patient, imaging with magnetic resonance imaging, CT or other modality is typically not needed to confirm the diagnosis. Especially in cranial nerve III palsies, there is controversy whether imaging should occur in a diabetic patient with a classical papillary-sparing presentation [82, 83].

Mononeuropathies may be identified on testing with nerve conduction studies. This is more common in carpal tunnel syndrome, ulnar mononeuropathy, and fibular mononeuropathy which are often asymptomatic. Nerve conduction studies in compression mononeuropathies distally typically demonstrate slowing of conduction velocity across the compressed segment (ulnar, fibular, tibial nerve) or increased distal latency compared to nearby nerves (median nerve). Multiple nerves are often compared, or side to side comparisons are made to exclude underlying DSP.

For carpal tunnel syndrome, nerve ultrasound has become a more common procedure, demonstrating enlarged median nerve cross sectional area in the wrist in affected individuals compared to controls [84]. Thus far, no differentiation between ultrasound appearance of diabetic vs. non-diabetic nerves have been found [85]. Another study suggested a larger cross-sectional area of the tibial nerve at the tarsal tunnel in diabetic patients [86]. Further studies are still needed on the utility of this measure for diabetic patients. Magnetic resonance imaging is also used for assessment of carpal tunnel syndrome, but data in diabetes vs. control patients is lacking and cost is significantly higher than nerve conduction studies or ultrasound [87].

4.4. Treatment

Treatment of compression induced mononeuropathies is aimed at relieving the site of trauma. Bracing, avoiding extenuating activity, and changing postures are initial non-surgical approaches. Data for surgical approach to compressive neuropathy is better known in median mononeuropathies at the wrist (carpal tunnel syndrome) because of larger reported cohort studies. However, data are conflicting in regards to outcome of carpal tunnel syndrome surgical release with some studies showing poorer outcomes and some not significantly different from non-diabetic patients [88, 89]. This may occur due to differences in patient selection. Results of surgical release of the ulnar nerve at the cubital tunnel, the second most common mononeuropathy (2.1%) are worse compared to carpal tunnel syndrome [81, 90]. It is not clear whether this is due to underlying diabetic polyneuropathy or due to patient selection bias (misdiagnosis).

Treatment of ischemic induced mononeuropathies is typically supportive. Pain management is often needed for thoracic radiculopathies, meralgia paresthetica (lateral femoral cutaneous nerve palsy). Prisms or patching can be used for diplopia in ocular motor cranial nerve palsies (cranial nerve 3, 4, and 6). Taping of the eyelid and lubrication may be needed in facial nerve palsies to prevent corneal abrasion. Little data are available for prognosis. Many patients improve over 3-6 months, but some may have permanent muscle weakness or ptosis [91, 92]. Treatment with intravenous alpha-lipoic acid has also been reported as improving outcomes but was not placebo controlled [93]. Otherwise, treatment for mononeuropathies in diabetes is not significantly different than in non-diabetics.

5. Diabetic autonomic neuropathy

5.1. Overview

Autonomic neuropathy is a form of peripheral neuropathy affecting the nerves of the autonomic nervous system. Autonomic neuropathy most commonly affects organs of the cardiovascular, gastrointestinal, urinary, and reproductive systems, although any system of the body may be affected. Its etiology is poorly understood, but as with other forms of peripheral neuropathy long exposure to hyperglycemia, advanced glycation end products, vascular hypoxia [94], and activation of the polyol pathway are thought to play major roles. Typical signs and symptoms depend on the organ affected, but include resting sinus tachycardia without sinus arrhythmia, orthostatic hypotension, delayed gastric emptying, diabetic diarrhea, constipation, erectile dysfunction, bladder dysfunction, hypoglycemia unawareness, distal hyperhidrosis or anhidrosis, facial sweating, and gustatory sweating. Cardiovascular autonomic neuropathy is life threatening and carries a high risk of mortality [2, 95, 96].

5.2. Epidemiology

The prevalence of autonomic neuropathy in type 1 diabetes populations varies widely depending on duration of diabetes and method of assessment, with prevalences ranging from 2.6% in individuals with short duration of diabetes [97] to 90% in pancreatic transplant candidates [98]. Defining autonomic neuropathy based on an abnormal heart rate response to deep breathing and the presence of at least two autonomic neuropathy symptoms, the prevalence ranged from 3.7% to 11.3%, with a decreasing trend with higher BMI, in the Pittsburgh Epidemiology of Diabetes Complications (EDC) when the mean duration of diabetes was approximately 20 years [96]. In a subgroup of this same cohort twenty years later, when mean diabetes duration was 40 years, the prevalence of autonomic neuropathy based on an abnormal response to deep breathing was 61% [99]. In the entire EDC cohort, the incidence of autonomic neuropathy based on an abnormal heart rate response to deep breathing and the presence of at least two autonomic neuropathy symptoms was 0.78 per 100 person years of duration of diabetes, with a lower incidence for a given duration of diabetes in more recently diabetes diagnosed cohorts in the Pittsburgh Epidemiology of Diabetes Complications study [100]. In the Diabetes Control and Complications Trial/ Epidemiology of Diabetes Interventions and Complications study population, which because of inclusion criteria was a healthier cohort at study baseline than the EDC population, the prevalence of autonomic neuropathy at the follow-up years 13/14 of Epidemiology of Diabetes Interventions and Complications study, representing approximately 27 years of duration of type 1 diabetes, was 29% and 35% in the former intensively treated and conventionally treated Diabetes Control and Complications Trial participants [10]. The presence of diabetic autonomic neuropathy is associated with poor prognosis. In the EDC study, mortality during 20 years of follow-up was increased 2.43-fold after controlling for age, sex, BMI, and other late complications [96].

5.3. Pathophysiology

Diabetic autonomic neuropathy is a neuropathic disorder of the peripheral nervous system in individuals with diabetes or prediabetes. The pathogenesis of diabetic autonomic neuropathy is poorly understood, but long exposure to hyperglycemia [94, 101], advanced glycation end products [2, 94, 101], vascular insufficiency [2, 94], and activation of the polyol pathway [2, 94, 101] have been long thought to play major roles. The nerves of the autonomic nervous system innervate every organ of the body and as such any organ system can be affected by diabetic autonomic neuropathy. Disorders resulting from damage to autonomic nerve fibers are typically classified into the following syndromes: cardiovascular autonomic neuropathy (CAN), gastrointestinal, genitourinary, hypoglycemia unawareness, and sudomotor.

5.3.1. Pathogenesis

Long exposure to hyperglycemia is one of the strongest hypotheses on the etiology of diabetic peripheral neuropathy. In individuals with type 1 diabetes, results from the Diabetes Control and Complications Trial showed significantly lower declines in the R-R interval over time in those in the intensive therapy arm of the trial [97]. Whether this was due to lower levels of hyperglycemia was not specified. There was a low incidence of CAN in both treatment arms (4% in the intensive group and 9% in the conventional group), with a 45% lower incidence in the treatment arm [10]. Follow-up of the entire cohort thirteen to fourteen years after the close-out of the trial revealed a marked increase in the prevalence of CAN in the entire cohort, which was significantly greater in the former conventional therapy group. Differences in HbA1c accounted for the majority of the group differences in the incidence of CAN [102]. The beneficial effect of former intensive therapy on the incidence of neuropathy appeared to be greater for CAN than for distal symmetrical polyneuropathy, suggesting that the detrimental effect of hyperglycemia may be greater on small nerve fibers than large nerve fibers [10]. Mechanisms by which hyperglycemia may cause nerve damage include activation of the polyol pathway and accumulation of advanced glycation end products [2, 94, 101].

5.3.2. Cardiovascular Autonomic Neuropathy (CAN)

Cardiovascular autonomic neuropathy results from damage to the nerves that innervate the heart and coronary blood vessels. Because of its clinical importance, it has been the most studied of all of the diabetic autonomic neuropathy syndromes. It is the most life threatening of all of the diabetic autonomic neuropathy syndromes and carries a high risk of mortality. Signs/symptoms of CAN include orthostatic hypotension, sinus tachycardia, exercise intolerance, silent myocardial infarction, and sudden death.

Autonomic nervous system innervation of the heart largely regulates heart rate variability. In diabetes, cardiac autonomic nervous system dysfunction generally progresses from the apex to the base of the heart [103]. Diabetic autonomic neuropathy appears to affect the long nerve fibers first [2]. In CAN, autonomic dysfunction is usually observed first as a decrease in parasympathetic activity, reflecting damage to the vagal nerve, the longest of the autonomic nerve fibers, and a compensatory increase in sympathetic autonomic nervous system activity

[103]. Sympathetic activity increases heart rate while parasympathetic activity decreases heart rate. The decline in parasympathetic activity is reflected in the decline in variation in heart rate with inspiration and expiration, where there is less of a decline in heart rate with expiration. A decline in heart rate variability is one of the earliest manifestations of CAN [103]. This compensatory increase in heart rate with parasympathetic denervation also manifests in an increased resting heart rate, and rates may reach greater than 100 beats per minute [103], resting sinus tachycardia.

Autonomic innervation of the heart also regulates blood pressure. The apparent early vagal denervation in CAN results in increased sympathetic nervous system activity, partially due to the counter-regulatory activity of the parasympathetic neurons, increasing blood pressure. During sleep, this is reflected in the "non-dipping" pattern of blood pressure often observed in individuals with type 1 diabetes [104, 105]. This lack of nocturnal bradycardia is associated with prolongation of the heart rate corrected Q-T interval in adolescents with type 1 diabetes [106], although Stella et al [105] observed no cross-sectional association between "non-dipping" and CAN in adults with type 1 diabetes. Later cardiac sympathetic denervation results in loss in the normal heart rate and blood pressure responses to exercise. The normal increase in heart rate and blood pressure and subsequent increased cardiac output is impaired, reducing exercise tolerance [2, 103]. Sympathetic cardiac denervation also manifests as orthostatic hypotension, a prolonged drop in blood pressure upon standing due to reduced baroreceptor stimulated sympathetic increase in heart rate and vasoconstriction of splanchnic vascular beds. Orthostatic hypotension may often be asymptomatic, but can result in dizziness, syncope, falls and fractures.

CAN is associated with silent myocardial ischemia and infarction [2, 107], and carries a high risk of mortality [95, 96]. The association of diabetic CAN with silent myocardial infarction is likely due to the higher frequency of silent myocardial ischemia in individuals with diabetic CAN [2]. Damage to the myocardial sensory afferent fibers may reduce the sensation of ischemic pain [2]. A meta-analysis of twelve studies of individuals with diabetes showed a 2-fold higher risk of silent ischemia in those with CAN [2]. In a population of middle-age and elderly individuals with type 1 diabetes, poorer cardiac autonomic function predicted future coronary heart disease events [108]. Perhaps due to its association with silent myocardial ischemia, cardiovascular disease, resting tachycardia, and exercise intolerance, CAN greatly increases the risk of sudden death [109-111]. We have shown in individuals with long-standing type 1 diabetes that CAN as diagnosed based on heart rate variability and in the presence of at least one other symptom of autonomic neuropathy was a significant predictor of mortality, independently of distal symmetrical polyneuropathy and other late complications of diabetes [96].

5.3.3. Gastrointestinal autonomic neuropathy

Diabetic autonomic neuropathy affecting the gastrointestinal system may result in gastroparesis, esophageal dysfunction, diarrhea, fecal incontinence, or constipation. Gastroparesis, or delayed gastric emptying, is common in type 1 diabetes, with prevalence rates from approximately 30 to 50% [4, 112-114] and appears to be more prevalent in type 1 than in type 2 diabetes

[115]. Symptoms of gastroparesis include nausea, vomiting, anorexia, bloating, early satiety, and wide swings in blood sugar [112]. hyperglycemia delays gastric emptying [116] while hypoglycemia accelerates it [117]. Esophageal dysfunction is thought to result from a combination of impairment of vagal nerve and enteric nervous system innervation of esophageal smooth muscle cells regulating peristalsis [117]. Symptoms of esophageal dysfunction include difficulty swallowing (dysphagia) and heartburn. Peristalsis dysmotility of the lower gastrointestinal track can result in diarrhea or constipation, both very commonly observed in type 1 diabetes. The diarrhea may be due to bacteria overgrowth resulting from bowel stasis, very rapid peristalsis, or both. Very slow peristalsis activity may result in constipation. Fecal incontinence results from poor anal sphincter tone and impaired rectal sensation [2].

5.3.4. Genitourinary autonomic neuropathy

Autonomic nerve dysfunction or damage affecting the genitourinary system may manifest as erectile and/or ejaculation dysfunction or failure in males, dyspareunia in females, and bladder dysfunction, in both genders. Autonomic neuropathy affecting the reproductive organs manifests as erectile and ejaculation failure in males and reduced sexual arousal, reduced vaginal lubrication and painful intercourse in females. Autonomic neuropathy affecting the urinary tract may result in decreased frequency of urination and increased urinary tract infections, increased post void residual volume, dribbling, and urinary incontinence [118, 119].

Erectile dysfunction in diabetes may be due to one or any combination of the following: neuropathy, atherosclerosis, changes in corporal erectile tissue including deposition of AGEs, anti-hyperglycemic medications, and psychological factors, although neuropathy appears to be the predominate cause [119]. The corpus cavernosum is innervated by both sympathetic and parasympathetic nerve fibers and sensory and somatic nerve fibers [120, 121]. The neurogenic basis of erectile dysfunction is a decrease in smooth muscle relaxation of the corpus cavernosum [119, 122], inadequate nitric oxide synthase activity [119, 122], impaired sensation of the glans penis [119, 120], and abnormal motor function of erectile tissue [119].

Little is known about the pathogenesis of sexual dysfunction in women. It is characterized by reduced sexual arousal, atrophic vaginitis and subsequent painful intercourse. It is poorly related to glycemic control, age, duration of diabetes, or diabetes complications [123], but appears to be related to depression and to improve with estrogen creams [118]. In a substudy of the Diabetes Control and Complications Trial/ Epidemiology of Diabetes Interventions and Complications cohort examining female sexual dysfunction in 424 women with type 1 diabetes and a mean age of 42.8 years, the prevalence of female sexual dysfunction was 35% [124].

Bladder dysfunction is one of the most common complications of diabetes, affecting a large proportion of the type 1 diabetic population [117] and occurring early in the disease process. The diabetic neurogenic bladder is caused by degeneration of both afferent myelinated and efferent non-myelinated nerve fibers to the bladder. Afferent nerve fiber degeneration results in reduced sensation of a full bladder [125]. Efferent nerve fiber degeneration results in reduced frequency of micturition, incomplete emptying of the bladder, i.e. increased post-void residual volume, and eventually urinary incontinence [125]. The neurogenic bladder is associated with recurrent urinary tract infections [125] and may lead to renal failure/disease.

5.3.5. Hypoglycemia unawareness and associated autonomic failure

Autonomic neuropathy is associated with more severe hypoglycemic events [126, 127] and the loss of symptoms prompting awareness of hypoglycemia [128, 129]. However, the jury is still out on whether autonomic neuropathy actually causes a loss of counter-regulatory responses to hypoglycemia [130]. Hypoglycemia associated autonomic failure (HAAF) can occur in the absence of autonomic neuropathy [126, 131, 132]. Conversely, diabetic autonomic neuropathy is observed in the absence of hypoglycemia symptom loss [131, 133]. Additionally, reversal of hypoglycemia symptom awareness is observed after strict avoidance of hypoglycemia for a relative short period of times, i.e. several weeks to months [134-136]. This would all appear to suggest that autonomic neuropathy is not a causative factor in hypoglycemia unawareness, i.e. the loss of the counter-regulatory responses to hypoglycemia. However, in the presence of autonomic neuropathy and in combination with HAAF a greater reduction in counterregulatory response hypoglycemia is observed than in hypoglycemia unawareness without autonomic neuropathy [130]. Furthermore, the recovery of hypoglycemia awareness symptoms with strict avoidance of hypoglycemia is not as complete in those with autonomic neuropathy [128]. Even with the recovery of awareness symptoms, the epinephrine response to hypoglycemia is only partially recovered and even less so in those with autonomic neuropathy [130]. In aggregate, this suggests that autonomic neuropathy is not the predominate cause of hypoglycemia unawareness but does enhance its severity and may play a partial etiologic role.

5.3.6. Sudomotor autonomic neuropathy

Abnormalities in thermoregulation are common in type 1 diabetes [137, 138]. The sweat glands are innervated by sudomotor postganglionic unmyelinated sympathetic c-fibers. Autonomic neuropathy affecting sudomotor nerve function results in both anhidrosis and hyperhidrosis. Sudomotor dysfunction manifests symptomatically as dry scaly skin of the limbs and appendages, heat intolerance, and gustatory sweating. With increasing duration of diabetes, anhidrosis becomes more severe, progressing in a distal to proximal direction [118]. Gustatory sweating, in which there is excessive sweating in the face and trunk in response to eating is thought to result from imperfect reinnervation of postganglionic sudomotor C-fibers following denervation [118].

5.4. Assessment

Assessment of cardiovascular autonomic nervous system function can be done by measuring heart rate variability, the heart rate response in postural change from lying or sitting to standing, the blood pressure change from lying or sitting to standing, and the diastolic blood pressure response to a sustained hand grip. Heart rate variability can be assessed my measuring the heart rate response to paced deep breathing, the Valsava maneuver, and spectral analysis. The heart rate response to deep breathing and the heart rate response to a change in posture to the standing position predominately reflect parasympathetic function [2]. The heart rate response to the Valsalva maneuver reflects both parasympathetic and sympathetic function fairly equally [2]. The change in blood pressure from a lying or sitting position to a standing position and the blood pressure response to a sustained hand grip reflects sympathetic nervous system function [2].

Assessment of autonomic neuropathy affecting the gastrointestinal track can be done by endoscopy and scintographic measurement of esophageal bolus transit time for esophageal dysfunction; scintography, isotope breath tests, and ultrasonography for gastroparesis; hydrogen breath test for diabetic diarrhea; barium enema for constipation; and anorectal manometry, endoanal ultrasonography, colon transit tests, digital examination of the rectum, protoscopy and sigmoidoscopy for fecal incontinence [2, 139].

Erectile dysfunction can be assessed by taking a case history, such as with the International Index of Erectile Dysfunction, by physical examination including examining of external genitalia, blood tests including measurement of testosterone levels, measurement of nocturnal penile tumescence, and Doppler studies [2, 117, 140]. The Female Sexual Function Index has been used to evaluate sexual dysfunction in women with type 1 diabetes [124]. Vaginal plethysmography has also been used to directly assess vaginal lubrication in women with diabetes [141].

Post void residual volume can be assessed by transurethral catherization or non-invasively via ultrasound [142]. Bladder sensation and upper urinary tract dilation can be assessed with cystometry and voiding cystometrogram. Uroflometry can be used to assess urinary flow rate and sphincter function. A urine culture should also be done to assess bacteria cystitis. In women, a urogynecological examination should be done in order to exclude pelvic prolapse.

Assessment of sudomotor function can be done with the Quantitative Sudomotor Axon Reflex Test (QSART), thermoregulatory sweat test, or the sympathetic skin response. The thermoregulatory sweat test can be used to assess the pattern and distribution of anhydrosis [143]. The QSART is used to assess postganglionic sudomotor nerve function [119, 143]. The sympathetic skin response assesses postganglionic sudomotor sympathetic nerve fibers [144].

5.5. Management

Treatment and management of diabetic autonomic neuropathy includes tight glycemic control [4]; however, the primary focus is on alleviation of symptoms [4, 101]. Management of orthostatic hypotension consists of educating the patient in strategies to avoid or address reversible causes of hypotension, increased fluid and salt consumption supplemented with mineralocorticoid therapy, pharmacotherapy with sympathomimetic agents, and wearing clothing such as compression stockings that increase venous return [2, 101, 118]. Antioxidants and cardioselective beta-blockers may be beneficial in cardiac autonomic neuropathy [2].

For patients with esophageal dysmotility, proton pump therapy is conventionally used [119]. Fluid consumption immediately after consumption of medications should be advised in order to avoid pill-induced esophagitis in these patients [119]. Diets low in fat and soluble fiber may be beneficial in patients with gastroparesis [2, 119], although pharmacotherapy with prokinetic agents is the mainstay of therapy [119]. Insulin pump therapy may also help to improve symptoms in type 1 diabetic patients with gastroparesis [119]. Antibiotic therapy is beneficial in the treatment of diarrhea [2, 119].

Treatment of bladder dysfunction may be behavioral, pharmacological, or surgical. Behavioral management includes pelvic floor exercises to strengthen the muscles of the pelvic floor that support the bladder and urethretha. It also includes a program of scheduled fluid intake and micturition, manual procedures such as the Crede's maneuver, pelvic tapping, the Valsava maneuver, and clean intermittent self-catheterization. Pharmacotherapy includes the use of antimuscarinic agents, cholinergic agents, and tricyclic antidepressants. In cases refractory to non-pharmacological and pharmacological treatment, surgical procedures such as vesicle neck resection, selective pudendal nerve block, unilateral pudendal neurectomy, and sacral neuromodulation may be beneficial [2, 119, 142, 145].

Treatment and management of erectile dysfunction should include psychological counseling; however, pharmacotherapy with the PDE5 inhibitors (sildenafil, vardenafil, tadalafil) is the mainstay of therapy. Intracavernous or intraurethral injections with vasoactive medication, vacuum constriction devices, and penile prosthesis implantation are also options [2, 119]. Vaginal estrogen creams in has been shown to be beneficial in diabetic women with female sexual dysfunction [118].

6. Conclusion

Peripheral and autonomic neuropathy is a common complication of type 1 diabetes with significant morbidity and mortality. Fortunately, aggressive hyperglycemia control can delay the onset and minimize the severity of neuropathy in this population. The pathophysiology of neuropathy is complex and likely involves multiple mechanisms, which may be the reason for lack of efficacious treatments beyond glucose control. Early recognition of peripheral and autonomic neuropathy is also important to decrease amputation risk and mortality.

Author details

Baqiyyah Conway[1*] and Amanda Peltier[2]

*Address all correspondence to: baqiyyah@yahoo.com

1 Department of Epidemiology, School of Public Health, West Virginia University, Morgantown, West Virginia, USA

2 Division of Neurology, Department of Medicine, Vanderbilt University, Nashville, TN, USA

References

[1] Dyck PJ, Albers JW, Anderson H, Arezzo JC, Biessels GJ, Bril V, et al. Diabetic Polyneuropathies: Update on Research Definition, Diagnostic Criteria and Estimation of Severity. Diabetes Metab Res Rev. 2011. Epub Jun 21, 2011.

[2] Vinik AI, Maser RE, Mitchell BD, Freeman R. Diabetic Autonomic Neuropathy. Diabetes Care. 2003;26:1553-79.

[3] Coppini DV, Bowtell PA, Weng C, Young PJ, Sonksen PH. Showing neuropathy is related to increased mortality in diabetic patients-a survival analysis using an accelerated failure time model. J Clin Epidemiol. 2000;53(5):519-23.

[4] Boulton AJ, Vinik AI, Arezzo JC, Bril V, Feldman EL, Freeman R, et al. Diabetic Neuropathies: a statement by the American Diabetes Association. Diabetes Care. 2005;28(4):956-62.

[5] Tesfaye S, Stevens LK, Stephenson JM, Fuller JH, Plater M, Ionescu-Tirgoviste C, et al. Prevalence of diabetic peripheral neuropathy and its relation to glycaemic control and potential risk factors: the EURODIAB IDDM Complications Study. Diabetologia. 1996;39(11):1377-84.

[6] Fagerberg SE. Studies on the pathogenesis of diabetic neuropathy. III. Diabetic neuropathy in relation to diabetic vessel complications. Acta Med Scand. 1957;157(5): 401-6.

[7] Albers JW, Herman WH, Pop-Busui R, Martin CL, Cleary P, Waberski B. Subclinical neuropathy among Diabetes Control and Complications Trial participants without diagnosable neuropathy at trial completion: possible predictors of incident neuropathy. Diabetes Care. 2007;30(10):2613-8.

[8] England JD, Gronseth GS, Franklin G, Miller RG, Asbury AK, Carter GT, et al. Distal symmetric polyneuropathy: a definition for clinical research: report of the American Academy if Neurology, the Amerian Association of Electrodiagnostic Medicine, and the American Academy of Physical Medicine and Rehabilitation. Neurology. 2005;65(2):199-207.

[9] Dyck PJ, Kratz KM, Karnes JL, Litchy WJ, Klein R, Pach JM, et al. The prevalence by staged severity of various types of diabetic neuropathy, retinopathu, and nephropathy in a population-based cohort: the Rochester Diabetic Neuropathy Study. Neurology. 1993;43(4):817-24.

[10] Pop-Busui R, Herman WH, Feldman EL, Low PA, Martin CL, Cleary PA, et al. DCCT and EDIC Studies in Type 1 Diabetes: Lessons for Diabetic Neuropthy Regarding Metabolic Memory and Natural History. Curr Diab Rep. 2010;10:276-82.

[11] Dyck PJ, O'Brien PC, Litchy WJ, Harper CM, Klein CJ, Dyck PJB. Monotonocity of nerve tests in diabetes: subclinical nerve dysfunction precedes diagnosis of polyneuropathy. Diabetes Care. 2005;28(9):2192-200.

[12] Intensive blood-glucose control with sulphonylureas or insulin compared with conventional treatment and risk of complications in patients with type 2 diabetes (UKPDS 33). Lancet. 1998;352:837-53.

[13] The effect of intensive treatment of diabetes on the development and progression of long-term complications in insulin-dependent diabetes mellitus. The Diabetes Control and Complications Trial Research Group. N Engl J Med. 1993;329(14):977-86.

[14] Albers JW, Herman WH, Pop-Busui R, Feldman EL, Martin CL, Cleary PA, et al. Effect of prior intensive treatment during the Diabetes Control and Complications Trial (DCCT) on peripheral neuropathy in Type 1 diabetes during the Epidemiology of Diabetes Interventions and Complications (EDIC) Study. Diabetes Care. 2010;33(5): 1090-6.

[15] Dyck PJ, Windebank AJ. Diabetic and nondiabetic lubosacral radiculoplexus neuropathies: new insights into pathophysiology and treatment. Muscle Nerve. 2002;25(4): 477-91.

[16] Laughlin RS, Dyck PJ, Melton LJ 3rd, Leibson C, Ransom J, Dyck PJB. Incidence and prevalence of CIDP and the association of diabetes mellitus. Neurology. 2009;73(1): 39-45.

[17] Vinik A. Approach to the Management of the Patient with Neuropathic Pain. J Clin Endocrinol Metab. 2010;95(11):4802-11.

[18] Stamboulis E, Voumvourakis K, Andrilopoulou A, Koutsis G, Tentolouris N, Kodoounis A, et al. Association between asymptomatic median mononeuropathy and diabetic polyneuropathy severity in patients with diabetes mellitus. J Neurol Sci. 2009;278(1-2):41-3.

[19] Singh R, Gamble G, Cundy T. Lifetime risk of symptomatic carpal tunnel syndrome in Type 1 diabetes. Diabet Med. 2005;22(5):625-30.

[20] Gabbay KH, Spack N, Loo S, Hirsch HJ, Ackil AA. Aldose reductase inhibition: studies with alrestatin. Metabolism. 1979;28(4 S1):471-6.

[21] Sugimoto K, Nishizawa Y, Horiuchi S, Yagihashi S. Localization in human diabetic peripheral nerve of NE-carboxymethyllysine-protein adducts, an advanced glycation endproduct. Diabetologia. 1997;40:1380-7.

[22] Jack M, Wright D. Role of advanced glycation endproducts and glyoxidase I in diabetic peripheral sensory neuropathy. Transl Res. 2012;159(5):355-65.

[23] Cameron NE, Cotter MA, Maxfield EK. Anti-oxidant treatment prevents the development of peripheral nerve dysfunction in streptozotocin-diabetic rats. Diabetologia. 1993;36(4):299-304.

[24] Lupachyk S, Shevalye H, Maksimchyk Y, Drel VR, Obrosova IG. PARP inhibition alleviates diabetes-induced systemic oxidative steress and neural tissue 4-hydoxynonenal adduct accumulation: correlation with peripheral nerve function. Free Radic Biol Med. 2011;50(10):1400-9.

[25] Cameron NE, Cotter MA, Jack AM, Basso MD, Hohman TC. Protein kinase C effects on nerve function, perfusion, NA(+), K(+)-ATPase activity and glutathione content in diabetic rats. Diabetologia. 1999;42(9):1120-30.

[26] Ahlgren SC, Levine JD. Protein kinase C inhibitors decrease hyperalgesia and C-fiber hyperexcitability in the streptozotocin-diabetic rat. J Neurophysiol. 1994;72(2):684-92.

[27] Apfel SC, Arezzo JC, Brownlee M, Federoff H, Kessler JA. Nerve growth factor administration protects against experimental diabetic sensory neuropathy. Brain Res. 1994;634(1):7-12.

[28] Feradji V, Sotelo J. Low serum levels of nerve growth factor in diabetic neuropathy. Acta Neurol Scand. 1990;81(5):402-6.

[29] Obrosova I. Diabetes and the peripheral nerve. Biochemica et Biophysica Acta. 2009;1792:931-40.

[30] Callaghan BC, Hur J, Feldman EL. Diabetic neuropathy: one disease or two? Curr Opin Neurol. 2012;25(5):536-41.

[31] Wiggin TD, Sullivan KA, Pop-Busui R, Amato A, Sima AA, Feldman EL. Elevated triglycerides correlate with progression of diabetic neuropathy. Diabetes. 2009;7(1634-1640).

[32] Vincent AM, Edwards JL, McLEan LL, Hong Y, Cerri F, Lopez I, et al. Mitochondrial biogenesis and fission in axons in cell culture and animal models of diabetic neuropathy. Acta Neuropathol. 2010;120(4):477-89.

[33] Ludvigson MA, Sorenson RL. Immunohistochemical localization of aldose reductase. I. Enzyme purification and antibody preparation--localization in peripheral nerve, artery, and testis. Diabetes. 1980;29(6):438-49.

[34] Bradley JL, Thomas PK, King RH, Muddle JR, Ward JD, Tesfaye S, et al. Myelinated nerve fibre regeneration in diabetic sensory polyneuropathy: correlation with type of diabetes. Acta Neuropathol. 1995;90(4):403-10.

[35] Tosaki T, Kamiya H, Yasuda Y, Naruse K, Kato K, Kozakae M, et al. Reduced NGF secretion by Schwann cells under the high glucose condition decreases neurite outgrowth of DRG neurons. Exp Neurol. 2008;213(3):381-7.

[36] Polydefkis M, Hauer P, Sheth S, Sirdofsky M, Griffin JW, McArthur JC. The time course of epidermal nerve fibre regeneration: studies in normal controls and in people with diabetes, with and without neuropathy. Brain. 2004;127(Pt 7):1606-15.

[37] Miranda-Palma B, Sosenko JM, Bowker JH, Mizel MS, Boulton AJM. A comparison of the monofilament with other testing modalities for foot ulcer susceptibility. Diabetes Res Clin Pract. 2005;70(1):8-12.

[38] Wang Y, Goodrich JM, Werner R, Gillespie B, Basu N, Franzblau A. Agreement between clinical screening procedures for neuropathy in the feet. Muscle Nerve. 2012;45(5):653-8.

[39] Dyck PJ, Davies JL, Litchy WJ, O'Brien PC. Longitudinal assessment of diabetic polyneuropathy using a composite score in the Rochester Diabetic Neuropathy Study cohort. Nuerology. 1997;49(1):229-39.

[40] Shy ME, Frohman EM, Arezzo JC, Cornblath DR, Giuliani MJ, Kincaid JC, et al. Quantitatve sensory testing. Report of the Therapeutics and Technology Assessment Subcommittee of the American Academy of Neurology. Neurology. 2003;60:898-904.

[41] Arendt-Nielsen L, Yarnitsky D. Experimental and clinical applications of quantitative sensory testing applied to skin, muscles and viscera. J Pain. 2009;10(6):556-72.

[42] Freeman R, Chase KP, Risk MR. Quantitative sensory testing cannot differentiate simulated sensory loss from sensory neuropathy. Neurology. 2003;60(3):465-70.

[43] Ziegler D, Low PA, Litchy WJ, Boulton AJ, Vinik AI, Freeman R, et al. Efficacy and safety of antioxidant treatment with a-lipoic acid over 4 years in diabetic polyneuropathy: the NATHAN 1 trial. Diabetes Care. 2011;34(9):2054-60.

[44] Bird SJ, Brown MJ, Spino C, Watling S, Foyt HL. Value of repeated measures of nerve conduction and quantitative sensory testing in a diabetic neuropathy trial. Muscle Nerve. 2006;34(2):214-24.

[45] Ahmed A, Bril V, Orszag A, Paulson J, Yeung E, Ngo M, et al. Detection of Diabetic Sensorimotor Polyneuropathy by Conreal Confocal Microscopy in Type 1 Diabetes. Diabetes Care. 2012;35(4):821-8.

[46] Herrmann DN, Boger JN, Jansen C, Alessi-Fox C. In vivo confocal microscopy of Meissner corpuscles as a measure of sensory neuropathy. Neurology. 2007;69(23):2121-7.

[47] Almodovar JL, Ferguson M, McDermott MP, Lewis RA, Shy ME, Herrmann DN. In vivo confocal microscopy of Meissner corpuscles as a novel sensory measure in CMT1A. J Peripher Nerv Syst. 2011 09/01;16(3):169-74. eng.

[48] Tracy JA, Englestad JK, Dyck PJB. Microvasculitits in diabetic lumbosacral radiculoplexus neuropathy. J Clin Neuromusc Dis. 2009;11(1):44-8.

[49] Zochodne DW, Isaac D, Jones C. Failure of immunotherapy to prevent, arrest or reverse diabetic lubosacral plexopathy. Acta Neurol Scand. 2003;107(4):299-301.

[50] Peltier AC, Donofrio PD. Chronic inflammatory demyelinating polyradiculoneuropathy: from bench to bedside. Semin Neurol. 2012;32(3):187-95.

[51] Waaijman R, Arts MLJ, Haspels R, Busch-Westbroek TE, Nollet F, Bus SA. Pressure-reduction and preservation in custom-made footware of patients with diabetes and a history of plantar ulceration. Diabet Med. 2012.

[52] Daousi C, MacFarlane IA, Woodward A, Nurmikko TJ, Bundred PE, Benbow SJ. Chronic painful peripheral neuropathy in an urban community: a controlled comparisonof people with and without diabetes. Diabet Med. 2004;21(9):976-82.

[53] Abbott CA, Malik RA, van Ross ER, Kulkarni J, Boulton AJ. Prevalence and characteristics of painful diabetic neuropathy in a large community-based diabetic population in the UK. Diabetes Care. 2011;34(10):2220-4.

[54] Sosenko JM, Boulton AJ, Kubrusly DB, JK W, Skyler JS. The vibratory perception threshold in young diabetic patients: associations with glycemia and puberty. Diabetes Care. 1985;8:605-7.

[55] Arnold R, Kwai N, Lin CS, Poynten AM, Kiernan MC, Krishnan AV. Axonal dysfunction prior to neuropathy onset in type 1 diabetes. Diabetes Metab Res Rev. 2012. Epub Sept 25, 2012.

[56] Pabbidi RM, Shuang-Quan Y, Peng S, Khardori R, Pauza ME, Premkumar LS. Influence of TRPV1 on diabetes-induced alterations in thermal pain sensitivity. Mol Pain. 2008 March 1, 2008. Epub March 1, 2008.

[57] Hong S, Wiley JW. Early painful diabetic neuropathy is associated with differential changes in the expression and function of vanilloid receptor 1. J Biol Chem. 2005;280(1):618-27.

[58] Cheng HT, Dauch JR, Hayes JM, Hong Y, Feldman EL. Nerve growth factor mediates mechanical allodynia in a mouse model of Type 2 diabetes. J Neuropathol Exp Neruol. 2009;68(11):1229-43.

[59] von Hehn CA, Baron R, Woolf CJ. Deconstructing the neuropathic pain phenotype to reveal neural mechanisms. Neuron.73(4):638-52.

[60] Galer BS, Gianas A, Jensen MP. Painful diabetic polyneuropathy: epidemiology, pain description, and quality of life. Diabetes Res Clin Pract. 2000;47(2):123-8.

[61] Watson CP, Moulin D, Watt-Watson J, Gordon A, Eisenhoffer J. Controlled-release oxycodone relieves neuropathic pain: a randomized controlled trial in painful diabetic neuropathy. Pain. 2003;105:71-8.

[62] Jarvis B, Coukell AJ. Mexiletine. A review of its therapeutic use in painful diabetiv neuropathy. Drugs. 1998;56:691-707.

[63] Backonja M, Beydoun A, Edwards KR, Schwartz SL, Fonseca V, Hes M, et al. Gabapentin for the symptomatic treatment of painful neuropathy in patients with diabetes mellitus: a randomized controlled trial. JAMA. 1998;280(21):1831-6.

[64] Arezzo JC, Rosenstock J, LaMoreaux L, Pauer L. Efficacy and safety of pregabalin 600 mg/d for treating painful diabetic peripheral neuropathy: A double-blind placebo-controlled trial. BMC Neurol. 2008;8. Epub Sept. 16, 2008.

[65] Goldstein DJ, Lu Y, Detke MJ, Lee TC, Iyengar S. Duloxetine vs. placebo in patients with painful diabetic neuropathy. Pain. 2005;116(1-2):109-18.

[66] Max MB, Lynch SA, Muir J, Shoaf SE, Smoller B, Dubner R. Effects of desimipramine, amitriptyline, and fluoxetine on pain in diabetic neuropathy. N Engl J Med. 1992;326:1250-6.

[67] Forst T, Pohlmann T, Kunt T, Goitom K, Schulz G, Lobig M, et al. The influence of local capsaicin treatment on small nerve fibre function and neurovascular control in symptomatic diabetic neuropathy. Acta Diabetol. 2002;39(1):196.

[68] Wilker SC, Rucker JC, Newman NJ, Biousse V, Tomsak RL. Pain in ischaemic ocular motor cranial nerve palsies. Br J Ophthalmol. 2009;93:1657-9.

[69] Kikta DG, Breuer AC, Wilbourn AJ. Thoracic root pain in diabetes: The spectrum of clinical and electromyographic findings. Ann Neurol. 2004;11(1):80-5.

[70] Azad N, Emanuele NV, Abraira C, Henderson WG, GColwell J, Levin SR, et al. The effects of intensive glycemic control on neuropathy in the VA cooperative study on type II diabetes mellitus. J Diabetes Complications. 1999;13(5-6):307-13.

[71] Parisi TJ, Mandrekar J, Dyck JB, Klein CJ. Meralgia paresthetica: Relation to obesity, advanced age, and diabetes mellitus. Neurology. 2011;77:1538-42.

[72] Karpitskaya Y, Novak C, Mackinnon S. Prevalence of Smoking, Obesity, Diabetes Mellitus, and Thyroid Disease in Patients with Carpel Tunnel Syndrome. Ann Plast Surg. 2002;48(3):269-73.

[73] Perkins BA, Olaleye D, Bril V. Carpal Tunnel Syndrome in Patients with Diabetic Polyneuropathy. Diabetes Care. 2002;25:565-9.

[74] Makepeace A, Davis WA, Bruce DG, Davis TME. Incidence and determinants of carpal tunnel decompression surgery in Type 2 diabetes. The Fremantle Diabetes Study. Diabetes Care. 2008;31:498-500.

[75] Duru NS, Acar H, Ayta S, Elevli M. Bilateral carpal tunnel syndrome in a child with type 1 diabetes mellitus. Neurol India. 2010;58(1):136-7.

[76] Kelkar P, Parry GJ. Mononeuritis multiplex in diabetes mellitus: evidence for underlying immune pathogenesis. J Neurol Neurosurg Psychiatry 2003;74:803-6.

[77] Albers JW, Brown MB, Sima AA, Greene DA. Frequency of median mononeuropathy in patients with mild diabetic neuropathy in the early diabetes intervention trial (ED-

IT). Tolrestat Study For EDIT (Early Diabetes Intervention Trial). Muscle Nerve. 1996;19(2):140-6.

[78] Gupta R, Rowshan K, Chao T, Mozaffar T, Steward O. Chronic nerve compression induces local demyelination and remyelination in a rat model of carpal tunnel syndrome. Exp Neurol. 2004;187(2):500-8.

[79] Mhoon JT, Juel VC, Hobson-Webb LD. Median nerve ultrasound as a screening tool in carpal tunnel syndrome: Correlation of cross-sectional area measures with electrodiabgnostic abnormality. Muscle Nerve. Epub Oct. 5, 2012.

[80] Chaudhuri KR, Davidson AR, Morris IM. Limited joint mobility and carpal tunnel syndrome in insulin-dependent diabetes. Rheumatology. 1989;28(3):191-4.

[81] Vinik A, Mehrabyan A, Colen L, Boulton A. Focal Entrapment Neuropathies in Diabetes. Diabetes Care. 2004;27(7):1783-8.

[82] Kupersmith MJ, Heller G, Cox TA. Magnetic resonance angiography and clinical evaluation of third nerve palsies and posterior communicating artery aneurysms. J Neurosurg. 2006;105(2):228-34.

[83] Yanovitch T, Buckley E. Diagnosis and management of third nerve palsy. Curr Opin Opthalmol. 2007;18(5):373-8.

[84] Cartwright MS, Hobson-Webb LD, Boon AJ, Alter KE, Hunt CH, Flores VH, et al. Evidence-based guideline: Neuromuscular ultrasound for the diagnosis of carpal tunnel syndrome. Muscle Nerve. 2012;46(2):287-93.

[85] Hobson-Webb LD, Massey JM, Juel VC. Nerve ultrasound in diabetic polyneuropathy: Correlation with clinical characteristics and electrodiagnostic testing.Muscle Nerve. Epub Aug. 13, 2012.

[86] Riazi S, Bril V, Perkins BA, Abbas S, Chan VWS, Ngo M, et al. Can ultrasound of the tibial nerve detect diabetic peripheral neuropathy. Diabetes Care. Epub Oct. 1, 2012.

[87] Kerasnoudis A. Ultrasound and MRI in Carpal Tunnel Sydrome: The Dilemma of Simplifying the Approach to a Complex Disease or Making Complex Assessments of a Simple Problem. J Hand Surg 37(10):2200-1.

[88] Thomsen NOB, Rosen I, Dahlin LB. Neurophysiologic recovery after carpal tunnel release in diabetic patients. Clinical Neurophysiology. 2010;121(9):1569-73.

[89] Mondelli M, Padua L, Reale F, Signorini AM, Romano C. Outcome of surgical release among diabetics with carpal tunnel syndrome. Arch Phys Med Rehabil. 2004;85(1): 7-13.

[90] Wake DJ, Wright RJ, Love SC, Campbell IW. Ulnar mononeuropathy in diabetes mellitus. British J of Diabetes and Vascular Disease. 2005;5:171-2.

[91] Kanazawa A, Haginomori S, Takamaki A, Nonaka R, Araki M, Takenaka H. Prognosis for Bell's palsy: a comparison of diabetic and nondiabetic patients. Acta Otolaryngol. 2007;127:888-91.

[92] Berlit P. Isolated and combined pareses of cranial nerves II, IV, and VI. a retrospective study of 412 patients. J Neruol Sci. 1991;103:10-5.

[93] Tankova T, Cherninkova S, Koev D. Treatment for diabetic mononeuropathy with a-lipoic acid. Int J Clin Pract. 2005;59(6):645-50.

[94] Podwall D, Gooch C. Diabetic neuropathy: clinical features, etiology, and therapy. Curr Neurol Neurosci Rep. 2004;4(1):55-61.

[95] Maser RE, Mitchel BD, Vinik AI, Freeman R. The association between cardiovascular autonomic neuropathy and mortality in individuals with diabetes: a meta-analysis. Diabetes Care. 2003;26:1895-901.

[96] Conway B, Miller RG, Costacou T, Fried L, Kelsey S, Evans RW, et al. Adipostiy and mortality in type 1 diabetes. Int J Obes. 2009;33(7):796-805.

[97] The Diabetes Control and Complications Trial Research Group. The effect of intensive diabetes therapy on measures of autonomic nervous system function in the Diabetes Control and Complications Trial (DCCT). Diabetologia. 1998;41:416-23.

[98] Kennedy WR, Navarro X, Sutherland DER. Neuropathy profile of diabetic patients in a pancreatic transplantation program. Neurology. 1995;45:773-80.

[99] Conway B, Aroda V, Maynard JD, Matter N, Fernandez S, Ratner RE, et al. Skin Intrinsic Fluorescence Correlates with Autonomic and Distal Symmetrical Polyneuropathy in Individuals with Type 1 Diabetes. Diabetes. 2011;34(4):1000-5.

[100] Pambianco G, Costacou T, Ellis D, Becker DJ, Klein R, Orchard TJ. The 30-Year Natural History of Type 1 Diabetes Complications: The Pittsburgh Epidemiology of Complications Study Experience. Diabetes. 2006;55:1463-9.

[101] Dejgaard A. Pathophysiology and Treatment of Diabetic Neuropathy. Diabetic Medicine. 1998;15:97-112.

[102] Pop-Busui R, Low PA, Waberski BH, Martin CL, Albers JW, Feldman EL, et al. Effects of prior intensive therapy on cardiac autonomic nervous system function in type 1 diabetes mellitus: the Diabetes Control and Complications Trial/Epidemiology of Diabetes Intreventins and Complications study (DCCT/EDIC). Circulation. 2009;119(22):2886-93.

[103] Pop-Busui R. Cardiac Autonomic Neuropathy in Diabetes: A clinical perspective. Diabetes Care. 2010;33:434-41.

[104] Spallone V, Gambardella S, Maiello MR, Barini A, Frontoni S, Menzinger G. Relationship between autonomic neuropathy, 24-h blood pressure profile, and nephropathy in normotensive IDDM patients. Diabetes Care. 1994;17(6):578-84.

[105] Stella P, Tabak AG, Zgibor JC, Orchard TJ. Late diabetes complications and non-dipping phenomenon in patients with Type 1 diabetes. Diabetes Res Clin Pract. 2006;71(1):14-20.

[106] Karavanaki K, Kazianis G, Kakleas K, Konstantopoulos I, Karayianni C. QT interval prolongation in associateion with impaired circadian variation of blood pressure and heart rate in adolescents with Type 1 diabetes. Diabet Med. 2007;24(11):1247-53.

[107] Niakan E, Harati Y, Rolak LA, Comstock JP, Rokey R. Silent myocardial infarction and diabetic cardiovascular autonomic neuropathy. Arch Intern Med. 1986;146(11): 2229-30.

[108] May O, Arildsen H, Damsgaard EM, Mickley H. Cardiovascular autonomic neuropathy in insulin-dependent diabetes mellitus: prevalence and estimated risk of coronary heart disease in the general population. J Int Med. 2000;248:483-91.

[109] Suarez GA, Clark VM, Norell JE, Kottke TE, Callahan MJ, O'Brien PC, et al. Sudden cardiac death in diabetes mellitus: risk factors in the Rochester diabetic neuropathy study. J Neurol Neurosurg Psychiatry. 2005;76(2):240-5.

[110] Ewing DJ, Boland O, Neilson JM, Cho CG, Clark BF. Autonomic neuropathy, QT lengthening, and unexpected deaths in male diabetic patients. Diabetologia. 1991;34(3):182-5.

[111] Vinik AI, Ziegler D. Diabetic cardiovascular autonomic neuropathy. Circulation. 2007;115(3):387-97.

[112] Sfarti C, Trifan A, Hutanasu C, Cojocariu C, Singeap A, Stanciu C. Prevalence of Gastroparesis in Type 1 Diabetes Mellitus and its Relationship to Dsypeptic Symptoms. J Gastrointestin Liver Dis. 2010;19(3):279-84.

[113] De Block CEM, De Leeuw IH, Pelckmans PA, Callens D, Maday E, Van Gaal LF. Delayed Gastric Emptying and Gastric Autoimmunity in Type 1 Diabetes. Diabetes Care. 2002;25(5):912-7.

[114] Jebbink HJ, Bravenboer B, Akkermans LM, vanBerge-Henegouwen GP, Smout AJ. Relationships between dyspeptic symptoms and gastrointestinal motility in patients with type 1 (insulin-dependent) diabetes mellitus. Diabetologia. 1993;36(10):948-54.

[115] Matsumoto M, Yoshimura R, Akiho H, Higuchi N, Kobayashi K, Matsui N, et al. Gastric emptying in diabetic patients by the (13)C-octanoic acid breath test: role of insulin in gastric motility. J Gastroenterol. 2007;42(6):469-74.

[116] Schvarcz E, Palmer M, Aman J, Horowitz M, Stridsberg M, Berne C. Physiological hyperglycemia slows gastric emptying in normal subjects and patients with insulin-dependent diabetes mellitus. Gastroenterology. 1997;113(1):60-6.

[117] Tesfaye S, Boulton AJ, Dyck PJ, Freeman R, Horowitz M, Kempler P, et al. Diabetic neuropathies: update on definitions, diagnostic criteria, estimation of severity, and treatments. Diabetes Care. 2010;33(10):2285-93.

[118] Freeman R. Autonomic peripheral neuropathy. Lancet. 2005;365:1259-70.

[119] Kempler P, Amarenco G, Freeman R, Frontoni S, Horowitz M, Stevens M, et al. Management strategies for gastrointestinal, erectile, bladder, and sudomotor dysfuntion in patients with diabetes. Diabetes Metab Res Rev. 2011;27:665-77.

[120] Bleustein CB, Arezzo JC, Eckholdt H, Melman A. The neuropathy of erectile dysfunction. Int J Impot Res. 2002;14(6):433-9.

[121] Hamdan FB, Al-Matubsi HY. Assessment of erectile dysfuntion in diabetic patients. Int J Androl. 2008;32(2):176-85.

[122] de Tejada IS, Goldstein I, Azadzoi K, Krane RJ, Cohen RA. Impaired Neurogenic and Endothelium-mediated Relaxation of Penile Smooth Muscle from Diabetic Men with Impotence. N Engl J Med. 1989;320(16):1025-30.

[123] Enzlin P, Mathieu C, Van Den Bruel A, Vanderschueren D, Demyttenaere K. Prevalence and Predictors of Sexual Dysfunction in Patients with Type 1 Diabetes. Diabetes Care. 2003;26:409-14.

[124] Enzlin P, Rosen R, Wiegel M, Brown J, Wessells H, Gatcomb P, et al. Sexual Dysfuntion in Women with Type 1 Diabetes: Long-term findings from the DCCT/EDIC study cohort. Diabetes Care. 2009;32:780-5.

[125] Ziegler D, Stief C. Genitourinary Complications. In: Veves A, Malik RA, editors. Diabetic Neuropathy. 2nd ed. Totowa, New Jersey: Humana Press; 2007. p. 453-72.

[126] Freeman R. Hypoglycemia and the Autonomic Nervous System. In: Veves A, Malik RA, editors. Diabetic Neuropathy: Clinical Management. Contemporary Diabetes. 2nd ed. Totowa, New Jersey: Humana Press; 2007. p. 379-88.

[127] Stephenson JM, Kempler P, Perin PC, Fuller JH. Is autonomic neuropathy a risk factor for severe hypoglycaemia? The EURODIAB IDDM Complications Study. Diabetologia. 1996;39(11):1372-6.

[128] Fanelli C, Pampanelli S, Lalli C, Del Sindaco P, Ciofetta M, Lepore M, et al. Long-term intensive therapy of IDDM patients with clinically overt autonomic neuropathy: effets on hypoglycemia awareness and counterregulation. Diabetes. 1997;46(7): 1172-81.

[129] Bottini P, Boschetti E, Pampanelli S, Ciofetta M, Del Sindaco P, Scionti L, et al. Contribution of autonomic neuropathy to reduced plasma adrenaline responses to hypoglycemia in IDDM: evidence for a non-selective defect. Diabetes. 1997;46(5):814-23.

[130] Bolli GB, Fanelli CG, Porcellati F, Pampanelli S. Diabetic Autonomic Neuropathy: Response to Hypoglycemia. In: Gries FA, Cameron NE, Low PA, Ziegler D, editors.

http://dx.doi.org/10.5772/55372

Textbook of Diabetic Neuropathy. Stuttgart, Germany: Georg Thieme Verlag; 2003. p. 286-94.

[131] Ryder RE, Owens DR, Hayes TM, Ghatei MA, Bloom SR. Unawareness of hypoglycaemia and inadequate hypoglycaemic counterregulation: no causal relation with diabetic autonomic neuropathy. BMJ. 1990;301(6755):783-7.

[132] Dagogo-Jack SE, Craft S, Cryer PE. Hypoglycemia-induced autonomic failure in insulin-dependent diabetes mellitus. Recent antecedent hypoglycemia reduces autonomic responses to, symptoms of, and defense against subsequent hypoglycemia. J Clin Invest. 1993;91(3):819-28.

[133] Hepburn DA, Patrick AW, Eadington DW, Ewing DJ, Frier BM. Unawareness of hypoglycaemi in insulin-treated diabetic patients: prevalence and relationship to autonomic neuropathy. Diabet Med. 1990;7(8):711-7.

[134] Fanelli C, Pampanelli S, Epifano L, Rambotti AM, Di Vincenzo A, Modarelli F, et al. Long-term recovery from unawareness, deficient counterregulation and lack of cognitive dysfuntion during hypoglycaemia, following institution of rational, intensive thereapy in IDDM. Diabetologia. 1994;37:1265-76.

[135] Cranston I, Lomas J, Maran A, Macdonald I, Amiel SA. Restoration of hypoglycaemia awareness in patients with long-duration of insulin-dependent diabetes. Lancet. 1994;344(8918):283-7.

[136] Dagogo-Jack S, Rattarasarn C, Cryer PE. Reversal of hypoglycemia unawareness, but not defective glucose counterregulation, in IDDM. Diabetes. 1994;43:1426-34.

[137] Hoeldtke RD, Bryner KD, Horvath GG, Phares RW, Broy LF, Hobbs GR. Redistribution of sudomotor responses is an early sign of sympathetic dysfunction in type 1 diabetes. Diabetes. 2001;50(2):436-43.

[138] Maggs DC, Macdonald IA, Tattersall RB. Thermoregulatory responses to hyperinsulinaemic hypoglycaemia and euglycaemia in IDDM. Diabetologia. 1994;37(7):689-96.

[139] O'Donovan D, Samson M, Feinle C, Jones KL, Horowitz M. Diabetic Autonomic Neuropathy: Gastrointesitnal Tract. In: Gries FA, Cameron NE, Low PA, Ziegler D, editors. Textbook of Diabetic Neuropathy. New York, New York: Thieme; 2003. p. 246-62.

[140] Stief CG, Ziegler D. Diabetic Autonomic Neuropathy: Urogenital System. In: Gries FA, Cameron NE, Low PA, Ziegler D, editors. Textbook of Diabetic Neuropathy. Stuttgart, Germany: Georg Thieme Verlag; 2003. p. 262-78.

[141] Wincze JP, Albert A, Bansal S. Sexual arousal in diabetic females: physiological and self-report measures. Arch Sex Behav. 1993;22(6):587-601.

[142] Dorsher PT, McIntosh PM. Neurogenic Bladder. Adv in Urol. 2012. Epub February 8, 2012.

[143] Low PA. Postural Hypotension and Anhydrosis. In: Veves A, Malik RA, editors. Diabetic Neuropathy: Clinical Management. 2nd ed. Totowa, New Jersey: Humana Press, Inc.; 2007. p. 413-32.

[144] Kucera P, Goldenberg Z, Kurca E. Sympathetic skin response: review of the method and its clinical use. Bratisl Lek Listy. 204;105(3):108-16.

[145] Golbidi S, Laher I. Bladder dysfunction in diabetes mellitus. Frontiers in Pharmacology. 2010 November 16, 2010;1.

Chapter 14

Diabetic Autonomic Neuropathy and Circadian Misalignment in Type 1 Diabetes

Elena Matteucci and Ottavio Giampietro

Additional information is available at the end of the chapter

http://dx.doi.org/10.5772/52033

1. Introduction

Misalignment of circadian rhythms has been evidenced in patients with type 1 diabetes and there is a close relationship between alterations in neuroendocrine sleep architecture, circadian clock oscillations, glucose metabolism, autonomic function, and diurnal profiles of blood pressure and heart rate [1-5]. In turn, circadian misalignment may modify the peak incidence of cardiovascular events in diabetic people [6-9]. Diabetic autonomic neuropathy, particularly cardiac autonomic neuropathy, is considered an important potential factor involved in the disruption of circadian cardiovascular rhythms [10]. This serious chronic complication is rarely diagnosed because it remains for a long times asymptomatic; contrariwise, it seems to have a significant prognostic value [10-12]. The review summarises the battery of non-invasive autonomic function tests available for diabetic autonomic neuropathy diagnosis as well as cross-sectional and follow-up studies supporting their importance in risk stratification for diabetic micro-vascular complications and cardiovascular morbidity/mortality.

2. A bit of history and a bit of anatomy

In 1973, the British Medical Journal and the Lancet published three articles on diabetic autonomic neuropathy [13-15], which would then be followed over the years by an unbroken series of studies and publications. Wheeler and Watkins identified vagal denervation of the heart as a feature of diabetic autonomic neuropathy that could be evaluated by monitoring beat-to-beat variation in heart rate [14]. Ewing et al. found the vascular responses to the Valsalva manoeuvre and sustained handgrip useful in providing an objective assessment of the integrity of the autonomic nervous system in diabetes [15]. Ewing himself later developed the cardiovascular autonomic function test battery still in use to provide an objective diagnosis of autonomic nervous system involvement [16]. The battery included: Valsalva manoeuvre, heart rate response to standing up, heart rate response to deep breathing, blood pressure response to standing up, and blood pressure response to sustained handgrip (Appendix 1).

Brief description of the five non invasive cardiovascular reflex tests used by Ewing et al. [15] to assess autonomic function in diabetic subjects.

Valsalva manoeuvre: the subject sits quietly and then blows in a mouthpiece at a pressure of 40 mmHg for 15 s. The heart rate normally increases during the manoeuvre and decreases after release. The ratio of the longest R-R interval shortly after the manoeuvre to the shortest R-R interval during the manoeuvre is measured.

Heart rate response to standing up: the subject lies quietly and then stands up unaided. The heart rate normally increases with a maximum at about the 15th beat after starting to stand and thereafter decreases with a minimum around the 30th beat. Electrocardiogram tracings are used to determine the 30:15 ratio, calculated as the ratio of the longest R-R interval around the 30th beat to the shortest R-R interval around the 15th beat.

Heart rate response to deep breathing: the subject sits quietly and then breathes deeply at a rate of six breaths per minute. The maximum and the minimum heart rate during each breathing cycle are measured, and the mean of the differences during successive breathing cycles is measured.

Blood pressure response to standing up: the blood pressure is measured using a sphygmomanometer while the subject is lying down and after standing. The difference in systolic blood pressure is a measure of postural blood pressure change.

Blood pressure response to sustained handgrip: handgrip is maintained at 30% of the maximum voluntary contraction up to a maximum of five minutes and the blood pressure is measured each minute. The difference between the diastolic blood pressure just before release of handgrip, and before starting, is measured.

Based on his 10-yr experience, Ewing et al. 1) stressed the fallacy of relying on a single test, particularly heart rate variation during deep breathing, to make diagnosis of autonomic neuropathy, and 2) stated that the previous classification of tests into parasympathetic and sympathetic (Table 1), although clinically useful, should not be considered physiologically precise because of the complexity of the autonomic pathways [16].

Blood flow adjustments are achieved by local vascular control mechanisms (mechanical forces and chemical stimuli) but require to be coordinated by a remote central neural control [17]. Autonomic motor control is effected by long parasympathetic preganglionic fibres and short sympathetic preganglionic fibres that originate within the central nervous system. The former synapse on short postganglionic fibres arising from ganglia located close to the effector targets, the latter synapse on long postganglionic fibres arising from the paravertebral chain ganglia or collateral ganglia. Parasympathetic neurons limit their influence mainly to the control of cardiac function, whereas sympathetic neurons innervate the heart, blood ves-

http://dx.doi.org/10.5772/52033

sels, adrenal glands, and kidneys [17]. The arterial baroreflex modulates beat-to-beat blood pressure oscillations: afferent baroreceptor discharge from the carotid sinus and aortic arch is relayed to the nucleus tractus solitarius in the dorsomedial region of the medulla. As a result, changes in the efferent sympathetic and parasympathetic outflow to the heart and blood vessels adjust cardiac output and vascular resistance to return blood pressure to baseline. Similarly, the cardiopulmonary baroreceptors minimise changes in arterial blood pressure in response to changes in blood volume.

Cardiovascular tests in diagnosing diabetic autonomic neuropathy	
Parasympathetic	**Sympathetic**
Resting heart rate	Resting heart rate
Heart rate response to deep breathing	Blood pressure response to standing up
Heart rate response to standing up	Blood pressure response to sustained handgrip
Valsalva manoeuvre	Blood pressure response to cold
Spectral analysis of heart rate variation (high frequency component)	Spectral analysis of heart rate variation (very low frequency component)

Table 1. Classification of cardiovascular tests for the diagnosis of diabetic neuropathy.

The complexity of the autonomic pathways is exemplified by the following quotations. The act of breathing modulates autonomic neural outflow from the brainstem, but the mechanisms underlying the respiratory sinus arrhythmia are still unclear [18]: only fluctuations in efferent cardiac vagal activity or combined vagal/sympathetic heart rate modulation? Moreover, is respiratory sinus arrhythmia driven by respiratory synchronous oscillations in blood pressure via the arterial baroreflex or both respiratory sinus arrhythmia and blood pressure are independently related to respiration via nonbaroreflex mechanisms?

Small negative changes of central volume reduce cardiac output without significant alterations of arterial blood pressure: 1) short-term cardiovascular control through respiratory sinus arrhythmia and baroreflex feedback are optimised at mild hypervolemia; 2) both the time and frequency domain data support the presence of a Bainbridge reflex (i.e. hypervolemia-induced tachycardia) at moderately elevated levels of central volume, to reduce cardiac preload under volume loading conditions. Finally, mild to moderate levels of hypovolemia do not cause significant reductions in arterial pressure, explained in part by a mild tachycardia and increased feed forward gain from heart rate to arterial pressure [19].

Physical activity produces intensity-dependent increases in arterial blood pressure that are mediated by central signals arising from higher brain centres and by peripheral feedback from skeletal muscle (exercise pressor reflex) with further modulation provided by the arterial baroreflex. The sensory component of the exercise pressor reflex is comprised of myelinated group III and unmyelinated group IV skeletal muscle afferents that respond to both mechanical (mechanoreflex) and metabolic (metaboreflex) stimuli. However, the receptors activating muscle afferent fibres as well as the factors contributing to a decrease in reflex activity in oxidative muscle are still not precisely characterised [20].

3. Current standards of medical care in diabetes

Up to 70% of people with diabetes experience nervous system damage in their lifetime. Diabetic neuropathy compromises quality of life being a major contributing cause of lower limb amputation (http://www.diabetes.org/diabetes-basics/diabetes-statistics/) [11, 21-22].

Diabetic neuropathy is considered to be a multifactorial process whose contributing factors, yet not completely understood, are metabolic, vascular, autoimmune, oxidative and nitrosative stress, and neuro-hormonal growth factor deficiency [20-21].

The classification of diabetic neuropathy that was originally proposed by Thomas [23] has been recently adapted by Vinik [22, 24] (Table 2).

Clinical Presentation and Diagnosis		**Differential Diagnosis**
Focal neuropathies	Mononeuritis	
	Entrapment syndromes	
Diffuse neuropathies	Proximal motor (amyothrophy)	Co-existing chronic inflammatory demyelinating polyneuropathy
		Monoclonal gammopathy of undetermined significance
		Circulating GM1 antibodies and antibodies to neuronal cells
		Inflammatory vasculitis
Generalised symmetric polyneuropathies	Acute sensory	
	Chronic sensorimotor	
	- Large fibre	
	- Small fibre	
	Autonomic	

Table 2. Classification of diabetic neuropathy proposed by Vinik et al. [22].

Diabetic autonomic neuropathy is the least recognised and understood diabetic complication: clinical symptoms generally do not appear until long after the onset of diabetes, but subclinical autonomic dysfunction can occur within one year of diagnosis in type 2 diabetes and within two years of diagnosis in type 1 diabetes [24]. Diabetic autonomic neuropathy can involve the entire autonomic nervous system leading to a wide range of symptoms

[21-22, 24]. Cardiac autonomic neuropathy can manifest as tachycardia (heart rate > 100 bpm), decreased exercise tolerance, orthostatic hypotension (a fall in systolic blood pressure > 20 mmHg upon standing without appropriate heart rate response), cardiac denervation syndrome with silent myocardial infarction, paradoxical supine or nocturnal hypertension, intra- and peri-operative cardiovascular instability, left ventricular diastolic dysfunction.

Peripheral diabetic autonomic neuropathy can manifest as decreased thermoregulation, decreased sweating, altered blood flow, impaired vasomotion, and oedema. From the metabolic point of view, there may be hypoglycaemia unawareness with decreased counter-regulatory catecholamine responses as well as hypoglycaemia unresponsiveness with reduction in glucagon and epinephrine secretion in response to hypoglycaemia. Gastrointestinal diabetic autonomic neuropathy can manifest as oesophageal dysmotility, gastro-paresis diabeticorum, diarrhoea or constipation, faecal incontinence. Genitourinary symptoms include erectile dysfunction, retrograde ejaculation, neurogenic bladder and cystopathy, female sexual dysfunction. Sudomotor diabetic autonomic neuropathy may manifest as anhidrosis, hyperhidrosis, heat intolerance, gustatory sweating, and dry skin. Pupillomotor function impairment and pseudo-Argyll-Robertson pupil have also been described.

The American Diabetes Association [11] recommends that:

1. a comprehensive diabetes evaluation should include a history of diabetes related micro-vascular complications: retinopathy, nephropathy, and neuropathy (sensory, including history of foot lesions; autonomic, including sexual dysfunction and gastro-paresis);

2. a comprehensive diabetes evaluation should include presence/absence of patellar and Achilles reflexes as well as determination of proprioception, vibration, and monofilament sensation;

3. all patients should be screened for distal symmetric polyneuropathy at diagnosis of type 2 diabetes and 5 years after the diagnosis of type 1 diabetes and at least annually thereafter, using simple clinical tests. Electrophysiological testing is rarely needed, except in situations where clinical features are atypical;

4. screening for signs or symptoms of cardiac autonomic neuropathy should be instituted at diagnosis of type 2 diabetes and 5 years after the diagnosis of type 1 diabetes. Special testing is rarely needed;

5. medications for relief of specific symptoms related to distal symmetric polyneuropathy or diabetic autonomic neuropathy are recommended as they improve the quality of life of the patient;

6. foot examination should include testing for loss of protective sensation, i.e. 10-g monofilament plus testing for any one of the following: vibration using 128-Hz tuning fork, pinprick sensation, ankle reflex, vibration sensation threshold.

4. Diagnostic tests of cardiovascular autonomic neuropathy

The presence of cardiac autonomic neuropathy may be indicated by resting tachycardia (heart rate > 100 bpm) that is due to an imbalance of the sympathetic/parasympathetic tone. Because neuropathy is seen first in the longest fibres, early in the natural history of diabetes there is impairment of parasympathetic function, followed later by sympathetic denervation that progresses from the apex of the ventricles towards the base of the heart and increases the propensity to dysrhythmias [10, 25]. Moreover, cardiac autonomic neuropathy reduces exercise tolerance by impairing heart rate, blood pressure, and cardiac output responses to exercise. Indeed, subjects with diabetes and suspected cardiac autonomic neuropathy should perform a cardiac stress test before undertaking an exercise program. The assumption of upright posture results in gravity-mediated displacement of blood into the veins of the pelvis and lower limbs, reducing venous return to the heart. In healthy people, this leads to a reflex increase in sympathetic nervous system activity, increasing peripheral vascular resistance and heart rate such that arterial pressure is maintained [26]. In diabetic people, sympathetic vasomotor denervation may lead to orthostatic hypotension that is aggravated when combined with orthostatic bradycardia [25]. Moreover, a large proportion of diabetic patients receive multi-drug therapy that potentially contributes to the fall in blood pressure on assuming the upright posture [24]. Table 3 provides a list of drugs, which may interfere with autonomic function tests.

In diabetes, analysis of 24-h ambulatory blood pressure monitoring (ABPM) showed altered characteristics of blood pressure rhythm [1]. In particular, diabetic patients had a high prevalence of increased night time blood pressure or non-dipping profile [27-32] that could reflect a) the presence of autonomic neuropathy [32-33] resulting in sympathetic predominance during sleep, but also b) the circadian misalignment due to obstructive sleep apnoea in obese subjects with type 2 diabetes [34]. Chronobiologically interpreted ambulatory blood pressure monitoring uncovered that midline estimate statistic of rhythm (MESOR) and mean of systolic blood pressure and diastolic blood pressure were higher in diabetic patients than in healthy subjects [35-42]. Figures 1-2 show the relationship between heart rate response to deep breathing and the circadian blood pressure rhythm parameters midline estimate statistic of rhythm and acrophase.

Abnormalities in respiration-related heart rate variability can be evaluated in a number of different ways, from the simple bedside tests of short-term heart rate differences previously listed to the spectral analysis of heart rate variability, taking into account that normative values of heart rate variability indices are affected mainly by age [10]:

1. Heart rate response to deep breathing, which measures sinus arrhythmia during quiet respiration and primarily reflects parasympathetic function.

2. Heart rate response to standing up induces reflex tachycardia followed by bradycardia and is both vagal and baroreflex mediated.

3. Valsalva manoeuvre evaluates cardio-vagal function in response to a standardized increase in intrathoracic pressure, primarily parasympathetic mediated.

4. Time domain measures of heart rate variability are summarised in Table 4[43]. In a continuous ECG record, each QRS complex is detected, and the normal-to-normal (NN) in-

tervals (that is, all intervals between adjacent QRS complexes resulting from sinus node depolarisations) or the instantaneous heart rate is determined.

5. Frequency domain measures of heart rate variability evaluate how power (variance) distributes as a function of frequency using power spectral density (PSD) analysis (Table 5) [43]. Vagal activity is thought to contribute mainly to the high frequency (HF, 0.15-0.4 Hz) component, which is related to respiratory activity, while the sympathetic system is thought to modulate the lower-frequency heart rate variability components. The very low frequency (VLF, <0.04 Hz) components are related to fluctuations in vasomotor tone associated with thermoregulation, and the low frequency (LF, 0.04-0.15 Hz) components are considered to be associated with the baroreceptor reflex [10, 44].

6. QT interval prolongation in the ECG has been used to diagnose cardiac autonomic neuropathy with reasonable sensitivity, specificity and positive predictive value [12, 45] although there is no universal agreement on 1) QT measurement and correction techniques, and 2) normality range [46]. Age dependency of cardiovascular autonomic responses is exemplified in Figure 3. Figures 4-6 show the heart rate variability with deep breathing, lying to standing, and Valsalva manoeuvre, respectively, in patients with type 1 diabetes and control subjects.

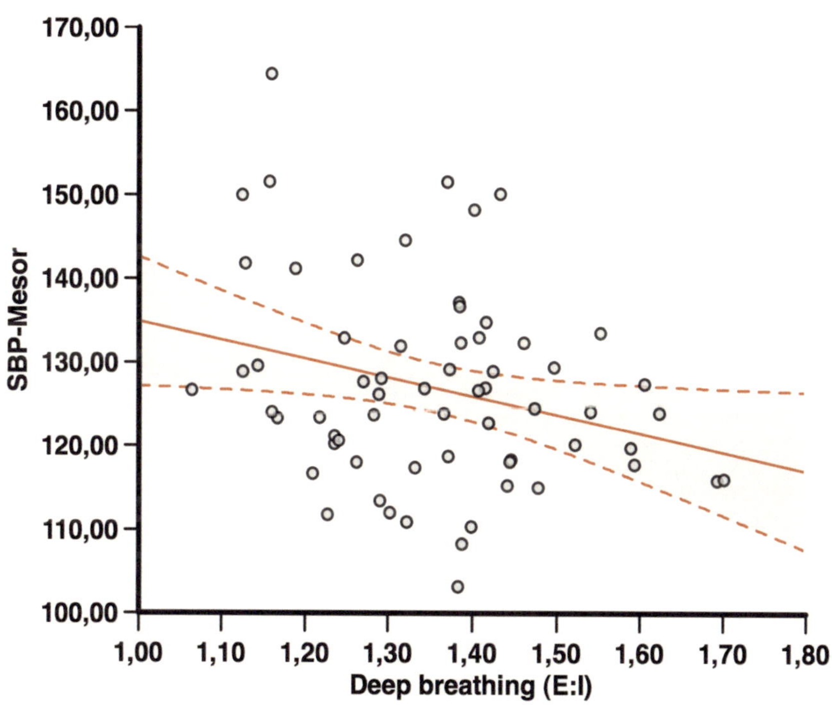

Figure 1. The linear relationship between age and heart rate response to deep breathing expressed as expiratory/inspiratory (E:I) ratio and systolic blood pressure (SBP)midline estimate statistic of rhythm (MESOR) in 20 patients with type 1 diabetes and 25 age-matched control subjects.

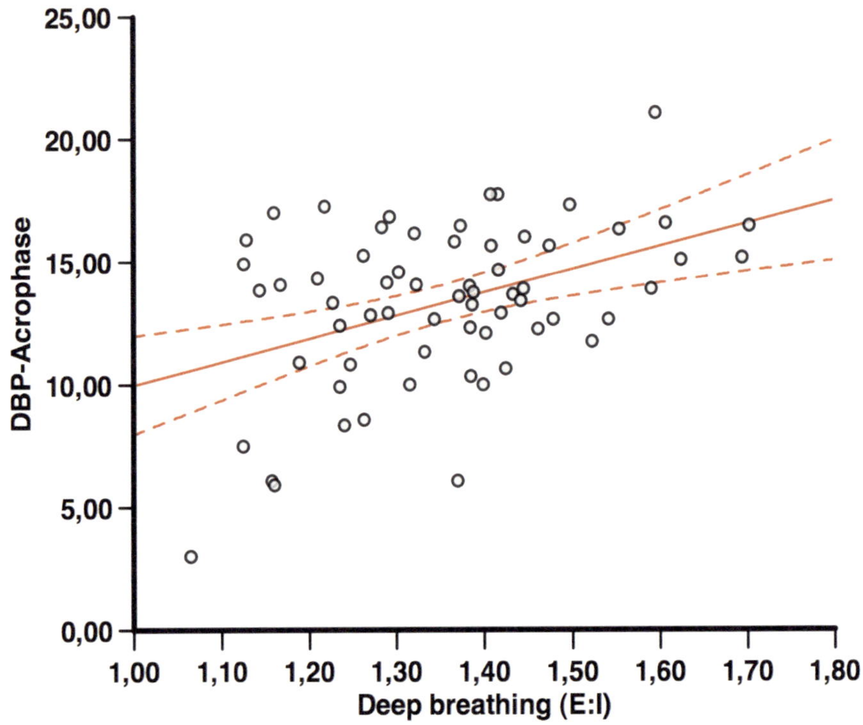

Figure 2. The linear relationship between age and heart rate response to deep breathing expressed as expiratory/ inspiratory (E:I) ratio and diastolic blood pressure (DBP) acrophase in the same subjects as in Figure 1.

Drug class	Medication	Effect on heart rate	Effect on blood pressure
Anti-inflammatory drugs	acetylsalicylic acid	x	
Angiotensin converting enzyme inhibitors	captopril	x	
	enalaprin	x	
	lisinopril	x	
	quinalapril	x	
	trandolapril	x	
Angiotensin II type 1 receptor blockers	eprosartan	x	
	losartan	x	
α-adrenoceptor antagonists	doxazosin		x
β-blockers	atenolol	x	
	bisoprolol	x	
	metoprolol	x	
	nebivolol	x	

http://dx.doi.org/10.5772/52033

Drug class	Medication	Effect on heart rate	Effect on blood pressure
Calcium channel blockers	diltiazem	x	
	nifedipine	x	
	verapamil	x	
Cardiac glycosides	digoxin	x	
Diuretics	furosemine, thiazides		x
	spironolactone	x	
Psychoactive drugs		x	
Benzodiazepines	alprazolam	x	x
	diazepam	x	
	lorazepam		
	midazolam	x	
Tricyclic antidepressants	amitriptyline	x	x
	carbamazepine	x	
	desipramine	x	x
	doxepin	x	x
	fluvoxamine	x	x
	imipramine	x	x
	nortriptyline	x	x

Table 3. Drug classes which may interfere with autonomic function tests and some examples of medications [12].

Variable	Units	Description
STATISTICAL MEASURES		
SDNN	ms	Standard deviation (SD) of all normal-to-normal (NN) intervals
SDANN	ms	Standard deviation (SD) of the averages of normal-to-normal (NN) intervals in all 5-minute segments of the entire recording
RMSSD	ms	Root-mean square of the differences of successive normal-to-normal (NN) intervals
SDNN index	ms	Mean of the standard deviations (SDs) of all normal-to-normal (NN) intervals for all 5-minute segments of the entire recording
SDSD	ms	SD of differences between adjacent normal-to-normal (NN) intervals
NN50 count	ms	Number of pairs of adjacent normal-to-normal (NN) intervals differing by more than 50 ms in the entire recording (counting all such NN intervals pairs or only pairs in which the first or the second interval is longer)
pNN50	%	NN50 count divided by the total number of all normal-to-normal (NN) intervals

Variable	Units	Description
GEOMETRIC MEASURES		
Heart rate variability triangular index		Total number of all normal-to-normal intervals divided by the height of the histogram of all normal-to-normal (NN) intervals measured on a discrete scale with bins of 7.8125 ms (1/128 seconds)
Triangular interpolation (TINN)	ms	Baseline width of the minimum square difference triangular interpolation of the highest peak of the histogram of all normal-to-normal (NN) intervals
Differential index	ms	Difference between the widths of the histogram of differences between adjacent normal-to-normal intervals measured at selected heights
Logarithmic index	ms	Coefficient ϕ of the negative exponential curve $k \cdot e^{-\phi t}$, which is the best approximation of the histogram of absolute differences between adjacent NN intervals

Table 4. Time domain measures of heart rate variability described by the Task Force of the European Society of Cardiology and the North American Society of Pacing and Electrophysiology. The four measures marked in grey were recommended for time domain heart rate variability assessment [43].

Variable	Units	Description
ANALYSIS OF SHORT-TERM RECORDINGS		
5-min total power	ms^2	The variance of normal-to-normal (NN) intervals over the temporal segment
VLF	ms^2	Power in very low frequency (VLF) range
LF	ms^2	Power in low frequency (LF) range
LF norm	nu	LF power in normalized units LF/(total power-VLF)x100
HF	ms^2	Power in high frequency (HF) range
HF norm	nu	HF power in normalized units HF/(total power-VLF)x100
LF/HF	ms^2	Ratio LF [ms^2]/HF[ms^2]
ANALYSIS OF ENTIRE 24 HOURS		
Total power	ms^2	Variance of all normal-to-normal (NN) intervals
ULF	ms^2	Power in the ultra low frequency (ULF) range
VLF	ms^2	Power in the VLF range
LF	ms^2	Power in the LF range
HF	ms^2	Power in the HF range
α		Slope of the linear interpolation of the spectrum in a log-log scale

Table 5. Frequency domain measures of heart rate variability described by the Task Force of the European Society of Cardiology and the North American Society of Pacing and Electrophysiology [43].

http://dx.doi.org/10.5772/52033

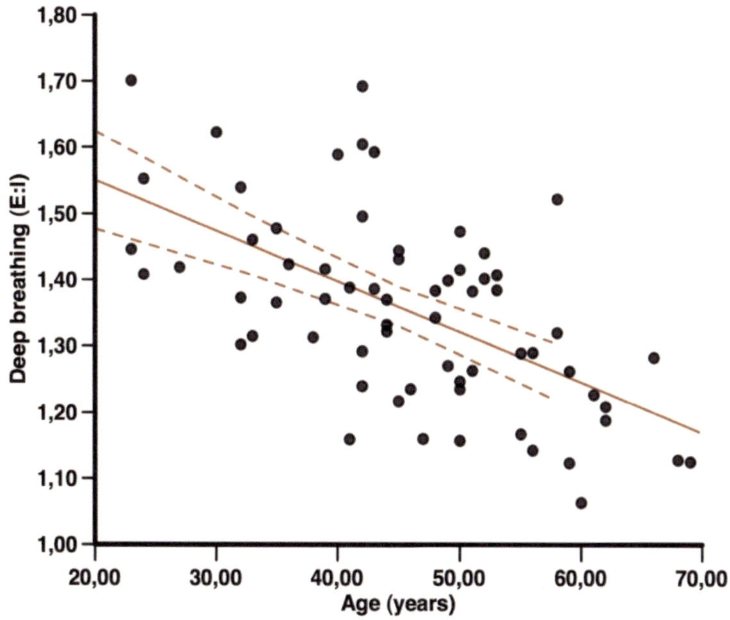

Figure 3. The linear relationship between age and heart rate response to deep breathing expressed as expiratory/inspiratory (E:I) ratio.

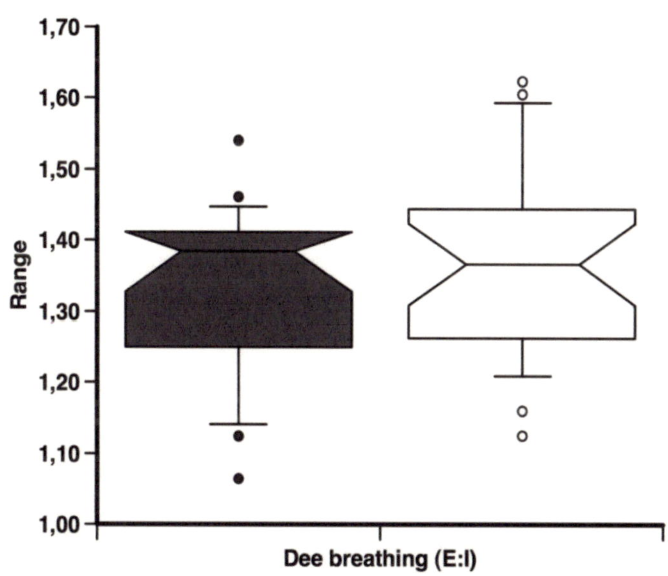

Figure 4. Two-way box percentile plots of heart rate response to deep breathing expressed as expiratory/inspiratory (E:I) ratio in 20 patients with type 1 diabetes (black box) and 25 age-matched control subjects (white box).

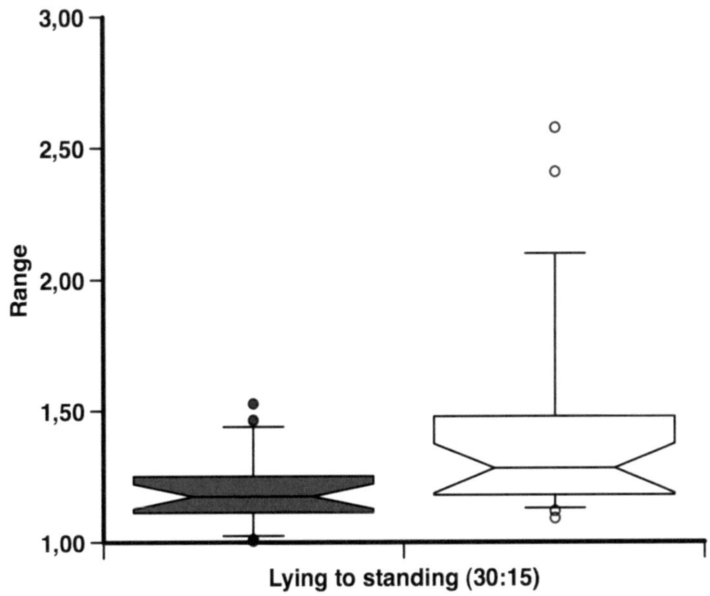

Figure 5. Two-way box percentile plots of heart rate response to standing upcalculated as the ratio of the longest R-R interval around the 30th beat to the shortest R-R interval around the 15th beat in 20 patients with type 1 diabetes (black box) and 25 age-matched control subjects (white box).

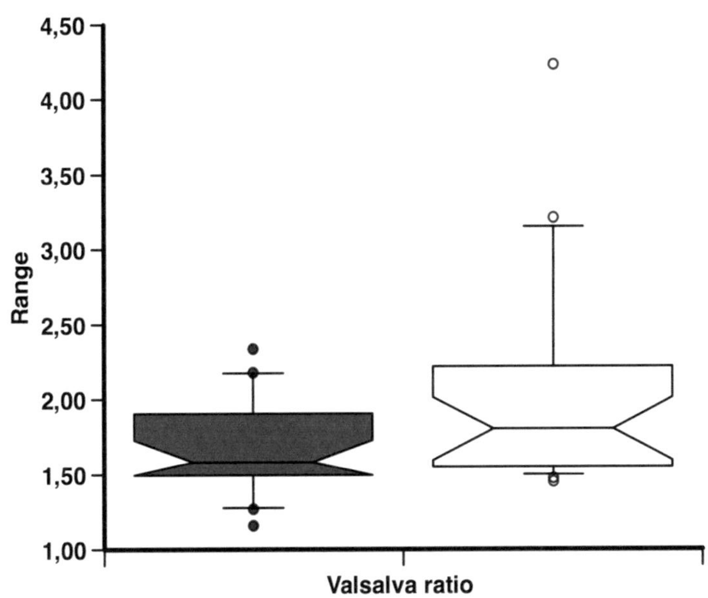

Figure 6. A two-way box percentile comparison plot of heart rate response to Valsalva manoeuvre expressed as the ratio of the longest R-R interval shortly after the manoeuvre to the shortest R-R interval during the manoeuvre in 20 patients with type 1 diabetes (black box) and 25 age-matched control subjects (white box)

http://dx.doi.org/10.5772/52033

5. What kind of relationship is between cardiac autonomic neuropathy, cardiovascular mortality, and albuminuria

Chronic misalignment between the endogenous circadian timing system and the behavioural cycles may increase the risk of diabetes, obesity, cardiovascular disease and cancer [5] as well as the presence of diseases may affect circadian rhythms. While cardiovascular events generally occur in the early morning hours [47-48], abnormalities in the circadian pattern of cardiovascular events in the diabetic population has been attributed to differences in the duration of diabetes and supposedly the variable extent of underlying diabetic autonomic neuropathy [6-9, 49]. In 1989 Hjalmarson et al. observed two peaks of symptom onset of acute myocardial infarction for patients with diabetes: a peak, 28%, was discernible between 6:01 AM and 12:00 noon and a secondary peak, 25%, between 6:01 PM and midnight. In patients over 70 years of age, smokers, diabetics, those receiving β-blockers, and women, the morning and the evening peaks were of the same size [6]. Moreover, angina has long been considered an unreliable index of myocardial infarction in diabetic patients with coronary artery disease [50-51]. The prolonged anginal perception threshold in diabetic patients was suggested to be partly the result of damage to the sensory innervation of the heart [52]. In the same 1990, to investigate the incidence and mechanism of painless myocardial ischemia on exercise testing in diabetic patients, Murray et al. performed two studies: 1) retrospectively, all exercise tests carried out in the hospital during the past 5 years were reviewed for silent ischemia; 2) prospectively, diabetic patients with known or suspected coronary artery disease underwent autonomic function testing and a second exercise test. They concluded that silent myocardial ischemia on exercise testing was common among patients with diabetes mellitus and was associated with severe autonomic dysfunction [53].

Ambulatory electrocardiographic monitoring in 60 patients with diabetes and coronary artery disease, 25 of whom underwent also autonomic nervous system testing, evidenced that 1) silent ischemia was highly prevalent since 91% of all ischemic episodes were silent, and 2) time of onset of ischemia followed a circadian distribution with a peak incidence in the morning hours, except in patients with moderate to severe autonomic nervous system dysfunction who did not demonstrate such a peak [7]. Using harmonic regression model to evaluate the circadian variation of myocardial infarction symptom onset in patients (n = 3882) who were enrolled in the Onset Study, it was then confirmed that patients with type 1 diabetes and those with type 2 diabetes for 5 or more years had an attenuation of the morning peak in acute myocardial infarction [9]. Authors concluded that inconsistency in observation of such an effect in patients with diabetes in the past might well have been due to differences in the duration of diabetes and thus the variable extent of underlying autonomic dysfunction [9]. To exemplify inconsistencies among clinical observations, the time of onset of ischemic pain in patients enrolled in the Thrombolysis in Myocardial Ischemia (TIMI) III Registry Prospective Study and in the TIMI IIIB trial showed a circadian variation with a peak in the morning hours between 6 AM and 12 noon. This circadian variation was observed both in patients with unstable angina and in those with evolving non-Q-wave acute myocardial infarction and in all subgroups tested, diabetics included [8]. On the contrary, Li et al. showed there was no a significant morning peak of incidence of acute myocardial infarction in patients with diabetes but was obvious in control subjects; however, disappear of morning peak was not associated with duration of diabetes [49].

Mechanisms through which cardiovascular circadian rhythms may be altered in diabetes are under current investigation. The tight crosstalk between components of circadian and metabolic cycles in mammals suggests that changes in nutrient-dependent signalling pathways such as in metabolic disorders may transmit cues that affect cardiovascular rhythmicity through transcriptional and non-transcriptional mechanisms [1, 54]. Moreover, a functional antagonism between melatonin and insulin has been supposed on the basis of animal and clinical studies. Melatonin inhibits insulin release through both the pertussis-toxin-sensitive membrane receptors MT_1 and MT_2 and the second messengers 3',5'-cyclic adenosine monophosphate, 3',5'-cyclic guanosine monophosphate and inositol 1,4,5-trisphosphate. In turn, increased insulin levels exert an inhibitory effect on the pineal gland and melatonin[55].

The relationship between cardiovascular prognosis and cardiac autonomic neuropathy has been investigated for a long time since the rate of deaths within a mean follow-up of 5.8 years had been found five times higher in the diabetic patients with cardiac autonomic neuropathy than in the diabetic patients free from cardiac autonomic neuropathy; most of these deaths were from cardiac causes [56]. The reasons why cardiac autonomic neuropathy affects quality and length of life are not well established, but cardiac autonomic neuropathy has been found to be associated with exercise intolerance, silent myocardial ischemia, prolongation of QT interval that may cause arrhythmias, decreased myocardial perfusion reserve, left ventricular hypertrophy and diastolic dysfunction [24, 57-59]. The variability of mortality rates revealed in the studies could be related to the study population, the modality for assessing cardiac autonomic neuropathy, the criteria used to define the presence of cardiac autonomic neuropathy, and the length of follow-up [60]. In 2003, Maser et al. examined by meta-analysis this relationship: 15 studies published from 1966 to 2001 could be included whose follow-up ranged from 0.5 to 16 years. The study-specific relative risks for individuals with cardiac autonomic neuropathy ranged from 0.91 to 9.20 with a pooled relative risk for mortality of 3.45 for studies that used two or more measures to define cardiac autonomic neuropathy, and of 1.20 for those studies defining cardiac autonomic neuropathy with one measure of autonomic function [60].

Our Table 6 summarises the main studies of cardiac autonomic neuropathy and mortality/ morbidity in patients with diabetes mellitus restarting from the year 2001 onwards. In that year, a 3-7 year (mean 4.5) follow up was obtained in 107 diabetic patients with no history of myocardial infarction or angina, a normal ECG, and two or more additional risk factors, who underwent ECG stress test, a thallium-201 myocardial scintigraphy with dipyridamole, and 48-h ECG monitoring to assess silent myocardial ischemia. In addition, cardiac autonomic neuropathy was searched for by standardized tests evaluating heart rate variations [61]. The study confirmed that 1) the prevalence of type 1 silent myocardial ischemia was high (about 30%) and significant coronary stenoses were found in approximately one-third of those patients with silent myocardial ischemia; 2) there was only a trend of higher risk of major cardiac events in the diabetic patients with silent myocardial ischemia than in the dia-

http://dx.doi.org/10.5772/52033

betic patients without silent myocardial ischemia; 3) cardiac autonomic neuropathy was significantly associated with an increased risk of major cardiac events. According to the Kaplan-Meier method, the increase in the risk of major cardiac events linked to cardiac autonomic neuropathy was significant after adjusting for silent myocardial ischemia, but the highest rate was found in patients who had silent myocardial ischemia and cardiac autonomic neuropathy. Authors concluded that the poor cardiovascular prognosis related to cardiac autonomic neuropathy in previous studies was probably associated with undetected silent myocardial ischemia in many patients [61].

Ref.	Follow up (years)	Sample size	Tests of CAN	Definition of CAN	Results	Comments
61	4.5	107 patients (of whom 17 with T1DM) and normal ECG	HR variability during deep breathing, Valsalva and lying to standing tests	The results were compared with those from an age-matched control series	CAN was a better predictor of major cardiac events (odds ratio 4.30, 1.07-17.31) than silent myocardial ischemia (evaluated by ECG stress test, myocardial scintigraphy with dipyridamole, and 48-h ECG monitoring)	Limited number of asymptomatic patients with predominantly T2DM
62	3.5	532 patients with DM (483 with T2DM)	HR variability during deep breathing; SBP decrease during standing	Not stated	Increased all-cause mortality associated with the lowest quintile of HR variability (hazard ratio 1.49, 1.01-2.19)	The cohort was predominantly male; no direct adjustment for use of cardio-active medications
63	2.5	715 survivors of AMI (117 with DM)	Spectral analysis of HR variability (24-h Holter ECG)	According to cutpoints previously established	Decreased HR variability remains predictive also in diabetic patients (hazard ratio for SDNN < 50 ms 2.56, 1.26-5.19)	Moderate power due to the small number of death in diabetic patients; DM was not classified
65	5.3	872 of 950 patients with T2DM underwent baseline neuropathy assessment	HR variability during deep breathing	According to age-related range values	Borderline or abnormal expiratory/ inspiratory ratio at baseline was associated with the occurrence of stroke (hazard ratio 2.3, 1.17-4.70)	Only one autonomic test instead of a battery
66	3.8	146 patients with T2DM with suspected coronary artery disease	Deep breathing, Valsalva manoeuvre, lying to standing, postural systolic blood pressure change, handgrip test	Three or more of the tests were abnormal	Although perfusion defects remained a strong predictor of cardiac risk, CAN predicted the occurrence of death and cardiac events independent of perfusion defects	Retrospective design; limited number of subjects; symptomatic diabetic patients
67	15	311 patients with T2DM and 151 patients with T1DM	Quantitative sudomotor axon reflex test, HR response to deep breathing and to the Valsalva manoeuvre, BP responses during tilt and the Valsalva manoeuvre	According to the 10 point score composite autonomic severity scale (CASS)	Sudden cardiac death relates more directly to coronary ischemia, cardiac arrhythmia, or nephropathy than it does to diabetic autonomic neuropathy	Northern European sample; unavailable serial data obtained before and during sudden cardiac death; not all applicable risk factors could be modelled

Ref.	Follow up (years)	Sample size	Tests of CAN	Definition of CAN	Results	Comments
68	10.1	388 patients with T1DM of whom 197 with diabetic nephropathy	HR variability during deep breathing	HR variability < 10 bpm	CAN predicted cardiovascular mortality and morbidity in patients with diabetic nephropathy (hazard ratio 6.4, 1.5-26.3), but not all-cause mortality	CAN determined by only one test, but well characterised population
69	9.2	104 patients with T2DM of whom 51 with diabetic nephropathy	HR variability during deep breathing	Not stated	Non-dipping phenomenon predicted all-cause mortality (1% increase in dipping was associated with a lower risk 0.97, 0.94-0.998); HR variability was confirmed to be a predictor also in T2DM (1 bpm increase 0.92, 0.87-0.98)	Low patient number, but well characterised population
70	9.0	1560 non diabetic and 160 diabetic subjects (MONIKA/ KORA Study)	Time domain measures, corrected QT interval, and QT dispersion were obtained from a 12-lead resting ECG	Not stated	The relative risk of mortality in subjects with corrected QT > 440 ms increased by twofold and threefold in the non diabetic and diabetic group, respectively; prolonged QT interval predicted cardiovascular mortality only in the non diabetic group (risk ratio 4.47, 2.44-9.22)	Short period of ECG recording (20s) without control for respiration
71	7.1	1458 patients with T2DM	HR variability during deep breathing, Valsalva manoeuvre and postural change	According to age-related reference values (total maximum CAN score of 3)	Hazard ratio for acute stroke events in patients with abnormal CAN scores was 2.7 compared with patients with normal scores; a CAN score of 3 was significantly associated with a new ischaemic stroke event in patients with diabetes	Lack reference values for CAN tests specific for Korean people; the effect of glycaemic control status on the development of stroke has not been assessed; limited number of events
71	13.6	490 individuals from a population-based cohort (Hoorn Study) of whom 135 with T2DM	HR variability during deep breathing and standing up, 5 tests of spectral analyses of HR variability, and one baroreflex sensitivity measurement	Cardiovascular autonomic dysfunction total score	Both microalbuminuria and CAN are independently associated with cardiovascular mortality, and the excess mortality attributable to microalbuminuria cannot be explained by CAN	Moderate level of reproducibility of autonomic function parameters; CAN total score evaluated at baseline only; spectral analyses performed during 3 min; albumin/creatinine ratio measured in one urine sample only
72	15.5	178 diabetic patients of whom 110 with T2DM	HR variability during deep breathing, Valsalva manoeuvre, and lying to standing, postural systolic blood pressure change, diastolic blood pressure response to handgrip test	Two or more abnormal tests	The relative risk of all-cause mortality associated with CAN was 2.85, 1.75-4.65; Valsalva ratio and handgrip had an independent predictive value	Sources of lower sample representativeness: 1) 26% of invited subjects refused to participate (older than responders), 2) patients' ability to cooperate to the function tests
73	15.5	165 diabetic patients of	Time and frequency domain parameters	Not stated	The low frequency band in the frequency domain was the most powerful predictor of all-	Sources of lower sample representativeness: 1) only patients who completed all

Ref.	Follow up (years)	Sample size	Tests of CAN	Definition of CAN	Results	Comments
		whom 97 with T2DM	based on 24-hour ECG recordings		cause mortality (estimated relative risk of death with an increase by 1 standard deviation 0.65)	5 function tests and had an acceptable 24-hour ECG recording could be analysed, 2) ECG was recorded during normal daily activity
74	15.5	136 diabetic patients of whom 77 with T2DM	Five autonomic function tests together with time and frequency domain parameters based on 24-hour ECG recordings	Not stated	Three simple autonomic function tests (Valsalva, 30:15, and handgrip) were superior to HR variability in predicting all-cause mortality in the diabetic population	Sources of lower sample representativeness: 1) percentage of invited subjects who refused to participate (older than responders), 2) patients' ability to cooperate to the function tests and to have an acceptable 24-hour ECG recording

Table 6. Studies that evaluated mortality and morbidity in patients with diabetes mellitus and cardiovascular autonomic neuropathy (CAN) from 2001 onward. AMI, acute myocardial infarction; DM, diabetes mellitus; SBP, systolic blood pressure; SDNN, standard deviation of normal RR intervals; T2DM, type 2 diabetes mellitus; T1DM, type 1 diabetes mellitus.

Wheeler et al. evaluated short-term all-cause mortality in an elderly cohort of predominantly male veteran patients with diabetes [62]. Among the 532 patients with RR variability measures (evaluated by heart rate response to timed deep breathing), subjects who died (n = 120) had significantly lower heart rat variability than survivors. The lowest quintile of heart rate variability with deep breathing was found to be associated with a 50% increase in mortality. After adjusting for age, smoking status, creatinine, pack-year of cigarettes smoked, diabetes duration, race, history of ischemic heart disease, and hypertension, the hazard ratio was 1.49 with a 95% confidence interval 1.01-2.19 [62].

Whang et al. used data from the Multicenter Post Infarction Program (MPIP, a longitudinal observational study of 715 survivors of acute myocardial infarction, including 117 diabetic patients, enrolled from 1979 to 1980) to test two hypotheses: 1) RR interval variability was lower in diabetic patients, and 2) low RR interval variability was less predictive of mortality in diabetic patients [63]. Six frequency-domain measurements and one time-domain measurement of RR interval variability were evaluated on the basis of 24-hour Holter electrocardiographic recordings. Reduced RR interval variability was significantly more frequent in diabetic patients than in non-diabetic patients for all measurements except high frequency power. Moreover, in diabetic patients, the association between reduced RR interval variability and all-cause mortality was at least as strong as it was in non-diabetic patients for all measurements except high frequency power [63].

Since the risk of fatal and non-fatal strokes were increased in diabetic patients compared with non-diabetic patients over a 7-year follow up period [64], Cohen et al. evaluated the relationship between a number cardiovascular risk factors in normotensive and hypertensive type 2 diabetic patients (enrolled in the Appropriate Blood Pressure Control in Diabetes trial) on the incidence of stroke [65]. Cardiovascular risk factors included also autonomic function testing, and automated electrocardiographic measure of heart rate response to deep breathing. Expiratory/inspiratory (E:I) ratio was categorised as normal (53.6%), borderline (9.5%), or abnormal (36.9%) based on age-related range values. The presence of a borderline or abnormal expiratory/inspiratory ratio at baseline was significantly associated with the occurrence of stroke in the follow up period (hazard ratio 2.3, 1.17-4.70). Thus, diabetic autonomic neuropathy was a significant independent risk factor also for the occurrence of stroke [65].

In order to investigate the prognostic value of cardiac autonomic neuropathy in relation to myocardial perfusion defects, Lee et al. evaluated 146 consecutive patients with type 2 diabetes mellitus who underwent thallium-201 single photon emission computed tomography (SPECT) for suspected coronary artery disease and who tested for autonomic nerve function within three months of the single photon emission computed tomography study [66]. Cardiac autonomic function tests included deep breathing, Valsalva manoeuvre, lying to standing, postural systolic blood pressure change, and handgrip test; cardiac autonomic neuropathy was defined by the presence of ≥ 3 abnormal tests. Patients were followed up for 46±24 months to record deaths and major cardiac events. Significant predictors of death were perfusion defects, cardiac autonomic neuropathy, and older age; significant predictors of cardiac events were perfusion defects, cardiac autonomic neuropathy, hypertension, and longer history of diabetes [66].

Suarez et al. investigated the risk factors for sudden cardiac death in the prospective, population based, Rochester Diabetic Neuropathy Study (RDNS) cohort: 462 diabetic patients (of whom 115 with type 1 diabetes) were followed up over 15 years [67]. At baseline, patients underwent 1) neuropathy assessment by the neuropathy impairment score, neuropathy symptoms and change score, nerve conduction studies, and quantitative sensation; 2) autonomic neuropathy assessment by quantitative sudomotor axon reflex test, heart rate variability to deep breathing and to the Valsalva manoeuvre, beat to beat blood pressure responses during tilt and the Valsalva manoeuvre; 3) assessment of other putative risk factors, metabolic control, diabetic retinopathy and nephropathy; 4) recording of a 12-lead ECG every two years. The medical records, death certificates, and necropsy reports of all deaths were reviewed and 21 cases of sudden cardiac death were identified. In bivariate analysis of risk covariates, evolving and previous myocardial infarction, bundle branch block or pacing, and nephropathy stage were stronger risk covariates than were indicators of diabetic autonomic neuropathy and HDL cholesterol. In bivariate analysis and adjusting for nephropathy, diabetic autonomic neuropathy was not statistically significant factor [67].

In a prospective observational follow up study, Astrup et al. evaluated the predictive value of cardiac autonomic neuropathy for cardiovascular mortality and morbidity (primary end point), all cause mortality and progression of diabetic nephropathy (secondary end points) in 197 patients with type 1 diabetes and diabetic nephropathy and 191 patients with long standing diabetes and normoalbuminuria who were followed for 10.1 years [68]. After adjustment for cardiovascular risk factors, autonomic dysfunction was a predictor of cardiovascular mortality and morbidity in type 1 diabetic patients with diabetic nephropathy (hazard ratio 6.4, 1.5-26.3), whereas the impact of heart rate variability on all-cause mortality was not significant. Moreover, there was no correlation between abnormal heart rate variability and rate of decline of glomerular filtration rate [68]. One year later, Astrup et al. published the results of a study aimed at evaluating the prognostic significance of cardiovascular risk factors, including cardiac autonomic neuropathy and 24-hour blood pressure level and rhythm, for all-cause mortality in type 2 diabetic patients (n = 104) with and without diabetic nephropathy [69]. In a Cox regression analysis, predictors of all-cause mortality included cardiac autonomic neuropathy (1 beat/min increase 0.92, 0.87-0.98) together with age, male sex, left ventricular hypertrophy, haemoglobin A1c, daytime systolic blood pressure, glomerular filtration rate (or albuminuria, alternatively) and dipping (1% increase in dipping was associated with a lower risk 0.97, 0.94-0.998). After adjusting for traditional cardiovascular risk factors, non-dipping of night blood pressure remained a significant predictor of all-cause mortality [69].

Prolonged QT corrected (QTc > 440 ms) interval was an independent predictor of mortality over 9 years in the non-diabetic (n = 1560) and diabetic (n = 160) elderly general population of the Monitoring of Trends and Determinants in Cardiovascular Disease (MONICA) study, whereas QT dispersion did not predict mortality in non-diabetic or diabetic subjects. On the contrary, reduced heart rate variability appeared to be a more specific marker only in the diabetic elderly general population [70]. Ko et al. investigated whether cardiac autonomic neuropathy was associated with acute ischaemic stroke in 1458 patients with type 2 diabetes during 7.1 year follow up [71]. At follow-up, 131 patients (11.6%) had developed newly diagnosed acute ischaemic stroke. Baseline cardiac autonomic neuropathy score was significantly associated with the development of ischaemic stroke in patients with type 2 diabetes. Indeed, the hazard ratio for acute stroke events in patients with abnormal cardiac autonomic neuropathy scores was 2.7 compared with patients with normal scores [71]. In order to investigate whether cardiac autonomic neuropathy could explain the relationship between microalbuminuria and cardiovascular mortality, 490 individuals from a population-based cohort (Hoorn Study) were followed for a median period of 13.6 years [72]. At baseline, were evaluated glucose tolerance status, HbA1c, and albuminuria. Cardiovascular autonomic function tests included four tests that reflected heart rate or blood pressure changes due to deep breathing or standing up, five tests of spectral analyses of heart rate variability, and one baroreflex sensitivity measurement. Both microalbuminuria and cardiac autonomic neuropathy were independently associated with cardiovascular mortality. However, after adjustment for age, sex, glucose tolerance status, and other cardiovascular risk factors, microalbuminuria (relative risk 1.33, 0.83–2.13), in contrast to cardiovascular autonomic dysfunction total score (1.52, 1.11–2.09), was not independently associated with all-cause mortality. The excess of mortality attributable to microalbuminuria could not be explained by cardiac autonomic neuropathy [72].

Finally, May and Arildsen have evaluated long-term predictive power on all-cause mortality of five function tests for cardiac autonomic neuropathy as well as of heart rate variability based on 24-hour ECG recordings (both time domain analyses and frequency domain analyses were performed) in the same sample during a 15.5-year follow up period [73-75]. When considering the five function tests for cardiac autonomic neuropathy (heart rate variability during deep breathing, Valsalva manoeuvre, and lying to standing, postural systolic blood pressure change, diastolic blood pressure response to handgrip test) it was apparent that the relative risk of all-cause mortality associated with cardiac autonomic neuropathy was 2.85, 1.75-4.65; Valsalva ratio, heart rate response to standing up (30;15 ratio), and handgrip had an independent predictive value with regard to long-term all cause mortality [73]. When considering separately time and frequency domain parameters of heart rate variability calculated on the basis of a 24-hour ECG recording, the power in the low frequency band was the only heart rate variability parameter with an independent predictive value on all-cause mortality [74]. When considering long-term predictive power of heart rate variability together with a battery of five autonomic function tests, the latter ones were superior to the former ones; particularly, Valsalva, 30:15 ratio, and handgrip were independent predictors of death [75].

6. Concluding remarks

Several studies have evaluated the predictive value of various cardiac autonomic neuropathy parameters for all cause mortality and/or cardiovascular mortality and morbidity. They almost all agree that cardiac autonomic dysfunction is associated with a high-risk excess mortality/morbidity in diabetic patients. Toward a general consensus, however, many challenges remain to be addressed by the research community. Drawbacks and limitations mainly concern the following features that deserve attention and discussion [76]:

1. Establishing appropriate study design for evaluating the particular association. Prospective cohort studies are considered less vulnerable to bias than retrospective studies, because the outcomes have not occurred when the cohort is assembled and the exposures are assessed. In cohort studies the population may be fixed or open: undoubtedly, in long-term follow ups, the prevalence of cardiac autonomic neuropathy progressively increases in a direct proportion to age, duration of diabetes, and poor glycaemic control.

2. Defining clear health outcomes that should require confirmation by masked investigators in order to guarantee their accuracy.

3. Establishing the length of follow up interval, which depends on the particular outcome under study. It has been shown that the longer the follow up, the higher the likelihood of attrition.

4. Calculating the required sample size on the basis of anticipated differences between the groups, the background rate of the outcome, and the probability of making some statistical errors.

5. Using suitable cardiovascular autonomic reflex tests to diagnose cardiac autonomic neuropathy taking into account that a) the diagnostic definition of cardiac autonomic neuropathy based on several tests (of both vagal and sympathetic functions) reduces the probability of false positives, b) the gold standard for clinical autonomic testing includes heart rate response to deep breathing, standing, and Valsalva manoeuvre, and blood pressure response to standing [12].

6. Identifying in advance the various cardiovascular prognostic factors (how many and which ones?) to reasonably adjust for in the analysis. Risk adjustment is essential to making fair comparisons and first requires strict definition of each specific outcome, particularly in diabetic people provided the complex association of traditional, non-traditional and disease-specific risk factors with mortality/morbidity.

Author details

Elena Matteucci* and Ottavio Giampietro*

*Address all correspondence to: elena.matteucci@med.unipi.it

Department of Clinical and Experimental Medicine, Italy

References

[1] Matteucci, E., & Giampietro, O. (2012). Circadian Rhythm of blood pressure in diabetes mellitus: evidence, mechanisms and implications. *Current Diabetes Reviews*, in press.

[2] Huang, W., Ramsey, K. M., Marcheva, B., & Bass, J. (2011). Circadian rhythms, sleep, and metabolism. *The Journal of Clinical Investigation*, 121(6), 2133-2141.

[3] Froy, O. (2011). The circadian clock and metabolism. *Clinical Science*, 120(2), 65-72.

[4] Takeda, N., & Maemura, K. (2011). Circadian clock and cardiovascular disease. *Journal of Cardiology*, 57(3), 249-256.

[5] Litinski, M., Scheer, F. A., & Shea, S. A. (2009). Influence of the circadian system on disease severity. *Sleeps Medicine Clinics*, 4(2), 143-163.

[6] Hjalmarson, A., Gilpin, E. A., Nicod, P., Dittrich, H., Henning, H., Engler, R., Blacky, A. R., Smith, S. C., Jr Ricou, F., Ross, J., & Jr , . (1989). Differing circadian patterns of symptom onset in subgroups of patients with acute myocardial infarction. *Circulation*, 80(2), 267-275.

[7] Zarich, S., Waxman, S., Freeman, R. T., Mittleman, M., Hegarty, P., & Nesto, R. W. (1994). Effect of autonomic nervous system dysfunction on the circadian pattern of myocardial ischemia in diabetes mellitus. *Journal of the American College of Cardiology*, 24(4), 956-962.

[8] Cannon, C. P., Mc Cabe, C. H., Stone, P. H., Schactman, M., Thompson, B., Theroux, P., Gibson, R. S., Feldman, T., Kleiman, N. S., Tofler, G. H., Muller, J. E., Chaitman, B. R., & Braunwald, E. (1997). Circadian variation in the onset of unstable angina and

non-Q-wave acute myocardial infarction (the TIMI III Registry and TIMI IIIB). *The American Journal of Cardiology*, 79(3), 253-258.

[9] Rana, J. S., Mukamal, K. J., Morgan, J. P., Muller, J. E., & Mittleman, . (2003). Circadian variation in the onset of myocardial infarction: effect of duration of diabetes. *Diabetes*, 52(6), 1464-1468.

[10] Pop-Busui, R. (2010). Cardiac autonomic neuropathy in diabetes. *Diabetes Care*, 33(2), 434-441.

[11] American Diabetes Association. (2012). Standards of medical Care in diabetes- 2012. *Diabetes Care*, 35(1), 11-63.

[12] Spallone, V., Ziegler, D., Freeman, R., Bernardi, L., Frontoni, S., Pop-Busui, R., Stevens, M., Kempler, P., Hilsted, J., Tesfaye, S., Low, P., & Valensi, P. (2011). Cardiovascular autonomic neuropathy in diabetes: clinical impact, assessment, diagnosis, and management. *Diabetes/Metabolism Research and Reviews*, 27(7), 639-653.

[13] Watkins, P. J. (1973). Facial sweating after food: a new sign of diabetic autonomic neuropathy. *British Medical Journal*, 1(5853), 583-587.

[14] Wheeler, T., & Watkins, P. J. (1973). Cardiac denervation in diabetes. *British Medical Journal*, 4(5892), 584-586.

[15] Ewing, D. J., Campbell, I. W., & Burt, Clarke. B. F. (1973). Vascular reflexes in diabetic autonomic neuropathy. *Lancet*, 2(7842), 1354-1356.

[16] Ewing, D. J., Martyn, C. N., Young, R. J., & Clarke, B. F. (1985). The value of cardiovascular autonomic function tests: 10 years experience in diabetes. *Diabetes Care*, 8(5), 491-498.

[17] Thomas, G. D. (2011). Neural control of the circulation. *Advances in Physiology Education*, 35(1), 28-32.

[18] Sin, P. Y. W., Galletly, D. C., & Tzeng, Y. C. (2010). Influence of breathing frequency on the pattern of respiratory sinus arrhythmia and blood pressure: old questions revisited. *American Journal of Physiology. Heart and Circulatory Physiology*, 298(5), 1588-1599.

[19] Barbieri, R., Triedman, J. K., & Saul, J. P. (2002). Heart rate control and mechanical cardiopulmonary coupling to assess central volume: a systems analysis. *American Journal of Physiology Regulatory, Integrative and Comparative Physiology*, 283(5), 1210-1220.

[20] Mitchell, J. H., & Smith, S. A. (2008). Unravelling the mysteries of the exercise pressor reflex at the cellular level. *The Journal of Physiology*, 586(13), 3025-3026.

[21] Boulton, A. J., Vinik, A. I., Arezzo, J. C., Bril, V., Feldman, E. L., Freeman, R., Malik, R. A., Maser, R. E., Sosenko, J. M., & Ziegler, D. (2005). Diabetic neuropathies: a statement by the American Diabetes Association. *Diabetes Care*, 28(4), 956-962.

[22] Vinik, A. I., Strotmeyer, E. S., & Nakave, Patel. C. V. (2008). Diabetic neuropathy in older adults. *Clinics in Geriatric Medicine*, 24(3), 407-435.

[23] Thomas, P. K. (1997). Classification, differential diagnosis, and staging of diabetic peripheral neuropathy. *Diabetes*, 46(2), 54-57.

[24] Vinik, A. I., Maser, R. E., & Mitchell, Freeman. R. (2003). Diabetic autonomic neuropathy. *Diabetes Care*, 26(5), 1553-1579.

[25] Vinik, A. I., Maser, R. E., & Ziegler, D. (2011). Autonomic imbalance: prophet of dome or scope for hope? *Diabetic Medicine*, 28(6), 643-651.

[26] Jacob, G., Ertl, A. C., Shannon, J. R., Furlan, R., Robertson, R. M., & Robertson, D. (1998). Effect of standing on neurohumoral responses and plasma volume in healthy subjects. *Journal of Applied Physiology*, 84(3), 914-921.

[27] Cohen, C. N., Filho, F. M., de Fátima, Gonçalves. M., & de Brito, Gomes. M. (2001). Early alterations of blood pressure in normotensive and normoalbuminuric Type 1 diabetic patients. *Diabetes Research and Clinical Practice*, 53(2), 85-90.

[28] Lengyel, Z., Rosivall, L., Németh, C., Tóth, L. K., Nagy, V., Mihály, M., Kammerer, L., & Vörös, P. (2003). Diurnal blood pressure pattern may predict the increase of urinary albumin excretion in normotensive normoalbuminuric type 1 diabetes mellitus patients. *Diabetes Research and Clinical Practice*, 62(3), 159-167.

[29] Cuspidi, C., Meani, S., Lonati, L., Fusi, V., Valerio, C., Sala, C., Magnaghi, G., Maisaidi, M., & Zanchetti, A. (2006). Short-term reproducibility of a non-dipping pattern in type 2 diabetic hypertensive patients. *Journal of Hypertension*, 24(4), 647-653.

[30] Felício, J. S., Pacheco, J. T., Ferreira, S. R., Plavnik, F., Moisés, V. A., Kohlmann, O., Jr Ribeiro, A. B., & Zanella, M. T. (2006). Hyperglycemia and nocturnal systolic blood pressure are associated with left ventricular hypertrophy and diastolic dysfunction in hypertensive diabetic patients. *Cardiovascular Diabetolology*, 5, 19 EOF.

[31] Eguchi, K., Pickering, T. G., Hoshide, S., Ishikawa, J., Ishikawa, S., Schwartz, J. E., Shimada, K., & Kario, K. (2008). Ambulatory blood pressure is a better marker than clinic blood pressure in predicting cardiovascular events in patients with/without type 2 diabetes. *American Journal of Hypertension*, 21(4), 443-450.

[32] Cardoso, C. R., Leite, N. C., Freitas, L., Dias, S. B., Muxfeld, E. S., & Salles, G. F. (2008). Pattern of 24-hour ambulatory blood pressure monitoring in type 2 diabetic patients with cardiovascular dysautonomy. *Hypertension Research*, 31(5), 865-872.

[33] Spallone, V., Maiello, M. R., Morganti, R., Mandica, S., & Frajese, G. (2007). Usefulness of ambulatory blood pressure monitoring in predicting the presence of autonomic neuropathy in type I diabetic patients. *Journal of Human Hypertension*, 21(5), 381-386.

[34] Sharma, S., & Kavuru, M. (2010). Sleep and metabolism: an overview. *International Journal of Endocrinology*, 2010 270832.

[35] Guntsche, Z., Saraví, F. D., Reynals, E. A., Rauek, B., Rauek, M., & Guntsche, E. M. (2002). Parental hypertension and 24 h-blood pressure in children prior to diabetic nephropathy. *Pediatric Nephrology*, 17(3), 157-64.

[36] Zhao, Z. Y., Zhao, Z. Y., Wang, Y. Q., Yan, Z. H., Cui, J., & Li, Y. Y. (2005). Quantitative study of circadian variations of ambulatory blood pressure in Chinese healthy, hypertensive, and diabetes subjects. *Clinical and Experimental Hypertension*, 27(2-3), 187 EOF-94 EOF.

[37] Mannucci, E., Lambertucci, L., Monami, M., Fedeli, A., Chiasserini, V., Marchionni, N., Masotti, G., & Ungar, A. (2006). Pulse pressure and mortality in hypertensive type 2 diabetic patients. A cohort study. *Diabetes/Metabolism Research and Reviews*, 22(3), 172-175.

[38] Darcan, S., Goksen, D., Mir, S., Serdaroglu, E., Buyukinan, M., Coker, M., Berdeli, A., Köse, T., & Cura, A. (2006). Alterations of blood pressure in type 1 diabetic children and adolescents. *Pediatric Nephrology*, 21(5), 672-676.

[39] Leitão, C. B., Canani, L. H., Kramer, C. K., Moehlecke, M., Pinto, L. C., Ricardo, E. D., Pinotti, A. F., & Gross, J. L. (2008). Blood pressure means rather than nocturnal dipping pattern are related to complications in Type 2 diabetic patients. *Diabetic Medicine*, 25(3), 308-313.

[40] Chatterjee, M., Speiser, P. W., Pellizzarri, M., Carey, D. E., Fort, P., Kreitzer, P. M., & Frank, G. R. (2009). Poor glycemic control is associated with abnormal changes in 24-hour ambulatory blood pressure in children and adolescents with type 1 diabetes mellitus. *Journal of Pediatric Endocrinology & Metabolism*, 22, 1061-1067.

[41] Kramer, C. K., Leitão, C. B., Canani, L. H., & Gross, J. L. (2011). Afternoon blood pressure increase: a blood pressure pattern associated with microvascular complications in type 2 diabetes mellitus. *American Journal of Hypertension*, 24(1), 64-69.

[42] Vílchez-López, F. J., Carral-Sanlaureano, F., Coserria-Sánchez, C., Nieto, A., Jiménez, S., & Aguilar-Diosdado, M. (2011). Alterations in arterial pressure in patients with Type 1 diabetes are associated with long-term poor metabolic control and a more atherogenic lipid profile. *Journal of Endocrinological Investigation*, 24-9.

[43] Task Force of the European Society of Cardiology and the North American Society of Pacing and Electrophysiology. (1996). Heart rate variability: standards of measurement, physiological interpretation and clinical use. *Circulation*, 93(5), 1043-1065.

[44] Vinik, A. I., & Ziegler, D. (2007). Diabetic cardiovascular autonomic neuropathy. *Circulation*, 115(3), 387-397.

[45] Pappachan, J. M., Sebastian, J., Bino, B. C., Jayaprakash, K., Vijayakumar, K., Sujathan, P., & Adinegara, L. A. (2008). Cardiac autonomic neuropathy in diabetes mellitus: prevalence, risk factors and utility of corrected QT interval in the ECG for its diagnosis. *Postgraduate Medical Journal*, 84(990), 205-210.

[46] Rowlands, D. J. (2012). Graphical representation of QT rate correction formulae: an aid facilitating the use of a given formula and providing a visual comparison of the impact of different formulae. *Journal of Electrocardiology*, 45(3), 288-293.

[47] Pell, S., & D'Alonzo, . (1963). Acute myocardial infarction in a large industrial population: report of a 6-year study of 1,356 cases. *The Journal of the American Medical Association*, 185(11), 831-838.

[48] Muller, J. E., Stone, P. H., Turi, Z. G., Rutherford, Czeisler., Parker, C., Poole, W. K., Passamani, E., Roberts, R., Robertson, T., Sobel, B. E., Willerson, J. T., Braunwald, E., the, M. I. L. I. S., & Study, Group. (1985). Circadian variation in the frequency of onset of acute myocardial infarction. *The New England Journal of Medicine*, 313(21), 1315-1322.

[49] Li, J., Hua, Q., Pi, L., Tan, J., & Li, B. (2010). Circadian variation on the onset of acute ST segment elevation myocardial infarction in diabetic subjects. *Journal of Cardiovascular Disease Research*, 1(1), 23-26.

[50] Bradley, R. F., & Schonfeld, A. (1962). Diminished pain in diabetic patients with acute myocardial infarction. *Geriatrics*, 17-322.

[51] Nesto, R. W., Phillips, R. T., Kett, K. G., Hill, T., Perper, E., Young, E., Leland, O. S., & Jr , . (1988). Angina and exertional myocardial ischemia in diabetic and nondiabetic patients: assessment by exercise thallium scintigraphy. *Annals of Internal Medicine*, 108(2), 170-175.

[52] Ambepityia, G., Kopelman, P. G., Ingram, D., Swash, M., Mills, P. G., & Timmis, A. D. (1990). Exertional myocardial ischemia in diabetes: a quantitative analysis of anginal perceptual threshold and the influence of autonomic function. *Journal of American College of Cardiology*, 15(1), 72-77.

[53] Murray, D. P., O'Brien, T., Mulrooney, R., & O'Sullivan, D. J. (1990). Autonomic dysfunction and silent myocardial ischaemia on exercise testing in diabetes mellitus. *Diabetic Medicine*, 7(7), 580-584.

[54] Froy, O. (2010). Metabolism and circadian rhythms-implications for obesity. *Endocrine Reviews*, 31(1), 1-24.

[55] Espino, J., Pariente, J. A., & Rodríguez, A. B. (2011). Role of melatonin on diabetes-related metabolic disorders. *World Journal of Diabetes*, 2(6), 82-91.

[56] Ziegler, D. (1994). Diabetic cardiovascular autonomic neuropathy: prognosis, diagnosis and treatment. *Diabetes/Metabolism Reviews*, 10(4), 339-383.

[57] Taskiran, M., Fritz-Hansen, T., Rasmussen, V., Larsson, H. B., & Hilsted, J. (2002). Decreased myocardial perfusion reserve in diabetic autonomic neuropathy. *Diabetes*, 51(11), 3306-3310.

[58] Taskiran, M., Rasmussen, V., Rasmussen, B., Fritz-Hansen, T., Larsson, H. B., Jensen, G. B., & Hilsted, J. (2004). Left ventricular dysfunction in normotensive Type 1 diabetic patients: the impact of autonomic neuropathy. *Diabetic Medicine*, 21(6), 524-530.

[59] Nishimura, M., Hashimoto, T., Kobayashi, H., Fukuda, T., Okino, K., Yamamoto, N., Nakamura, N., Yoshikawa, T., Takahashi, H., & Ono, T. (2004). Association between cardiovascular autonomic neuropathy and left ventricular hypertrophy in diabetic haemodialysis patients. *Nephrology, dialysis, transplantation*, 19(10), 2532-2538.

[60] Maser, R. E., Mitchell, Vinik. A. I., & Freeman, R. (2003). The association between cardiovascular autonomic neuropathy and mortality in individuals with diabetes. *Diabetes Care*, 26(6), 1895-1901.

[61] Valensi, P., Sachs, Harfouche. B., Lormeau, B., Paries, J., Cosson, E., Paycha, F., Leutenegger, M., & Attali, J. R. (2001). Predictive value of cardiac autonomic neuropathy in diabetic patients with or without silent myocardial ischemia. *Diabetes Care*, 24(2), 339-343.

[62] Wheeler, S. G., Ahroni, J. H., & Boyko, E. J. (2002). Prospective study of autonomic neuropathy as a predictor of mortality in patients with diabetes. *Diabetes Research and Clinical Practice*, 58(2), 131-138.

[63] Whang, W., & Bigger, J. T. (2003). Coparison of the prognostic value of RR-interval variability after acute myocardial infarction in patients with versus those without diabetes mellitus. *The American Journal of Cardiology*, 92(3), 247-251.

[64] Haffner, S. M., Lehto, S., Rönnemaa, T., Pyörälä, K., & Laakso, M. (1998). Mortality from coronary heart disease in subjects with type 2 diabetes and in nondiabetic subjects with and without prior myocardial infarction. *The New England Journal of Medicine*, 339(4), 229-234.

[65] Cohen, J. A., Estacio, R. O., Lundgren, R. A., Esler, A. L., & Schrier, R. W. (2003). Diabetic autonomic neuropathy is associated with an increased incidence of strokes. *Autonomic neuroscience*, 108(1-2), 73 EOF-8 EOF.

[66] Lee, K. H., Jang, H. J., Kim, Y. H., Lee, E. J., Choe, Y. S., Choi, Y., Lee, M. G., Lee, S. H., & Kim, B. T. (2003). Prognostic value of cardiac autonomic neuropathy independent and incremental to perfusion defects in patients with diabetes and suspected coronary artery disease. *The American Journal of Cardiology*, 92(12), 1458-1461.

[67] Suarez, G. A., Clark, V. M., Norell, J. E., Kottke, T. E., Callahan, O'Brien. P. C., Low, P. A., & Dyck, P. J. (2005). Sudden cardiac death in diabetes mellitus: risk factors in the Rochester diabetic neuropathy study. *Journal of Neurology, Neurosurgery, and Psychiatry*, 76(2), 240-245.

[68] Astrup, A. S., Tarnow, L., Rossing, P., Hansen, B. V., Hilsted, J., & Parving, H. H. (2006). Cardiac autonomic neuropathy predicts cardiovascular morbidity and mortality in type 1 diabetic patients with diabetic nephropathy. *Diabetes Care*, 29(2), 334-339.

[69] Astrup, A. S., Nielsen, F. S., Rossing, P., Ali, S., Kastrup, J., Smidt, U. M., & Parving, H. H. (2007). Predictors of mortality in patients with type 2 diabetes with or without diabetic nephropathy: a follow-up study. *Journal of Hypertension*, 25(12), 2479-2485.

[70] Ziegler, D., Zentai, Perz. S., Rathmann, W., Haastert, B., Döring, A., & Meisinger, C. (2008). Prediction of mortality using measures of cardiac autonomic dysfunction in the diabetic and nondiabetic population: the MONICA/KORA Augsburg Cohort Study. *Diabetes Care*, 31(3), 556-561.

[71] Ko, S. H., Song, K. H., Park, S. A., Kim, S. R., Cha, B. Y., Son, H. Y., Moon, K. W., Yoo, K. D., Park, Y. M., Cho, J. H., Yoon, K. H., & Ahn, Y. B. (2008). Cardiovascular autonomic dysfunction predicts acute ischaemic stroke in patients with Type 2 diabetes mellitus: a 7-year follow-up study. *Diabetic Medicine*, 25(10), 1171-1177.

[72] Beijers, H. J., Ferreira, I., Bravenboer, B., Dekker, J. M., Nijpels, G., Heine, R. J., & Stehouwer, C. D. (2009). Microalbuminuria and cardiovascular autonomic dysfunction are independently associated with cardiovascular mortality: evidence for distinct pathways: the Hoorn Study. *Diabetes Care*, 32(9), 1698-1703.

[73] May, O., & Arildsen, H. (2011). Long-term predictive power of simple function tests for cardiovascular autonomic neuropathy in diabetes: a population-based study. *Acta Diabetologica*, 48(4), 311-316.

[74] May, O., & Arildsen, H. (2011). Long-term predictive power of heart rate variability on all-cause mortality in the diabetic population. *Acta Diabetologica*, 48(1), 55-59.

[75] May, O., & Arildsen, H. (2012). Simple function tests for autonomic neuropathy have a higher predictive value on all-cause mortality in diabetes compared to 24-h heart rate variability. *Journal of Diabetes and its Complications*, 26(3), 246-250.

[76] Aschengrau, A., Seage, G. R., & 3rd , . (2008). Essentials of epidemiology in public health. London; Jones & Bartlett Publishers;.

Chapter 15

Antioxidants in Decelerating Diabetic Nephropathy

Wen-Chin Lee, Chau-Jong Wang and Huei-Jane Lee

Additional information is available at the end of the chapter

http://dx.doi.org/10.5772/45927

1. Introduction

Diabetes mellitus (DM) is a group of metabolic diseases characterized with inappropriate hyperglycemia due to either a deficiency of insulin secretion or a combination of insulin resistance and inadequate insulin secretion (Masharani, 2008). Type 1 diabetes is caused by absolute deficiency of insulin secretion. Individuals at risk of developing this type of diabetes are found with serologic evidence of an autoimmune process occurring in the pancreatic islets and by genetic markers. In type 2 diabetes, it is a combination of resistance to insulin action and an inadequate compensatory insulin secretion response (American Diabetes Association, 2008). Diabetic nephropathy, one of the common complications of diabetes, has become the leading cause of end-stage renal failure in many countries (Chen et al., 2005). In general, about 1 out of 3 patients with type 1 or type 2 diabetes proceed to developing significant diabetic nephropathy (Zipp and Schelling, 2003). It is believed that the pathophysiologic mechanisms of renal disorder are similar in both types of diabetes (Kern et al., 1999). The pathogenesis and clinical course of diabetic nephropathy can be monitored by structural and hemodynamic changes. The earliest changes is an increase in glomerular filtration rate (GFR), also call "hyperfiltration" stage, which is followed by detectable glomerular lesions with normal albumin excretion rate. The next change is the development of microalbuminuria. Once microalbuminuria persist, both changes in glomerular structure, such as mesangial expansion and basement membrane thickening, and permeability happened, which is referred as "incipient nephropathy". Diabetic subjects with persistent microalbuminuria are at increased risk for "overt diabetic nephropathy". At this stage, prominent proteinuria, hypertension, and renal insufficiency progressed. The pathological findings in this stage are glomerular basement membrane (GBM) thickening, mesangial expansion and resulting in diffuse and/or nodular glomerulosclerosis, afferent and efferent arteriolar hyalinosis, and tubulointerstitial fibrosis (Cooper and Gilbert, 2003). After several years of persistent proteinuria, progression to end-stage renal disease will occur (Caramori and Mauer, 2001).

Advanced diabetic glomerulopathy is commonly characterized by diffuse glomerulosclerosis and may sometimes exhibit a distinctive morphological appearance, namely, the nodular form of glomerulosclerosis, as first described by Kimmelstiel and Wilson in 1936 (Kimmelstiel and Wilson, 1936; Kern et al., 1999). The stages of diabetic nephropathy are shown in Table 1 (Vora and Ibrahim, 2003).

Stage	Renal manifestation
1	Renal hyperfiltration (GFR↑) Renal hypertrophy
2	Silent stage Renal hyperfiltration (GFR*↑); Normal UAER*, blood pressure Early histologic changes: non-specific increase in basement membrane thickness, increase mesangial matrix
3	Microalbuminuria (UAER 30-300mg/24 h) or incipient nephropathy GFR may elevated or reduced into normal range. Histology: mesangial expansion, glomerular basement membrane thickening, arteriolar hyalinosis
4	Established or overt nephropathy (Proteinuria, nephrotic syndrome) GFR decline, Hypertension Histology: mesangial nodules (Kimmelstiel-Wilson lesions), tubulointerstitial fibrosis
5	ESRD***

* GFR, glomerular filtration rate

**UAER, urine albumin excretion rate

***ESRD, end stage renal disease

Table 1. Natural course of diabetic nephropathy in type 1 diabetes

The current strategies to treat diabetic nephropathy include intensive glycemic control, antihypertensive treatment with a particular focus on the interruption of renin-angiotensin-aldosterone system (RAS), restriction of dietary protein, and treatment of hyperlipidemia. There are several new approaches to the treatment of diabetic nephropathy based on an ever-growing mechanistic understanding of the causes of diabetic nephropathy by the specific pathogenic roles. These agents include pharmacologic inhibitors of advanced glycation end products (AGEs) formation, protein kinase C (PKC), oxidative stress, and transforming growth factor β (TGF-β) (Williams and Stanton, 2005).

2. Animal models of diabetes mellitus

Type 1 diabetes mellitus is typically an immune mediated destruction of the pancreatic

http://dx.doi.org/10.5772/45927

β cells. Type 2 diabetes mellitus is characterized by insulin resistance and insulin secretion impairment. Animal models have been used extensively in the field of diabetes study. The current available animal models of type 1 and type 2 diabetes are shown in Table 2 (Rees and Alcolado, 2005).

Type 1	BB (Bio breeding) rat
	Chinese hamster
	Celebes black ape
	Keeshond dog
	LETL (Long Evans Tokushima lean) rat
	New Zeland white rabbit
	NOD (non-obese diabetic) mouse
	Streptozotocin-induced rats
Type 2	CBA/Ca mouse
	db/db mouse
	Diabetic Torri rat
	GK (GotoKakizaki) rat
	Israeli sand rat
	KK mouse
	New Zeland obese mouse
	NSY (Nagoya-Shibata-Yasuda) mouse
	Ob/Ob mouse
	OLETF (Otsuka Long-Evans Tokushima fatty) rat
	Zucker rat

Table 2. Animal models of type 1 and 2 diabetes mellitus

3. The molecular mechanism of oxidative stress in diabetic nephropathy

There are four major biochemical pathways considered to lead to the development of diabetic complications associated with hyperglycemia, (1) the polyol pathway, glucose is converted to sorbitol and then metabolized to fructose. Advanced glycation end products (AGE) and reactive oxygen species (ROS) formation also occurs via this pathway, (2) the hexosamine pathway, fructose-6-phosphate is converted to glucosamine intermediates and the production of ROS is subsequently increased, (3) the protein kinase C (PKC) pathway, glucose is converted to glyceraldehyde-3-phosphate and leads to the formation of diacylglycerol (DAG). The elevation of intracellular DAG levels activate PKC, and then activate NADPH oxidase to induce ROS, (4) the formation of advanced glycation end products (AGEs), interaction of AGEs with the receptors of advanced glycation end-products (RAGE) results in ROS activation (Stirban et al., 2008; Shah et al., 2009; Forbes et al., 2008; Brownlee, 2005; Kanwar et al., 2008; Singh et al., 2011).

Increased oxidative stress has been a widely accepted participant in the development and progression of diabetes and its complications (Maritim et al., 2003). ROS are activated in glomerular mesangial and tubular epithelial cells by high glucose, AGE, and cytokines (Park et al., 1999). Hyperglycemia activates the glycolytic pathway and excess generation of mitochondrial ROS initiates a vicious circle by activating several signaling to increase protein kinase C (PKC), and stimulating NADPH oxidase to induce ROS generation (Johansen et al., 2005). Free radicals has been found to be formed disproportionately increase in diabetic subjects by glucose oxidation, nonenzymaticglycation of proteins, and then oxidative degradation of glycated proteins. Excessively amount of free radicals induce damage to cellular proteins, membrane lipids, nucleic acids, and then cell death (Maritim et al., 2003). Besides, increased ROS can cause vascular endothelium abnormalities, reacting directly with nitric oxide (NO) to produce cytotoxic peroxynitrite and increasing reactivity to vasoconstrictors and modification of extracellular matrix proteins (Schnackenberg, 2002). ROS can also damage endothelial cells indirectly by stimulating expression of various genes involved in inflammatory pathway (Baldwin, 1996). Previous study finds that high glucose induces ROS and then up-regulates TGF-β1 and extracellular matrix (ECM) expression in the glomerular mesangial cell (Lee et al., 2003). There are also evidences that antioxidants can effectively inhibit high glucose induced TGF-β1 and fibronectin up-regulation (Ha et al., 1997). Ha et al. (2002) reported that ROS mediate high glucose-induced activation of NF-κB and NF-κB dependent monocyte chemoattractant protein (MCP)-1 expression. NF-κB, a nuclear transcription factor, can initiate the transcription of genes associated with inflammatory response. It is induced by various cell stress-associated stimuli including growth factors, vasoactive agents, cytokines, and oxidative stress (Kuhad and Chopra, 2009). Advanced glycation end products induced by hyperglycemia stimulate NF-κB activation, which sustains the activation of NF-κB in diabetes (Gao et al., 2006). Increased steady-state mRNA levels of inflammatory genes have been shown to associate with interstitial fibrosis and progressive human diabetic nephropathy (Kuhad and Chopra, 2009).

TGF-β plays an important role in the development of renal hypertrophy and accumulation of extracellular matrix (ECM) components in diabetes mellitus (Wolf and Ziyadeh, 1999). The expression of TGF-β was found increased in diabetic nephropathy of experimental animals and in humans (Park et al., 1997; Yamamoto et al., 1993; Sharma et al., 1997; Shankland et al., 1994). Treatment with anti-TGF-β antibody has been documented that it attenuated the effect of high glucose induced cellular hypertrophy *in vitro* and in streptozotocin-induced diabetic mice (Wolf et al., 1992; Ziyadeh et al., 1994; Sharma et al., 1996). TGF-β is also the key regulator of ECM remodeling in mesangium causing mesangial expansion and inducing the process of epithelial-mesenchymal transition (EMT) causing tubulointerstitial fibrosis (Ziyadeh et al., 2000; Oldfield et al., 2001). As the accumulation of ECM and persistence of tubulointerstitial fibrosis, the renal function progress to end-stage renal disease (ESRD). The relation between oxidative stress and diabetic nephropathy are shown in Figure 1 (Shah et al, 2007).

http://dx.doi.org/10.5772/45927

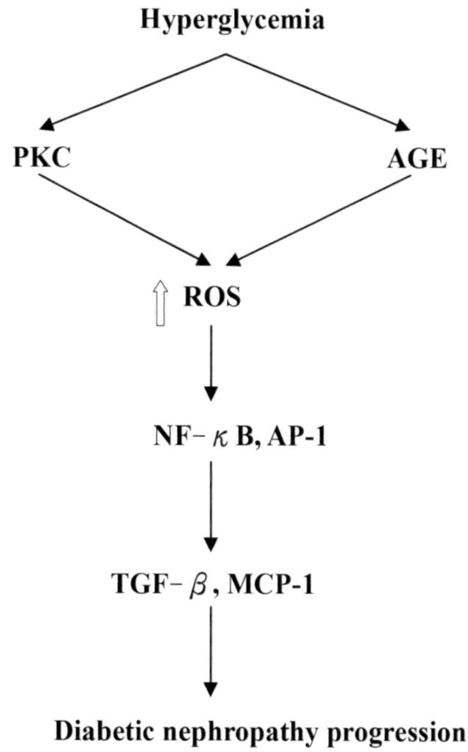

Figure 1. The relation between oxidative stress and diabetic nephropathy* *PKC, protein kinase C; AGE, advanced glycation end products; ROS, reactive oxygen species; NF-κB, nulcear factor-kappa B; AP-1,activator protein-1; TGF-β, transforming growth factor-beta; MCP-1, monocyte chemotactic protein-1

4. Improvement of antioxidantive status in diabetic nephropathy

There are many evidences suggest that ROS play an important role in the pathogenesis of diabetic nephropathy (Rosen et al., 2001). To prevent the development and progression of diabetic nephropathy, it would be effective in combing the strategies to prevent overproduction of ROS and to increase the removal of preformed ROS. (Ha et al., 2008). Some natural products were proved to possess the ability to decelerate diabetic nephropathy via reducing oxidative status. The flower of *Hibiscus sabdariffa*Linnaeus calyx (family Malvaceae, local name Karkaday) is commonly used in cold and hot beverages and as a supplement due to its perceived potential of health benefits. The flower extract has been reported to decrease blood pressure, and have antitumor characteristics as well as immune-modulating and anti-leukemic effects (Haji Faraji and Haji Tarkhani, 1999; Tseng et al., 2000). *Hibiscus sabdariffa*L. extract contains polyphenolic acids, flavonoids, protocatechuic acid (PCA) and anthocyanins. *Hibiscus sabdariffa*L. extract has been found to contain various polyphenols and was shown to have antioxidative potential to inhibit the development of atherosclerosis in cholesterol-fed rabbits, LDL oxidation and ox-LDL-mediated macrophage apoptosis (Chen et al., 2003; Chang et al., 2006). Wang et al. (2009) demonstrated that aqueous extract of *Hibiscus sabdariffa* L. (HSE) is capable of increasing catalase and glutathione activities significantly in diabetic kidney. In histological examination, HSE improves hydropic change of renal proximal convoluted tubules in diabetic rats. HSE was also revealed to up-regulate Akt/Bad/ 14-3-3 ▪ and NF-κB-mediated transcription in diabetic nephropathy. Luteolin is a plant-derived flavonoid, it has various biological activities including anti-inflammatory (Jang et al., 2008), antimutagenic, and antitumorigenic properties (Ross and Kasum, 2002). It also possesses direct antioxidant activity (L´opez-L´azaro, 2009), and may be useful in treatment of many chronic disease associated with oxidative stress, such as cardiovascular diseases (McCord, 1985; Jeroudi et al., 1994), liver diseases (Comporti, 1985; Poli et al., 1987), diabetes (Oberley, 1988), and aging (Harman, 1981). Wang et al. (2011) demonstrated that luteolin has protecting effect against development of diabetic nephropathy by changing the superoxide dismutase (SOD) activity, the malondialdehyde (MDA) content, and expression of Heme Oxygenase-1 (HO-1) protein.

On the other hand, some evidences show the exogenous or endogenous antioxidants also can reduce diabetic nephropathy. Oxidative stress via nicotinamide adenine dinucleotide phosphate (NADPH) oxidase and vascular endothelial growth factor (VEGF) pathway are documented to play important roles in the development of diabetic nephropathy. Nam et al. (2009) showed the effects of apocynin, a NADPH oxidase inhibitor, on diabetic nephropathy. They found that apocynincan not significantly decrease serum glucose levels but reduce urinary protein and albumin excretions. It is improved in glomerular and mesangial expansion as the apocynin treatment. Apocynin also decreased glomerular VEGF expression and reduced the concentration of 24 h urinary 8-OHdG and MDA. Additionally, Lee et al. (2005) demonstrated that antioxidant taurine prevented glomerular hypertrophy, mesangial expansion, and proteinuria in diabetic rats. Overexpression of catalytic antioxidants was also shown to protect against diabetic injury in several transgenic animals. Craven et al. (2001) showed that diabetic mice transgenic for Cu/Zn SOD had significantly lower urinary albumin excretion, glomerular hypertrophy, and glomerular expression of TGF-β1 and collagen IV protein compared to non-transgenic mice. Hamada et al. (2007) demonstrated that overexpression a small antioxidant, thioredoxin 1, effectively inhibited 8-OHdG in the kidney, albuminuria, mesangial expansion, and tubular injury in diabetic mice. Du et al. (2003) found that overexpression of MnSOD in bovine aortic endothelial cells prevented high glucose-induced activation of PKC, NK-kB, hexosamine, and advanced glycation end product (AGE) pathways. Brezniceanu et al. (2007) demonstrated that renal catalase overexpression in db/db mice attenuated ROS generation, angiotensinogen, proapoptotic gene expression and apoptosis in the kidneys of diabetic mice *in vivo*.

Although strict glycemic control is very important in DM patients, many of the current standard therapeutic approaches may also ameliorate oxidative stress as pleiotropic effects (Singh et al., 2011), such as angiotensin-2 converting enzyme (ACE) inhibitors(Kobayashi et al., 2006), angiotensin-2 receptor blockers (ARB) (Ogawa et al., 2006) and aldosterone blockers (spironolactone) (Takebayashi et al., 2006). They activate eNOS to increase bioavailability of nitric oxide, inhibit synthesis of angiotensin 2 and TGF-β and to decelerate or prevent tubulointerstitial fibrosis in diabetic nephropathy, accompanied with control of systemic and intrarenal blood pressure. Cilostazol is a specific inhibitor of phosphodiesterase 3 (PDE 3). Its major effects are prevention of platelet aggregation and dilation of blood vessels via an increase in tissue cAMP levels (Matsumoto et al., 2005). Cilostazol was shown to inhibit vascular smooth muscle cell proliferation *in vitro* as well as suppress neointimal formation in balloon-injured rat carotid arteries due to its antiplatelet and vasodilator properties (Takahashi et al., 1992; Ishizaka et al., 1999). Our previous study showed that cilostazol decreases reactive oxygen species activity significantly in the kidneys of diabetic rats and improves urine albumin/creatinine ratio. Cilostazol also can improve the diabetes-caused increasing glomerular size, TGF-β, and NF-kB in early diabetic nephropathy (Lee et al., 2010). The lipid-lowering agents such as statins, which can inhibit HMG-CoA reductase to be demonstrated to activate eNOS, maintain glomerular filtration rate and renal cortical blood flow, and further to ameliorate glomerular lesions(Usui et al., 2003; Endres and Laufs, 2004). Benfotiamine was used in the treatment of diabetic nephropathy, it was also demonstrated to reduce ROS formation and may decrease hyperfiltration and proteinuria in patients with diabetic nephropathy(Babaei-Jadidi et al., 2003). Potential therapies in these ideal antioxidants would influence the pathways of ROS generation to decelerate diabetic nephropathy.

Author details

Wen-Chin Lee[1,2*], Chau-Jong Wang[3] and Huei-Jane Lee[3]

1 Division of Nephrology, Department of Internal Medicine, Show Chwan Memorial Hospital, Changhua, Taiwan

2 General Education Center, Central Taiwan University of Science and Technology, Taichung, Taiwan

3 Institute of Biochemistry and Biotechnology, Medical College, Chung Shan Medical University, Taichung, Taiwan

References

[1] American Diabetes Association(2008). Diagnosis and classification of diabetes mellitus.Diabetes Care31: SS60., 55.

[2] Babaei-Jadidi, R., Karachalias, N., Ahmed, N., Battah, S., & Thornalley, P. J. (2003). Prevention of incipient diabetic nephropathy by high-dose thiamine and benfotiamine. *Diabetes*, 52, 2110-2120.

[3] Baldwin AS Jr(1996). The NF-KB and IKB proteins: new discoveries and insights. Annu Rev Immunol, 14, 649-683.

[4] Brezniceanu, M. L., Liu, F., Wei, C. C., Tran, S., Sachetelli, S., Zhang, S. L., Guo, D. F., Filep, J. G., Ingefinger, J. R., & Chan, J. S. (2007). Catalase overexpression attenuates angiotensinogen expression and apoptosis in diabetic mice. Kidney Int, 71, 912-923.

[5] Brownlee, M. (2005). The pathobiology of diabetic complications: a unifying mechanism. *Diabetes*, 54, 1615-1625.

[6] Caramori, M. L., & Mauer, M. (2001). Diabetic nephropathy. in Primer on kidney diseases,3rd edition (Greenberg A, Cheung AK, Coffman TM, Falk RJ, and Jennette JC eds) National Kidney Fundation, Florida., 212-218.

[7] Chang YC, Huang KX, Huang AC, Ho YC, and Wang CJ(2006). Hibiscus anthocyanins- rich extract inhibited LDL oxidation and oxLDL-mediated macrophages apoptosi. s. Food ChemToxicol, 44, 1015-1023.

[8] Chen CC, Hsu JD, Wang SF, Chiang HC, Yang MY, Kao ES, Ho YC, and Wang CJ(2003). Hibiscus sabdariffaExtract inhibits the development of atherosclerosis in cholesterol-fed rabbits. J Agric Food Chem, 51, 5472-5477.

[9] Chen HC, Guh JY, Chang JM, Hsieh MC, Shin SJ, and Lai YH(2005). Role of lipid control in diabetic nephropathy. Kidney IntSuppl94: SS62., 60.

[10] Comporti, M. (1985). Lipid peroxidation and cellular damage in toxic liver injury.Lab Invest, 53, 599-623.

[11] Cooper ME, and Gilbert RE(2003). Pathogenesis, prevention, and treatment of di. abetic nephropathy, In Comprehensive clinical nephrology 2nd edition (Johnson RJ, and Feehally J, eds) Mosby, Edinburgh., 439-450.

[12] Craven PA, Melhem MF, Phillips SL, and DeRubertis FR. (2001). Overexpression of Cu2+/Zn2+ superoxide dismutase protects against early diabetic glomerular injury in transgenic mice. *Diabetes*, 50, 2114-2125.

[13] Du, X., Matsumura, T., Edelstein, D., Rossetti, L., Zsengelle´, r. Z., Szabo´, C., & Brownlee, M. (2003). Inhibition of GAPDH activity by poly(ADP-ribose) polymerase activates three major pathways of hyperglycemic damage in endothelial cells. J Clin Invest, 112, 1049-1057.

[14] Endres, M., & Laufs, U. (2004). Effects of statins on endothelium and signaling mechanisms. Stroke35 (Suppl 1): , 2708 EOF-11 EOF.

[15] Forbes JM, Coughlan MT, and Cooper ME. (2008). Oxidative stress as a major culprit in kidney disease in diabetes. *diabetes*, 1446-1454.

[16] Gao, L., Wang, F., Wang, B., Gong, B., Zhang, J., Zhang, X., & Zhao, J. (2006). Cilostazol protects diabetic rats from vascular inflammation via nuclear factor-KB-dependent down-regulation of vascular cell adhesion molecule-1 expression. J PharmacolExpTher, 318, 53-58.

[17] Ha, H., Lee, S. H., & Kim, K. H. (1997). Effects of rebamipide in a model of experimental diabetes and on the synthesis of transforming growth factor-β and fibronec-

tin, and lipid peroxidation induced by high glucose in cultured mesangial cells. J PharmacolExpTher, 281, 1457-1462.

[18] Ha, H., Yu, M. R., Choi, Y. J., Kitamura, M., & Lee, H. B. (2002). Role of high glucose-induced nuclear factor-KB activation in monocyte chemoattractant protein-I expression by mesangial cells. J Am SocNephrol, 13, 894-902.

[19] Ha, H., Hwang, I. A., Park, J. H., & Lee, H. B. (2008). Role of reactive oxygen species in the pathogenesis of diabetic nephropathy. Diabetes Res ClinPract82 Suppl 1: S, 42-5.

[20] Haji, Faraji. M., & Haji, Tarkhani. A. (1999). The effect of sour tea (Hibiscus sabdariffa) on essential hypertension. J Ethnopharmacol, 65, 231-236.

[21] Hamada, Y., Miyata, S., Nii-Kono, T., Kitazawa, R., Kitazawa, S., Higo, S., Fukunaga, M., Ueyama, S., Nakamura, H., Yodoi, J., Fukagawa, M., & Kasuga, M. (2007). Overexpression of thioredoxin1 in transgenic mice suppresses development of diabetic nephropathy. Nephrol Dial Transplant, 22, 1547-1557.

[22] Harman, D. (1981). The aging process. ProcNatlAcadSci USA, 78, 7124-7128.

[23] Ishizaka, N., Taguchi, J., Kimura, Y., Ikari, Y., Aizawa, T., Togo, M., Miki, K., Kurokawa, K., & Ohno, M. (1999). Effects of a single local administration of cilostazol on neointimal formation in balloon-injured rat carotid artery. *Atherosclerosis*, 142, 41-46.

[24] Jang, S., Kelley, K. W., & Johnson, R. W. (2008). Luteolin reduces IL-6 production in microglia by inhibiting JNK phosphorylation and activation of AP-1. ProcNatlAcadSci USA, 105, 7534-7539.

[25] Jeroudi, M. O., Hartley, C. J., & Bolli, R. (1994). Myocardial reperfusion injury: role of oxygen radicals and potential therapy with antioxidants. Am J Cardiol73: , 2B EOF-7B EOF.

[26] Johansen, J. S., Harris, A. K., Rychly, D. J., & Ergul, A. (2005). Oxidative stress and the use of antioxidants in diabetes: linking basic science to clinical practice. CardiovascDiabetol4: 5.

[27] Kanwar, Y. S., Wada, J., Sun, L., Xie, P., Wallner, E. I., Chen, S., Chugh, S., & Danesh, F. R. (2008). Diabetic nephropathy: mechanisms of renal disease progression. ExpBiol Med, 233, 4-11.

[28] Kern, W. F., Laszik, Z. G., Nadasdy, T., Silva, F. G., Bane, B. L., & Pitha, J. V. (1999). The kidney in metabolic disorder-- diabetes mellitus, hyperuricemia, oxalosis, nephrocalcinosis, and nephrolithiasis. in Atlas of renal pathology (Kern WF, Laszik ZG, Nadasdy T, Silva FG, Bane BL, and Pitha JV, eds) W.B. Saunders company, Philadelphia., 97-112.

[29] Kimmelstiel, P., & Wilson, C. (1936). Intercapillary lesions in glomeruli of the kidney. Am. J Pathol, 12, 83-97.

[30] Kobayashi, N., Honda, T., Yoshida, K., Nakano, S., Ohno, T., Tsubokou, T., Matsuoka, H., & (200, . (2006). Critical role of bradykinin-eNOS and oxidative stress-LOX-1 pathway in cardiovascular remodeling under chronic angiotensin-converting enzyme inhibition. *Atherosclerosis*, 187, 92-100.

[31] Kuhad, A., & Chopra, K. (2009). Attenuation of diabetic nephropathy by tocotrienol: involvement of NF-KB signaling pathway. Life Sci, 84, 296-301.

[32] Lee, E. A., Seo, J. Y., Jiang, Z., Yu, M. R., Kwon, M. K., Ha, H., & Lee, H. B. (2005). Reactive oxygen species mediate high glucose-induced plasminogen activator inhibitor-1 upregulation in mesangial cells and in diabetic kidney. Kidney Int, 67, 1762-1771.

[33] Lee, H. B., Yu, M. R., Yang, Y., Jiang, Z., & Ha, H. (2003). Reactive oxygen species-regulated signaling pathways in diabetic nephropathy.J Am SocNephrol14: S, 241-245.

[34] Lee, W. C., Chen, H. C., Wang, C. Y., Lin, P. Y., Ou, T. T., Chen, C. C., Wen, M. C., Wang, J., & Lee, H. J. (2010). Cilostazol ameliorates nephropathy in type 1 diabetic rats involving mprovement of oxidative stress and regulation of TGF-β and NF-B.BiosciBiotechnolBiochem, 74, 1355-1361.

[35] L´opez-L´azaro, M. (2009). Distribution and biological activities of the flavonoid luteol in Mini Rev Med Chem, 9, 31-59.

[36] Maritim AC, Sanders RA, and Watkins JB 3rd(2003). Diabetes, oxidative stress, and antioxidants: A review. J BiochemMolToxicol, 17, 24-38.

[37] Masharani, U. (2008). Diabetes Mellitus and hypoglycemia, in Current medical diagnosis and treatment, 47. th edition (McPhee SJ, Papadakis MA, and Tierney LM, eds), McGraw-Hill, New York., 1032-1073.

[38] Matsumoto, T., Kobayashi, T., Wakabayashi, K., & Kamata, K. (2005). Cilostazol improves endothelium-derived hyperpolarizing factor-type relaxation in mesenteric arteries from diabetic rats. Am J Physiol Heart CircPhysiol289: HH1940., 1933.

[39] McCord JM(1985). Oxygen-derived free radicals in postischemic tissue injury. N Engl J Med, 312, 159-163.

[40] Nam SM, Lee MY, Koh JH, Park JH, Shin JY, Shin YG, Koh SB, Lee EY, and Chung CH(2009). Effects of NADPH oxidase inhibitor on diabetic nephropathy in OLETF rats: The role of reducing oxidative stress in its protective property. Diabetes Res ClinPract, 83, 176-182.

[41] Oberley LW(1988). Free radicals and diabetes.Free RadicBiol Med, 5, 113-124.

[42] Ogawa, S., Mori, T., Nako, K., Keto, T., Takeuchi, K., & Ito, S. (2006). Angiotensin II type 1 receptor blockers reduce urinary oxidative stress markers in hypertensive diabetic nephropathy. *Hypertension*, 47, 699-705.

[43] Oldfield, Bach. L. A., Forbes, J. M., Nikolic-Paterson, D., Mc Robert, A., Thallas, V., Atkins, R. C., Osicka, T., Jerums, G., & Copper, . (2001). Advanced glycation end products cause epithelial-myofibroblast transdifferentiation via the receptor for advanced glycation end products (RAGE). J Clin Invest, 108, 1853-1863.

[44] Park, I. S., Kiyomoto, H., Abboud, S. L., & Abboud, H. E. (1997). Expression of transforming growth factor-β and type IV collagen in early streptozotocin- induced diabetes. Diabetes, 46, 473-480.

[45] Park JY, Ha SW, and King GL(1999). The role of protein kinase C activation in the pathogenesis of diabetic vascular complications.Perit Dial Int19: SS227., 222.

[46] Poli, G., Albano, E., & Dianzani, M. U. (1987). The role of lipid peroxidation in liver damage. ChemPhys Lipids, 45, 117-142.

[47] Rees DA and Alcolado JC(2005). Animal models of diabetes mellitus. Diabet Med , 22, 359-370.

[48] Ro°, sen. P., Nawroth, P. P., King, G., Mo°, ller. W., Tritschler, H. J., & Packer, L. (2001). The role of oxidative stress in the onset and progression of diabetes and its complications: a summary of a Congress Series sponsored by UNESCO-MCBN, the American Diabetes Association and the German Diabetes Society. Diabetes Metab Res Rev, 17, 189-212.

[49] Ross JA, and Kasum CM(2002). Dietary flavonoids: bioavailability, metabolic effects, and safety. Annu Rev Nutr, 22, 19-34.

[50] Schnackenberg CG(2002). Physiological and pathophysiological roles of oxygen radicals in the renal microvasculature.Am J PhysiolRegulIntegr Comp Physiol282: RR342., 335.

[51] Shah IM, Mackay SP, and McKay GA(2009). Therapeutic strategies in the treatment of diabetic nephropathy- a translational medicine approach. Curr Med Chem, 16, 997-1016.

[52] Shah, S. V., Baliga, R., Rajapurkar, M., & Fonseca, V. A. (2007). Oxidants in chronic kidney disease. J Am SocNephrol, 18, 16-28.

[53] Shankland, S. J., Scholey, J. W., Ly, H., & Thai, K. (1994). Expression of transforming growth factor-β1 during diabetic renal hypertrophy.Kidney Int, 46, 430-442.

[54] Sharma, K., Jin, Y., Guo, J., & Ziyadeh, F. N. (1996). Neutralization of TGF-beta by anti-TGF-beta antibody attenuates kidney hypertrophy and the enhanced extracellular matrix gene expression in STZ-induced diabetic mice. *Diabetes*, 45, 522-530.

[55] Sharma, K., Ziyadeh, F. N., Alzahabi, B., Mc Gowan, T. A., Kapoor, S., Kurnik, B. R., Kurnik, P. B., & Weisberg, L. S. (1997). Increased renal production of transforming growth factor-beta 1 in patients with type II diabetes. Diabetes, 46, 854-859.

[56] Singh, D. K., Winocour, P., & Farrington, K. (2011). Oxidative stress in early diabetic nephropathy: fueling the fire. Nat Rev Endocrinol, 7, 176-184.

[57] Stirban, A., Rosen, P., & Tschoepe, D. (2008). Complications of type 1 diabetes: new molecular findings. Mt Sinai J Med, 75, 328-351.

[58] Takahashi, S., Oida, K., Fujiwara, R., Maeda, H., Hayashi, S., Takai, H., Tamai, T., Nakai, T., & Miyabo, S. (1992). Effect of cilostazol, a cyclic AMP phosphodiesterase inhibitor, on the proliferation of rat aortic smooth muscle cells in culture. J Cardiovasc Pharmacol , 20, 900-906.

[59] Takebayashi, K., Matsumoto, S., Aso, Y., & Inukai, T. (2006). Aldosterone blockade attenuates urinary monocyte chemoattractant protein-1 and oxidative stress in patients with type 2 diabetes complicated by diabetic nephropathy. J Clin Endocrinol Metab , 91, 2214-2217.

[60] Tseng TH, Kao TW, Chu CY, Chou FP, Lin WL, and Wang CJ(2000). Induction of apoptosis Hibiscus protocatechuic acid in human leukemia cells via reduction of retinoblastoma (RB) phosphorylation and Bcl-2 expression. Bi. ochemPharmacol, 60, 307-315.

[61] Usui, H., Shikata, K., Matsuda, M., Okada, S., Ogawa, D., Yamashita, T., Hida, K., Satoh, M., Wada, J., & Makino, H. (2003). HMG-CoA reductase inhibitor ameliorates diabetic nephropathy by its pleiotropic effects in rats. Nephro. Dial Transplant , 18, 265-272.

[62] Vora JP, and Ibrahim HAA(2003). Clinical manifestations and natural history of diabetic nephropathy, in Comprehensive clinical nephrology, 2nd edition (Johnson RJ, and Feehally J, eds), Mosby, Edinburgh., 425-437.

[63] Wang, G. G., Lu, X. H., Li, W., Zhao, X., & Zhang, C. (2011). Protective effects of luteolin on diabetic nephropathy in STZ-Induced diabetic rats. Evid Based Complement Alternat Med doi:10.1155/2011/ .

[64] Wang SC, Lee SF, Wang CJ, Lee CH, Lee WC, and Lee HJ(2009). Aqueous Extract from Hibiscus sabdariffa Linnaeus Ameliorate Diabetic Nephropathy via Regulating Oxidative Status and Akt/Bad/14-3-3{gamma} in an Experimental Animal Model. eCAM 10.1093/ecam/nep181.

[65] Williams ME, and Stanton RC(2005). Management of diabetic kidney disease, in Joslin's Diabetes Mellitus (Kahn CR, Weir GC, King GL, Jacobson AM, Moses AC, and Smith RJ, eds) Lippincott Williams & Wilkins, Philadelphia., 925-949.

[66] Wolf, G., Sharma, K., Chen, Y., Ericksen, M., & Ziyadeh, F. N. (1992). High glucose-induced proliferation in mesangial cells is reversed by autocrine TGF-β. Kidney Int, 42, 647-656.

[67] Wolf, G., & Ziyadeh, F. N. (1999). Molecular mechanisms of diabetic renal hypertrophy. Kidney Int, 56, 393-405.

[68] Yamamoto, T., Nakamura, T., Noble, N. A., Ruoslahti, E., & Border, W. A. (1993). Expression of transforming growth factor-β is elevated in human and experimental diabetic nephropathy. ProcNatlAcadSci USA, 90, 1814-1818.

[69] Zipp, T., & Schelling, J. R. (2003). Diabetic nephropathy, in Nephrology secrets 2nd edition (Hricik DE, Miller RT, Sedor JR, eds) Hanley &Belfus Inc. Medical Publishers, Philadelphia., 105-111.

[70] Ziyadeh, F. N., Hoffman, B. B., Han, D. C., Iglesias La, Cruz. M. C., Hong, S. W., Isono, M., Chen, S., Mc Gowan, T. A., & Sharma, K. (2000). Long-term prevention of renal insufficiency, excess matrix gene expression, and glomerular mesangial matrix expansion by treatment with monoclonal anti-transforming growth factor-beta antibody in db/db diabetic. mice. ProcNatlAcadSci USA, 97, 8015-8020.

[71] Ziyadeh, F. N., Sharma, K., Ericksen, M., & Wolf, G. (1994). Stimulation of collagen gene expression and protein synthesis in murine mesangial cells by high glucose is mediated by activation of transforming growth factor-β. J Clin Invest , 93, 536-542.

Chapter 16

The Effect of Type 1 Diabetes Mellitus on the Dento-Craniofacial Complex

Mona Aly Abbassy, Ippei Watari,
Ahmed Samir Bakry and Takashi Ono

Additional information is available at the end of the chapter

http://dx.doi.org/10.5772/52973

1. Introduction

Diabetes mellitus (DM) is one of the systemic diseases affecting a considerable number of patients worldwide [1]. Numerous experimental and clinical studies on the complications of DM have demonstrated extensive alterations in bone and mineral metabolism, linear growth, and body composition [2]. Depletion of insulin in Type 1 Diabetes Mellitus (T1DM) causes a reduction of bone mineral density and decreases skeletal mass, thus altering linear growth, body composition and delaying fracture healing. A considerable sector of literature was dedicated to studying the effects of T1DM on long bones; however, fewer studies discussed the effects of T1DM type on the craniofacial complex which is regulated by hormones, nutrients, mechanical forces, and various local growth factors.

Bone metabolism in the craniofacial complex involves a mosaic growth sites that grow at different rates and mature at different times, its growth and by analogy, the response to growth disruption is much more complex than that of the appendicular skeleton. Previous studies showed that T1DM may significantly affect the bone remodeling process which is observed during conducting treatments involving the application of mechanical or functional forces to the craniofacial complex and the teeth as those applied during orthodontic movement. Moreover, it is expected that the T1DM may alter the general growth of patients due to insulin deficiency and consequently leads to delayed skeletal maturation.

Type 1 diabetes mellitus (T1DM) is an endocrine–metabolic syndrome of childhood and adolescence, characterized by hyperglycemia as a cardinal biochemical feature, with important consequences for physical and emotional development. Several mechanisms have been reported to explain the altered bone remodeling in diabetes, one of which is diminished bone formation as a result of decreased osteoblastic activity or enhanced apoptosis of osteoblastic cells. Another contributing factor may be increased bone resorptive activity. However, it is still controversial whether osteoclastic recruitment and function are altered in diabetes, because no change or decrease in the activity of osteoclasts has been reported [1].

Among researchers, there is lack of consensus about the impact of this disease on dental health. It has been suggested that hyperglycemia is associated with decreased salivary secretion and high salivary glucose levels, particularly in cases of severe insulin deficiency. Consequently, an increased cariogenic challenge in such individuals can be expected. However, no clear evidence has been found for an association between dental caries and diabetes mellitus [3].

The main aim of this chapter is to discuss the complexity of the dento-craniofacial system and how it is affected by T1DM condition. Moreover, the various detrimental effects of T1DM on the dento-craniofacial complex will be explored using the dynamic histomorphometric analysis and a histological study that will demonstrate that T1DM condition induced various detrimental effects on the quality of bone and on the bone turnover process observed in the dento-craniofacial complex.

2. Effect of T1DM on Bone

2.1. Types of Bone formation in craniofacial complex

Bone forms in two ways, resulting in two types of mature bone – intramembranous and cartilage. Cartilage bone forms in a replacement process within the cartilage models of the embryo and infant. Intramembranous bone forms through the activation of the osteoblast cell or specialized bone forming cells in one of the layers of fetal connective tissue. The bones of the cranial vault, the face, and the clavicle are intramembranous in origin. All other bones of the body form from cartilage. Intramembranous bone include the mandible, the maxilla, the premaxilla, the frontal bone, the palatine bone, the squamous part of temporal bone, the zygomatic bone, the medial plate of the pterygoid process, the vomer, the tympanic part of the temporal bone, the nasal bone, the lacrimal bone, and the parietal bone. The original pattern of intramembranous bone changes with progressive maturative growth when these bones begin to adapt to environmental influences. This accounts for deformities due to malfunction, disease and other environmental factors [4].

2.2. Causes of growth problems

Growth disturbances can be associated with specific anatomic or functional defects. They may be of endocrine or non endocrine origin and may result from genetic, nutritional or environmental factors. Disturbances in somatic growth show themselves in retardation or acceleration of the skeletal system, including the facial and cranial bones. Causes for growth problems usually fall into the following categories [5]:

- **Familial short stature**

  Familial short stature is a tendency to follow the family's inherited short stature (shortness).

- **Constitutional growth delay with delayed adolescence or delayed maturation**

  A child who tends to be shorter than average and who enters puberty later than average, but is growing at a normal rate. Most of these children tend to eventually grow to approximately the same height as their parents.

- **Illnesses that affect the whole body (Also called systemic diseases.)**

  Constant malnutrition, digestive tract diseases, kidney disease, heart disease, lung disease, hepatic disease, diabetes, and severe stress can cause growth problems.

- **Endocrine (hormone) diseases**

  Adequate production of the thyroid hormone is necessary for normal bone growth. Cushing's syndrome can be caused by a myriad of abnormalities that are the result of hypersecretion of corticosteroids by the adrenal gland. Growth hormone deficiency involves a problem with the pituitary gland (small gland at the base of the brain) that secretes several hormones, including growth hormone.

- **Congenital (present at birth) problems in the tissues where growth occurs**

  A condition called intrauterine growth restriction (IUGR), slow growth within the uterus occurs during a pregnancy. The baby is born smaller in weight and length than normal, in proportion to his/her short stature.

2.3. Effect of DM on Bone and Growth

Hand-wrist radiographs have been studied in juvenile diabetics [6]. There is delayed appearance or delayed development of a center of ossification, usually of a carpal bone. These defects occur twice as frequently in boys than in girls, and the total incidence of juvenile diabetics with anomalies and developmental defects is 24.3%. There is also retardation of bone growth in 60% of diabetic males and 51% of diabetic females. The longer the duration of diabetes, the greater the tendency to bone growth retardation. The decreased bone mass in diabetics has been explained by decreased proliferative capacity of the diabetic fibroblasts, and early senescence of all cells has been suggested as basic to the diabetic problem. This degeneration would lead to early osteopenia in bone [6]. The yearly bone loss was reported to be 1.35% in patients with T1DM [7]. In addition, the rate of bone mineral loss is significantly greater among patients with a deterioration of the metabolic state, despite increasing insulin dosage, when compared with patients with unchanged or improved insulin secretion. This may indicate that the exogenous insulin administration does not fully compensate for the decrease in endogenous insulin secretion. These studies also showed increased bone resorption in T1DM patients with no signs of vitamin D deficiency associated with the disease. Vertebral bone density has been studied in T1DM children [7]. It was found that diabetic children exhibited cortical bone density that was slightly, but significantly, lower than the controls. The decrease in cortical bone density in the diabetic group did not correlate with age, sex, duration of diabetes, or glycosylated hemoglobin levels. These results suggested that in children with uncomplicated T1DM, decreased vertebral bone density is a minor abnormality that affects only cortical bone [6].

2.4. Outline of studying the effect of diabetes mellitus on craniofacial growth

Approximately 60% of adult bone mass including craniofacial bone is gained during the peak of the growth period which coincides with the onset of T1DM condition affecting the bone formation process [8]. It is worth mentioning here that although T1DM condition exact etiological factors are totally unknown however; understanding the course of T1DM condition and its impact on craniofacial development may lead to improving the oral health for a large sector of the population worldwide.

Numerous experimental and clinical studies on the complications of DM have demonstrated extensive alterations in bone and mineral metabolism, linear growth, and body composition. Investigators in the fields of bone biology including orthodontics have long been interested in the general causes that affect the normal growth of the craniofacial region. T1DM has been shown to affect the general growth of patients with earlier onset of the disease, especially onset before or around the circumpubertal growth spurts [9].

In general, growth of the craniofacial complex is controlled by genetic and environmental factors [3, 10]. Regulatory mechanisms responsible for normal morphogenesis of the face and head involve hormones, nutrients, mechanical forces, and various local growth factors. The poor growth and alterations in bone metabolism have been associated with T1DM in both humans and experimental animals [3]. It is of prime importance investigating the changes in craniofacial bone structure and dynamic bone formation in DM condition to explore the impact of the diabetic condition on various mandibular growth elements and bone quality.

The following parts of this chapter are going to focus on these points:

- Investigating the effects of juvenile diabetes on general craniofacial growth and skeletal maturation.
- Analyzing the pattern of association between craniofacial morphology and skeletal maturation.
- Determination of the changes in bone morphology in diabetic rat mandible using micro-C.T.
- Determination of the mineral apposition rate and the bone formation rate in diabetic rat mandible using histomorphometric analysis.

2.5. Animal and Experimental diabetic Model

The animal studies using diabetic model presents various advantages when compared to studies carried out on human diabetic cases. Human studies can be limited by small sample sizes, cross-sectional designs, uncontrolled variables, and often retrospective nature, animal models have been used to yield more rigorous analyses [11].

http://dx.doi.org/10.5772/52973

2.6. Diabetic model

Experimental diabetic models include the streptozotocin-induced diabetic rat and the spontaneously diabetic BioBreeding [12] rat. The occurrence of different abnormalities indicating altered bone formation after inducing DM with streptozotocin (STZ) is well documented [3, 13, 14]. Streptozotocin-induced diabetes mellitus (STZ-DM), caused by the destruction of pancreatic β-cells and is similar to T1DM in human, is characterized by mild to moderate hyperglycemia, glucosuria, polyphagia, hypoinsulinemia, hyperlipidemia, and weight loss. STZ-DM also exhibits many of the complications observed in human DM including enhanced susceptibility to infection and cardiovascular disease, retinopathy, alterations in angiogenesis, delayed wound healing, diminished growth factor expression, and reduced bone formation [15].

2.7. Importance of testing the uncontrolled diabetic condition

In the usual clinical situation, although T1DM patient is treated with insulin, patient may still suffer from an overall poor diabetic metabolic state with an uncontrollable blood glucose level and a high and sometimes changing insulin requirement [16].

2.8. Inducing diabetic condition

All the experimental protocols followed had been approved by the Institutional Animal Care and Use Committee of Tokyo Medical and Dental University, and the experiments were carried out under the control of the University's Guidelines for Animal Experimentation. In our investigation we explored the various effects of DM using the streptozotocin DM model. Twelve 3-week old male Wistar rats were used for this study. They were randomly divided into two groups, the control group and the diabetes group (DM group), each group consists of 6 rats. The rats in the control group were injected intra-peritoneal with a single dose of 0.1M sodium citrate buffer (pH 4.5), while the rats in the DM group were injected intra-peritoneal with a single dose of citrate buffer containing 60mg/kg body weight of streptozotocin (Sigma Chemical Co., St. Louis, MO, USA). [13, 16 - 18] All animals were fed on standard Rodent diet (Rodent Diet CE-2; Japan Clea Inc., Shizuoka, Japan) with free access to water. Body weights, the presence of glucose in urine and blood glucose levels were recorded on day 0,2,7,14,21 and 28 after STZ injection.

Diabetes condition was determined by the presence of glucose in urine and blood. The urine of the rats was tested using reagent strips (Uriace Ga; TERUMO). [20, 21] Blood samples of the rats were obtained via vein puncture of a tail vein, and blood glucose levels were determined using a glucometer (Ascensia Brio. Bayer Medical). Positive urine test and a blood glucose level greater than 200 mg/dl was considered DM. [3]

Fig. 1. shows the weights of the rats (mean±SD) in both groups. DM group showed a significant decrease in weight. After STZ injection by 48 hours the urine test showed that the entire DM group had a high glucose level and this was confirmed by the high blood glucose measurements as shown in Fig. 2. A Student's t-test was used to compare the mean of weights and blood glucose levels in both groups.

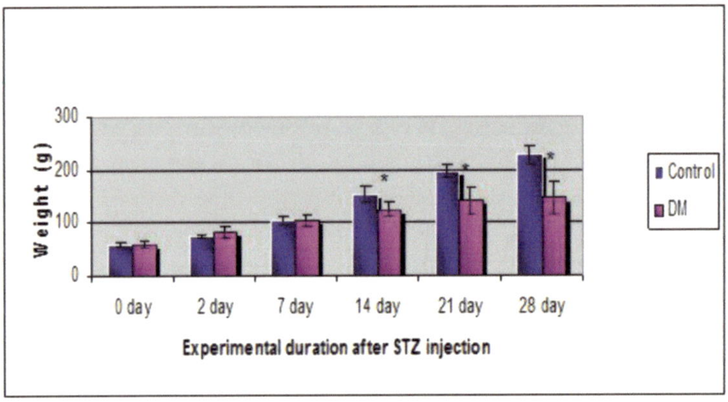

Figure 1. Comparison between the changes of the rat's weight in the control and DM group. * The weights of the DM group are significantly decreased as compared to the weights of the control group (*p<0.05*).

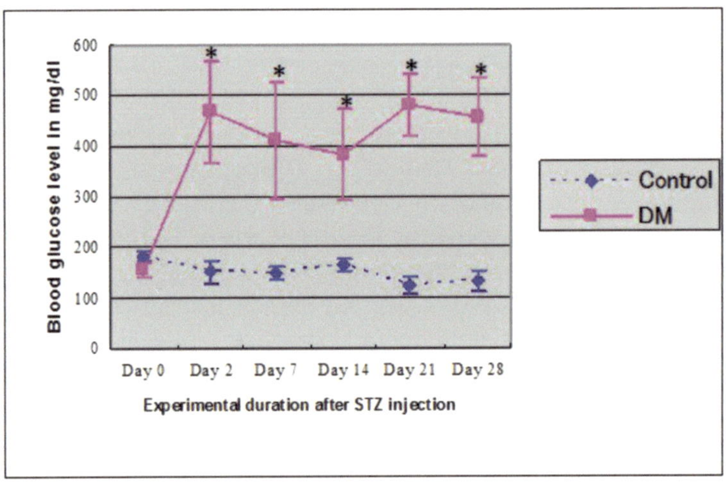

Figure 2. Line graph represents the blood glucose levels for the control and DM group. The blood glucose level in DM group increased significantly 48h post-STZ injection and during the entire experimental period. Values are mean±SD. Significant differences between the two groups are marked with asterisks ($p < 0.05$).

2.9. Analytic studies conducted to test the effect of diabetic condition on craniofacial growth

Cephalometric analysis

Cephalometric measurements are still one of the most widely spread diagnostic aids crucial for the diagnosis of various abnormalities in the craniofacial complex [22].

http://dx.doi.org/10.5772/52973

The protocol for examining the cephalometric measurements in DM rats involves the following steps:

- Prior to each radiographic session, the rats are anaesthetized with diethyl ether and intraperitoneal injection of 8% chloral hydrate using 0.5ml/100g of body weight.
- Each animal is then placed in this specially-designed apparatus (Fig. 3) to maintain standardized head posture and contact with the film (SGP-3, Mitsutoy, Tokyo, Japan) where the head of each rat is fixed firmly with a pair of ear rods oriented vertically to the sagittal plane and the incisors are fixed into a plastic ring.
- The settings of lateral and dorsoventral cephalometric radiographs are 50/55kVp, 15/10mA, and 20/60-sec impulses respectively.[11, 23]
- A 10 mm steel calibration rod is incorporated into the clear acrylic table on which the animals are positioned for the radiographs.
- All the radiographs are developed and scanned at high resolution by the same operator.[11]

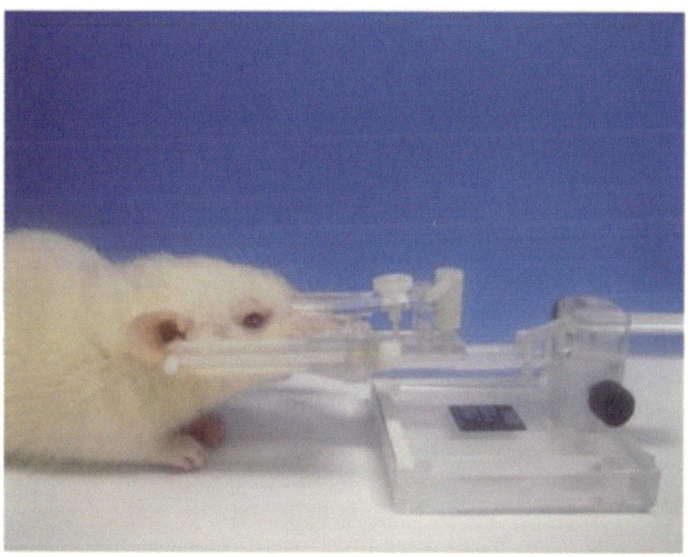

Figure 3. Apparatus for roentgenographic cephalometry

The cephalometric landmarks (Table 1; Fig. 4) were derived from previous studies on rodents.[11, 24-26] Selected linear measurements were then obtained (Table 2). To ensure reliability and replicability of each measurement, each distance was digitized twice and the two values were averaged.

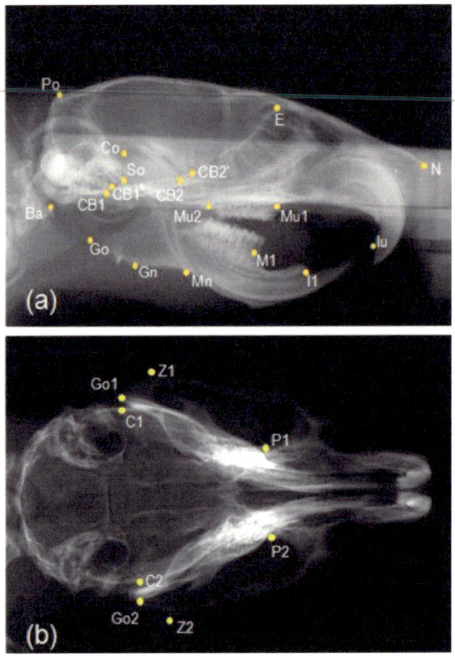

Figure 4. Location of cephalometric points on radiographs: (A) Sagittal and (B) transverse.

On the sagittal radiograph

N: The most anterior point on the nasal bone
E: The intersection of the frontal bone and floor of anterior cranial fossa
Po: The most posterior and superior point on the skull
Ba: The most posterior and inferior point on the occipital condyle
Co: The most posterior and superior point on the mandibular condyle
Go: The most posterior point on the mandibular ramus
Mn: The most concave portion of the concavity on the inferior border of the mandibular corpus
Gn: The most inferior point on the ramus that lies on a perpendicular bisector of the line Go-Mn
Il: The most anterior and superior point on the alveolar bone of the mandibular incisor
So: The intersection of the most anterior tympanic bulla and the superior border of the sphenoid bone
CB1: The most anterior point on the occipital bone at the spheno-occipital synchondrosis
CB1′ : The most posterior point on the sphenoid bone at the spheno-occipital synchondrosis
CB2: The most anterior point on the sphenoid bone at the spheno-basispheno synchondrosis
CB2′ : The most posterior point on the basisphenoid bone at the spheno-basispheno-synchondrosis
Ml: The junction of the alveolar bone and the mesial surface of the first mandibular molar
Mu1: The junction of the alveolar bone and the mesial surface of the first maxillary molar
Mu2: The junction of the alveolar bone and the distal surface of the third maxillary molar
Iu: The most anterior-inferior point on the maxilla posterior to the maxillary incisors

On the transverse radiograph

Z1 & Z2: The points on the lateral portion of the zygomatic arch that produce the widest width
Go1 & Go2: The points on the angle of the mandible that produce the widest width
P1 & P2: The most anterior and medial points within the temporal fossae that produce the most narrow palatal width
C1 & C2: The points on the cranium that produce the widest cranial width

Table 1. Definitions of radiographic points

http://dx.doi.org/10.5772/52973

Neurocranium
Po-N: total skull length
Po-E: cranial vault length
Ba-E: total cranial base length
So-E: anterior cranial base length
Ba-CB1: occipital bone length
CB1′ -CB2: sphenoid bone length
Ba-So: posterior cranial base length
Po-Ba: posterior neurocranium height
Viscerocranium
E-N: nasal length
Mu2-Iu: palate length
CB2-Iu: midface length
E-Mu1: viscerocranial height
Mandible
Go-Mn: posterior corpus length
Ml-Il: anterior corpus length
Co-Il: total mandibular length
Co-Gn: ramus height
Transverse X-ray
Go1-Go2: Bigonial width
C1-C2: Maximum cranial width
P1-P2: Palatal width
Z1-Z2: Bizygomatic width

Table 2. Measurements of craniofacial skeleton

In our studies, evaluation of the craniofacial growth of diabetic rats at the age of 7 weeks was done using lateral and dorsoventral cephalometric radiographs. All of the data in each experiment were confirmed the normal distribution, so a Student's t-test was used to compare the mean of each data recorded in the control group and in the DM group. All statistical analyses were performed at a 5% significance level using statistic software (v. 10; SPSS, Chicago, IL, USA).

2.9.1. Changes in the Total Skull

The size of total skull, denoted by Po-N, was significantly smaller in the DM group than in the control group.

2.9.2. Changes in the Neurocranium

Cranial vault length (Po-E), total cranial base length (Ba-E), anterior cranial base length (So-E), Occipital bone length (Ba-CB1), and posterior cranial base length (Ba-So) showed statistically significant decrease in DM group (Table 3, Fig. 5, 6), while other dimensions exhibited no significant differences.

Table 3: Significant changes in the Total skull and Neurocranium	
Po-N	total skull length
Po-E	cranial vault length
Ba-E	total cranial base length
So-E	anterior cranial base length
Ba-CB1	occipital bone length
Ba-So	posterior cranial base length

Table 3. Significant changes in the Total skull and Neurocranium

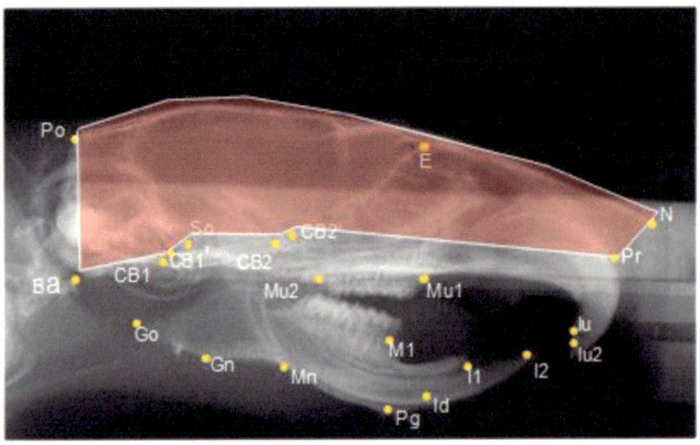

Figure 5. Neurocranium

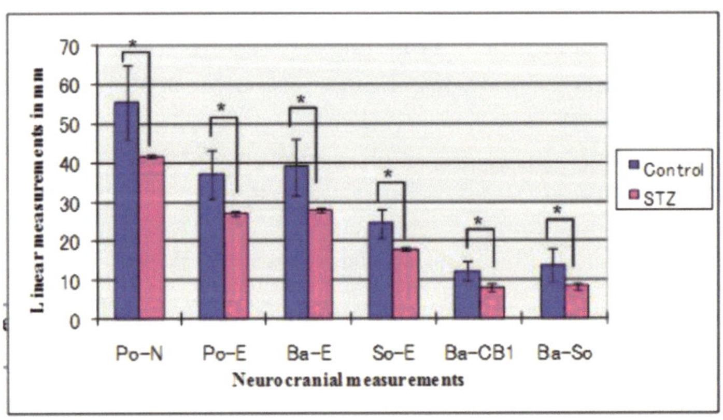

Figure 6. Changes in the neurocranial measurements of the control and DM group. All the significant measurements are shown in this figure. Values are mean±S.D. Significant differences between the two groups are marked with asterisks ($p<0.05$).

2.9.3. Changes in the Viscerocranium

All measurements of the viscerocranium, including the nasal length (E-N), palatal length (Mu2-Iu), midface length (CB2-Iu), and viscerocranial height (E-Mu1) showed a statistically significant decrease in DM group (Table 4, Fig. 7,8)

Table 4 : Significant changes in the Viscerocranium	
E-N	Nasal length
Mu2-Iu	Palate length
Cb2-Iu	midface length
E-Mu1	Posterior viscerocranial height

Table 4. Significant changes in the Viscerocranium

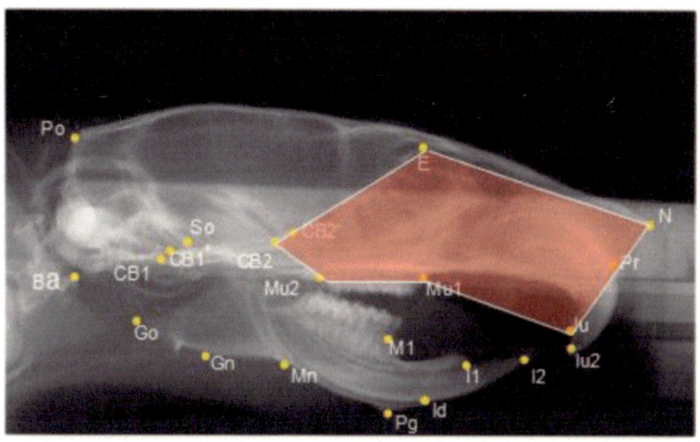

Figure 7. Viscerocranium

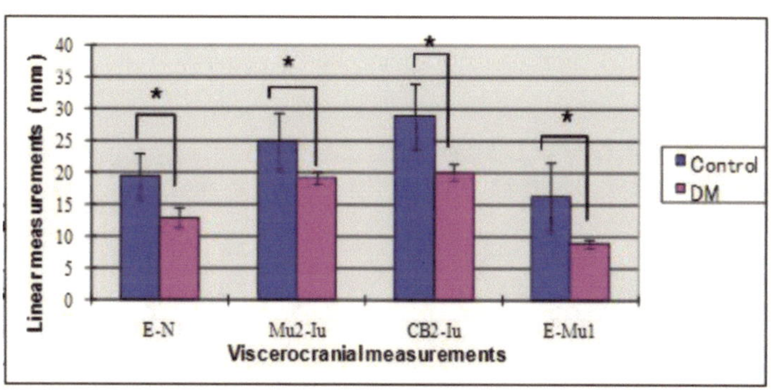

Figure 8. Changes in the viscerocranial measurements of the control and DM group. All the viscerocranial measurements are significant. Values are mean±S.D. Significant differences between the two groups are marked with asterisks ($p<0.05$).

2.9.4. Changes in the Mandible

In the DM group, the posterior corpus length (Go-Mn), total mandibular length (Co-Il) and the ramus height (Co-Gn) were significantly shorter than in the control group (Table 5, Fig. 9, 10), whereas no remarkable differences were found in the remaining dimensions.

Table 5: Significant changes in the Mandible	
Go-Mn	Posterior corpus length
Co-Il	Total mandibular length
Co-Gn	Ramus height

Table 5. Significant changes in the Mandible

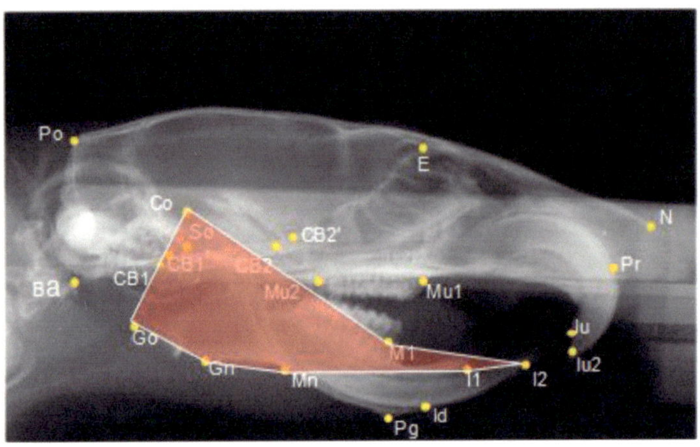

Figure 9. Mandible

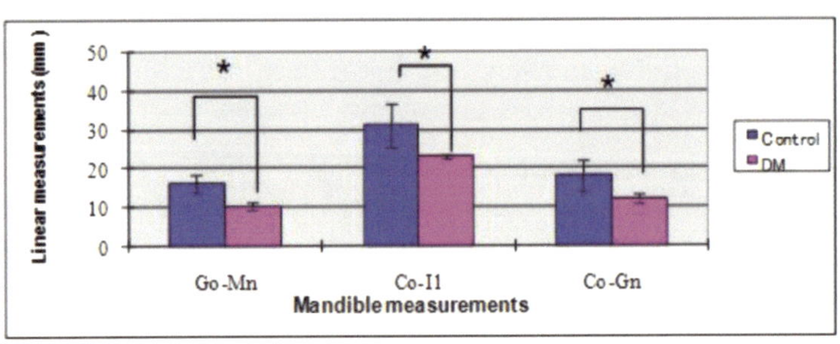

Figure 10. Changes in the mandible measurements of the control and DM group. Values are mean ± S.D.Significant differences between the two groups are marked with asterisks ($p<0.05$).

2.9.5. Changes in the Transverse X-ray

In transverse X-ray only the maximum cranial width (C1-C2) and the bizygomatic width (Z1-Z2) were statistically decreased in DM group (Table 6, Fig. 11, 12).

All other linear measurements showed no significant differences between both groups

Table 6: Significant changes in the transverse X-ray	
C1-C2	Maximum cranial width
Z1-Z2	Bizygomatic width

Table 6. Significant changes in the transverse X-ray

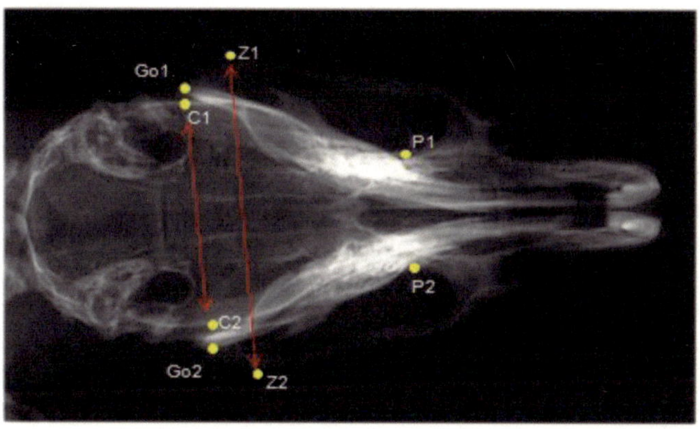

Figure 11. Transverse X-ray measurements

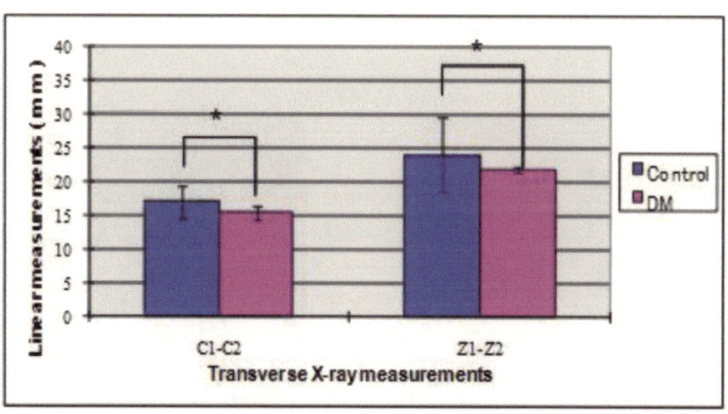

Figure 12. Changes in the transverse X-ray measurements of the control and DM group. Two measurements in the transverse X-ray were significant. Values are mean±S.D. Significant differences between the two groups are marked with asterisks ($p<0.05$)

2.10. Histomorphometric analysis

2.10.1. Fluorescent dyes used for double labeling in histomorphometric analysis

Fluorochromes are calcium binding substances that are preferentially taken up at the site of active mineralization of bone known as the calcification front, thus labeling sites of new bone formation. They are detected using fluorescent microscopy on undecalcified sections. Labeling bones with fluorochrome markers provides a means to study the dynamics of bone formation. The rate and extent of bone deposition and resorption can be determined using double and triple fluorochrome labeling sequences. The sequential use of fluorochromes of clearly contrasting colors permits a more detailed record of events relating to calcification. Flurochromes commonly used in mammals include tetracycline, calcein green, xylenol orange, alirazin red, and hematoporphyrin. Calcein is a fluoresces bright green when combined with calcium [27].

2.10.2. Calcein administrations and sections preparation

The steps needed for detecting the double labeling involves the following:

- Rats are subcutaneously injected with 50 mg/kg body weight calcein fluorescent marker on day 21 and day 28 after STZ injection [28]. The time difference between the 2 injections is one week to be able to compare the amount of bone formed during this period (Fig. 13).
- Sacrifice of all animals by transcardiac perfusion under deep anesthesia using 4% paraformaldehyde in 0.1 M phosphate buffer (pH 7.4).
- Mandibles are dissected and fixed in the same solution for 24 hours.
- All specimens are embedded in polystyrene resin (Rigolac, Nisshin EM Co. Ltd., Tokyo, Japan).
- Undemineralized ground frontal sections are processed to show the crown and both apices of buccal and lingual roots of the lower second molar [28].

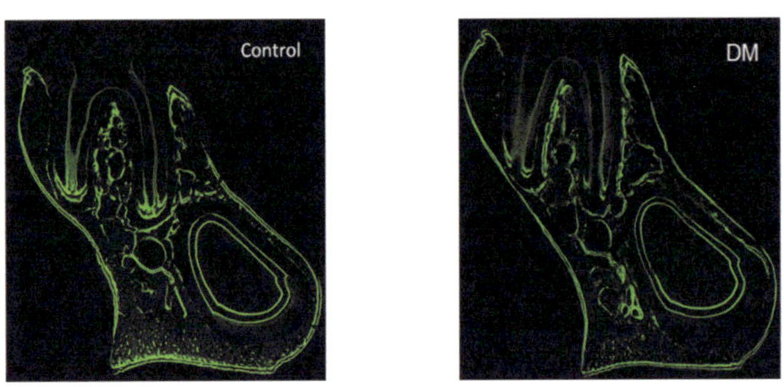

Figure 13. Frontal sections of the mandibular second molar area. (A) Control; (B) DM. Fluorescent labeling on the periosteal surface indicates new bone formation.

http://dx.doi.org/10.5772/52973

2.10.3. Method of analysis

The bone around the lower second molar is centrally located within the mandibular arch, and because of the parallel alignment of the buccal and lingual roots this made a precise reference when frontal sections are produced [29]. To conduct the histomorphometric analysis it is essential to use a digitizing morphometry system to measure bone formation indices. The system consists of a confocal laser scanning microscope (LSM510, Carl Zeiss Co. Ltd., Jena, Germany), and a morphometry program (LSM Image Browser, Carl Zeiss Co. Ltd., Jena, Germany). Bone formation indices of the periosteal surfaces of the alveolar/jaw bone include mineral apposition rate (μm/day) and bone formation rate ($\mu m^3/\mu m^2$/day), according to the standard nomenclature described by [30]. The calcein-labeled surface (CLS, in mm) is calculated as the sum of the length of double labels (Thomas *et al.*) plus one half of the length of single labels (sL) along the entire endosteal or periosteal bone surfaces; that is, CLS = dL + 0.5sL [31]. The mineral apposition rate (MAR, in μ / day) is determined by dividing the mean of the width of the double labels by the interlabel time (7 days). The bone formation rate (BFR) is calculated by multiplying MAR by CLS [32]. Based on the reference line along the long axis of the buccal root, the area superior to the root apex was considered alveolar bone, while the area inferior to the root apex was considered the jaw bone. The lingual side of the bone is excluded, because the existence of the incisor root may influence bone formation.

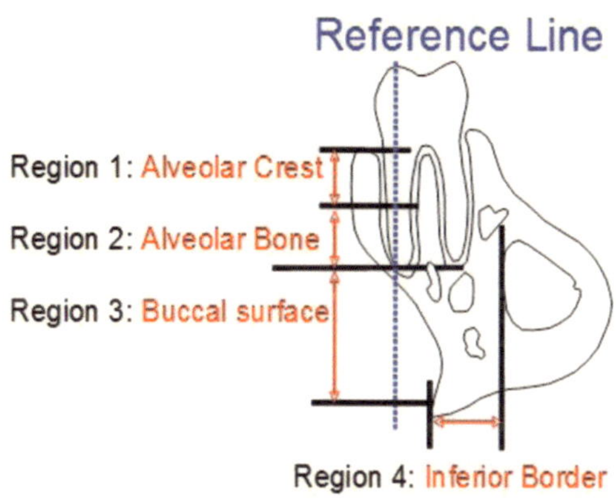

Figure 14. Schematic drawing of observation regions for dynamic bone histomorphometry. The periosteal surfaces were delimited into 4 areas as alveolar crest (region 1), alveolar bone (region 2), buccal surface of the jaw bone (region 3), and inferior border of the jaw bone (region 4).

The periosteal surfaces of the mandible are divided into four regions for analysis (Fig. 14.):

2.10.4. Histomorphometric indices

The obtained results in our study showed that in the alveolar bone (region 2), there was a significant decrease in the MAR (Fig. 15A) BFR (Fig.15B) recorded in the DM group compared to the control group. However, in the alveolar crest (region 1), the MAR and the BFR in the control and the DM groups were not significantly different. ($P < 0.05$). In the buccal surface (region 3) and inferior borders (region 4) of the jaw bone the MAR (Fig.15A) and BFR (Fig. 15B) were significantly suppressed compared with those in the control group ($P < 0.05$). Most of the periosteal surfaces in the mandibular regions of the control group showed significantly higher values recorded for the mineral apposition rate and the bone formation rate when compared to the DM group. These results agree with previous studies that recorded diminished lamellar bone formation in DM rats' femur and may suggest an association between the DM condition and the decreased number and function of osteoblasts [16, 19]. The alveolar crest region was the only region that did not show a significant difference in the mineral apposition rate and the bone formation rate parameters among the two groups; this may be attributed to the unique nature of this region exhibiting a highly intensive bone remodeling process especially during the teeth eruption that decreases toward the base of the socket [33], however further studies are needed to elaborate the detailed pattern of bone growth at the alveolar crest region.

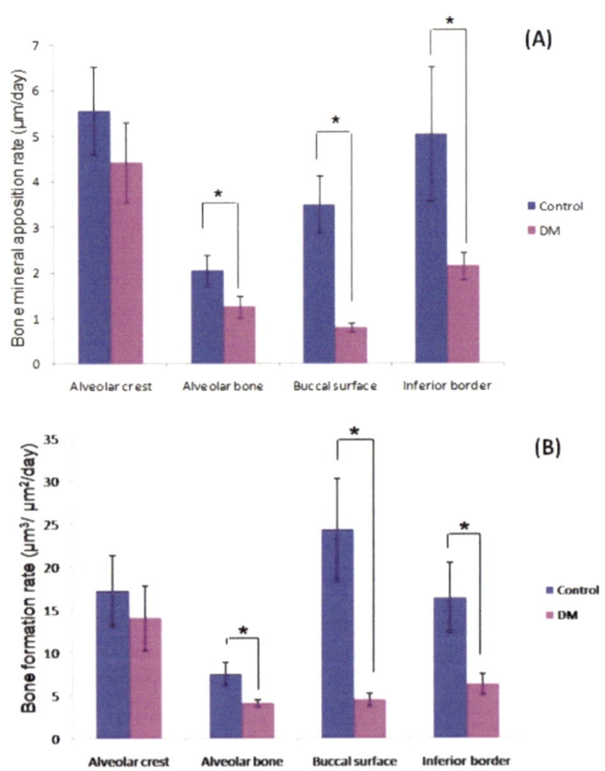

Figure 15. A) The changes in mineral apposition rate (MAR) of the mandible between the control group and the DM group. Alveolar crest (region 1, upper 1/2 of the tooth root, near the tooth crown). Alveolar bone (region 2, lower 1/2 of the tooth root, near the root apex). Buccal surface of the jaw bone (region 3). Inferior border of the jaw bone (region 4). The data are expressed as means ± SD. N = 5 for each group. *Significantly different from controls, with ($p<0.05$). (B) The changes in the bone formation rate (BFR/BS) of the mandible between the control group and the DM group. Alveolar crest (region 1, upper 1/2 of the tooth root, near the tooth crown). Alveolar bone (region 2, lower 1/2 of the tooth root, near the root apex). Buccal surface of the jaw bone (region 3). Inferior border of the jaw bone (region 4). The data are expressed as means ± S.D. N = 5 for each group. *Significantly different from controls, with ($p<0.05$).

http://dx.doi.org/10.5772/52973

2.10.5. Microtomography of the mandible (Micro-CT)

Micro-computed tomography (micro-CT) has rapidly become a standard technique for the visualization and quantification of the 3D structure of trabecular bone. Bone architecture and mineralization are generally considered to be important components of bone quality, and determine bone strength in conjunction with bone mineral density.

2.10.6. Protocol adopted to examine the mandible using Micro-CT

In our study all specimens were imaged by micro-CT (inspeXio SMX-90CT; Shimadzu Science East Corporation, Tokyo, Japan)

- After removing only the soft tissue, the mandibular plane is set orthogonal to the sample stage.
- Three dimensional images of each hemi mandible are acquired with a resolution voxel size of 15 μm / pixel.
- Raw data are obtained by rotating the sample stage 360 degrees. Then, slice images are prepared using multi-tomographic image reconstruction software (MultiBP; Imagescript, Tokyo, Japan).
- The resulting gray-scale images are segmented using a low-pass filter to remove noise and a fixed threshold to extract the mineralized bone phase.
- The volume of interest (VOI) is drawn on a slice-based method starting from the first slice containing the crown of the first molar and moving dorsally 100 slices [34, 35], in the area of the alveolar crest (Between the buccal and lingual roots of the second molar at the cervical region); and the buccal surface of the jaw bone [29]. Trabecular bone was carefully contoured on the first and the last slice, while the intermediate slices were first interpolated by morphing.
- For observation and analysis of reconstructed 3D images, 3D trabecular structure analysis software (TRI/3D-BON; RATOC System Engineering, Tokyo, Japan) is used [36]. Reconstructed 3D images were prepared from slice images using the volume rendering method, to analyze the microstructure of the bone (Fig. 16).
- The following parameters are measured: tissue volume (TV), bone volume (BV), bone surface (BS), bone surface / bone volume (BS/BV), bone-volume fraction (BV/TV).
- Four properties of the trabeculae are evaluated: trabecular thickness (Tb.Th), trabecular number (Tb.N), trabecular separation (Tb.Sp), and Trabecular space (Tb.S) [36].

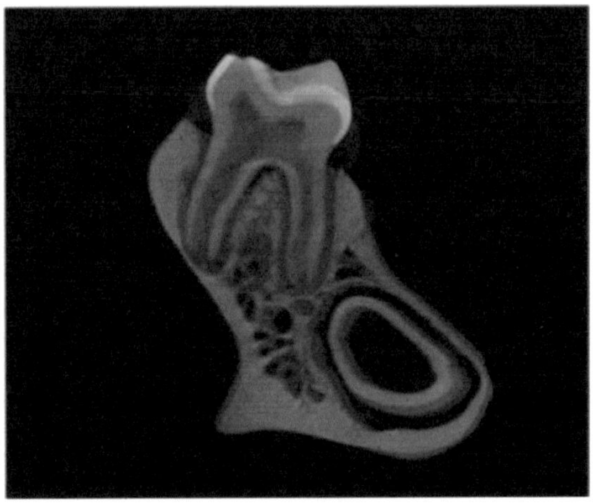

Figure 16. The left mandible was imaged by micro-CT

2.10.7. Microtomography of the DM mandible

The quantification of micro-CT trabecular bone changes (mean±SD) is shown for the DM and the control groups in (Table 4). All trabecular parameters in both alveolar bone and buccal surface of jaw bone showed significant changes. Compared with the control group, bone volume fraction (BV/TV) was significantly decreased only in the alveolar bone; however, trabecular thickness (Tb.Th) and trabecular numbers (Tb.N) were significantly decreased both in alveolar and buccal surface of jaw bone, in the DM group. Correspondingly, significantly higher trabecular separation (Tb.Sp) and trabecular space (Tb.S) were revealed both in alveolar and buccal surface of jaw bone for the DM group when compared with that of the control group. Also, the bone surface / bone volume (BS/BV) was significantly increased only in alveolar bone (P< 0. 05). These findings indicate deterioration of the bone quality in the DM group. These results agree with other research work suggesting that the glycaemic levels play an important role in modulating the trabecular architecture especially in mandibular bone [15].

The DM condition resulted in alteration of the trabecular distance and thickness as compared to the control group indicating profound impact on the histological integrity of the bone. The reduction in trabecular bone volume accompanied by the expansion of the bone marrow space is in agreement with another investigation [37]. In this context, these results may describe a state of osteopenia in experimental diabetic rats, which might be the result of an imbalance between bone formation and resorption

2.10.8. Procedure for preparing mandibles for histological analysis

- Mandibles for all groups were decalcified in 10% EDTA solution pH 7.4 for 5 weeks at 4ºC [38].

- Specimens are then dehydrated in an ascending ethanol series and embedded in paraffin (Fig. 17).
- Serial horizontal sections (5 μm thick parallel to the occlusal plane) are prepared using a microtome (Leica RM 2155,Nussloch,Germany)(Fig.17)

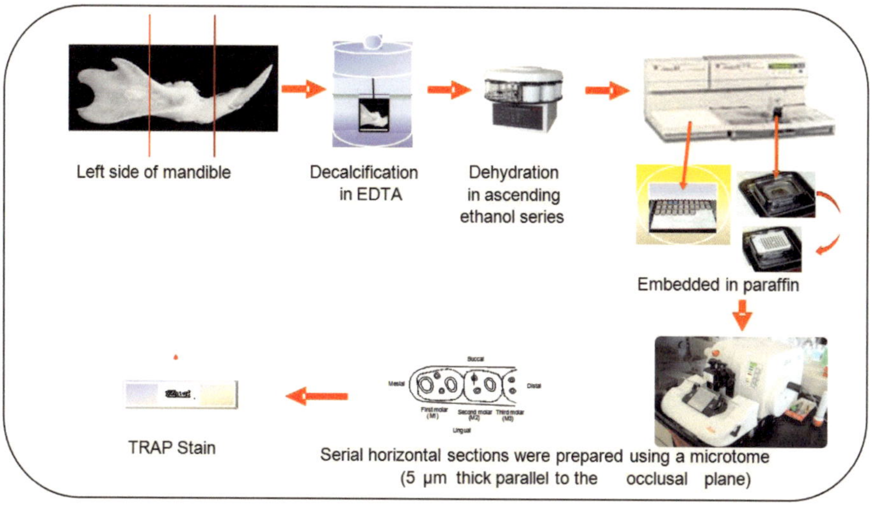

Figure 17. Experimental procedure for histological section preparation

2.10.9. *TRAP staining*

Histological sections are incubated for 30–60 min at 37ºC in a mixture of 0.8% naphthol AS-BI phosphate (Sigma, St Louis, MO, USA), 0.7% fast red violet salt (Sigma, St Louis, MO, USA) and 50mM sodium tartate diluted in 0.2M sodium acetate buffer (pH 5.4). Sections were examined under a light microscope. For the histomorphometric assessment of resorption, the number of tartrate-resistant acid phosphatase-positive multinucleated cells (osteoclasts) on the distal surface of the alveolar bone adjacent to the mesio-buccal root of the second molar were counted in each 540 μm x 120 μm area in five consecutive sections, at the middle third of the root selected at least 25μm apart from each specimen (n = 5) of each group [39, 40].

2.10.10. *Histological analysis*

Bone-resorption activity was assessed by counting the number of tartrate-resistant acid phosphatase-positive multinucleate cells (osteoclasts) on the distal surface of the alveolar bone adjacent to the mesio-buccal root of the second molar (Fig. 18A-D). Statistical analysis demonstrated a significantly higher number of osteoclast cells in the control group when compared with the DM group ($P < 0.05$) (Fig. 18 E). Results revealed that the number of osteoclasts was significantly lower in the DM rats than in the controls, in line with previous studies on DM rats' mandible [40] and long bones [41, 42]. These results confirm that the decreased rate of bone turnover may be associated with the DM condition.

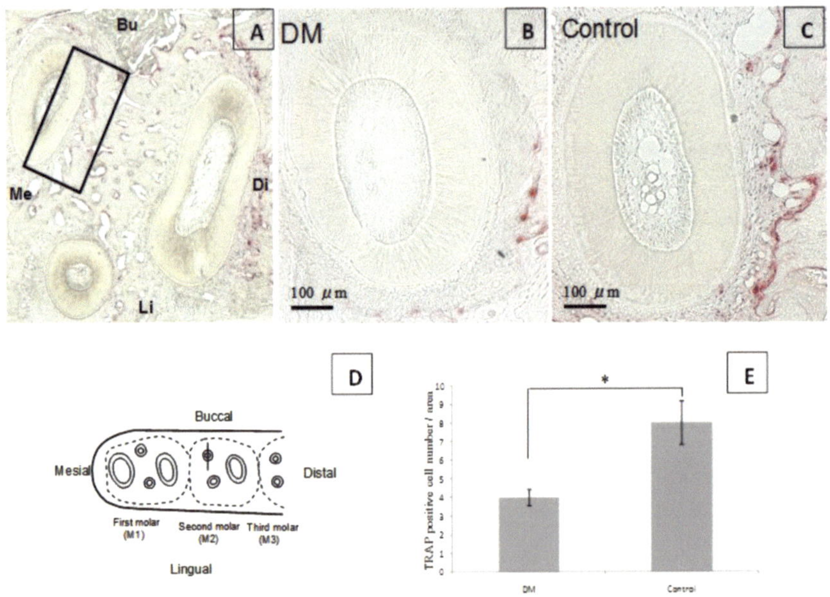

Figure 18. Osteoclast counts in a horizontal section of the mandibular second molar region stained with Tartarate-resistant acid phosphatase (TRAP). (A) Low magnification photograph of the three roots of the second molar stained with TRAP stain. The black rectangle (540 X 120 μm) indicates the area on the distal surface of the alveolar bone adjacent to the middle third of the mesio-buccal root of the second molar in which the osteoclast cells were counted. Bu, buccal; Li, lingual; Me, mesial; Di, distal. (B) The mesio-buccal root of the control rat (original magnification 100X). (C) The mesio-buccal root of the DM rat (original magnification 100X). (D) A schematic drawing showing the observation area on the distal surface of the alveolar bone adjacent to the mesio-buccal root of the second molar in which the osteoclast cells were counted. (E) Statistical analysis demonstrated a significantly higher number of osteoclast cells in the control group when compared with the DM group ($P < 0.05$).

2.11. Suggested mechanisms for the effect of diabetic condition on craniofacial complex

Growth of the craniofacial complex is controlled by genetic and environmental factors [2, 10]. Regulatory mechanisms responsible for normal morphogenesis of the face and head involve hormones, nutrients, mechanical forces, and various local growth factors. The poor growth and alterations in bone metabolism have been associated with T1DM in both humans and experimental animals [2]. Because human studies can be limited by small sample sizes, cross-sectional designs, uncontrolled variables, and often retrospective nature, animal models have been used to yield more rigorous analyses [10]. In our studies we observed the rat growth from the age of 3 weeks old till 7 weeks old. This time period is corresponding to early growth stage in human according to previous craniofacial growth studies [43, 44]. Consequently, in the current study STZ-DM model was used to investigate the effect of T1DM on craniofacial growth.

The studied STZ-DM rats showed significantly reduced growth in most of the craniofacial skeletal units but no significant differences were observed between controls and DM group as regards the remaining craniofacial skeletal units (Sphenoid bone length, posterior neurocranium height, anterior corpus length, bigonial width and palatal width). Craniofacial growth as a whole was also significantly lower in DM group compared to controls in all three dimensions. Previous study investigated the DM effect exclusively on the growth of the mandible and suggested that the diabetic condition had a differential effect on the osseous components and / or its associated non-skeletal tissues. They found that the disharmonious growth of the mandible was due to DM condition and might not be associated with diabetic condition complications such as renal failure, anemia, body weight change or alteration in the food intake qualities [2]. Thus we hypothesize that the deficiency in the craniofacial growth in our experiment might be attributed to the diabetic condition in the DM group as it was reported that specific alterations in bone metabolism are associated with DM. Moreover, several pathogenic possibilities have been proposed, such as insulinopenia, bone microangiopathy, impaired regulation of mineral metabolism, alterations in local factors that regulate bone remodeling, and even an intrinsic disorder associated with T1DM [37, 45]. The aforementioned insulin hormone deficiency that is associated with T1DM cases may have direct effect on bone metabolism. It was mentioned in literature that normal insulin hormone level exerts direct anabolic effects on bone cells [37]. Multiple osteoblast-like cell lines express insulin receptors on the cell surface and have a high capacity for insulin binding [46]. Moreover, osteoclasts exhibit reduced bone resorption in response to insulin stimulation [47]. These findings support the idea that the actions of insulin in bone could be mediated directly via stimulation of osteoblasts in combination with inhibition of osteoclasts, [15, 47] and this mechanism of action may explain the retardation of craniofacial growth in STZ-DM.

Diabetes has a deleterious effect on osseous turnover due to decreased osteoblast and osteoclast activities and numbers and, a lower percentage of osteoid surface and osteocalcin synthesis, as well as increased time for mineralization of osteoid [37]. It was reported that the influence of diabetes on discrete stages of matrix-induced endochondral bone formation could have profound effects on the biomechanical behavior of bone. Also, chondrogenesis and calcification of bone were reduced by 50% in diabetic animals [48]. This was evident in the current study results that showed a significant decrease in the craniofacial linear measurements of the DM group.

In addition to this, insulin may exert synergistic effects with other anabolic agents in bone, such as parathyroid hormone (PTH) [15, 47]. An animal model of T1DM has frequently demonstrated alteration in bone turnover, retarded growth, increased concentration of PTH, and reduced concentration of 1,25-dihydroxivitamin D [37, 49]. The effects of PTH on the bones are complex; it stimulates resorption or bone formation depending on the concentration used, the duration of the exhibition, and the administration method [37, 48, 49, 50]. Also, 1,25-dihydroxivitamin D, like PTH, belongs to the most important group of bone regulatory hormones. It regulates osteoclastic differentiation from hematopoietic mononuclear cells, and osteoblastic functions and activity [37, 51].

Moreover, Insulin may indirectly regulate the enhancement of growth hormone (GH) serum concentration by direct regulation of the hepatic growth hormone receptor, this results in abnormalities in the insulin growth factor-1 (IGF-1) in T1DM [52] which consequently may have lead to the retarded growth in uncontrolled DM in the current study.

In the present study most of the periosteal surfaces in the mandibular regions of the control group showed significantly higher values recorded for the mineral apposition rate and the bone formation rate when compared to the DM group. These results agree with previous studies that recorded diminished lamellar bone formation in DM rats' femur and may suggest an association between the DM condition and the decreased number and function of osteoblasts [16, 19]. The alveolar crest region was the only region that did not show a significant difference in the mineral apposition rate and the bone formation rate parameters among the two groups; this may be attributed to the unique nature of this region exhibiting a highly intensive bone remodeling process especially during the teeth eruption that decreases toward the base of the socket [33].

A significant decrease of bone volume fraction, trabecular thickness, and trabecular numbeis confirmed by Micro-CT analysis in DM rats, there was Also, it showed a significant increase of the trabecular separation and the trabecular space in the DM group when compared with the control group. This finding indicates deterioration of the bone quality in the DM group. These results agree with other research work suggesting that the glycaemic levels play an important role in modulating the trabecular architecture especially in mandibular bone [15]. In this context, these results may describe a state of osteopenia in experimental diabetic rats, which might be the result of an imbalance between bone formation and resorption.

A histometric evaluation of bone resorption was performed by counting the number of osteoclast cells on the distal surface of the alveolar bone adjacent to the mesio-buccal root of the second molar. These evaluations revealed that the number of osteoclasts was significantly lower in the DM rats than in the controls, in line with previous studies on DM rats' mandible [40] and long bones [41, 42]. These studies confirm that the decreased rate of bone turnover may be associated with the DM condition.

This deteriorating effect on mandibular bone structure and dynamic bone formation might be be attributed to several pathogenic possibilities, such as insulinopenia, bone microangiopathy, impaired regulation of mineral metabolism, alterations in local factors that regulate bone remodeling, and even an intrinsic disorder associated with DM [12, 37]. However, the detrimental effects observed may not be associated with the significant loss of rats` weights observed in the diabetic group starting from day 14 because previous research [2, 12, 15, 42] showed that the mandibular growth was not affected in normal rats supplied with restricted diet and having same pattern of weight loss resembling weight loss pattern observed in DM rats.

3. Effect of Type 1 Diabetes on teeth susceptibility to caries

3.1. Tooth formation

Tooth growth begins before birth and continues throughout adolescence. The dental development is a continuous process of tooth initiation, matrix secretion, crown mineralization, dental eruption, and root completion. Primate dental development begins before birth with initiation of the deciduous dentition, followed by initiation of the permanent dentition. During the process of dental eruption the tooth must move past the bone margin (alveolar eruption) and the gum (gingival eruption) in order to emerge into the oral cavity and eventually into functional occlusion. Dentine is formed when odontoblasts secrete a collagenous matrix predentine which rapidly undergoes mineralization to form primary dentine. Dentine formation begins at the dentine horn underlying the future cusp tip and progresses inward through secretion and downward through extension until it reaches the apex of the root. Enamel is formed when ameloblasts secrete enamel matrix proteins that mineralize into long, thin bundles of hydroxyapatite crystallites known as enamel prisms. As the secretory cells progress outward toward the future tooth surface, additional adjacent cells are activated through extension until the forming front reaches the cervix of the crown [3].

The resistance of the dental tissues to caries is determined by the quantitative content of the inorganic and organic matrices. Numerous reports have showed that teeth with a correct macro- and microstructure and a proper degree of mineralization are more resistant to the activity of external cariogenic factors [3].

Several biological complications in patients suffering from type 1 diabetes mellitus have been widely investigated over the previous years, however, the scientific data available on the possible effects of T1DM on teeth are scant. These data suggest that T1DM condition may be associated with a change in the chemical composition of the teeth or alteration in the total thickness of enamel or dentin.

Various clinical studies on children reported high caries prevalence in diabetic children when compared with healthy controls [3]. This high caries prevalence may be associated with factors affecting the tooth structure itself or due to some changes in the oral environment causing the increase of the susceptibility of the teeth to dental caries.

3.2. Effects of Type 1 Diabetes on tooth mineral composition

Proper mineralization of teeth during its development is the key factor for the proper resistance of teeth to cariogenic challenge and thus any metabolic disorder affecting the teeth mineralization during its development may render these teeth more prone to be involved by caries. Rat experimental model provides an excellent model for the study of the various metabolic disorders on the mineralization of teeth hard tissues due the fact that the rats incisors are continuously growing and erupting during its life and thus it is possible to study various effects of metabolic disorders which can be induced artificially during the growth period of these rats [53]. The results obtained from the aforementioned experimental rat model can be compared to the results obtained from control rats living under identical situations and thus can easily eliminate many variables that can affect the outcome of the results of any experiments conducted on humans.

In vitro studies on animal models affected by the streptozotocin induced diabetic condition showed that there is a low concentration of calcium and fluoride in the growing rats` incisors after inducing the diabetic condition by the streptozotocin injection [54]. Moreover, there was a concomitant increase in the concentration of calcium in blood serum and a decrease in fluoride concentration in blood serum. It was suggested that the decrease of calcium concentration in the teeth structure in this study was due to decrease of the cellular activity of ameloblasts during the enamel development [54]. This suggestion may be backed by the results obtained from a similar streptozotocin induced diabetic rat model which showed that the diabetic condition is associated with a decrease in the calcium deposition in bone due to a generalized metabolic activity decrease [12, 28]. The recorded increase in calcium in blood serum was attributed to the absence of insulin which aids in the transfer of calcium from the blood serum to the body tissues. The low concentration of fluoride observed in the tooth structure and in the blood serum may be attributed to the incorporation of the fluoride in bone matrix which is induced by the high concentration of the estrogen observed in the blood serum [54]. Moreover, the increase in fluoride elimination in urine may have caused this decrease in fluoride concentration in the diabetic rats.

3.3. Effects of Type 1 Diabetes on salivary status

The saliva contents and rate of flow are among the critical factors that predict the caries incidence in the oral cavity. Type 1 DM is among the endocrine disease that elevates the glucose level concentration in saliva and decreases the salivary rate of flow.

The mechanism by which the glucose level may increase in saliva may be explained by previous research showed that the increase of blood glucose level in T1DM cases is associated with a concomitant increase of glucose level in saliva. Moreover, it was previously suggested that T1DM causes an increase in the permeability of the basement membrane of the parotid gland that favors the transfer of glucose from the parotid gland to the saliva in the oral cavity [3].

The mechanism by which T1DM decreases the salivary flow may be attributed to the detrimental effects induced by the T1DM condition on the salivary gland tissues itself causing a generalized decrease in the saliva in the oral cavities.

The factors of increased glucose level and decrease in salivary flow cause the improper clearance of glucose from the oral cavity and impairs the buffering capacity of saliva rendering it more acidic, these aforementioned effects consequently increase the metabolic activities of the bacterial biofilm in the oral cavity and render teeth more susceptible to dental caries [3].

Previous research work [3] showed that the dietary habits conducted by the diabetic patients do not have a significant effect on the prevalence of caries in these patients when compared to normal individuals and thus it may be concluded that the increase in caries prevalence in diabetic patients is likely associated with factors affecting the development of teeth or due to some detrimental effects induced by the oral environment that increases the risk of caries occurrence in oral cavities of T1DM patients.

http://dx.doi.org/10.5772/52973

4. Conclusions

It is obvious that the T1DM condition significantly affects craniofacial growth, bone formation mechanism and the quality of the bone formed which may alter many aspects of planning and treatment of orthodontic patients affected by this globally increasing hormonal disturbance. Moreover, T1DM condition impairs the proper tooth development and alters the oral environment rendering teeth more susceptible to dental caries.

There should be a new strategy for treating orthodontic patients suffering from metabolic disorders specially those disorders having direct and indirect effects on bone growth as the diabetic condition. The orthodontic craniofacial linear measurements were significantly decreased in the T1DM cases when compared to normal cases. Moreover, greater risks of developing dental caries and possible tooth loss are associated with patients suffering from T1DM; these risks may complicate the outcome of orthodontic treatment which is associated with less ability of orthodontic patients to implement proper oral hygiene measures due to increased areas of bacterial biofilm formation around orthodontic brackets

These comprehensive studies done on bone and craniofacial growth suggest that planning the treatment in craniofacial region for patients affected with hormonal disorders is a more complex procedure when compared to the treatment of normal patients, moreover it is suggested that it is of prime importance to keep close attention to the general systemic condition of these patients and administer the proper hormonal therapy for these patients when needed to avoid any detrimental effects on bone resulting from any hormonal imbalance. Moreover, it is highly recommended to closely monitor the salivary and the dental conditions of these patients to allow early intervention for treating any developing dental caries.

Within the limitations of this *in vitro* study, it was concluded that:

1. T1DM reduces craniofacial growth, resulting in retardation of skeletal development.

2. DM in the rat affects the bone architecture, as shown by Micro-CT, and impairs the rate of the mandibular bone formation, as examined by the dynamic histomorphometric analysis.

3. All of these results were verified on the cellular level by a histological study that showed the diminished number of osteoclasts on the alveolar wall, suggesting that the early stage of DM resulted in low bone turnover.

4. These findings should be considered when conducting any treatment in the craniofacial region in T1DM since the better understanding of how diabetes affects bone will improve our ability to protect bone health in diabetic patients.

5. The tooth structure and the saliva condition are negatively influenced by the T1DM condition and thus strict oral hygiene measures should be conducted with orthodontic patients suffering from T1DM condition to decrease the risk of developing dental caries in these patients.

6. Good control of diabetes mellitus should be considered before orthodontic treatment by a long time inorder to obtain the best outcome.

Author details

Mona Aly Abbassy[1,2,3,4*], Ippei Watari[1], Ahmed Samir Bakry[5,6,7] and Takashi Ono[1]

*Address all correspondence to: monaabbassy@gmail.com

1 Orthodontic Science, Department of Orofacial Development and Function, Division of Oral Health Sciences, Graduate School, Tokyo Medical and Dental University, Japan

2 Global Center of Excellence Program; International Research Center For Molecular Science in Tooth and Bone Disease at Tokyo Medical and Dental University, Tokyo Medical and Dental University, Japan

3 Orthodontic Department, Faculty of Dentistry, King Abdulaziz University, Saudia Arabia

4 Alexandria University, Alexandria, Egypt

5 Cariology and Operative Dentistry Department, Graduate School of Medical and Dental Sciences, Tokyo Medical & Dental University, Japan

6 Conservative Dentistry Department, Faculty of Dentistry, Alexandria University, Egypt

7 Conservative Dentistry Department, Faculty of Dentistry, King Abdulaziz University, Saudia Arabia

References

[1] Bensch, L., Braem, M., Van Acker, K., & Willems, G. (2003). Orthodontic treatment considerations in patients with diabetes mellitus. *American Journal of Orthodontics and Dentofacial Orthopedics,*, 123(1), 74-78.

[2] Giglio, M. J., & Lama, M. A. (2001). Effect of experimental diabetes on mandible growth in rats. *European Journal of Oral Sciences*, 109(3), 193-197.

[3] Siudikiene , J., Machiulskiene, V., Nyvad, B., Tenovuo, J., & Nedzelskiene , I. (2006). Dental caries and salivary status in children with type 1 diabetes mellitus, related to the metabolic control of the disease. *European Journal of Oral Sciences*, 114(1), 8-14.

[4] Salzmann, J. A. (1979). Practice of orthodontics under public health guidance. *American Journal of Orthodontics*, 76(1), 103-104.

[5] Kumar, P., & Clark, M. (2009). *Kumar and Clark's Clinical Medicine* (7th edition), Elsevier.

[6] El -Bialy, T., Aboul-Azm, S. F., & El -Sakhawy, M. (2000). Study of craniofacial morphology and skeletal maturation in juvenile diabetics (Type I). *American Journal of Orthodontics and Dentofacial Orthopedics*, 118(2), 189-195.

[7] Roe, T. F., Mora, S., Costen, G., Kaufman, F., Carlson, M., & Gilsanz, V. (1991). Vertebral bone density in insulin-dependent diabetic children. *Metabolism*, 40(9), 967-971.

[8] Eastell, R., & Lambert, H. (2002). Diet and healthy bones. *Calcified Tissue International*, 70(5), 400-404.

[9] Chew, F. S. (1991). Radiologic manifestations in the musculoskeletal system of miscellaneous endocrine disorders. *Radiologic Clinics of North America*, 29(1), 135-147.

[10] Yonemitsu, I., Muramoto, T., & Soma, K. (2007). The influence of masseter activity on rat mandibular growth. *Archives of Oral Biology,*, 52(5), 487-493.

[11] Singleton, D. A., Buschang, P. H., Behrents, R. G., & Hinton, R. J. (2006). Craniofacial growth in growth hormone-deficient rats after growth hormone supplementation. *American Journal of Orthodontics and Dentofacial Orthopedics*, 130(1), 69-82.

[12] Abbassy, M. A., Watari, I., & Soma, K. (2008). Effect of experimental diabetes on craniofacial growth in rats. *Archives of Oral Biology*, 53(9), 819-825.

[13] Hough, S., Avioli, L. V., Bergfeld, M. A., Fallon, M. D., Slatopolsky, E., & Teitelbaum, S. L. (1981). Correction of abnormal bone and mineral metabolism in chronic streptozotocin-induced diabetes mellitus in the rat by insulin therapy. *Endocrinology*, 108(6), 2228-2234.

[14] Tein, MS, Breen, S. A., Loveday, B. E., Devlin, H., Balment, R. J., Boyd, R. D., et al. (1998). Bone mineral density and composition in rat pregnancy: effects of streptozotocin-induced diabetes mellitus and insulin replacement. *Experimental Physiology*, 83(2), 165-174.

[15] Thrailkill, K. M., Liu, L., Wahl, E. C., Bunn, R. C., Perrien, D. S., Cockrell, G. E., et al. (2005). Bone formation is impaired in a model of type 1 diabetes. *Diabetes*, 54(10), 2875-2881.

[16] Follak, N., Kloting, I., Wolf, E., & Merk, H. (2004). Histomorphometric evaluation of the influence of the diabetic metabolic state on bone defect healing depending on the defect size in spontaneously diabetic BB/OK rats. *Bone*, 35(1), 144-152.

[17] Alkan, A., Erdem, E., Gunhan, O., & Karasu, C. (2002). Histomorphometric evaluation of the effect of doxycycline on the healing of bone defects in experimental diabetes mellitus: a pilot study. *Journal of Oral and Maxillofacial Surgery*, 60(8), 898-904.

[18] Mc Cracken-Wesson, MS, Aponte., R., Chavali, R., & Lemons, J. E. (2006). Bone associated with implants in diabetic and insulin-treated rats. *Clinical Oral Implants Research*, 17(5), 495-500.

[19] Shyng, Y. C., Devlin, H., & Sloan, P. (2001). The effect of streptozotocin-induced experimental diabetes mellitus on calvarial defect healing and bone turnover in the rat. *International Journal of Oral and Maxillofacial Surgery*, 30(1), 70-74.

[20] Abdus, Salam. M., Matsumoto, N., Matin, K., Tsuha, Y., Nakao, R., Hanada, N., & Senpuku, H. (2004). Establishment of an animal model using recombinant NOD.B10.D2 mice to study initial adhesion of oral streptococci. *Clinical and Diagnostic Laboratory Immunology*, 11(2), 379-386.

[21] Matin, K., Salam, M. A., Akhter, J., Hanada, N., & Senpuku, H. (2002). Role of stromal-cell derived factor-1 in the development of autoimmune diseases in non-obese diabetic mice. *Immunology*, 107(2), 222-232.

[22] Chidiac, J. J., Shofer, F. S., Al-Kutoub, A., Laster, L. L., & Ghafari, J. (2002). Comparison of CT scanograms and cephalometric radiographs in craniofacial imaging. *Orthodontics and Craniofacial Research*, 5(2), 104-113.

[23] Vande Berg, J. R., Buschang, P. H., & Hinton, R. J. (2004b). Absolute and relative growth of the rat craniofacial skeleton. *Archives of Oral Biology*, 49(6), 477-484.

[24] Engstrom, C., Jennings, J., Lundy, M., & Baylink, D. J. (1988). Effect of bone matrix-derived growth factors on skull and tibia in the growing rat. *Journal of Oral Pathology*, 17(7), 334-340.

[25] Kiliaridis, S. E. C., & Thilander, B. (1985). The relationship between masticatory function and craniofacial morphology. I. A cephalometric longitudinal analysis in the growing ratfed a soft diet. *European Journal of Orthodontics*, 7, 273-283.

[26] Vandeberg, J. R., Buschang, P. H., & Hinton, R. J. (2004a). Craniofacial growth in growth hormone-deficient rats. *The Anatomical Record. Part A, Discoveries in Molecular, Cellular and Evolutionary Biology*, 278(2), 561-570.

[27] Stuart, A., & Smith, D. (1992). Use of the Fluorochromes xylenol orange, calcein green, and tetracycline to document bone deposition and remodeling in healing fractures in chickens. *Avian diseases*, 36, July, 447-449.

[28] Abbassy, M. A., Watari, I., & Soma, K. (2010). The effect of diabetes mellitus on rat mandibular bone formation and microarchitecture. *European Journal of Oral Sciences*, 118(4), 364-369.

[29] Shimomoto, Y., Chung, C. J., Iwasaki-Hayashi, Y., Muramoto, T., & Soma, K. (2007). Effects of occlusal stimuli on alveolar/jaw bone formation. *Journal of Dental Research*, 86(1), 47-51.

[30] Parfitt, A. M. (1988). Bone histomorphometry: standardization of nomenclature, symbols and units (summary of proposed system). *Bone*, 9(1), 67-69.

[31] Keshawarz, N. M., & Recker, R. R. (1986). The label escape error: comparison of measured and theoretical fraction of total bone-trabecular surface covered by single label in normals and patients with osteoporosis. *Bone*, 7(2), 83-87.

[32] Sheng, M. H., Baylink, D. J., Beamer, W. G., Donahue, L. R., Rosen, C. J., Lau, K. H., et al. (1999). Histomorphometric studies show that bone formation and bone mineral apposition rates are greater in C3H/HeJ (high-density) than C57BL/6J (low-density) mice during growth. *Bone*, 25(4), 421-429.

[33] Gerlach, R. F., Toledo, D. B., Fonseca, R. B., Novaes, P. D., Line, S. R., & Merzel, J. (2002). Alveolar bone remodelling pattern of the rat incisor under different functional conditions as shown by minocycline administration. *Archives of Oral Biology,*, 47(3), 203-209.

[34] Ding, M., Odgaard, A., & Hvid, I. (1999). Accuracy of cancellous bone volume fraction measured by micro-CT scanning. *Journal of Biomechanics*, 32(3), 323-326.

[35] Laib, A., & Ruegsegger, P. (1999). Calibration of trabecular bone structure measurements of in vivo three-dimensional peripheral quantitative computed tomography with 28-microm-resolution microcomputed tomography. *Bone*, 24(1), January, 35-39.

[36] Takada, H., Abe, S., Tamatsu, Y., Mitarashi, S., Saka, H., & Ide, Y. (2006). Three-dimensional bone microstructures of the mandibular angle using micro-CT and finite element analysis: relationship between partially impacted mandibular third molars and angle fractures. *Dent Traumatol*, 22(1), 18-24.

[37] Duarte, V. M., Ramos, A. M., Rezende, L. A., Macedo, U. B., Brandao-Neto, J., Almeida, M. G., & Rezende, A. A. (2005). Osteopenia: a bone disorder associated with diabetes mellitus. *Journal of Bone and Mineral Metabolism*, 23(1), 58-68.

[38] Yokoyama, M., Atsumi, T., Tsuchiya, M., Koyama, S., & Sasaki, K. (2009). Dynamic changes in bone metabolism in the rat temporomandibular joint after molar extraction using bone scintigraphy. *Europen Journal of Oral Sciences,*, 117(4), 374-379.

[39] Misawa, Y., Kageyama, T., Moriyama, K., Kurihara, S., Yagasaki, H., Deguchi, T., Ozawa, H., & Sahara, N. (2007). Effect of age on alveolar bone turnover adjacent to maxillary molar roots in male rats: A histomorphometric study. *Archives of Oral Biology*, 52(1), 44-50.

[40] Mishima, N., Sahara, N., Shirakawa, M., & Ozawa, H. (2002). Effect of streptozotocin-induced diabetes mellitus on alveolar bone deposition in the rat. *Archives of Oral Biology*, 47(12), 843-849.

[41] Glajchen, N., Epstein, S., Ismail, F., Thomas, S., Fallon, M., & Chakrabarti, S. (1988). Bone mineral metabolism in experimental diabetes mellitus: osteocalcin as a measure of bone remodeling. *Endocrinology*, 123(1), 290-295.

[42] Shires, R., Teitelbaum, S. L., Bergfeld, M. A., Fallon, M. D., Slatopolsky, E., & Avioli, L. V. (1981). The effect of streptozotocin-induced chronic diabetes mellitus on bone and mineral homeostasis in the rat. *Journal of Laboratory Clinical Medicine*, 97(2), 231-240.

[43] Losken, A., Mooney, M. P., & Siegel, M. I. (1994). Comparative cephalometric study of nasal cavity growth patterns in seven animal models. *Cleft Palate Craniofacial Journal*, 31(1), 17-23.

[44] Siegel, M. I., & Mooney, M. P. (1990). Appropriate animal models for craniofacial biology. *Cleft Palate Journal*, 27(1), 18-25.

[45] Ward, D. T., Yau, S. K., Mee, A. P., Mawer, E. B., Miller, CA, Garland, H. O., et al. (2001). Functional, molecular, and biochemical characterization of streptozotocin-induced diabetes. *Journal of the American Society of Nephrology*, 12(4), 779-790.

[46] Pun, K. K., Lau, P., & Ho, P. W. (1989). The characterization, regulation, and function of insulin receptors on osteoblast-like clonal osteosarcoma cell line. *Journal of Bone and Mineral Research*, 4(6), 853-862.

[47] Thomas, D. M., Udagawa, N., Hards, D. K., Quinn, J. M., Moseley, J. M., Findlay, D. M., et al. (1998). Insulin receptor expression in primary and cultured osteoclast-like cells. *Bone*, 23(3), 181-186.

[48] Reddy, G. K., Stehno-Bittel, L., Hamade, S., & Enwemeka, C. S. (2001). The biomechanical integrity of bone in experimental diabetes. *Diabetes Research and Clinical Practice*, 54(1), 1-8.

[49] Tsuchida, T., Sato, K., Miyakoshi, N., Abe, T., Kudo, T., Tamura, Y., et al. (2000). Histomorphometric evaluation of the recovering effect of human parathyroid hormone (1-34) on bone structure and turnover in streptozotocin-induced diabetic rats. *Calcified Tissue International*, 66(3), 229-233.

[50] Toromanoff, A., Ammann, P., Mosekilde, L., Thomsen, J. S., & Riond, J. L. (1997). Parathyroid hormone increases bone formation and improves mineral balance in vitamin D-deficient female rats. *Endocrinology*, 138(6), 2449-2457.

[51] Collins, D., Jasani, C., Fogelman, I., & Swaminathan, R. (1998). Vitamin D and bone mineral density. *Osteoporosis International,*, 8(2), 110-114.

[52] Chiarelli, F., Giannini, C., & Mohn, A. (2004). Growth, growth factors and diabetes. *European Journal of Endocrinology,*, 151(3), U109-U117.

[53] Ozbek, M., Dural, S., Kanli, A., Tuncel, M., & Orhan, K. (2009). Morphological evaluation of rat incisor enamel and dentin induced by pregnancy and lactation using a scanning electron microscope. *Journal of Veterinary Medical Science*, 71(10), 1273-1277.

[54] Balint , E., Marshall , C. F., & Sprague, S. M. (2001). Glucose-induced inhibition of in vitro bone mineralization. *Bone*, 28(1), 21-28.

Section 5

Patient Care

Chapter 17

Type I Diabetes in Children: Facilitating Adherence to Medical Regimens

Laura Nabors and Jenny Bartz

Additional information is available at the end of the chapter

http://dx.doi.org/10.5772/52283

1. Introduction

Approximately 1 in every 400 to 600 children has Type I diabetes. The care of children with Type I diabetes involves complex procedures including daily blood glucose testing, dietary monitoring, intensive insulin therapy, and physical activity to maintain metabolic control in the face of pancreatic failure. The aforementioned procedures as well as adjustment of insulin doses based on blood glucose monitoring are critical areas for adherence to the medical regimen. The work and complexity of maintaining a diabetes regimen can lead to adherence issues for children and their families [4,5]. Adhering to diabetes regimens, however, is related to long-term positive health outcomes. If children do not take care of their diabetes they can experience problems with their vision as well cardiovascular issues and circulation problems. This chapter reviews critical issues for adherence for children and adolescents. Ideas for improving adherence also are presented.

Only about 50% of adults and children with chronic illnesses follow or adhere to their medical regimens. Adherence is a very important area of study for adolescents with Type I diabetes, because managing this disease involves multiple strategies including diet, exercise, and glucose monitoring as well as administering medication [9,10]. The early teenage years also are a peak time in terms of incidence rates for developing diabetes, and puberty is a difficult time to manage insulin levels, because adolescents may have decreased insulin sensitivity and poor self-management skills [11]. In this chapter we use the terms adherence and self-management to discuss a child's diabetes care and how well a child's medical regimen is followed. The terms are similar, but it is important to define self-management as a broader concept that involves diabetes management activities by the child and his or her caregivers. Adherence is often more narrowly defined as following one's medical regimen. Both terms are important and critical as adherence and good self-management lead to positive health outcomes for youth who have diabetes.

2. Children and diabetes management

Caregivers of preschool-age children may feel that they need to be vigilant and constantly monitor their child's diabetes. Sullivan-Bolyai, Knafl, Deatrick, and Gray found that mothers of preschoolers valued education from health care professionals that would provide them with solutions to diabetes management dilemmas [12]. Mothers said that they valued being able to contact health care professionals by telephone when they had a question about their child's diabetes. As they become more comfortable with diabetes management for their child, mothers appreciate being able to converse about methods for maintaining their child's medical regimen and "good" care while at the same time working to find ways to fit diabetes care into the framework of family routines and the daily life of the family. Health care professionals can support caregivers by helping them identify their strengths and by providing affirmations and encouragement if their confidence for managing their child's diabetes decreases [12].

Chisholm and colleagues studied predictors of adherence in children ages two- to eight-years-old who had Type I diabetes. Mothers were primary informants and participants resided in Britain. Mothers provided data by telephone interview about the foods consumed by their child in the last 24 hours. Other information was collected through a review of the child's medical chart. Results of this study indicated that mothers were following medical recommendations. Also, increased education of mothers was related to higher or better levels of adherence, such as more frequent blood glucose monitoring and lower glycosated hemoglobin levels for children. Monitoring of injections was more consistent than monitoring blood glucose testing and diet, which were more difficult to consistently record and review. The authors concluded that parents may benefit from repeated education sessions to review information related to adherence, especially ideas related to nutrition and diet. The aforementioned studies provide some evidence of the importance of assessing adherence in younger children. Prospective, longitudinal studies are needed with younger children, to determine strategies for improving adherence.

Davis and her colleagues found that younger children, in the preschool- and elementary school-age range have adherence problems [13]. Davis et al. found that parental warmth was related to better adherence for children between the ages of four and ten years. In contrast, parents who were characterized as being overly strict with their child tended to have children with poorer glycemic control. Davis et al. concluded that parental warmth is related to better family cohesion and reduced family conflict, which are variables that are associated with better adherence in children. Results of the study by Davis et al. also revealed that children residing in low-income families were likely to have poorer adherence. Overall, there is a paucity of research on adherence for young children as compared to adolescents, and we believe that this is an area for further research. Habits from childhood continue to

http://dx.doi.org/10.5772/52283

the later years and good management in childhood can also transfer to the adolescent years, making good adherence practices a pattern of behavior that is a resilience factor for a child throughout his or her life.

The clinician or health care provider should assess parent reactions and strategies for coping with misbehavior during mealtime, when he or she is working with parents of younger children. Wilson, DeCourcey, and Freeman found that over-reaction and over-correction of mealtime problems was associated with relatively poor parental coping and management of the child's diabetes. These researchers speculated that, "parents who perceive themselves as over-reactive may be removing themselves from oversight of the illness (p. 220)." Children, in turn, appear to benefit from parental guidance and education. Patton et al. assessed young children's mealtime behaviors with parents [15]. Children were between the ages of two and eight years, with a mean age of approximately five and a half years. Children who were in poorer control, with relatively poorer diabetes management, had mealtime relationships with their parents that were characterized by rigidity and coercive feeding behaviors on the part of parents. Increasing positive and open communication between children with Type I diabetes and their parents or caregivers also may lead to improved parent-child interactions and positive diabetes management. Wilson et al. proposed that longitudinal studies should be conducted to gain a greater understanding of the ways that parent-child interactions support diabetes management. Health professionals and clinicians should strive to advise parents about and assist them in developing a pattern of positive mealtime interactions with their child.

3. Adolescents and diabetes management

Self-efficacy for diabetes management is grounded in a social cognitive approach, which emphasizes a "can do" attitude toward managing problem situations [16]. The adolescent should be encouraged to think of him- or herself as being able to complete diabetes management tasks that he or she is capable of managing, and be encouraged to gain expertise and master new skills, such as administering his or her own insulin. The tasks assigned to the adolescent should be commensurate with his or her abilities so that he or she can master the self-management task and move to a higher level of self-efficacy for working with his or her diabetes. Berg et al. also stated that high feelings of self-efficacy for managing diabetes may be especially helpful for adolescents with "acting out" behavior problems or *externalizing* problems [17].

Another important thing to address is fear of hypoglycemia or hyperglycemia, especially with adolescents and their parents. Battista, Hart, Greco, and Gloizer assessed adolescent report of diabetes management for youth with Type I Diabetes for adolescents between the ages of thirteen to eighteen [18]. The youth in their sample were experiencing social anxiety. These authors thought it was important to assess social anxiety as it might be a factor contributing to poor diabetes management and because social anxiety might contribute to poor diabetes management when an adolescent was in social situations with peers. Their findings indicated some support for these notions. They also reported that fears of hypoglycemic or hyperglycemic episodes might "drive" adolescent behavior and fears could lead to poor diabetes management. We also have found that fear of either type of episode can be related to poor diabetes management in adolescents and older children (i.e., children in late elementary school). Hence, it is important to discuss management of diabetes in cases of both hypo- and hyperglycemia with youth. Additionally, it is important to discuss how fears of either type of episode can influence poor management choices in order to provide advance guidance and opportunities to discuss fears related to either type of problem.

Di Battista et al. found that social anxiety may be an important indicator of poor diabetes management in adolescent boys as opposed to girls [18]. They concluded that socially anxious boys may have difficulty managing their diabetes in mid- to older-adolescence. Health care providers should ask questions about anxiety and diabetes management in social situations in order to determine if anxiety about peer reactions is influencing choices adolescents, especially males, make in terms of diabetes management. Practicing explaining the need for good management to peers is one way to prepare adolescents to go through stressful peer situations. Another idea is to teach the adolescent who has diabetes to educate his or her peers about what could happen if he or she is in "poor" metabolic control. Finally, teaching relaxation and other anxiety management techniques may assist the adolescent in managing diabetes related anxiety in social situations. When a young male has diabetes, clinicians should inquire about diabetes management in social situations in order to determine if the young man is struggling to manage his diabetes when he is interacting with peers. We believe that asking about management of diabetes in front of peers may be important for girls too, because there is a tendency for girls to administer limited insulin or lower insulin doses as a weight management strategy [19].

4. Parents and diabetes management

Findings from previous studies have indicated that support from family and friends may facilitate self-management for adolescents with Type I diabetes [20]. For example, Drew et al. proposed that parental warmth and acceptance of the child, within a relationship that is open and where communication is high fostered independence for adolescents with diabetes [21]. Berg et al. also supported the importance of parental involvement and monitoring as a key ingredient for successful diabetes management by adolescents [17]. In a sense both the parent and child are collaborators working to reach high positive levels of communication and adherence to the diabetes care regimen for the child. As a coach the parent can also work to encourage adolescent self-efficacy for diabetes management.

High levels of family conflict and a lack of cohesion in family relationships have been related to poor metabolic control (higher glycosated hemoglobin levels) [22]. Similarly, good family relationships may have a positive effect on adherence [23]. Arguably, the most important relationship that may drive the aforementioned results about the "family" is the parent-child or caregiver-child relationship. Parents' and adolescents' perceptions of family functioning are related to adolescents' adherence, management, and metabolic control, which are critical components of adolescent diabetes care [22,24]. A warm, caring, and supportive relationship with parents or caregivers appears to be a protective factor, supporting adherence, irrespective of the child's age [15]. A good quality relationship will be marked by regular communication about diabetes management as well as warmth and encouragement [21]. The role of the parent or caregiver changes with the age of the child. The parent plays a more direct role in diabetes management for younger children, while for adolescents the role could be described as a mentoring or coaching relationship, with the adult being a member of a "team" with the child to support his or her diabetes management. We recommend a "rubber-band" approach for adolescents, based on need. The parent helps more and pulls tight when the adolescent requests or really needs help (e.g., eating irresponsibly) and then relaxes when the adolescent is exhibiting good self-management skills. A rubber band approach also may be appropriate for younger children. However, the parent or caretaker does play a relatively larger role, in terms of caregiver contribution or share of diabetes management tasks, when the child is younger.

One idea to help in building a strong child-caregiver management unit is to describe a team approach to diabetes management. In this approach, parents can be coaches and help monitor and guide their child's increasing responsibility for diabetes management as he or she passes through adolescence [17]. Both the parent and child could take turns coaching the team or finding ideas to help the child improve his or her "game plan" for self-management of diabetes. This promotes a shared leadership and responsibility framework in the cooperative relationship between parents or caregivers and children who have Type I Diabetes. Vesco et al. proposed that a "shared responsibility" framework provides the adolescent with the support he or she needs to optimize diabetes management [25]. A spirit of cooperation between parents and child, who are both part of a team working to achieve the highest level of diabetes care for the child, can be an optimal framework for a shared responsibility approach [21]. Involvement of mothers and fathers is important to positive coping with diabetes; however, more information is needed on the relative contributions of each parent or caregiver, and on the role that each should take in helping a child manage diabetes.

Parents or caregivers serve as "monitors" of their child's diabetes management and in this role report on the child's management to the medical team. Health professionals need to ask questions and remain cognizant of the fact that premature transfer of diabetes management to the child can have deleterious effects. Both health care professionals and caregivers need to remain aware of the balancing act – between monitoring and direct assistance – that is needed to help children and adolescents manage their diet and other aspects of their medical regimen. Premature transfer of diabetes self-management, in the absence of child skills or readiness to manage his or her diabetes, has been associated with poor outcomes [25]. Caregivers may need to remain involved, on some level, throughout the adolescent period [17]. Vesco et al. found that youth-caregiver conflict over "direct" management tasks, such as testing and insulin administration, is indicative of or a marker of potential difficulties in diabetes management [25]. Stress and conflict over indirect management, such as planning meals, can also be a negative influence on management, but is less likely to be related to poor management than conflict over direct management tasks.

Parents may encourage a child to find benefits related to having diabetes or find benefits associated with going through the trials associated with maintaining good diet, exercise, glucose monitoring, and insulin administration habits. Tran and colleagues found that young adolescents, between the ages of ten to fourteen years, provided higher ratings of positive reactions to diabetes stress if they were also reporting high levels of benefit finding [26]. Benefit-finding was likened to making a positive meaning as one copes with adverse life events. They speculated that those adopting a benefit-finding approach could positively reframe trials and tribulations related to diabetes management; therefore, lowering children's stress levels. Interestingly, they also reported that benefit-finding was associated with higher levels of negative reactions to diabetes-related stress. One idea they had about this was that children who are "benefit-finders" are more attuned to their emotional experiences in general, which allows them to process and move through troubling emotions so that they adapt or move on with their lives. Because they process and deal with negative affect, it becomes *less* disruptive in their lives. Unfortunately, benefit-finding was not related to changes in blood glucose levels; future research may uncover reasons for this.

It is important to assess both parent/caregiver and child views of "who should be responsible for what" in terms of diabetes management tasks [21]. This can be especially important to uncover for direct management tasks or factors related to direct management tasks, such as those questions listed in Table 1.

- Who reminds about or remembers the injection or bolus (insulin administration for those on a pump) schedule?
- Who gives the injection or administers the bolus?
- Who adjusts the bolus or insulin dose based on documented blood glucose monitoring?
- Who remembers to monitor blood glucose?
- Who does blood glucose checks?
- Is there any conflict or trouble among parents/child related to blood glucose monitoring or insulin checks?
- Who records or "counts" carbs at mealtimes?
- Who is responsible for making sure the child has snacks easily available in case of an insulin reaction?
- Who notices and monitors for "highs" and "lows?"
- Does your child or do you have any fears about *hyperglycemic* or *hypoglycemic* episodes?
- What do you and your child know about *hyperglycemic* or *hypoglycemic* episodes? (your child's triggers or warning signs, what happens)
- What is your knowledge of the signs to signal an insulin reaction?
- Who decides about and rotates the site for an insulin injection or bolus?
- What are your and your child's fears related to managing diabetes?
- What are your and your child's ideas about who should be "in charge" of diabetes management?
- Is there any conflict about diabetes management between your child and you?
- What does your child think that you should be doing to help with diabetes management?
- Does your child have anxiety about diabetes management tasks in social situations with peers?

Table 1. Questions to Uncover Information about Diabetes Management

http://dx.doi.org/10.5772/52283

Assessing the adolescents' perceptions of parental involvement, in terms of level of involvement (e.g., "too much" or "too little") can provide key information about the adolescent's perspective; assessing family members' perspectives provides key information too. Finally, asking about diabetes management in social situations with peers can provide other key information [18]. When armed with data from the types of questions listed in Table 1, the health professional can take the adolescent's and caregivers' perspectives into account when discussing diabetes management. Health professionals should help the child and caregivers work toward a model of shared decision making that is a best fit for each individual child and caregiver unit.

Haugstvedt et al. reported that both mothers and fathers worry about the long-term health outcomes that their child may face [27]. Care is a burden for both parents, especially fear of nocturnal hypoglycemia for the child. There can be differences in mothers' and fathers' perceptions of their child's diabetes. Mothers may play a greater role in their child's care and subsequently feel more distressed about their child's illness compared to fathers [27, 28]. Being more involved with their child's care may be related to mothers feeling more confident about their ability to manage their child's diabetes, although both mothers and fathers may feel confident about their ability to manage their child's diabetes [29]. Leonard et al. found that mothers reported higher confidence for managing their child's diabetes when their child was away from home or experienced changes in activity levels compared to fathers [29]. Mothers and fathers may also have different styles of coping, with mothers being more emotional and fathers being more likely to seek and discuss medical information with their child [28]. Fathers may express hesitancy toward being in support groups, which mothers can find to be of value [29]. Although more research about father involvement is needed, we believe that involvement of fathers in care can provide support for mothers and children. Their involvement has the potential to improve diabetes management.

5. Peer factors and diabetes management

Peers are integral to adolescents' diabetes management. Adherence behaviors and self-care may suffer in social situations with peers, because adolescents are hesitant to appear different from the norm and perform diabetes management tasks. Adolescents also may report feeling pressure from their peers to eat "junk food" that is not healthy for them [30]. Adolescents may benefit from "problem-solving" with diabetes educators or counselors in order to learn how to cope and follow their regimen during stressful social situations with peers, such as parties. Children also may benefit from learning refusal skills to help them say "no thank you" to junk food, and to request opportunities to eat foods which are low in carbohydrates and are consistent with their meal and snack plans for optimal management of their diabetes. Salamon et al. developed a four-item "Self-Care Around Friends" (SCF) measure that examines adolescent perceptions of worry in social situations [30]. Questions are rated on 7-point Likert scales. The questions are:

(1) Over the past month, how many times did you have to do your diabetes care around other kids?, (2) How stressful was it to do your care around your friends during this time?, (3)

How worried were you about your friends' reactions to you doing your self-care in front of them?, and (4) How open were you in doing your care in front of your friends? (p. 53).

These questions, or similar ones, may assist health care professionals in learning about stress experienced by adolescents when interacting with their friends and needing to manage their diabetes.

Salamon et al. also used items from the "Diabetes Stress Questionnaire" (*DSQ*), which is another measure that can assess adolescent stress [31]. This measure has subscales, "Peer Stress" and "Adverse Interpersonal Effects," that have questions addressing stress in social situations. Examples of questions on these subscales that might be relevant are, I am able to…

(1) have friends tell me foods I shouldn't eat. (2) talk with my friends about my diabetes, (3) eat or snack when my friends are not eating. (4) test and administer insulin while with friends. (p. 54) [31].

Health care professionals and clinicians can use adolescents' responses to these types of questions as a starting point for asking more questions to better understand problem situations with peers. Then problem-solving can occur, and the adolescent and health care professional can discuss ideas for managing stressful social situations. Consequently, the *DSQ* is another measure that is useful for assessment of stress related to adherence [31]. We believe that the types of questions in this paragraph and the preceding one also can be used to assess how older elementary school-age children interact with peers to assist them with diabetes management.

Skinner et al. assessed children's perceptions of their diabetes. They recruited adolescents with Type I Diabetes from outpatient clinics in four regional hospitals in south England [23]. Participants completed questionnaires measuring well-being, self-management, social support, diabetes-specific support, and peer support. Girls had more severe diabetes and reported greater levels of depression and anxiety, lower positive well-being, and more support from friends than boys. Social support was positively related to perceived control and total well-being. However, none of the social support measures were related to perceived seriousness or perceived impact of diabetes. They concluded that perceptions of diabetes "well-being" were more positive if adolescents believed they were receiving peer support. Skinner et al. stated that "adolescents need a supportive peer group, whose lifestyle does not radically conflict with the demands of diabetes, for dietary self-care and well-being to be optimal (265)."

Schroff-Pendley and her fellow researchers found that peer support was very important to adolescents with Type I diabetes [11]. They suggested that education for peers would allow them to support diabetes management for their friends with Type I Diabetes. Without education and training, they cautioned that peers might not be able to provide support that would be related to higher levels of adherence. Greco et al. conducted a study that showed the value of education in enhancing positive peer support [32]. Greco et al. developed a program for best friends and children with Type I Diabetes to increase support for diabetes management. Participants were children with diabetes between the ages of 10 to18 years

http://dx.doi.org/10.5772/52283

and their friends. They found that education received during sessions was effective in improving friends' knowledge about diabetes. Their findings indicated that friends who attended the groups were able to offer guidance and emotional support to peers who had diabetes. Much of the research on peer support focuses on adolescents. Extending research to assess the importance and function of peer support for children is an area where further study is needed.

6. Summary

Children and adolescents with Type I Diabetes struggle with adhering to a complex medical regimen. Flexible regimens, which include the use of insulin pumps and adjustments using the pumps, termed basal-boluses, require frequent decisions about diabetes management and heighten the importance of adherence. Family and peer support can be critical to positive diabetes management and low glycosated hemoglobin levels. Improving control over the child's diabetes management also leads to positive health outcomes.

Guidance and support from caregivers or parents also is important. The role of the parent may shift over the course of a child's development, with the caregiver directing management in early childhood, and then shifting his or her role to one of support and coaching as the child enters the teenage years. All things being equal, it is beneficial for parents to remain aware of their child's management and be ready to assist when needed. In this way, the parent can form a band of support around the child that facilitates his or her adherence and self-efficacy for managing his or her diabetes. Encouraging children with diabetes to discuss their self-management needs also may improve the involvement of family and peers. Educating peers, so that they know how to be supportive, can increase their positive influence on the child's diabetes management [32]. In the future, interventions targeting increasing peer support and defining critical issues for parents in terms of when to act as a coach and when to increase monitoring will have practical implications that will facilitate children's diabetes management. Moreover, conducting longitudinal studies to assess factors related to adherence in various populations (e.g., children with diabetes and celiac disease versus children with only diabetes; children in single parent versus nuclear families) will shed light on variations in factors related to adherence both within and between populations. This will be important in improving our understanding of ways to facilitate diabetes management for children in special populations.

Author details

Laura Nabors* and Jenny Bartz

University of Cincinnati, USA

References

[1] Centers for Disease Control and Prevention. National Diabetes Fact Sheet: General Information and National Estimates on Diabetes in the United States, 2002. Atlanta, GA. U.S. Department of Health and Human Services, Centers for Disease Control and Prevention, 2003. Government Doc. No. HE 20.7002:D 54/6.

[2] Anderson B, Auslander WF, Jung KC, Miller JP, Santiago JV. Assessing Family Sharing of Diabetes Responsibilities. Journal of Pediatric Psychology 1990;15(4) 477-492.

[3] Chisholm V, Atkinson L, Donaldson C, Noyes K, Payne A, & Kelnar C. Predictors of Treatment Adherence in Young Children with Type I Diabetes. Journal of Advanced Nursing 2007; 57 82-493.

[4] Chang C-W, Yeh C-H, Lo F-S, Shih Y-L. Adherence behaviors in Taiwanese Children and Adolescents with Type 1 Diabetes Mellitus. Journal of Nursing and Healthcare of Chronic Illness in Association with Journal of Clinical Nursing 2007; 16(7b) 207-214.

[5] Schilling LS, Dixon JK, Knafl, KA, Lynn MR, Murphy K, Dumser S, Grey M. A New Self-Report Measure of Self-Management of Type I Diabetes for Adolescents. Nursing Research 2009;58(4) 228-236.

[6] Bui H, Perlman K, Daneman D. Self-monitoring of Blood Glucose in Children and Teens with Diabetes. Pediatric Diabetes 2005; 6 50-62.

[7] Frey MA, Ellis D, Templin T, Naar-King S, Gutai JP. Diabetes Management and Metabolic Control in School-Age Children with Type 1 Diabetes. Children's Health Care 2006;35 349-363.

[8] Rapoff, MA. Adherence to Pediatric Medical Regimens, Second Edition. Issues in Clinical Child Psychology. New York: Springer; 2009.

[9] Silverstein J, Klingensmith G, Copeland K, Plotnick L, Kaufman R, Laffel L, Deeb L, Grey M. et al. Care of Children and Adolescents with Type I Diabetes: A Statement of the American Diabetes Association. Diabetes Care 2005;28(1) 186-212.

[10] La Greca AM, Schuman WB. Adherence to Prescribed Medical Regimens. In Michael Roberts (Editor) Handbook of Pediatric Psychology: Second Edition. New York: Guilford Press; 1995, pp. 55-83.

[11] Shroff-Pendley J, Kasmen LJ, Miller DL, Donze J, Swenson C, Reeves G. Peer and Family Support in Children and Adolescents with Type I Diabetes. Journal of Pediatric Psychology, 2002;27(5) 429-438.

[12] Sullivan-Bolyai S, Knafl K, Deatrick J, Grey M. Maternal Management Behaviors for Young Children with Type I Diabetes. Maternal and Child Nursing 2003;28(3) 160-166.

[13] Davis CL, Delamater AM, Shaw KH, La Greca AM, Eidson MS, Perez-Rodriguez JE, Nemery R. Brief Report: Parenting Styles, Regimen Adherence, and Glycemic Control in 4- to 10-year-old Children with Diabetes. Journal of Pediatric Psychology 2001; 26(2) 123-129.

[14] Wilson AC, DeCourcey WM, Freeman KA. The Impact of Managing School-Aged Children's Diabetes: The Role of Child Behavior Problems and Parental Discipline Strategy. Journal of Clinical Psychology in Medical Settings 2009;16 216-222.

[15] Patton SR, Piazza-Waggoner C, Modi AC, Dolan LM, Powers SW. Family Functioning at Meals Relates to Adherence in Young Children with Type I Diabetes. Journal of Pediatrics and Child Health 2009;45 736-741.

[16] Bandura A. Social Cognitive Theory. In Vasta R. (ed.). Annals of Child Development. Vol. 6. Six theories of child development. Greenwich, CT: JAI Press. 1989. p 1-60.

[17] Berg CA, King PS, Butler JM, Pham P, Palmer D, Wiebe DJ. Parental Involvement and Adolescents' Diabetes Management: The Mediating Role of Self-Efficacy and Externalizing and Internalizing Behaviors. Journal of Pediatric Psychology 2011;36(3) 329-339.

[18] Di Battista AM, Hart TA, Greco L, Gloizer J. Type I Diabetes among Adolescents: Reduced Diabetes Self-Care Caused by Social Fear and Fear of Hypoglycemia. Diabetes Educator 2009;35(3) 465-475.

[19] Hoagen B, Ruth-Sahd LA, Schneider M. Diabulimia: What It Is and How to Recognize It In Critical Care. Dimensions of Critical Care Nursing 2009;28(4) 147-153.

[20] Wysocki T, Harris MA, Greco P, Harvey LM, McDonnell K, Danda CL, Bubb J, White N H. Social Validity of Support Group and Behavior Therapy Interventions for Families of Adolescents with Insulin Dependent Diabetes Mellitus. Journal of Pediatric Psychology 1997;22 635-649.

[21] Drew LM, Berg C, Wiebe DJ. The Mediating Role of Extreme Peer Orientation in the Relationships Between Adolescent-Parent Relationship and Diabetes Management. Journal of Family Psychology 2010;24(3) 299-306.

[22] Hauser ST, Jacobson AM, Lavori P, Wolfsdorf JI, Herskowitz RD, Milley JE, Bliss R, Gelfand E. Adherence among Children and Adolescents with Insulin Dependent Diabetes Mellitus Over a 4-year Longitudinal Follow-up: II. Immediate and Long-Term Linkages with Family Milieu. Journal of Pediatric Psychology 1990;15 527-542.

[23] Skinner TC, John M, Hampson SE. (2000). Social Support and Personal Needs Models of Diabetes as Predictors of Self-Care and Well-Being: A Longitudinal Study of Adolescents with Diabetes. Journal of Pediatric Psychology 2000;25 257-267.

[24] Wysocki T, Greco P, Harris MA, Bubb J, White NH. Behavior Therapy for Families of Adolescents with Diabetes: Maintenance of Treatment Effects. Diabetes Care 2001;24 441-446.

[25] Vesco AT, Anderson BJ, Laffel LMB, Dolan LM, Igerski LM, Hood KK. Responsibility Sharing Between Adolescents with Type I Diabetes and Their Caregivers: Importance of Adolescent Perceptions of Diabetes Management and Control. Journal of Pediatric Psychology 2010;35(10) 1168-1177.

[26] Tran W, Wiebe DJ, Fortenberry KT, Butler JM, Berg CA. Benefit Finding, Affective Reactions to Diabetes Stress, and Diabetes Management Among Early Adolescents. Health Psychology 2011;30(2) 212-219.

[27] Haugstvedt A, Wentzel-Larsen T, Rokne B, Graue M. Perceived Family Burden and Emotional Distress: Similarities and Differences Between Mothers and Fathers of Children with Type 1 Diabetes in a Population-Based Study. Pediatric Diabetes 2011;12 107-114.

[28] Hansen JA. Dissertation: Paternal Contribution to Disease Care in Parenting a Child with Type 1 Diabetes. 2010; American University UMI 3421618.

[29] Leonard BJ, Kratz BJ, Skay CL, Rheinberger MM. Comparison of Mother-Father Perceptions of Their Child's Self-Management of Diabetes. Issues in Comprehensive Pediatric Nursing 1997;20 69-87.

[30] Salamon KS, Hains AA, Fleischman KM, Davies WH, Kichler J. Improving Adherence in Social Situations for Adolescents with Type 1 Diabetes Mellitus (T1DM): A Pilot Study. Primary Care Diabetes 2010;4 47-55.

[31] Boardway RH, Delamater AM, Tomakowsky J, Gutai JP. Stress Management Training for Adolescents with Diabetes. Journal of Pediatric Psychology 1993;18 29-45.

[32] Greco P, Pendley JS, McDonald K, Reeves G. A Peer Group Intervention for Adolescents with Type I Diabetes and Their Best Friends. Journal of Pediatric Psychology 2001;28(8) 485-490.

Chapter 18

The Influence of Family Support, Parental Coping and School Support on Adherence to Type 1 Diabetes' Self-Care in Adolescents

A. Cristina Almeida, M. Graça Pereira and
Engrácia Leandro

Additional information is available at the end of the chapter

http://dx.doi.org/10.5772/53062

1. Introduction

Diabetes Mellitus is a globe and a growing serious public health problem. Type 1 Diabetes is estimated to be one of the five most prevalent chronic diseases in children and adolescents, corresponding to 5-10% of all cases worldwide [1, 2]. Type 1 diabetes is an autoimmune chronic disease resulting from total absence of insulin secretion. In order to replace the absence of insulin production by the cells in the islets of Langerhans, located in the pancreas, it is necessary to administer exogenous insulin [3-5].

Nutrition and physical exercise also play fundamental roles in managing type 1 diabetes, in association with insulin therapy. The nutrition of an adolescent with diabetes should be guided by the principles of healthy eating and by the regular practice of physical exercise, in order to facilitate the control of blood glucose levels, prevent associated complications, maintain body weight within the normal standards and reduce cardiovascular diseases risk factors, providing psychosocial and familiar well-being [6-9]. However, diet and physical activity are the type of self-care activities that adolescents with diabetes are less concerned with [10].

Type 1 diabetes has a multifactorial etiology, in which genetic factors are important, due to modifications in the HLA complex (Human Leukocite Antigen Complex), behavioral factors, which can include viral infections (enteroviruses, coxsackie virus, congenital rubella) and environmental borne toxins, such as nitrosamines or even food such as the early exposure to cow's milk proteins, cereals or gluten, and in this case, the antibodies produced by the immune system's T cells to destroy these potentially invading agents also act on the pancreas β cells, destroying them [11-13].

Self-management and self-care is of critical importance for the control of this type of diabetes in children and adolescents. In fact, the responsibility of regularly monitoring the disease and its symptoms and the compliance with the treatment lies with the family and later, in accordance with the growth and the development phase, are gradually transferred to the child/adolescent [14-17]. Therefore, the main goals for type 1 Diabetes Mellitus's treatment, in children and adolescents, emphasize the prevention of symptoms and their severity, the prevention of short and long term complications, and the appropriate growth and development of the adolescent allowing the suitable maintenance of daily activities such as those related to family dynamics, school and social life [15, 18-20].

However, the multiple physiological and psychosocial modifications occurring during adolescence compromise diabetes treatments during this developmental period [15, 21, 22] and often, the adolescent show serious difficulties in adhering to self-care management of diabetes and the prevention of its complications. The conflicts arising from the demands and complexities involved in the self-management of diabetes, and the adolescent's expectations regarding their own experiences, in this developmental phase, may account for this scenario [23, 24].

According to the World Health Organization (WHO), adolescence is placed between 10-19 years, during which the individual is subjected to changes of biological nature, determined by puberty that will produce a rapid growth with consequently distinct body transformations; changes of cognitive nature, with a higher complexity in reasoning skills, through the attainment of autonomy and identity construction and also changes of social nature with the experience of new and different roles [25-27]. However, the constant need to declare autonomy and independence leads the adolescent to idealize feelings of invulnerability, inconsistent with the acceptance of a chronic disease such as type 1 diabetes that may encourage non-adherence to self-care [22].

Parental involvement, communication, cohesion and family conflicts that arise when managing diabetes self-care, are good examples of the type of family support available to the adolescent. A higher level of family conflict and less involvement account for worse outcomes of adherence to diabetes self-care in adolescents [28]. In turn, schools with staff and peers also account from other sources of social support that the adolescent with type 1 diabetes may count on, in daily life, that may influence metabolic control and quality of life [29]. Peer pressure and the demands of the social environment (school, recreational activities and family) may hinder adherence to self-care in adolescents with diabetes [30, 31].

This chapter's main goal is to describe the relationship among family support, school support and parental coping in adolescents with type 1 diabetes on adherence to self-care in order to inform the development of interventions programs to meet adolescents' needs regarding diabetes management.

2. Adherence to self-care in the adolescent with type 1 diabetes

The diagnosis of a chronic condition such as diabetes involves a change in lifestyle as well as the use of therapeutic methods that, at times, adolescents may not have the will or capacity to integrate into their daily lives resulting in risks to their health [32-35]. Considering that the prescribed treatment regimen can be complex, the role of health professionals involved with patient's care is of crucial relevance and intervention should emphasize symptoms' control and the promotion of quality of life [36-38].

There are strong evidences that individuals with chronic diseases, such as diabetes, present difficulties in adhering to the prescribed therapeutic regimes, with the consequent complexities of managing and controlling the disease [39, 40]. However, the literature shows that some adolescents have problems in adhering to a self-administrate treatment regardless of the type of disease or its severity [41].

Non-adherence to treatment of a chronic disease, particularly in type 1 diabetes, embodies a problem of multifactorial etiology and indeed different attempts to explain adherence behavior to prescribed treatments have been proposed [32]. According to the World Health Organization [41], different factors affecting adherence can be classified into five groups: 1) social, economic and cultural factors; 2) factors related to the health services and professionals; 3) factors underlying the disease and the comorbidity; 4) factors related to the treatment and 5) factors related to the patient.

Adolescents with diabetes, in particular, go through a phase of strong psychosocial changes and have to deal simultaneously with the changes of adolescence itself and as well as coping with the demands of controlling the disease treatment specificities [16, 42-45]. The hormonal changes occurring during puberty that cause insulin resistance, the rebelliousness characteristic of this phase, and almost total absence of residual insulin secretion by the pancreas, may complicate diabetes treatment, particularly, adherence [15, 46, 47].

The stigma associated with chronic disease, the need for self-care in social contexts and the risk of hypoglycemia, reinforces the idea that adolescents with diabetes are different from their colleagues and friends, which can lead to a feeling of inferiority and negatively influence adherence to self-care behaviors outside their family and personal context [46, 48, 49]. Since adolescence corresponds to the transition between childhood and adulthood, both families and health professionals encourage and stimulate the independence of these youngsters regarding the management of their diabetes [46, 48, 49]. However, this rapid transition can lead to personal and family conflicts, probably because the adolescent has not developed the necessary maturity to assume this type of responsibility [16]. In fact, management of diabetes can be considered a major challenge for adolescents, worsened by physical and hormonal changes, characteristic of this developmental phase which may lead to frequent changes in the therapeutic regimen [50]. Living with a chronic disease, during adolescence is hard and the adolescent may experience more difficulties in adapting to diabetes [2, 17]. Very often, adolescents with diabetes mention their frustration, stress and anxiety, with a lack of motivation regarding the management of the disease, which may negatively influence their adherence to self-care. This set of emotions may also hinder the behaviors necessary for adherence to treatment [51, 52].

A chronic condition, such as diabetes, implies a permanent process of compliance with self-care in order to minimize the effects of its progression and, as a result, is often associated with lower therapeutic adherence [14, 49, 53, 54]. The methods aimed at increasing the success of therapeutic adherence can be classified into four main groups: 1) patient education; 2) existing communication between healthcare professionals and patient; 3) dosage and type of drugs and 4) the accessibility of health services to attend the patient [55]. However, evidence showed that through a multidisciplinary approach comprising educational and behavioral interventions, treatment adherence rates can significantly improve, when compared to the strategies that use each intervention separately [56, 57]. So, taking in consideration the different variables that contribute to noncompliance, it is fundamental to consider a multifactorial approach, to the extent that a single approach will not successfully improve patients' adherence to treatment [55].

Adherence to diabetes self-care involves a complex set of daily behaviors that require the frequent monitoring of blood glucose, insulin administration, recommendations about nutrition and physical exercise [58] as well as making changes and adjustments whenever one of these factors changes [47, 59]. Therefore, the complexity of self-care behaviors may explain low adherence rates and may lead to significant suffering, although compliance significantly reduces the incidence and progression of associated complications [60-62]. Positive outcomes regarding adherence may be related to how each adolescent interprets, learns and draws conclusions regarding the meaning of the disease and its treatment [17]. However, some adolescents with diabetes may lie about their self-care behaviors to avoid being reprimanded by their parents or physician [63, 64].

Good adherence to self-care, in adolescents, may be explained by feelings of social acceptance, distorted or optimistic perception of their behavior or by minimizing the importance of strict compliance with the treatment [51, 65]. On the other hand, non-adherence may be related to specific psychosocial characteristics of adolescent's developmental phase [15, 43, 47, 50, 58]. Peer pressure and fear of a negative reaction from the group can lead to loss of support from colleagues, thus increasing the risk of diabetes complications [58]. The demands associated with self-care does not facilitate the adolescent's growing desire for autonomy and both diabetes and its treatment may result and be perceived as limitations in physical activities, and one's lifestyle [44, 66, 67].

Whereas the responsibility for diabetes self-care increases with adolescent's age, compliance follows in the opposite direction, indicating that adolescents show better adherence when they are more in tune with the guidelines and values of their parental figures [50, 66, 68, 69]. In fact, in the late adolescence stage, older adolescents show a greater concern with the body, sexuality and with independence from parents and authority figures what may explain poor results regarding adherence compared to younger adolescents [50, 65, 70-72].

The increase of emotional distress and autonomy and less acceptance of diabetes, due to a higher awareness of the impact of diabetes on the adolescent's identity and psychosocial development, may also negatively influence adherence to self-care [59, 72-75]. Generally, adolescents tend to have worse outcomes regarding the administration of insulin, the practice of physical exercise, nutrition care and self-monitoring of blood glucose, when compared to children [39, 76]. However, a greater knowledge of diabetes and long experience with the disease decreases attitudes of denial, allowing the adolescent to gradually begin to accept the therapeutic regimen with better results [77, 78]. Also, adolescents who are more responsible for their treatment will have their task of identity formation and psychosocial development facilitated due to the management of their diabetes [65].

Male adolescents have worse adherence to self-care than female adolescents [69], but the latter show higher incidence of depression, eating disorders and psychosocial implications, which may interfere with the process of body image's acceptance [43, 51, 79]. However, literature is controversial regarding gender. A study [80] found male adolescent to present higher levels of adherence to self-care. In other gender related studies, the differences in adherence to self-care were minimal, which may suggest that there are many similarities in the reactions and behaviors of adolescents of both genders regarding their performance in diabetes self-care, meaning that gender may not be considered a risk factor [41, 79, 81].

3. The family support in adherence to self-care

Family impacts on its members' health and the opposite is also true [82]. Family support consists of the individual perception regarding the availability and the caregiving received from their family that allows the development of greater resilience and psychological well-being in the face of stress-inducing events [83-85]. Family support is a complex multidimensional concept associated with the individual's mental health and in direct relation to support received from family members [84, 86, 87]. Hence, family support relates to the behaviors of affection, sensitivity, cooperation and trust, encouraging the autonomy and independence amongst family members [86].

There are numerous types and qualities of support available to families: tangible family support, such as actions that cause well-being among family members; family emotional support, which has to do with empathy, listening, and attention to family members giving advice, which is vital in moments of great difficulties and important decision-making [86, 88]. However, the perception of family support is influenced by personal factors, stable traits and intrinsic changes, in each person, over time [86, 88].

The perception of high levels of family support is associated with a positive disposition [89] and, as a result, when family support is positively perceived, feelings of well being within the family members are promoted [86].

The concept of family support can also be defined as a part of one's informal and close relationship network, benefiting the individual with the exchanges among family members [85]. In this sense, the individual develops greater resilience and psychological well-being, that enables the development of more adjusted responses to stress-inducing events that are closely related to a better coping with a chronic disease [85, 90, 91]. Therefore, it is necessary for family dynamics to show a set of fundamental aspects which favor the development of family support among its members, such as: 1) congruent, directional, functional and emotional communication; 2) consistent and flexible rules; 3) democratic leadership shared with the offspring; 4) self-esteem, 5) integrated couple's relationship, allowing the family to act as a whole but ensuring each individual's personality [92]. The accomplishment of these functions, in association with the perception of the family as loving, cohesive and with clear boundaries, provides members with important tools for individual growth as well as providing its members with a support system [92].

In situations of chronic disease, family support proves to be an important resource in self-care behaviors for adolescent, with a direct correlation between the perception of family support and an increased motivation for self-care behaviors and health in general [82, 90, 93]. This support appears to be of greatest importance in children and adolescents who experience high levels of stress due to a chronic condition and may also affect their development and the quality of their social relationships within their family system [94-96]. However, on one hand, some families become so close that its members are attached, in a way that may affect the autonomy of the patient and, on the other hand, there are families who may become more distant due to the strain that the disease imposes on the family [82]. Within this perspective, a family providing support, affection, guidance and adjusted strategies to solve problems, establishes and promotes best conditions for adherence to self-care, evidencing its responsibility in sharing diabetes' self-care activities with the adolescent [14, 97]. In fact, the family is the main source of support in chronic disease, whether through tangible support, such as preparing meals, administering the medication and in the daily care or through emotional and social support ([82, 90]. Both family and friends influence the control of diabetes, regarding compliance with the medical treatment, diet and the practice of physical exercise [98, 99].

Family support represents an important factor in understanding treatment adherence in adolescents with type 1 diabetes, helping the adolescent to adapt to the demands of the disease and consequently to diabetes self-care. A low family support is a good predictor of poor adherence to self-care in diabetes [73, 100, 101].

Family organization significantly affects family health behaviors in the same way that individual's health also affects the family. Therefore, the family is a resource of strategic importance, since it may or may not help the adolescent with diabetes to properly manage the disease and to achieve treatment's goals [90]. Family support entails emotional and behavioral benefits for its members and is therefore, a reciprocal and proactive process with both parties benefiting from its positive effects, which are particularly important in adolescents who experience high levels of stress, such as in the process of a chronic disease [94, 99]. In the case of diabetes, a direct relationship between family support, characteristics of adolescents with diabetes and therapeutic adherence has been found [70, 82]. The family can act as a support unit for the adolescent's daily self-care tasks, such as motivating physical activity and compliance with the nutrition plan and encouraging insulin administration, after receiving proper guidance, [71, 90].

http://dx.doi.org/10.5772/53062

Regarding diabete's treatment, parents are considered the major providers of social support, even more than peers. Those adolescents, whose parents are less involved and therefore less supportive, show lower adherence to self-care behaviors [70, 102, 103]. The existence of good communication, good skills for an effective resolution of problems and conflicts and flexibility among family members are essential conditions for the adolescent to effectively adapt to the demands of diabetes [17]. Therefore, parental support is positively associated with adolescents' adherence to the prescribed therapeutic regimen [98, 104-106]. In a study involving adolescents with diabetes, a higher family support was a good indicator of adherence to self-care, suggesting the influence that perceived family support has on the implementation and management of diabetes in the daily life of adolescents [107]. In fact, family support appears to have a direct effect on adolescents' adherence to self-care through direct parental supervision on self-care activities. The authors found family support to be a moderator between adolescents' adherence to self-care and quality of life i.e. when family support was high, a positive relationship between adherence and quality of life was found [108]. However, the adolescent may sometimes perceive family support as invasive [109, 110]. In fact, diabetes may modify the process of adolescent's development and family dynamics, and the psychosocial tasks of progressively acquiring autonomy and independence, on the part of the adolescent, may be affected. Therefore, the family's challenge relies on allowing the adolescent to acquire independence with the consequent constraints associated with diabetes, without being super-protective [111].

Given the specific tasks and behaviors in managing diabetes self-care, family support was significantly higher among younger children and in those where the disease was more recently diagnosed [70, 82].

Diabetes requires from the adolescent, family and health professionals a set of efforts in order to achieve a good metabolic control and reduce future complications [112]. Family's participation and collaboration play an important role when it comes to ensure the well-being of the adolescent with diabetes [111].

4. Adherence to self-care and parental coping

Coping is related to efforts, whether cognitive or behavioral, used by the individual to face internal or external demands caused by a specific stress-inducing situation [113, 114]. Coping also implies a dynamic process depending on individual differences and circumstances occurring throughout life [115-117].

Given that coping is a changing process, the individual is not limited to a single coping strategy, since changes will occur resulting from the assessment of stressful situations [116-118]. For this reason, the individual can begin the process by using a strategy and later keep the same strategy, change it or use a combination of different strategies, as the relationship with the environment changes [119, 120].

Coping strategies represent actions, thoughts or behaviors to cope with a stress-inducing event that may, according to their function, be subdivided into two types: emotion-focused coping and problem-focused coping [119, 121, 122]. Emotion-focused coping concerns the efforts to regulate the emotional state that is associated with stress or results from stressful events ([17, 119]. These efforts are directed to somatic sensations or feelings, in order to transform the emotional state manifested by the individual; this type of strategies seeks to minimize the unpleasant physical sensation caused by a state of stress. Problem-focused coping consists of making an effort to act upon a stressful situation, by trying to change it [119, 122, 123]. This type of strategy aims to modify the existing problems in the relationship between the individual and the context that caused the tension [17, 124]. Therefore, coping actions can be directed either inwardly or outwardly [125, 126]. The first type includes strategies such as cognitive restructuring and the latter includes negotiation strategies to resolve an interpersonal conflict or request help from other individuals [125, 126]. In this sense, the process of coping is considered a mediator between the stressful situation and its consequences, whether by focusing on the problem or on the emotion, and its main purpose is to improve the emotional state that results from the confrontation with the stressor [123].

In the case of a chronic disease, coping presents itself as a dynamic process that changes over time, according to the objective demands and the subjective assessments of the situation involving changes in thoughts and actions [115-117, 127]. In addition to personal requirements, defined goals, external resources, such as social support from family, friends and health professionals, economic resources and internal resources, such as intelligence, resilience and locus of control and the characteristics of the disease and treatment are also factors that impact the disease evaluation process that is stress-inducing [118, 120]. As a result, each person has a subjective understanding of the disease, personal attitudes and behavior towards the illness that corresponds to coping mechanisms behind the biomedical factors influencing the course of the disease. Disease severity does not seem to have a consistent relation with the coping used by an individual in adjusting to a chronic disease but coping systems are significantly influenced by psychological and social factors [128].

As a chronic disease, diabetes implies adaptations in terms of physical exercise, food and socializing with peers, that are considered stressful triggering a process of psychological adaptation, with consequent changes in family dynamics [129]. The entire adapting process depends on both the complexity and the severity of the disease, impacting on the stability of the family structure and the development of coping strategies. However, in most cases, parents of children and adolescents with diabetes develop effective coping strategies to manage the diabetes' demands, even if some may show more difficulties and problems adapting to this disease [130, 131].

Chronic disease can be understood as a stress-inducing event affecting the normal development of the child and disturbing the social relations within the family system, changing family routines with constant medical consultations, medication and hospital admissions [96, 132]. Thus, parents and adolescents' psychological resources and the family structure interact and contribute to the adolescent's adaptation to diabetes [96]. The inadequacy of the adolescent can be related more with how the family deals with the sick adolescent, than with the behaviors of the adolescent [96, 132]. As a result, family routines change and the family must adapt to living with a sick child, since strict relationship patterns may influence the

http://dx.doi.org/10.5772/53062

adolescent's emotional development. Parents should be enlightened and aware of the specific diabetes' treatment demands, so that the adolescent does not become depressive and/or distressed [129]. Some studies show, after the diagnosis, that some mothers of children or adolescents with a chronic disease, have trouble sleeping and present a significant emotional impact with associated feelings of concern, fear and responsibility [133].

There is a greater responsibility for mothers in the daily care of a child with diabetes. Often, is up to the mother to accompany the child/adolescent to the medical consultation, keep monitoring records of the blood glucose, guide the child regarding diet and care about the daily insulin administration [134, 135]. Sometimes, when a child is diagnosed with diabetes, parents' responses can lead to a family breakdown that may consequently influence the whole process of adapting and adjusting, by family members, to a chronic disease [133]. This situation can occur after the diagnosis, when the family ceases to participate in social events trying to avoid the ingestion of sweets and cakes hiding from the discomfort of having to relate to others in social situations [135]. Thus, parents who intensify the relationship of dependence and protection regarding the adolescent, as a coping strategy, start to lead their lives according to the child's needs and this process may become very tiresome for parents after a while [136].

Sharing specific tasks for diabetes management between the family and the adolescent, increases the later's knowledge about diabetes. The use of assertive behavior, in social contexts, is considered to be an adjusted strategy to cope with the disease and encourages adaptation. Disease management in diabetes can be stress-inducing, both for the adolescent and for the family, and disturb the harmony of the family dynamics [131].

In most cases, either the adolescent or the family may not act appropriately regarding diabetes, and ultimately fail to accomplish self-care tasks and may even lie regarding blood glucose monitoring if afraid of the disapproval or criticism from health professionals [135].

5. School support in adhering to self-care

School plays an important role in controlling diabetes, in adolescents, given the association between keeping proper self-care during normal school activities and good disease management and quality of life [29, 137, 138]. The school context can contribute to improve the acceptance of diabetes and adolescent' self-esteem and, consequently, have a positive influence on diabetes self-care, due to the continuity of diabetes care during school activities, allowing the adolescent to actively participate in school, reducing school interruptions and absences and ensuring the safety and the prevention of diabetes associated complications [138-140]. However, many adolescents tend to feel uncomfortable in pursuing diabetes self-care in the school environment, because they do not feel safe and properly supported, which could be one of the possible barriers, to adhere to diabetes self-care tasks [138, 141-144]. Also, the lack of knowledge of school teachers and other professionals about diabetes, unhealthy and limited food choices, the unfavorable school organization and class rules unfriendly for diabetes management may have a negative impact on adherence and cause feelings of discrimination among adolescents with diabetes [138, 141, 142, 145, 146]. Along with these barriers, the lack of private places for administering the insulin, which has to be done often in inappropriate places such as the bathroom, the absence of locations for adolescents with diabetes to keep the materials needed for diabetes self-care and the indifference of school staff regarding symptoms and difficulties expressed by these adolescents, may also negatively influence adherence [142, 147, 148].

For parents of teenagers with diabetes, the existence of well-informed teachers regarding diabetes and a proper school structure to receive students with this health condition, are considered the main support that school needs to provide for diabetes management in adolescents [29]. In a school environment, the strongest support comes from teachers and peers [107, 141]. Consequently, it is essential to improve communication between the family and the school, to improve the education of school professionals, to develop healthy menus in the canteen and cafeteria and also to have nurses available to take care of adolescents with diabetes or other chronic diseases, when needed, as well as promoting the education of school staff, students and teachers regarding diabetes, the same way as the school has learned how to care and accommodate students with special education needs [149].

Social support from the peer group has been rated as one of the most important resources for adolescents with diabetes, given that friends tend to provide more companionship and emotional support for self-care behaviors than family members [29, 106, 47, 150, 51]. Social support from peers significantly influences adolescent's adherence to self-care, with strong evidence suggesting that this support improves metabolic outcomes [31]. Despite the differences between the type of support provided by the family and peers, both types of support are also complementary, since the family provides more support in daily tasks, such as insulin administration and meal preparation, while friends provide more emotional support in relation to the practice of physical exercise and glucose monitoring contributing to a better psychological adjustment to diabetes [150, 152-155]. In fact, friends and peers allow the adolescent to enjoy moments of fun and relaxation, contributing to the successful management of diabetes. However, conflict situations between the adolescent with diabetes and peers, although normal and appropriate for psychosocial development, are associated with worse metabolic results, especially in female adolescents [156-158]. In turn, older adolescents, despite having better skills in problem solving, are more vulnerable and prone to peer group pressure regarding diabetes self-care which is associated with worse metabolic outcomes [159, 160]. The way adolescents cope with the need to be part of the group and treated the same way as other members may explain the secrecy regarding diabetes and its symptoms, in an attempt to avoid a negative impact on their social image if significant others find out about their disease [105, 161, 162].

A study on the influence of school and family support on self-care, in adolescents, found that these two types of support act as moderators in the relationship between the quality of life and adherence to the treatment, so when school support and family support were perceived as high, in adolescents with type 1 diabetes, good quality of life was positively related to good adherence [108].

http://dx.doi.org/10.5772/53062

Young people report having more difficulty in adhering to self-care activities in the school context and with their peer group [31, 138, 153, 154, 160, 163, 164]. The anticipation of peer pressure and the fear of being discriminated influence adolescents not to follow adherence to diabetes regimen, which means higher risks regarding their health [165]. In fact, interaction with the peer group and the social context influence adherence to self-care either through positive attitudes, such as the companionship of friends, or through negative attitudes, such as prejudices related to the adolescent's food choices [153, 160, 166]. However, a study on the relationship between adherence and peer support did not reveal a strong relationship probably due to the role that cognitive attributions and evaluations play: if positive, they may be considered a protective factor, if negative, adolescent adjustment to chronic disease may be negatively influenced [152]. Yet another study found that support from peers and teachers, as well as satisfaction with the support received, were associated with good metabolic control, in diabetes [137].

6. Conclusion

Psychosocial and physiological demands, typical of the adolescent's developmental phase and the intensive and demanding characteristics of diabetes treatment influence adherence to diabetes self-care. However, the support from family, peers and school play, an important role in managing and controlling diabetes by adolescents, who tend to present better adherence to self-care behaviors when support is perceived as appropriate. Therefore, intervention programs designed to promote adherence to diabetes self care in adolescents should also include family members and take in consideration the social context of adolescents.

In terms of family support, it is important for adolescent to have access to tangible support from the family in preparing food, monitoring the levels of glycemia and in administering insulin. However, if a high family support is associated with good adherence to the self-care, sometimes too much family involvement can entail a negative influence if the adolescent perceives this support to be a barrier to the development of his/her identity and autonomy. Consequently, it is also important for intervention, in diabetes, to include conflict resolution skills, self-efficacy and stress management strategies for both the adolescent and the family.

Coping strategies adopted by parents in order to deal with daily tasks and challenges, that diabetes management implies, interfere with the organization of family dynamics and impact on adherence to diabetes self-care. Given that the effectiveness of coping strategies influence adherence, it becomes important for parents and adolescents to integrate self-help groups or even family therapy, when they have trouble adapting to diabetes management.

Diabetes is a disease that requires constant monitoring and surveillance even within social contexts outside the family environment, as in the case of peer group activities. The support from both the school and the peer group impacts on adherence outcomes in adolescents. As a result, education regarding diabetes in schools is important, in order to improve knowledge about the management of diabetes and also to make support and resources more efficient and appropriate regarding diabetes self care's behaviors in the school context.

Finally, psychological interventions must also acknowledge the implications of diabetes on the adolescent's lifestyle in order not to jeopardize the development of autonomy, independence and social skills and instead, promote normal psychosocial development of the adolescent in the family, school, and other significant social environments.

Author details

A. Cristina Almeida[1], M. Graça Pereira[2] and Engrácia Leandro[1]

1 University of Minho, Social Sciences Institute, Portugal

2 University of Minho, School of Psychology, Portugal

References

[1] Faulkner M, Chang L. Family Influence on Self-Care, Quality of Life, and Metabolic Control in School-Age Children and Adolescents with Type 1 Diabetes. Journal of Pediatric Nursing 2007;22(1) 59-68.

[2] Duarte R, Góis C. Diabetes na Adolescência. In: Duarte R. (ed.) Diabetologia Clínica. 3th ed. Lisboa: Lidel - Edições Técnicas; 2002. p243-250.

[3] Shah B, Zinman B. Insulin Regimens for Type 1 Diabetes. In: Sperling M. (ed.) Type 1 Diabetes. Etiology and Treatment. New Jersey: Humana Press; 2003. p199-214.

[4] Haller MJ, Silverstein JH, Rosenbloom AL. Type 1 Diabetes in the Child and Adolescent. In: Lifshitz F. (ed.) Pediatric Endocrinology. 5th ed. New York: Informa Healthcare; 2007. p63-82.

[5] Doliba NM, Matschinsky FM. The Metabolic Basis of Insulin Secretion. In: Sperling MA. (ed.) Type 1 Diabetes. Etiology and Treatment. New Jersey: Humana Press; 2003. p115-144.

[6] Smart C, Vliet EA-v, Waldron S. Nutritional management in children and adolescents with diabetes. Pediatric Diabetes 2009;10(Suppl. 12) 110-117.

[7] Beebe CA. Nutritional Management in Type 1 Diabetes. In: Sperling MA. (ed.) Type 1 Diabetes. Etiology and Treatment. New Jersey: Humana Press; 2003. p261-278.

[8] Robertson K, Adolfsson P, Riddell M, Scheiner G, Hanas R. Exercise in children and adolescents with diabetes. Pediatric Diabetes 2009;10(Suppl. 12) 154-168.

[9] Raine JE, Donaldson MD, Gregory J, Van-Vliet G. Practical Endocrinology and Diabetes in Children. 2nd ed. Massachusetts: Blackwell Publishing; 2006.

[10] Escobar O, Drash AL, Becker DJ. Management of the Child with Type 1 Diabetes. In: Lifshitz F. (ed.) Pediatric Endocrinology. 5th ed. New York: Informa Healthcare; 2007. p101-124.

[11] Thorsdottir I, Ramel A. Dietary Intake of 10- to 16-Year-Old Children and Adolescents in Central and Northern Europe and Association with the Incidence of Type 1 Diabetes. Annals of Nutricion & Metabolism 2003;47 267-275.

[12] Dorman JS, Laporte RE, Songer TJ. Epidemiology of Type 1 Diabetes. In: Sperling MA. (ed.) Type 1 Diabetes. Etiology and Treatment. New Jersey: Humana Press; 2003. p3-22.

[13] Lernmark Å, Chung CH. Molecular Biology of β-Cell Destruction by Autoimmune Processes. In: Sperling MA. (ed.) Type 1 Diabetes Etiology and Treatment. New Jersey: Humana Press; 2003. p71-92.

[14] Silva I, Pais Ribeiro J, Cardoso H. Adesão ao Tratamento da Diabetes Mellitus: A Importância das Características Demográficas e Clínicas. Revista Referência 2006;2(2) 33-41.

[15] Fagulha A, Santos I, Grupo de Estudo da Diabetes Mellitus. Controlo glicémico e tratamento da diabetes tipo 1 da criança e adolescente em Portugal. Acta Médica Portuguesa 2004;17(2) 173-179.

[16] Skinner TC, Channon S, Howells L, McEvilley A. Diabetes During Adolescence. In: Snoek FJ, Skinner TC. (eds.) Psychology in Diabetes Care. West Sussex: John Wiley & Sons; 2000. p25-59.

[17] Barros L. Psicologia Pediátrica. Perspectiva desenvolvimentista. 2nd ed. Lisboa: Climepsi Editores; 2003.

[18] Hanas R. Diabetes tipo 1 em crianças, adolescentes e jovens adultos. Lisboa: Lidel Editores; 2007.

[19] Pina R. Diabetes na Criança. In: Duarte R. (ed.) Diabetologia Clínica. 3th ed. Lisboa: Lidel Editores; 2002. p229-242.

[20] American Diabetes Association (ADA). Standards of Medical Care in Diabetes. Diabetes Care 2007;30(Suppl. 1) S4-S41.

[21] Anderson BJ. Family Conflict and Diabetes Management in Youth: Clinical Lessons from Child Development and Diabetes Research. Diabetes Spectrum. Diabetes Spectrum 2004;17(1) 22-26.

[22] Pereira M, Almeida P. Barreiras à Adesão ao Regime Terapêutico da Diabetes In: Machado C, Almeida L, Gonçalves M, Ramalho V, (eds.) X Actas da Conferência Internacional de Avaliação Psicológica: Formas e Contextos. Braga: Psiquilibrios; 2004. p170-179.

[23] La Greca A, Harrisson HM. Adolescent Peer Relations, Friendships, and Romantic Relationships: Do They Predict Social Anxiety and Depression? Journal of Clinical Child and Adolescent Psychology 2005;34(1) 49-61.

[24] Yeo M, Sawyer S. Chronic illness and disability 2005;330 721-723.

[25] Silva GR, Cruz NR, Coelho EB. Perfil nutricional, consumo alimentar e prevalência de sintomas de anorexia e bulimia nervosa em adolescentes de uma escola da rede pública no município de Ipatinga, M. G. Revista Digital de Nutrição 2008;2(3) 1-15.

[26] Ribeiro C, Rosendo I. Saúde do adolescente em Medicina Geral e Familiar. Revista Portuguesa Clinica Geral 2011;27 184-186.

[27] Almeida P, Pereira MG. Família, Suporte Social e diabetes tipo 1 na adolescência. In: Pereira MG. (ed.) Psicologia da Saúde Familiar: aspectos teóricos e investigação. Lisboa: Climepsi Editores; 2007. p135-162.

[28] Hilliard ME, Herzerb M, Dolanc LM, Hood KK. Psychological screening in adolescents with type 1 diabetes predicts outcomes one year later. Diabetes Research and Clinical Practice 2011;94(1) 39-44.

[29] Wagner JA, Abbott G, Lett S. Age related differences in individual quality of life domains in youth with type 1 diabetes. Health and Quality of Life Outcomes 2004;2(54). doi:10.1186/1477-7525-2-54.

[30] Schiffrin A. Psychosocial issues in pediatric diabetes. Current Diabetes Reports 2001;1(1) 33-40.

[31] Lehmkuhl HD, Merlo LJ, Devine K, Gaines J, Storch EA, Silverstein JH, et al. Perceptions of Type 1 Diabetes among Affected Youth and their Peers Journal of Clinical Psychology in Medical Settings 2009;16(3) 209-215.

[32] Dias AM, Cunha M, Santos A, Neves A, Pinto A, Silva A, et al. Adesão ao regime Terapêutico na Doença Crónica: Revisão da Literatura. Millenium 2011;40 201-219.

[33] Sousa S, Pires A, Conceição C, Nascimento T, Grenha A, Braz L. Polimedicação em doentes idosos: adesão à terapêutica. Revista Portuguesa de Clínica Geral 2011;27(2) 176-182.

[34] Leite M. Programa de promoção da adesão terapêutica em crianças diabéticas. In: Guerra M, Lima L. (eds.) Intervenção Psicológica em Grupos em Contextos de Saúde. Lisboa: Climepsi Editores; 2005. p155-174

[35] Kakleas K, Kandyla B, Karayianni C, Karav K. Psychosocial problems in adolescents with type 1 diabetes mellitus. Diabetes & Metabolism 2009;35(5) 339-350.

[36] Catela A, Amendoeira J. Viver a Adesão ao Regime Terapêutico – Experiências Vividas do Doente Submetido a Transplante Cardíaco. Pensar Enfermagem 2010;14(2) 39-54.

[37] Sousa M, Peixoto M, Martins T. Satisfação do doente diabético com os cuidados de enfermagem: influência na adesão ao regime terapêutico. Revista Referência 2008;2(8) 59-67.

[38] Silveira L, Ribeiro V. Grupo de adesão ao tratamento: espaço de "ensinagem" para profissionais de saúde e pacientes. Interface - Comunicação, Saúde e Educação 2005;9(16) 91-104.

[39] Gimenes H, Zanetti M, Haas V. Fatores relacionados à adesão do paciente diabético à terapêutica medicamentosa. Revista Latino-Americana de Enfermagem 2009;17(1) 46-51.

[40] Almeida H, Versiani E, Dias A, Novaes M, Trindade E. Adesão a tratamentos entre idosos. Comunicação em Ciências da Saúde 2007;18(1) 57-67.

[41] World Health Organization (WHO). Adherence to long-term therapies - Evidence for action. Switzerland: WHO; 2003.

[42] Fragoso L, Araújo M, Lima A, Freitas R, Damasceno M. Vivências cotidiana de adolescentes com diabetes mellitus tipo 1. Texto & Contexto Enfermagem 2010;19(3) 443-451.

[43] Court J, Cameron F, Berg-Kelly K, Swift P. Diabetes in adolescence. Pediatric Diabetes 2009;10(Suppl. 12) 185-194.

[44] Genuth S. Relationship Between Metabolic Control and Complications in Diabetes: Therapeutic Implications of the Diabetes Control and Complications Trial. In: Sperling MA. (ed.) Type 1 Diabetes. Etiology and Treatment. New Jersey: Humana Press; 2003. p215-232

[45] Kennedy L, Idris I, Gazis A. Problem Solving in Diabetes. Oxford: Atlas Medical Publishing; 2006.

[46] Novato T, Grossi S, Kimura M. Qualidade de Vida e Auto-estima de adolescentes com diabetes mellitus. Acta Paulista de Enfermagem 2008;21(4) 562-567.

[47] Werther GA, Cameron FJ, Court JM. The Adolescent with Type 1 Diabetes. In: Sperling MA. (ed.) Type 1 Diabetes. Etiology and Treatment. New Jersey: Humana Press. 2003. p307-320.

[48] Alencar D, Alencar A. O papel da família na adaptação do adolescente diabético. Revista Rene. 2009;10(1) 19-28.

[49] Kyngäs A. Predictors of good adherence of adolescents with diabetes (insulin-dependent diabetes mellitus). Chronic Illness 2007;3(1) 20-28.

[50] La Greca A. Issues in Adherence With Pediatric Regimens. Journal of Pediatric Psychology 1990;15(4) 423-436.

[51] Mulvaney S, Mudasiru E, Schlundt D, Baughman C, Fleming M, Vanderwoude A, et al. Self-management in Type 2 Diabetes: The Adolescent Perspective. Diabetes Educator 2008;34(4) 674-682.

[52] Tilden B, Charman D, Sharples J, Fosbury J. Identity and Adherence in a Diabetes Patient: Transformations in Psychotherapy. Qualitative Health Research 2005;15(3) 312-324.

[53] Assunção T, Ursine P. Estudo de factores associados à adesão ao tratamento não farmacológico em portadores de diabetes mellitus assistidos pelo Programa Saúde da Família, Ventosa, Belo Horizonte. Ciência & Saúde Colectiva 2008;13(2) 2189-2197.

[54] Pais Ribeiro JL. Introdução à Psicologia da Saúde. 2nd ed. Coimbra: Quarteto; 2007.

[55] Osterberg L, Blaschke T. Adherence to Medication. The new england journal of medicine 2005;353 487-497.

[56] Henriques M. Adesão ao regime medicamentoso em idosos na comunidade. Eficácia das intervenções de enfermagem. PhD thesis. University of Lisbon; 2011.

[57] Bugalho A, Carneiro AV. Intervenções para aumentar a adesão terapêutica em patologias crónicas. NOC de Adesão Terapêutica. Lisboa: CEMBE; 2004.

[58] Salamon S, Allen A, Fleischman M, Davies H, Kichler J. Improving adherence in social situations for adolescents with type 1 diabetes mellitus (T1DM): a pilot study. Primary care diabetes 2010;4(1) 47-55.

[59] Farrell P. Diabetes, Exercício Físico e Esportes de Competição. Sports Science Exchange 2004;16(3), Disponível em: http://www.gssi.com.br/. Accessed 30 June 2012]

[60] Carmo T. Melhoria da adesão ao tratamento medicamentoso por meio da atenção farmacêutica. In: UNIMEP. (ed.) 5th Amostra Académica UNIMEP 9º Seminário de Extensão: Educação Brasileira: Extinção ou Sustentabilidade na Universidade 23-25 de October 2007; Piracicaba. Brazil.

[61] Pietropaolo M, Trucco M. Genetics of Type 1 Diabetes. In: Sperling MA. (ed.) Type 1 Diabetes. Etiology and Treatment. New Jersey: Humana Press; 2003. p23-54.

[62] Masharani U. Diabetes Desmystified. A self-teaching guide. New York: McGraw-Hill; 2008.

[63] Kyngäs HA, Kroll T, Duffy ME. Compliance in Adolescents With Chronic Diseases: A Review. Journal of Adolescent Health 2000;26(6) 379-388.

[64] Civita M, Dobkin P. Pediatric Adherence as a Multidimensional and Dynamic Construct, Involving a Triadic Partnership. Journal of Pediatric Psychology 2004;29(3) 157-169.

[65] Garrett S. Adesão ao tratamento da diabetes em adolescentes: factores motivacionais. Master Thesis. University of Oporto; 2007.

[66] Shaw R. Treatment Adherence in Adolescents: Development and Psychopathology. Clinical Child Psychology and Psychiatry 2001;6(1) 1359–1045.

[67] Greening L, Stoppelbein L, Reeves C. A Model for Promoting Adolescents'Adherence to Treatment for Type 1 Diabetes Mellitus. Children's Health Care 2006;35(3) 247-267.

[68] Jacobson A, The Diabetes Control and Complications Trial Research Group. The Diabetes Quality of Life Measure. In: Bradley C. (ed.) Handbook of Psychology and Diabetes. New York: Psychology Press; 2006. p65-88.

[69] Dashiff C, McCaleb A, Cull V. Self-care of young adolescents with type 1diabetes. Journal Pediatric Nursing 2006;21(3) 222-232.

[70] Wysocki T, Taylor A, Hough BS, Linscheid TR, Yeates KO, Naglieri JA. Deviation From Developmentally Appropriate Self-Care Autonomy. Diabetes Care 1996;19(2) 119-125.

[71] Santos E, Zanetti M, Otero L, Santos M. O cuidado sob a ótica do paciente diabético e de seu principal cuidador. Revista Latino-Americana de Enfermagem 2005;13(3) 397-406.

[72] Alcântara K, Zanetti R, Oliveira S. O adolescentes diabético numa visão psicossomática. Revista Académica Digital do Grupo POLIS Educacional 2008;4(5) 15. ISSN 1679-8902

[73] Pereira MG, Berg-Cross L, Almeida P, Machado J. Impact of Family Environment and Support on Adherence, Metabolic Control, and Quality of Life in Adolescents with Diabetes. International Journal of Behavioral Medicine 2008;15 187-193.

[74] Kovacs M, Iyengar S, Goldston D, Stewart J, Obrosky DS, Marsh J. Psychological functioning of children with insulin-dependent diabetes mellitus: a longitudinal study. Journal of Pediatric Psychology 1990;15(5) 619-632.

[75] Holmbeck GN, Kendall PC. Introduction to the Special Section on Clinical Adolescent Psychology: Developmental Psychopathology and Treatment. Journal of Consulting and Clinical Psychology 2002;70(1: 3-5.

[76] Hirschberg SL. The self-regulation of health behavior in children with insulin-dependent diabetes mellitus. Master Thesis. Faculty of Pacific Graduate School of Psychology; 2001.

[77] Garay-Sevilla ME, Nava LE, Malacara JM, Huerta R, León JD, Mena A, et al. Adherence to treatment and social support in patients with non-insulin dependent diabetes mellitus. Journal of Diabetes and Its Complications 1995;9(2) 81-86.

[78] Silva I, Pais Ribeiro J, Cardoso H, Ramos H. Effects of treatment adherence on metabolic control and quality of life in diabetic patients. Psychosomatic Medicine 2002;64 (1) 125-125.

[79] Schwartz D, Cline V, Hansen J, Axelrad M, Anderson BJ. Early risk factors for nonadherence in pediatric type 1 diabetes: A review of the recent literature. Current Diabetes Reviews 2010;6(3) 167-183.

[80] Hanna KG, Guthrie DW. Parental Involvement in Adolescents' Diabetes Management. Diabetes Spectrum 2003;16(3) 184-187.

[81] Fitzgerald JT, Anderson RM, Davis WK. Gender differences in diabetes attitudes and adherence. Diabetes Educator 1995;21(6) 523-529.

[82] Ribeiro C. Família, Saúde e Doença. O que diz a investigação? Revista Portuguesa Clinica Geral 2007;23 299-306.

[83] Seidl EF, Zannon CC, Tróccoli BT. Pessoas Vivendo com HIV/AIDS: Enfrentamento, Suporte Social e Qualidade de Vida. Psicologia: Reflexão e Crítica 2005;18(2) 188-195.

[84] Castro R, Campero L, Hernández B. La investigación sobre apoyo social en salud: situación actual y nuevos desafíos. Revista de Saúde Pública 1997;31(4) 425-435.

[85] Baptista AD, Neves SV, Baptista MN. Correlação entre suporte familiar, saúde mental e crenças irracionais em idosos religiosos. PSIC - Revista de Psicologia da Vetor Editora 2008;9(2) 155-164.

[86] Baptista MN, Norona APP, Cardoso HF. Relações entre suporte familiar e interesses profissionais. Revista Salud & Sociedad 2010;1(1) 28-40.

[87] Procidano ME, Heller K. Measures of perceived social support from friends and from family: Three validation studies American Journal of Community Psychology 1983;11(1) 1-24.

[88] Pinkerton J, Dolan P. Family support, social capital, resilience and adolescent coping. Child & Family Social Work 2007;12(3) 219-228.

[89] Weinstein SM, Mermelstein RJ, Hedeker D, Hankin BL, Flay BR. The Time-Varying Influences of Peer and Family Support on Adolescent Daily Positive and Negative Affect. Journal of Clinical Child & Adolescent Psychology 2006;35(3) 420-430.

[90] Zanetti ML, Biagg MV, Santos MA, Péres DS, Teixeira CS. O cuidado à pessoa diabética e as repercussões na família. Journal of Clinical Child & Adolescent Psychology 2006;35(3) 420-430.

[91] Kirk RH. Family support: the roles of early years' centers. Children & Society 2003;17(2) 85-99.

[92] Souza MS, Baptista MN. Associações entre Suporte Familiar e Saúde Mental. Psicologia Argumento 2008;26(54) 207-215.

[93] Baptista MN. Inventário de Percepção de Suporte Familiar (IPSF): Estudo Componencial em duas Configurações. Psicologia Ciência e Profissão 2007;27(3) 496-509.

[94] Siqueira AC, Betts MK, Dell'Aglio DD. A Rede de Apoio Social e Afetivo de Adolescentes Institucionalizados no Sul do Brasil. Revista Interamericana de Psicología 2006;40(2) 149-158.

[95] Silver EJ, Westbrook LE, Stein RK. Relationship of Parental Psychological Distress to Consequences of Chronic Health Conditions in Children. Journal of Pediatric Psychology 1998;23(1) 5-15.

[96] Castro EK, Piccinini CA. Implicações da Doença Orgânica Crônica na Infância para as Relações Familiares: Algumas Questões Teóricas. Psicologia: Reflexão e Crítica 2002;15(3) 625-635.

[97] Fisher L, Chesla CA, Skaff MM, Gilliss C, Mullan JT, Bartz RJ, et al. The Family and Disease Management in Hispanic and European-American Patients With Type 2 Diabetes. Diabetes Care 2000;23(3) 267-272.

[98] Pace A, Nunes P, Ochoa-Vigo K. O Conhecimento dos Familares acerca da Problemática do Portador de Diabetes Mellitus. Revista Latino-Americana de Enfermagem 2003;11(3) 312-319.

[99] Santos MA, Alves RP, Oliveira VA, Ribas CP, Teixeira CS, Zanetti ML. Representações sociais de pessoas com diabetes acerca do apoio familiar percebido em relação ao tratamento. Revista da Escola de Enfermagem USP 2011;45(3) 651-658.

[100] Beveridge RM, Berg CA, Wiebe DJ, Palmer DL. Mother and Adolescent Representations of Illness Ownership and Stressful Events Surrounding Diabetes. Journal of Pediatric Psychology 2006;31(8) 818-827.

[101] Lewin AB, Heidgerken AD, Geffken GR, Williams LB, Storch EA, Gelfand KM, et al. The Relation Between Family Factors and Metabolic Control: The Role of Diabetes Adherence. Journal of Pediatric Psychology 2006;31(2) 174-183.

[102] La Greca AM, Thompson KM. Family and friend support for adolescents with diabetes. Análise Psicológica 1998;1(16) 101-113.

[103] Stern M, Zevon MA. Stress, Coping, and Family Environment: The Adolescent's Response to Naturally Occurring Stressors. Journal of Pediatric Psychology 1990;5(3) 290-305.

[104] Harris MA, Mertlich D, Rothweiler J. Parenting Children With Diabetes. Diabetes Spectrum 2001;14(4) 182-184.

[105] Maia F, Araújo LR. Aspectos Psicológicos e Controle Glicêmico de Um Grupo de Pacientes Com Diabetes Mellitus Tipo 1 em Minas Gerais. Arquivos Brasileiros Endocrinologia & Metabologia 2004;48(2) 261-266.

[106] Skinner TC, John M, Hampson SE. Social Support and Personal Models of Diabetes as Predictors of Self-care and Well-Being: a Longitudinal Study of Adolescents with Diabetes. Journal of Pediatric Psychology 2000;25(4) 257-267.

[107] Pereira M, Almeida A, Rocha L, Leandro E. Predictors of Adherence, Metabolic Control and Quality of Life in Adolescents with Type 1 Diabetes. In: Liu C-P, (ed.) Type 1 Diabetes – Complications, Pathogenesis, and Alternative Treatments. Rijeka: InTech; 2011. p119-140.

[108] Pereira MG, Almeida A, Leandro E. Papel do Apoio Escolar e Suporte Familiar em Crianças com Diabetes Tipo 1. In: Psicosoma. (ed.) VII Congresso Internacional de Neurociências e Educação Especial 19-20 May 2012; Viseu, Portugal.

[109] Mellin AE, Neumark-Sztainer D, Patterson JM. Parenting Adolescent Girls with Type 1 Diabetes: Parents' Perspectives. Journal of Pediatric Psychology 2004;29(3) 221-230.

[110] Weinger K, O'Donnell KA, Ritholz MD. Adolescent Views of Diabetes-Related Parent Conflict and Support: A Focus Group Analysis. Journal of Adolescent Health 2001;29(5) 330-336.

[111] Heleno MV, Vizzotto MM, Mazzotti T, Cressoni-Gomes R, Modesto SF. Acampamento de Férias para Jovens com Diabetes Mellitus tipo 1: Achados da Abrodagem Psicológica. Boletim de Psicologia 2009;59(130) 77-90.

[112] Piccinini CA, Castro EK, Alvarenga P, Vargas S, Oliveira VZ. A doença crônica orgânica na infância e as práticas educativas maternas. Estudos de Psicologia 2003;8(1) 75-83.

[113] Folkman S, Lazarus RS. If It Changes It Must Be a Process: Study of Emotion and Coping During Three Stages of a College Examination. Journal of Personality and Social Psychology 1985;48(1) 150-170.

[114] Pais-Ribeiro J, Santos C. Estudo conservador de adaptação do Ways of Coping Questionnaire a uma amostra e contexto portugueses. Análise Psicológica 2001;4(19) 491-502.

[115] Folkman S, Lazarus RS. Coping as a Mediator of Emotion. Journal of Personality and Social Psychology 1988;54(3) 466-475.

[116] Pais Ribeiro JL, Rodrigues AP. Questões àcerca do coping: a propósito do estudo de adaptação do Brief COPE. Psicologia, Saúde & Doenças 2004;5(1) 3-15.

[117] Vivan S, Argimon IL. Estratégias de enfrentamento, dificuldades funcionais e fatores associados em idosos institucionalizados. Cadernos de Saúde Pública 2009;25(2) 436-444.

[118] Correia AR. Coping e Auto-eficácia em Pais de Crianças e Adolescentes com Diabetes tipo 1. Master Thesis. University Fernando Pessoa; 2010.

[119] Tuncay T, Musabak I, Gok DE, Kutlu M. The relationship between anxiety, coping strategies and characteristics of patients with diabetes. Health and Quality of Life Outcomes 2008;6(79) 9. diabwte:10.1186/1477-7525-6-79.

[120] Sousa MG, Landeiro ML, Pires R, Santos C. Coping e adesão ao regime terapêutico. Revista de Enfermagem Referência 2011;3 (4) 151-160.

[121] Lisboa C, Koller SH, Ribas FF, Bitencourt K, Oliveira L, Porciuncula LP, et al. Estratégias de Coping de Crianças Vítimas e Não Vítimas de Violência Doméstica. Psicologia: Reflexão e Crítica 2002;15(2) 345-362.

[122] Folkman S. Personal Control and Stress and Coping Processes: A Theoretical Analysis. Journal of Personality and Social Psychology 1984;46(4) 839-852.

[123] Vaz Serra A. A vulnerabilidade ao stress. Psiquiatria Clínica 2000;21(4) 261-278.

[124] Barros DS. Estratégias de Coping em Crianças Vítimas de Abuso Sexual. Master Thesis. University Fernado Pessoa; 2009.

[125] Nascimento CM, Nunes S. O Conceito de Enfrentamento e a sua Relevância na Prática da Psiconcologia. Encontro: Revista de Psicologia 2010;13(19) 91-102

[126] Antoniazzi AS, Dell'Aglio DD, Bandeira DR. O conceito de coping: uma revisão teórica. Estudos de Psicologia 1998;3(2) 273-294.

[127] Monteiro M, Matos AP, Coelho R. A adaptação psicológica de mães cujos filhos apresentam Paralisia Cerebral: Revisão da literatura. Revista Portugesa de Psicossomática 2002;4(2) 149-178.

[128] Amorim ML. Para lá dos números... Aspectos psicossociais e qualidade de vida do indivíduo com diabetes mellitus tipo 2. PhD Thesis. Institute of Biomedical Sciences Abel Salazar, University of Oporto; 2009.

[129] Coletto M, Câmara S. Estratégias de coping e percepção da doença em pais de crianças com doença crônica: o contexto do cuidador. Revista Diversitas - Perspectivas en Psicología 2009;5(1) 97-110.

[130] Macrodimitris SD, Endlen NS. Coping, Control, and Adjustment in Type 2 Diabetes. Health Psychology 2001;20(3) 208-216.

[131] Kovacs M, Finkelstein R, Feinberg TL, Crouse-Novak M, Paulauskas S, PollockM. Initial Psychologic Responses of Parents to the Diagnosis of Insulin-dependent Diabetes Mellitus in Their Children. Diabetes Care 1985;8(6) 568-575.

[132] Manuel J. Risk and Resistance Factors in the Adaptation in Mothers of Children with Juvenile Rheumatoid Arthristis. Journal of Pediatric Psychology 2001;26(4) 237-246.

[133] Souza IB, Marques DA, Lacerda OM, Collet N. Percepção das Mães Frente ao Diagnóstico do Filho com Diabetes Mellitus tipo 1. Cogitare Enfermagem 2011;16(1) 43-48.

[134] Zanetti ML, Mendes IC. Análise das Dificuldades Relacionadas às Atividades Diárias de Crianças e Adolescente com Diabetes Mellitus tipo 1: Depoimento de Mães Revista Latino-Americana de Enfermagem 2001;9(6) 25-30.

[135] Nunes, Dupas. Entregando-se à vivência da doença com o filho: a experiência da mãe da criança/adolescente diabético. Texto & Contexto Enfermagem 2004;13(1) 83-91.

[136] Brito TB, Sadala MA. Diabetes mellitus juvenil: a experiência de familiares de adolescentes e pré-adolescentes. Ciência & Saúde Coletiva 2009;14(3) 947-960.

[137] Lehmkuhl H, Nabors L. Children with Diabetes: Satisfaction with School Support, Illness Perceptions and HbA1C Levels. Journal of Developmental and Physical Disabilities 2008;20 101-114.

[138] Wang Y-L, Brown SA, Horner SD. School-Based Lived Experiences of Adolescents With Type 1 Diabetes: A Preliminary Study. Journal of Nursing Research 2010;18(4) 258-265.

[139] Santana EA, Silva SS. Educação Física escolar para alunos com diabetes mellitus tipo 1. Motriz Revista de Educação Física UNESP 2009;15 (3) 669-676.

[140] Jameson PL. Developing Diabetes Training Programs for School Personnel. School Nurse News 2004;21(4) 14-17.

[141] Amillategui B, Mora E, Calle JR, Giralt P. Special needs of children with type 1 diabetes at primary school: perceptions from parents, children, and teachers. Pediatric Diabetes. 2009;10(1): 67-73.

[142] Hayes-Bohn R, Neumark-Sztainer D, Mellin AE, Patterson JM. Adolescents and Parent Assessments of Diabetes Mellitus Management at School. Journal of School Health 2004;74(5) 166-169.

[143] Wilson V, Beskine D. Children and young people with type 1 diabetes: Managing at school. Journal of Diabetes Nursing 2007;11(10) 392-398.

[144] Nascimento LC, Amaral MJ, Sparapani VC, Mara L, Fonseca M, Nunes MR, et al. Diabetes mellitus tipo 1: evidências da literatura para seu manejo adequado, na perspectiva de crianças. Revista da Escola de Enfermagem USP 2011;45(3) 764-769.

[145] Olson AL, Seidler AB, Goodman D, Gaelic S, Nordgren R. School Professionals' Perceptions About the Impact of Chronic Illness in the Classroom. Archives of Pediatrics & Adolescent Medicine 2004;158(1) 53-58.

[146] Nabors L, Troillett A, Nash T, Masiulis B. School Nurse Perceptions of Barriers and Supports for Children With Diabetes. Journal of School Health 2005;75(4) 119-124.

[147] Wagner JA, Abbott G, Lett S. Age related differences in individual quality of life domains in youth with type 1 diabetes. Health and Quality of Life Outcomes 2004;2(54): 9 doi:10.1186/1477-7525-2-54.

[148] Nabors L, Lehmkuhl H, Christos N, Andreone T. Children with Diabetes: Perceptions of Support for Self-Management at School. Journal of School Healt. 2003;73(6) 216-221.

[149] Brener ND, Wheeler L, Wolfe LC, Vernon-Smiley M, Caldart-Olson L. Health Services: Results From the School Health Policies and Programs Study 2006. Journal of School Health 2007;77(8) 464-485.

[150] La Greca A, Auslander WF, Greco P, Spetter D, Fisher EB Jr, Santiago JV. I Get by with a little help from my Family and Friends: Adolescents' Support for Diabetes Care. Journal of Pediatric Psychology 1995;20(4) 449-476.

http://dx.doi.org/10.5772/53062

[151] Greco P, Pendley JS, McDonell K, Reeves G. A Peer Group Intervention for Adolescents With Type 1 Diabetes and Their Best Friends. Journal of Pediatric Psychology 2001;26(8) 485-490.

[152] Bearman KJ, La Greca A. Assessing Friend Support of Adolescents' Diabetes Care: The Diabetes Social Support Questionnaire-Friends Version. Journal of Pediatric Psychology 2002;27(5) 417-428.

[153] Wysocki T, Greco P. Social Support and Diabetes Management in Childhood and Adolescence: Influence of Parents and Friends. Current Diabetes Reports 2006;6 117-122.

[154] Karlsson A, Arman M, Wikblad K. Teenagers with type 1 diabetes—a phenomenological study of the transition towards autonomy in self-management. International Journal of Nursing Studies 2008;45(4) 562-570.

[155] Ferreira BS, Garcia A. Aspectos da amizade de adolescentes portadores de diabetes e câncer. Estudos de Psicologia 2008;25(2) 293-301.

[156] Helgeson VS, Siminerio L, Escobar O, Becker D. Predictors of Metabolic Control among Adolescents with Diabetes: A 4-Year Longitudinal Study. Journal of Pediatric Psychology 2009;34(3) 254-270.

[157] Frey MA, Guthrie B, Loveland-Cherry C, Park PS, Foster CM. Risky Behavior and Risk in Adolescents with IDDM. Journal of Adolescent Health 1997;20(1) 38-45.

[158] Silverstein JH, Klingensmith G, Copeland K, Plotnick L, Kaufman F, Laffel L, et al. Care of Children and Adolescents With Type 1 Diabetes. A statement of the American Diabetes Association. Diabetes Care 2005;28(1) 186-212.

[159] Thomas AM, Peterson L, Goldstein D. Problem Solving and Diabetes Regimen Adherence by Children and Adolescents with IDDM in Social Pressure Situations: A Reflection of Normal Development. Journal of Pediatric Psychology 1997;22(4) 541-561.

[160] Hains AA, Berlin KS, Davies WH, Smothers MK, Sato AF, Alemzadeh R. Attributions of Adolescents with Type 1 Diabetes Related to Performing Diabetes Care around Friends and Peers: The Moderating Role of Friend Support. Journal of Pediatric Psychology 2007;32(5) 561-570.

[161] Davidson M, Penney ED, Muller B, Grey M. Stressors and Self-Care Challenges Faced by Adolescents Living With Type 1 Diabetes. Applied Nursing Research 2004;17(2) 72-80.

[162] Michaud P-A, Suris J-C, Thomas LR, Kahlert C, Rudin C, Cheseaux J-J. To Say or Not to Say: A Qualitative Study on the Disclosure of Their Condition by Human Immunodeficiency Virus–Positive Adolescents. Journal of Adolescent Health 2009;44(4) 356-362.

[163] Burke H, Dowling M. Living with diabetes: Adolescents' perspectives. Journal of Diabetes Nursing 2007;11(3) 90-96.

[164] Berlin KS, Davies WH, Jastrowski KE, Hains AA, Parton EA, Alemzadeh R. Contextual Assessment of Problematic Situations Identified by Insulin Pump Using Adolescents and Their Parents. Families, Systems, & Health 2006;24(1) 33-44.

[165] Di Battista AM, Hart TA, Greco L, Gloizer J. Type 1 diabetes among adolescents: reduced diabetes self-care caused by social fear and fear of hypoglycemia. Diabetes Educator 2009;35(3) 465-475.

[166] Sparapani VC, Borges AV, Dantas IO, Pan R, Nascimento LC. A criança com Diabetes Mellitus Tipo 1 e seus amigos: a influência dessa interação no manejo da doença. Revista Latino-Americana de Enfermagem 2012;20(1) 117-125.

Chapter 19

Nutritional Management in Type 1 Diabetes Mellitus

Snežana Marković- Jovanović

Additional information is available at the end of the chapter

http://dx.doi.org/10.5772/52465

1. Introduction

An optimal nutrition along with insulin therapy in pations with type 1 diabetes, is the prerequisite for normal growth and development, adequate pubertal development, and regular performance in school and extracurricular activities, including sports in diabetic patients. Moreover, a balanced and healthy diet prevents hyper- or hypoglycemia and delays development of microvascular diabetic complications, including diabetic nephropathy. (Kliegman M Robert et al., 2007)

Dietary recommendations for children with diabetes are based on healthy eating recommendations suitable for all children and adults and therefore the whole family. Nutritional advice must be adapted to cultural, ethnic and family traditions and the psychosocial needs of the individual child. Likewise the choice of insulin regimen should take into account the dietary habits and lifestyle of the child.(NICE, 2004., American Diabetes Association, 2003)

A meal plan based on the individual's usual food intake should be determined and insulin therapy integrated into the usual eating and exercise patterns. Individuals on insulin therapy need to eat at consistent times synchronized with the time-actions of insulin, monitor blood glucose levels, and adjust insulindoses for the amount o food usually eaten or required (Frany J. Marion et al., 1994).

2. Guidelines on energy balance, energy intake and food components

No nutrition recommendations can be made for the prevention of type 1 diabetes at this time. (Franz MJ, et al., 2002), but increasing overweight and obesity in youth appears to be related to the increased prevalence of type 2 diabetes, particularly in minority adolescents. Although there are insufficient data at present to warrant any specific recommendations for the prevention of type 2 diabetes in youth, interventions similar to those shown to be effective for prevention of type 2 diabetes in adults (lifestyle changes including reduced energy intake and regular physical activity) are likely to be beneficial. Clinical trials of such interventions are ongoing in children.

Individuals who have pre-diabetes or diabetes should receive individualized medical nutrition therapy (MNT); such therapy is best provided by a registered dietitian familiar with the components of diabetes MNT. Meta-analysis of studies in non-diabetic, free-living subjects and expert committees report that MNT reduces LDL cholesterol by 15–25 mg/dl. (Yu-Poth S. et al., 1999. Grundy SM., et al. 1997)

The prevalence of overweight children and adolescents with type I Diabetes mellitus has tripled over the past 20 years, which appears to correspond to the increasing prevalence of obesity in the general population. The authors (Kliegman M Robert et al., 2007), have observed patients with type I diabetes, normal-weight preschool children have better glycemic control than age-matched overweight children. This may mean that excess body weight status may impede achievement of therapeutic goals in this group of patients.

The basis for energy requirements calculations is the determination of ideal body-weight. It is assessed corresponding to the respective tables comprising child's age, gender and body size data.

Guidelines for daily caloric requirements in children

- *1000 Kcal + 100 Kcal/year age (for 0-12 year old)*
- *1500-2000 kcal + 100 Kcal/year of age > 12 (for females 12-15)*
- *2000-2500 Kcal+ 200 Kcal/year of age > 12 (for males 12-15)*

Age	**kcal/kg/d**	**Protein (in grams) kg/d**
6 months	115	2.2
12 months	105	2.0
3 years	100	1.8
6 years	85	1.5
10 years	86	1.2
Male		
11-14 years	60	1.0
15-18 years	42	0.85
19-22 years	41	0.80
Females		
11-14 years	48	1.0
15-18 years	38	0.84
19-22 years	38	0.80
Adapted from National Academy of Sciences Food and Nutrition Board		

Table 1.

http://dx.doi.org/10.5772/52465

A recommendations and plans on intake of certain kinds of foods depends on daily energy expenditure which is determined by the individual patient's age, gender and level of physical activity. (Lean, M.E. J et al. 1980) In reality, the practical assessment of energy intake relies on follow-up of the patients' growth and body mass gain. If the tendency towards obesity has been identified (which usually occurs in the puberty and after the growth spurt cessation, most often in female patients) the energy intake should be reduced to 80-90% of standard calculated intake. On the other hand, in children with insufficient body weight a body mass deficit can be corrected using foods with high energy content. (Stepanović R., et al. 1991)/ An adequate diet enables a pediatric patient to utilize ingested food effectively even though the spontaneous endogenous insulin secretion ceased and life depends on anabolic effects of exogenous insulin administered usually in 2-3 daily doses. Since the insulin doses are delivered in the regular diurnal manner, at the same time every day, the food intake must be adjusted according to the dosage schedule, amount and type of administered insulin. A meal should be placed 30-60 minutes after regular insulin dose (in fact, regular insulin has an onset of action 15–60 min after injection, a peak effect 2–4 h after injection, and a duration of action of ranging from 5 to 8 h) comparing to 15 min with the newer synthetic insulin analogues. Synthetic insulin analogues, both lispro and aspart have an onset of action within 15 min, a peak in activity at 60–90 min, and a duration of action of 3–5 h. Therefore, a total daily food intake should be divided into six meals. Breakfast/ lunch / supper ratio should comprise 20% / 30% / 20% of a total daily intake while two snacks and a bedtime meal should consist of 10% of the daily intake each. Also, it is important to ingest about the same amount of carbohydrates at the regullar time every day and to eat meals regullarily in order to avoid the occurrence of hypoglycemic episodes. (Stepanović R., et al. 1991)

3. Carbohydrate

Dietary carbohydrate has both chemical structural features and form which have gained in importance in recent years. The process of digestion of carbohydrate has been known for many years and instinctively it is held that a monosaccharide must be absorbed more readily than an oligosaccharide, which requires hydrolysis before absorption.

The recommended dietary allowance (RDA) for digestible carbohydrate is 130 g/day and is based on providing adequate glucose as the required fuel for the central nervous system without reliance on glucose production from ingested proteins and fats. Although brain fuel needs can be met on lower-carbohydrate diets, long-term metabolic effects of very-low-carbohydrate diets are unclear, and such diets eliminate many foods that are important sources of energy, fiber, vitamins, and minerals and are important in dietary palatability (Institute of Medicine:2002). There are no trials specifically in patients with diabetes restricting total carbohydrate to <130 g/day. However, 1-year follow-up data from a weight-loss trialamong the subset with diabetes indicated that the reduction in fasting glucose was 21 mg/dl (1.17 mmol/l) and 28 mg/dl (1.55 mmol/l) for the low-carbohydrate and low-fat diets, respectively, with no significant difference in A1C levels (Stern L., et al. 2004).

Department for Agriculture (USDA) reveal that – 43%-47% of calories are contributed by dietary carbohydrate, whereas 36-37% of calories are contributed by dietary fat, with 13% from saturated fatty acids, 14% from monosaturated, and 7% from polyunsaturated. A reduction in high dietary takes of saturated fats, trans-fatty acids and cholesterol (all of which contains cholesterol-raising fatty acids) is an important goal to reduce the risk of cardiovascular disease. Although diabetes mellitus is usually categorized as a disease of carbohydrate metabolism, abnormalities of lipoprotein metabolism and adipose tissue distribution are also common. Cardiovascular disease accounts for the majority of deaths in people with diabetes. Analysis of the Multiple Risk Factor Intervention Trial data for men with diabetes matched with non-diabetic men reported relative risk of death for men with diabetes was increased at a range from 2.83 to 4.46 depending on their level of serum cholesterol. (Stamler J. et al. 1993)

Approximately 70% of the carbohydrate content should be derived from complex such as starch; intake of sucrose and highly refined sugars should be limited.

An intake of simple carbohydrates with high fiber foods - such as complex grains (bran), vegetables (beans and peas containing galactomannan) and fruit (pectin) is recommended; this combination of food slows intestinal food absorption, reduce postprandial hyperglycemia and lowers serum cholesterol levels (Stepanović R., et al. 1991).

4. Glycemic index and glycemic load

By definition, the glycemic index (GI), compares equal quantities of available carbohydrate in foods and provides a measure of carbohydrate quality. Available carbohydrate can be calculated by summing the quantity of available sugars, starch, oligosaccharides, and maltodextrins. By definition, (Salmeron J. etal 1997), the glycemic load (GL) is the product of a food's GI and its total available carbohydrate content: glycemic load = [GI × carbohydrate (g)]/100.

Therefore, the GL provides a summary measure of the relative glycemic impact of a "typical" serving of the food. Foods with a GL ≤10 have been classified as low glycemic load and those with a value ≥20 as high glycemic load (Brand-Miller JC, Holt SHA, Petocz P: Reply to R. Mendosa. Am J ClinNutr 77: 994–995, 2003). In healthy individuals, stepwise increases in GL have been shown to predict stepwise elevations in postprandial blood glucose and/or insulin levels (Brand-Miller JC et al, 2003). It can be seen from the equation that either a low-GI/high-carbohydrate food or a high-GI/low-carbohydrate food can have the same GL. However, while the effects on postprandial glycemia may be similar, there is evidence that the two approaches will have very different metabolic effects, including differences in β-cell function, triglyceride concentrations, free fatty acid levels (Wolever TMS, et al. 2002), and effects on satiety (Ball SD, et al. 2003).

Hence, the distinction has important implications for the prevention and management of diabetes and cardiovascular disease. Our concern is that the use of the GL or "glycemic response" in isolation may lead to the habitual consumption of lower-carbohydrate diets.

The use of the glycemic index has been shown to provide additional benefit to glycemic control over that observed when total carbohydrate is considered alone (Brand-Miller. et al. 2003). This index compares glycaemic excursions after ingestion of a carbohydrate and compares it with the glycemic excursions after an equivalent amount of the monosaccharide glucose. Thus numerical values can be ascribed to potatoes, rice, bread, etc., which give a comparative indication of glycemic consequence.

Factors that affect the glycemic response of foods are feeding rate, the rate of food ingestion, food ingredients (fat, protein, fiber, starch) and methods of cooking and food processing. Influence on glycemic response and physiological mechanisms of degradation of consumed food (pre-gastric and gastric hydrolysis, gastric emptying rate, intestinal hydrolysis and reaction to pancreatic and intestinal hormones). Bread, crackers, grain, potatoes, millet, corn, and chips have a high GI (> 90). Bran, oatmeal, rice, buckwheat have medium glycemic index (e.g. 70-90). Black bread, pasta, barley and cooked rice have the lowest glycemic index(<70) (Dimitrijević- Srećković V. 2002).

A controlled study in children using the GI of foods found flexible dietary instruction based on the food pyramid and low-GI choices achieved significantly better glycemic control after 12 months than more traditional dietary advice. (Gilbertson H. et al. 2001). In their study, Miller JB et al confirmed the significant influence of the lower GI nutrition on postprandial glucose levels. However, the impact on long-term glycemic control and co-morbidity was less efficient than pharmacological treatment.

Choosing low-GI foods in place of conventional or high-GI foods has a small but clinically useful effect on medium-term glycemic control in patients with diabetes. The incremental benefit is similar to that offered by pharmacological agents that also target postprandial hyperglycemia. (Jennie Brand-Miller et al. 2003)

In addition, several prospective observational studies have found that the overall GI and glycemic load (GI × g carbohydrate) of the diet, but not total carbohydrate content, are independently related to the risk of developing type 2 diabetes (Salmeron J et al, 1997), cardiovascular disease (Liu S et al, 2000), and some cancers (Augustin L, 2001, Franceschi S et al, 2001)

Low GI carbohydrate foods (GI < 55) may lower post-prandial hyperglycemia when they are chosen to replace higher GI foods (GI > 70) (Brand-Miller J. et al. 2003) Examples of low GI food sources include wholegrain breads, pasta, temperate fruits and dairy products. (Foster-Powell K. et al. 2002) Glycemic load (GL) is another method of predicting the postprandial blood glucose response, which takes into account both the GI of the food and the portion size. (Colombani PC, 2004). There has been no assessment of its efficacy in children.

Artificial sweeteners are widely used among diabetic patients. Two kinds of sweeteners may be distinguished:nutritive sweeteners which contain calories (fructose, sorbitol, mannitol) and non-nutritive which are calories-free (saccharin, cyclamate, aspartame). Fructose has the advantage over sucrose; for its better taste, slow absorption from the digestive system; no insulin is required for itsutilization and it causes hyperglycemia less often The fructose intake should be limited to 25g/d. Saccharin is about 500 times the sweeter than sucrose; its use may be connected to the increased risk of bladder carcinoma (Dimitrijevic-Srećković V., 2002).

5. Fat

The proportion of fat content in total energy intake should be approximately 35% in young children, and 25-30% in older children.

The vegetable fats have clearly advantage over animal ones. Intake decreases during childhood from approximately 2 g/kg/day in early infancy to 1 g/kg/day for a ten year old and to 0.8–0.9 g/kg/day in late adolescence. (Kauffman FR, 2005). Substituting butter with margarine, vegetable oil for animal oil, and lean cuts of meat, poultry, and fish for fatty meats, such as bacon, is advisable. These simple measures reduce serum low-density lipoprotein cholesterol, a predisposing factor to atherosclerotic disease.

Uncontrolled type I diabetes is associated with elevated plasma lipids, but adequate insulin therapy usually restores lipid levels to normal. People with type I diabetes who are treated with insulin generally have plasma cholesterol, VLDL cholesterol and triglyceride concentrations similar to those of the general population of the same age and sex (Kern P, 1987). Although not all studies agree, it appears that blood glucose control may directly influence the levels of several plasma lipid components. Qualitative abnormalities such as changes in a density of lipoprotein composition may exist even when the usual clinical measurements of plasma lipids are normal (Dunn FL, 1992). Evidence that dietary fat and the development of atherosclerosis are linked is controversial and there is little sign that a reduction in dietary fat would reduce atherosclerotic disease. Epidemiological studies from Japan are often quoted and in other populations a fall in cardiovascular morbidity has coincided with alterations in eating habits. (Nattras M., 1996) The dietary contents of polyunsaturated / saturated fatty acids should optimally correspond to 1.2: 1.0 ratios.

The primary goal regarding management of dietary fat is to decrease the intake of total fat, saturated fat, and trans-fatty acids (Franz MJ et al, 2002). Monounsaturated fatty acids (MUFA) and polyunsaturated fatty acids (PUFA) can be used as substitutes to keep lipid intake within recommended ranges or to improve the lipid profile.

Polyunsaturated fatty acids increase the production of lipid peroxides; some experimental studies considered their influence on occurrence of certain malignancies. They are rich in omega-6 fatty acids from sunflower oil and corn; moderate intake of these fatty acids lowers LDL cholesterol, while high intake lowers HDL cholesterol. Omega-3 fatty acids are found in deep sea blue fish (herring, mackerel, tuna and salmon). Their utilization from fish meat is more effective than the utilization from pharmacological supplements. The recommended intake of fish oil is 1.5-2.0 g / day. Omega-3 fatty acids moderately lower total cholesterol, significantly reduce triglyceride levels and reduce platelet aggregation, blood pressure and cardiovascular risk. However, they may increase hepatic glucose production, thus increasing blood glucose and hemoglobin A1-c levels. Therefore, in patients with impaired carbohydrate metabolism, the use of fish oil is not recommended; instead, blue sea fish meals should be taken 2-3 times a week.

Monounsaturated fatty acids are found in olive oil, walnuts and sesame. Studies have shown that application of these fatty acids for one month reduces insulin requirements and

http://dx.doi.org/10.5772/52465

improve insulin sensitivity; decreases blood glucose and triglyceride levels and arterial blood pressure as well. The Mediterranean diet, with increased use of olive oil-rich omega-9 fatty acids, reduces LDL cholesterol without affecting HDL cholesterol. Its intake improves insulin sensitivity, blood glucose and triglyceride levels and blood pressure. These mechanisms explain the reduction in coronary heart disease in Mediterranean countries. Monounsaturated fatty acids are more resistant to lipid peroxidation than the polyunsaturated fatty acids and less involved in the pathogenesis of atherosclerosis.

Trans-isomers of polyunsaturated fatty acids formed during the hydrogenation process may have potentially harmful effects. These trans-isomers are formed during solidification of vegetable oils. They are found in margarine and pastries, and intake of these foods increases LDL cholesterol and lowers HDL cholesterol. Therefore, in the UK and some European countries the intake of these trans-isomers in the amounts more than 5 g / day is not recommended. A consideration was given on intake of long chain omega-3 fatty acids. Epidemiological research studies have shown that prolonged use of concentrated fish oil may have an anti-atherogenic effect thanks to the high omega-3 acid contents (A. Simopoulos, 1991).

The existing nutritional recommendations of the European Association for the Study of Diabetes (EASD) and American Diabetes Association (ADA) on dietary composition promote greater flexibility in the proportions of energy derived from carbohydrate and from monounsaturated fat (MUFA). MUFA are promoted as the main source of dietary fat because of their lower susceptibility of lipid peroxidation and consequent lower atherogenic potential (Kratz M., et al. 2002).

In diabetes, cholesterol intake is limited to a maximum of 300 mg daily, in order to slow down the development of atherosclerotic process. This means that cholesterol-rich foods (brain, egg yolk) should be avoided, and lean meat (veal, beef, chicken) or fish should be used instead; instead of whole milk a milk containing 2.8% fat.

6. Proteins

Proteins are an essential nutrient, necessary for normal growth and development in childhood. Adequate protein ingestion is critical in normal muscle development. Proteins are an essential source of nitrogen.

The recommended intake is 15% of total caloric daily intake in older children and 20% in younger. The intake of proteins per kilogram of body weight should be higher in infants, children and adolescents in comparison to adults in order to support growth and development. The daily requirements are about 1.5g/kg for preschool children for and somewhat less -1g/kg for the children in school age –e.g., until the period of rapid growth during puberty, when the requirements increase again. (Stepanović R. et al 1991)

In diabetes variation in dietary protein may influence metabolic control by altering gluconeogenic substrate availability as well as insulin and contra-regulatory hormone secretion (Nuttall FQ., 1983).

Only in poorly controlled diabetes or in a period of recovering from ketoacidosis, the amount of protein should be greater than 2g/kg. The most important sources of protein are meat, fish and egg whites, but proteins are also represented in foods rich in carbohydrates (legumes, bread and cereals)

Excessive protein intake has also been implicated in the pathogenesis of diabetic renal disease and restricting its intake may retard the progression of nephropathy (Brenner BM., et al 1982)

The caloric mixture should comprise approximately 55% carbohydrate, 30% fat and 15% protein. A daily intake should be divided in 6-7 meals; breakfast and lunch should be represented with 20% of total caloric needs, dinner with 30% and each snack should contain 10% of daily calorie inputs. Each meal should be taken at certain time during the day with no major or frequent deviations. A bed time snack is considered an essential part of the regimen. This is necessary to prevent nocturnal hypoglycemia. The bed time snack includesat least 7-8g of protein, the amount equivalent to that in a meat or a milk exchange (7 to 8g). (Rudolph AM et al 1996)

7. Fiber

Dietary fibers may be divided into soluble (found in fruits, oats, barley, legumes and root vegetables) and insoluble (found in wheat, wheat bran, grains and some vegetables). Soluble fibers are mainly hemi-cellulose compounds that bind water, bile acids and build sequestered forms with monosaccharides and disaccharides; thus, they partially inhibit the action of digestive enzymes and slow down the process of absorption of food by increasing the time of intestinal passage. This action lowers postprandial glycemia and total cholesterol levels. These fibers also reduce the levels of lipids, cholesterol, LDL cholesterol and body mass. Soluble fiber supplements such as pectin, fiber from carob can improve metabolic regulation. Insoluble dietary fibers have little effect on blood glucose and no effects on lipids, but may increase satiety and inhibit hunger, and thus induce positive effects in obese patients with diabetes (Dimitrijevic-Srećković V., 2002).

8. Micronutrients: Vitamins and minerals

By complying with a proper and balanced diet, people with diabetes daily take adequate amount of vitamins and minerals, so there is usually no need for pharmacological supplements. The exceptions are some trace elements-copper, selenium and magnesium.

Individuals on weight –reducing diet, strict vegetarians patients with poor metabolic control and patients in critical care environments require special attention and assessment. A supplementation therapy containing vitamins and minerals is most often needed in these cases. In animal models it was shown that chromium deficiency was often associated with elevated blood glucose, cholesterol and triglyceride levels (Schrroeder HA, 1966;Wolscroft J et al,

1977). While serum zinc levels are generally lower in people with diabetes, zinc replacement is only suggested to be of benefit in helping to heal venous leg ulcer (Hoolbook T., et al 1979). There may be a need for magnesium replacement in patients with poor glycemic control or who are on diuretics. Magnesium depletion has been associated with decreased insulin sensitivity, which may improve with oral supplementation (Beaugerie L et al, 1990).

Some studies indicated that magnesium is a novel factor implicated to the pathogenesis of the diabetic complications. Magnesium plays a fundamental role as a cofactor in various enzymatic reactions of energy metabolism. Magnesium is a cofactor in cell membrane glucose – transporting mechanisms, as well as in various enzymes in carbohydrate oxidation. It is also involved, at multiple levels, in insulin secretion, binding and activity. Magnesium deficit has been described in patients with type I diabetes. Hypomagnesemia can also be the cause or a result of diabetes complications. If it is followed by diabetes, osmotic dieresis may play a role in the mechanisms responsible for magnesium deficiency. Magnesium loss may be linked to the development of diabetes complications via a reduction in the rate of inositol transport and its subsequent intracellular depletion that might enhance the development of complications. Magnesium is also taking part as a cofactor in many enzymes which are involved in lipid metabolism. Magnesium administration could decrease triglyceride, cholesterol and LDL cholesterol levels and also increase HDL cholesterol (Soltani N., 2011).

9. Sodium

The American Heart Association recommends that sodium intake should not exceed 3000 mg/day, while other authors (National High Blood Pressure Education Program, 1993) recommend not more than 2400mg/day. Individuals with mild to moderate hypertension should ingest no more than 2400mg of sodium daily (or less than 6 g/day of sodium chloride). A study performed in mildly hypertensive subjects with diabetes on moderate dietary sodium restriction showed a reduction of approximately 20 mmHg in systolic blood pressure. A difference in diastolic blood pressure was not achieved (Dodson PM., et al 1989).

Routine supplementation with antioxidants, such as vitamins E and C and carotene, is not advised because of lack of evidence of efficacy and concern related to long-term safety.

10. Recommended foods

A dietary intake of dark bread, rye, whole-meal bread, oats and barley flakes, porridge of maize flour, rice, spaghetti, potatoes, beans and lentils as a substitute for bread is recommended. Also, use of all kinds of vegetables (legumes, root and leafy vegetables) in the amount of 400-500 g/d (250g boiled, 250g fresh). All kinds of fruits are allowed, except for grapes, figs, prunes. The amount of fruit should be 500 g per day, divided into several installments. In addition, fresh fruit has an advantage over the pressed juice, since it is rich in dietary fibers.

Component	**Comment**
Protein	Not"/> 1g per body weight
Total fat	< 35% of energy intake
Saturated+trans-unsaturated fat	<10% of energy intake
n-6 Polyunsaturated fat	<10% of energy intake
n-3 Polyunsaturated fat	Eat fish, especially oily fish, once or twice weekly. Fish oil supplements-not recommended
cis-Monounsatureted fat	10-20% (60-70%) energy intake
Total carbohydrate	45-60%
Sucrose	Up to 10% of daily energy requirements, provided it is eaten within the healthy diet. Those who are overweight or who have hypertriglyceridemia should consider using not-nutritive sweeteners where appropriate
Fiber	No quantitative recommendation Soluble fiber"/> has beneficial effect on glycaemic and lipid metabolism Insoluble fiber"/> no direct effect on glycaemic and lipid metabolism but its high satiety content may benefit those trying to lose weight and its advantageous to gastrointestinal health
Vitamins and anti-oxidants	Encourage foods naturally rich in vitamins and anti-oxidants. With exception of some patients e.g. malnourishment, cancer etc. there is no evidence for the use supplements and some evidence that some are harmful
Salt	Approx 6 g sodium chloride per day

Table 2. (Connor H. et al. 2003)

The diet may contain dairy products - a skim milk, buttermilk, yogurt with 3.2% milk fat, cream, sour cream, butter, fatty cheeses and cheese. Lean meat (chicken, turkey, veal, beef, lamb, horse, deer, fish-river and sea), and cured meats from chicken, horse sausages, and sardines drained of oil are also recommended. Pork, duck, goose, sheep meat, fatty fish (catfish, perch, carp) should be avoided. The recommended intake is two poached eggs a week (in people with high cholesterol and triglyceride levels intake of yolk is not allowed). The use of vegetable fats is preferable (olive and sunflower oil) (Srećković V. Dimitrijevic, 2002).

The intake of starch should be provided by eating bread, grains, cereal, pasta, and starchy vegetables like corn and potatoes. They provide carbohydrate, vitamins, minerals, and fiber. Whole grain starches are healthier because they have more vitamins, minerals, and fiber.

The UK DAFNE Project (Dose Adjustment For Normal Eating) includes adults with type 1 diabetes participating in a group program. It is a kind of a group skills-based training with the aim to provide knowledge of flexible insulin meal–by-meal adjustments in order to match the carbohydrate content in a free diet.The groups consist of adult participants with type 1 diabetes of>2 years duration, without advanced complication, with HBA1c levels of 7.5-12%. DAFNE involves attending a 5-day training course plus a follow-up session around 8 weeks after the course and yearly half-day top-up sessions. The structured teaching program is delivered to groups of 6-8 participants and covers topics including carbohydrate estimation, blood glucose monitoring, insulin regimens, hypoglycemia, illness and exercise. A significant reductions in HbA1-c were found after 6 (-1.0%) and 12 months (-0.5%) of intervention, respectively. Also, a significant improvement in quality of life and well-being and satisfaction with treatment scores was registered (Nutrition Sub-Committee of the Diabetes Care Advisory Committee of Diabetes UK, 2003).

Exchange	**Calories**	**Grams of Carbohydrate**	**Grams of Protein**	**Grams of Fat**
Bread/starch	80	15	3	Trace
Fruit	60	15	-	-
		Meat		
Lean	55	7	3	-
Medium fat	75	-	7	3
High fat	100	-	7	8
Milk				
Skim	90	12	8	Trace
Low fat	120	12	8	5
Whole	150	12	8	8
Fat	45	-	-	5
Vegetable	25	5	2	-

Table 3. Nutrient composition of the exchanges

11. Nutrition recommendations for controlling diabetes complications

If there was a family history of hypercholesterolemia (total cholesterol >240 mg/dl) or a family cardiovascular event before age of 55 years, or if family history was unknown, a fasting lipid profile should be performed on children >2 years of age soon after diagnosis (after glucose control has been established). If family history is not of concern, then the first lipid screening should be considered at puberty (≥10 years). All children diagnosed with diabetes at or after puberty should have a fasting lipid profile performed soon after diagnosis (after glucose control has been established

Initial therapy should consist of optimization of glucose control and MNT using a Step 2 AHA diet (American Heart Association, 2010 Dietary Guidelines) aimed at a decrease in the amount of saturated fat in the diet. People diagnosed with type 1 diabetes in childhood have a high risk of early subclinical (Krantz JS et al, 2004, Järvisalo MJ et al, 2004, Haller MJ., 2004), and clinical (Orchard TJ., et al. 2001) CVD. Although intervention data are lacking, the AHA categorizes children with type 1 diabetes in the highest cardiovascular risk group and recommends both lifestyle and pharmacologic treatment for those with elevated LDL cholesterol levels (Kavey RE et al, 2006; McCrindle BW et al, 2007). Initial therapy should be with a Step 2 AHA diet, which restricts saturated fat to 7% of total calories and restricts dietary cholesterol to 200 mg/day. Data from randomized clinical trials in children as young as 7 months of age indicate that this diet is safe and does not interfere with normal growth and development

A proper nutrition and physical activity is essential for the prevention of arterial hypertension in diabetic patients. Hypertension, which is predictive of progression of micro- as well as macrovascular complications of diabetes, can be prevented and managed with interventions including weight loss, physical activity, moderation of alcohol intake, and diets such as DASH (Dietary Approaches to Stop Hypertension). The DASH diet emphasized fruits, vegetables, and low-fat dairy products; included whole grains, poultry, fish, and nuts; and was reduced in fats, red meat, sweets, and sugar-containing beverages Treatment of high-normal blood pressure (systolic or diastolic blood pressure consistently above the 90th percentile for age, sex, and height) should include dietary intervention and exercise aimed at weight control and increased physical activity, if appropriate(Chobanian AV., et al. 2003,*Sacks FM., et al. 2001, Appel LJ., et al. 2006).*

If target blood pressure is not reached with 3–6 months of lifestyle intervention, pharmacologic treatment should be considered (Standards of Medical Care in Diabetes—2012)

In individuals with diabetes and macroalbuminuria, reducing protein from all sources to 0.8 g/kg body wt/ day has been associated with slowing the decline in renal function (Franz MJ., et al 2002, Hansen H., et al 2002) ; however, such reductions in protein need to maintain good nutritional status in patients with chronic renal failure (Meloni C., et al 2002)

Although several studies have explored the potential benefit of plant proteins in place of animal proteins and specific animal proteins in diabetic individuals with microalbuninuria, the data are inconclusive. (Wheeler ML., et al 2002)

Medical nutrition therapy is important in preventing diabetes, managing existing diabetes, and preventing, or at least slowing, the rate of development of diabetes complications (Nutrition Recommendations and Interventions for Diabetes, 2008).

12. Nutritional management of exercise and sport

A regular physical activity improves glucose tolerance, increases muscle mass, reduces body fat mass and increases the number of insulin receptors and glucose entry into cells. A blood flow to the muscle and expansion of capillary space are stimulated during physical activity, which allows a better flow of insulin to muscle cells. (Zergollern Lj., et al., 1994) Regular physical exercise improves insulin resistance and reduction of triglyceride levels and increases total HDL and HDL2 concentration; it also helps in lowering blood pressure. It reduces mortality in type I diabetes and may reduce HbA1c up to 0.7% in type II diabetes (Ha TKK. et al., 1998).

The U.S. Department of Health and Human Services' Physical Activity Guidelines for Americans (U.S. Department of Health and Human Services, 2008), suggest that adults over age 18 years have up to 150 min/week of moderate-intensity, or 75 min/week of vigorous aerobic physical activity, or an equivalent combination of the two. In addition, the guidelines suggest that adults also do muscle-strengthening activities that involve all major muscle groups two or more days per week. Studies included in the meta-analysis of effects of exercise interventions on glycemic control (Boulé NG. et al., 2001). The DPP lifestyle intervention, which included 150 min/week of moderate intensity exercise, had a beneficial effect on glycemia in those with prediabetes. Therefore, it seems reasonable to recommend that people with diabetes try to follow the physical activity guidelines for the general population.

In patients who are in poor metabolic control, vigorous exercise may precipitate ketoacidosis because of the exercise-induced increase in the counter-regulatory hormones. On the other hand, there is an excessive amount of insulin in the body, the hepatic glucose production in response to excess muscle consumption could be insufficient, and symptoms of hypoglycemia might ensue.

When people with type 1 diabetes are deprived of insulin for 12–48 h and becomeketotic, exercise can worsen hyperglycemia and ketosis (Berger M, Berchtold P., et al., 1977); therefore, vigorous activity should be avoided in the presence of ketosis. However, it is not necessary to postpone exercise based simply on hyperglycemia, provided the patient feels well and urine and/or blood ketones are negative.

In individuals taking insulin and/or insulin secretagogues, physical activity can cause hypoglycemia if medication dose or carbohydrate consumption is not altered. For individuals on these therapies, additional carbohydrate should be ingested if pre-exercise glucose levels are <100 mg/dl (5.6mmol/l). Hypoglycemia is rare in diabetic individuals not treated with insulin or insulin secretagogues, and no preventive measures for hypoglycemia are usually advised in these cases.

It is therefore desirable that every person with diabetes planning or having physical exercise carry a glucose or sacharose preparation in form of tablets, jelly or candy or sugar in the form of cubes, candy, juice or soda. If hypoglycemias occur frequently, the entire dose insulin should be reduced by 10-15%.

The enhanced energy expenditure resulting from exercise increases the need for additional protein which should be met by increased consumption of nutritionally balanced diet. A small amount of additional protein may be required for muscle growth resulting from chronic physical conditioning.

Physical activity can acutely increase urinary protein excretion. However, there is no evidence that vigorous exercise increases the rate of progression of diabetic kidney disease, and there is likely no need for any specific exercise restrictions for people with diabetic kidney disease (Mogensen CE., 2002).

13. Conclusion

In conclusion, dietary recommendations for diabetic patients should be based on healthy eating recommendations suitable for all children and adults. Generally, the ideal diet for the normalization of glycemic control in people with diabetes has not yet been designed. In fact, there may be as many diets for diabetes as people with diabetes, and they could be based on the many individual manifestations, presentations, and complications of the disease. Individuals on insulin therapy need to eat at consistent times synchronized with the time-actions of insulin, monitor blood glucose levels, and adjust insulin doses for the amount of food usually eaten.

Medical nutrition therapy is important in preventing diabetes, managing existing diabetes, and preventing, or at least slowing, the rate of development of diabetes complications. No nutrition recommendations can be made for the prevention of type 1diabetes at this time. Although there are insufficient data at present to warrant any specific recommendations for the prevention of type 2 diabetes in youth, interventions similar to those shown to be effective for prevention of type 2 diabetes in adults are likely to be beneficial.

The caloric mixture should comprise approximately 55% carbohydrate, 30% fat and 15% protein. A flexible dietary instruction based on the food pyramid and low-glycemic index choices achieved significantly better glycemic control than more traditional dietary advice.

Several prospective observational studies have shown that the overall glycemic index and glycemic load of the diet, but not total carbohydrate content, are independently related to the risk of developing type 2 diabetes. An intake of simple carbohydrates with high fiber foods - such as complex grains, vegetables and fruit slows the intestinal absorption. It also reduces postprandial hyperglycemia and lowers serum cholesterol levels.

The primary goal regarding dietary fat is to decrease the intake of total fat, saturated fat, and trans-fatty acids. Monounsaturated fat should be promoted as the main source of dietary fat because of their lower susceptibility to lipid peroxidation and consequent lower atherogenic potential. Moderate intake of omega 3 and omega-9 fatty acids lowers LDL cholesterol.

If there was a family history of hypercholesterolemia or a family cardiovascular event before age of 55 years, or if family history was unknown, a fasting lipid profile should be performed on children >2 years of age soon after diagnosis (after glucose control has been established). All children diagnosed with diabetes at or after puberty should have a fasting lipid profile performed soon after diagnosis (after glucose control has been established. AHA categorizes children with type 1 diabetes in the highest for cardiovascular risk and recommends both lifestyle and pharmacologic treatment for those with elevated LDL cholesterol levels.

Proteins are an essential nutrient, necessary for normal growth and development in childhood. The recommended intake is 15% of total caloric daily intake in older children and 20% in younger children. The daily requirements are about 1.5g/kg for preschool children for and somewhat less -1g/kg for the children in school age –e.g., until the period of rapid growth during puberty, when the requirements increase again. Only in poorly controlled diabetes or in a period of recovering from ketoacidosis, the amount of protein should be greater than 2g/kg. Variable dietary proteins may influence metabolic control by altering gluconeogenic substrate availability as well as insulin and contra-regulatory hormone secretion. Excessive protein intake has also been implicated in the pathogenesis of diabetic renal disease. In individuals with diabetes and macroalbuminuria, reducing protein from all sources to 0.8 g • kg body wt−1 • day−1 has been associated with slowing the decline in renal function.

Hypertension can be prevented and managed with interventions including weight loss, physical activity, moderation of alcohol intake, and diets such as DASH (Dietary Approaches to Stop Hypertension. 2006). If target blood pressure is not reached with 3–6 months of lifestyle intervention, pharmacologic treatment should be considered. Insoluble dietary fibers have little effect on blood glucose and no effects on lipids, but they may increase satiety and inhibit hunger, thus inducing positive effects in obese diabetic patients.

By complying with a proper and balanced diet, people with diabetes take adequate amount of vitamins and minerals, so there is usually no need for pharmacological supplements. Zinc replacement is only suggested to be of benefit in helping to heal venous leg ulcer.

Author details

Snežana Marković- Jovanović

Medical Faculty, University of Prishtina, K. Mitrovica, Serbia

References

[1] American Diabetes Association. Nutrition principles and recommendations in diabetes (Position Statement). Diabetes Care 2003: 26(Suppl. 1): S51–S61.

[2] Appel LJ, Brands MW, Daniels SR, Karanja N, Elmer PJ, Sacks FM: Dietary approaches to prevent and treat hypertension: a scientific statement from the American Heart Association. 2006, Hypertension 47:296–308

[3] Augustin L: Dietary glycemic index and glycemic load in breast cancer risk: a case control study. Ann Oncol 12:1533–1538, 2001

[4] Ball SD, Keller KR, Moyer-Mileur LJ, Ding YW, Donaldson D, Jackson WD: Prolongation of satiety after low versus moderately high glycemic index meals in obese adolescents. Pediatrics, 2003: 111: 488–494

[5] Beaugerie L, Flourie B, Marteau P, Pellier P, et al. Digestion and apsorption in the human intestine of three sugar alcohols. Gastroenterology 99: 717-723, 1990.

[6] Berger M,Berchtold P, Cüppers HJ, DrostH,Kley HK, Müller WA, Wiegelmann W, Zimmerman-Telschow H, Gries FA, Krüskemper HL, Zimmermann H. Metabolic and hormonal effects of muscular exercise in juvenile type diabetics. Diabetologia 1977; 13: 355–365

[7] Boulé NG, Haddad E, Kenny GP, Wells GA, Sigal RJ. Effects of exercise on glycemic control and body mass in type 2 diabetes mellitus: a meta-analysis of controlled clinical trials. JAMA 2001; 286: 1218–1227

[8] Brand-Miller , Hayne S, Petocz P, Colagiuri S. Low-Glycemic Index Diets in the Management of Diabetes. A meta-analysis of randomized controlled trials. Diabetes Care 2003: 26: 2261–2267.

[9] Brand-Miller J, Hayne S, Petocz P, Colagiuri S. Low-Glycemic Index Diets in the Management of Diabetes. A meta-analysis of randomized controlled trials. Diabetes Care 2003: 26: 2261–2267

[10] Brand-Miller JC, Thomas M, Swan V, Ahmad ZI, Petocz P, Colagiuri S: Physiological validation of the concept of glycemic load in lean young adults. J Nutr. 2003: 133: 2728–2732

[11] Brenner BM, Mezer TW: Dietary protein intake and the progressive nature of kidney disease: the role of hemodynamically mediated glomerular injury in the pathogenesis of progressive glomerular sclerosis in aging renal ablation and intrinsing renal disease. N eng. J. Med 307:652-659, 1982

[12] Chobanian AV, Bakris GL, Black HR, Cushman WC, Green LA, Izzo JL Jr, Jones DW, Materson BJ, Oparil S, Wright JT Jr, Roccella EJ: The Seventh Report of the Joint National Committee on Prevention, Detection, Evaluation, and Treatment of High Blood Pressure: the JNC 7 report. JAMA 289:2560–2572, 2003

[13] Colombani PC. Glycemic index and load-dynamic dietary guidelines in the context of diseases.PhysiolBehav. 2004: 83(4): 603–10

[14] Connor H., Annan F., bunn E et al., The implementation of nutritional advice for people with diabetes . Diabetic Medicine 2003, Vol 20 p. 786-807

[15] Dimitrijević- Srećković V. : Dijetetskolečenje Tip I tip II dijebetesa, Dijabetes mellitus, inovacije znanja,2002: 57-65

[16] Dodson PM, Beevers M, Hallworth R, et al. Sodium restriction and blood pressure in hypertensive type 2 diabetes : randomized blind controlled and crossover studies of

moderate sodium restriction and sodium supplementation. Br Med J 298: 226-230, 1989

[17] Dunn FL: Plasma lipid and lipoprotein disorders in IDDM. 1992. Diabetes 41 (Suppl. 2): 102-106, 1992

[18] Foster-Powell K, Holt SH, Brand-Miller JC.International Table of Glycemic Index and Glycemic Load Values.Am J Clinical Nutrition 2002: 76: 5–56.

[19] Franceschi S, Dal Maso L, Augustin L, Negri E, Parpinel M, Boyle P, Jenkins DJ, La Vecchia C: Dietary glycemic load and colorectal cancer risk. Ann Oncol 12:173–178, 2001)

[20] Frany J. Marion, Horton S. Edwards, Bantle P John, et al. Nutrition Principles for the Management of Diabetes and Related Complications ; Diabetes care, 17, No5, 1994, 490-518

[21] Franz MJ, Bantle JP, Beebe CA, Brunzell JD, Chiasson JL, Garg A, Holzmeister LA, Hoogwerf B, Mayer-Davis E, Mooradian AD, Purnell JQ, Wheeler M: Evidence-based nutrition principles and recommendations for the treatment and prevention of diabetes and related complications. Diabetes Care , 2002: 25: 148–198

[22] Franz MJ, Bantle JP, Beebe CA, Brunzell JD, Chiasson JL, Garg A, Holzmeister LA, Hoogwerf B, Mayer-Davis E, Mooradian AD, Purnell JQ, Wheeler M: Evidence-based nutrition principles and recommendations for the treatment and prevention of diabetes and related complications. Diabetes Care 25: 148–198, 2002

[23] Gilbertson H, Brand-Miller J, Thorburn A et al. The effect of flexible low Glycemic index dietary advice versus measured carbohydrate exchange diets on glycemic control in children with type 1 diabetes. Diabetes Care 2001: 24: 1.

[24] Grundy SM, Balady GJ, Criqui MH, Fletcher G, Greenland P, Hiratzka LF, Houston-Miller N, Kris-Etherton P, Krumholz HM, LaRosa J, Ockene IS, Pearson TA, Reed J, Smith SC Jr, Washington R: When to start cholesterol-lowering therapy in patients with coronary heart disease: a statement for healthcare professionals from the American Heart Association Task Force on Risk Reduction. Circulation 1997: 95:1683–1685

[25] Ha TKK, Lean MEJ. Technical Review.Recommendation for the nutritional menagment of patient with diabetes. Eur. J ClinNutrituion 1998; 52: 647-481

[26] Haller MJ, Samyn M, Nichols WW, et al. . Radial artery tonometry demonstrates arterial stiffness in children with type 1 diabetes. Diabetes Care 2004; 27: 2911–2917

[27] Hansen HP, Tauber-Lassen E, Jensen BR, Parving HH: Effect of dietary protein restriction on prognosis in patients with diabetic nephropathy. Kidney Int 62:220–228, 2002

[28] Hoolbook T, Lanner E: serum zinc and healing of leg ulcer.1979, Lancet 2: 708-712

[29] Institute of Medicine: Dietary Reference Intakes: Energy, Carbohydrate, Fiber, Fat, Fatty Acids, Cholesterol, Protein, and Amino Acids. Washington, DC, National Academies Press, 2002

[30] Järvisalo MJ, Putto-Laurila A, Jartti L, et al..Carotid artery intima-media thickness in children with type 1 diabetes. Diabetes 2002; 51: 493–498;

[31] Jennie Brand-Miller, Susan Hayne, Peter Petocz, Stephen Colagiuri Low–Glycemic Index Diets in the Management of Diabetes,A meta-analysis of randomized controlled trial, Diabetes Care ,vol. 26 no. 8, 2003 : 2261-2267

[32] KAUFMANN FR. Surveillance and treatment for CVD in children with diabetes.ADA, Docnews 2005.

[33] Kavey RE, Allada V, Daniels SR, et al. American Heart Association Expert Panel on Population and Prevention Science, American Heart Association Council on Cardiovascular Disease in the Young, American Heart Association Council on Epidemiology and Prevention, American Heart Association Council on Nutrition, Physical Activity and Metabolism, American Heart Association Council on High Blood Pressure Research, American Heart Association Council on Cardiovascular Nursing, American Heart Association Council on the Kidney in Heart Disease, Interdisciplinary Working Group on Quality of Care and Outcomes Research. Cardiovascular risk reduction in high-risk pediatric patients: a scientific statement from the American Heart Association Expert Panel on Population and Prevention Science; the Councils on Cardiovascular Disease in the Young, Epidemiology and Prevention, Nutrition, Physical Activity and Metabolism, High Blood Pressure Research, Cardiovascular Nursing, and the Kidney in Heart Disease; and the Interdisciplinary Working Group on Quality of Care and Outcomes Research: endorsed by the American Academy of Pediatrics. Circulation 2006; 114: 2710–2738

[34] Kern P: Lipid disorders in diabetes mellitus, MT Sinai J Med, 1987: 54: 245-252,

[35] Kliegman M Robert, Behrman E Richard et al. Nelson Textbook of Pediatrics, The Endocrine system, Type 1 Diabetes mellitus ,2007: 2404-2425

[36] Krantz JS, Mack WJ, Hodis HN, Liu CR, Liu CH, Kaufman FR. Early onset of subclinical atherosclerosis in young persons with type 1 diabetes. J Pediatr 2004; 145: 452–457;

[37] Kratz M., Cullen P., kannenberg F., Kassner M., et al. Effect of dietary fatty acids on the composition and oxidizability of low density lipoprotein. Europian Journal of Clinical Nutrition 2002 56: 72-81

[38] Lean, M.E. J. And james, W.P.T. Prescription of diabetic diets in the 1980s. Lancet, i, 723-725.

[39] Liu S, Willett WC, Stampfer MJ, Hu FB, Franz M, Sampson L, Hennekens CH, Manson JE: A prospective study of dietary glycemic load, carbohydrate intake, and risk of coronary heart disease in US women. Am J ClinNutr 71:1455–1461, 2000

[40] McCrindle BW, Urbina EM, Dennison BA, et. Al.American Heart Association Atherosclerosis, Hypertension, and Obesity in Youth Committee, American Heart Association Council of Cardiovascular Disease in the Young, American Heart Association Council on Cardiovascular Nursing. Drug therapy of high-risk lipid abnormalities in children and adolescents: a scientific statement from the American Heart Association Atherosclerosis, Hypertension, and Obesity in Youth Committee, Council of Cardiovascular Disease in the Young, with the Council on Cardiovascular Nursing. Circulation 2007; 115: 1948–1967

[41] Meloni C, Morosetti M, Suraci C, Pennafina MG, Tozzo C, Taccone-Gallucci M, Casciani CU: Severe dietary protein restriction in overt diabetic nephropathy: benefits or risks? J RenNutr 12:96–101, 2002

[42] MogensenCE :Nephropathy. In Handbook of Exercise in Diabetes. 2nd ed. Ruderman N, Devlin JT, Kriska A Eds. Alexandria, VA, American Diabetes Association, 2002, p. 433–449

[43] National Hight Blood Pressure Education Program: Working Group Report on Primary Prevention of Hypertension . Bethesda, MD, U.S. Department of Health and Human Service , National Institutes of Health 1993, p.14

[44] Nattras M. Malims clinical diabetes:1996: Diet in Diabetes7: 117-132

[45] NICE. Type 1 diabetes diagnosis and treatment of type 1 diabetes in children and young people, 2004: (www.nice.org.uk/pdf/type1diabetes).

[46] Nutrition Recommendations and Interventions for Diabetes ;A position statement of the American Diabetes Association ;American Diabetes Association, Diabetes Care January 2008 vol. 31 no. Supplement 1 S61-S78

[47] Nutrition Subcommitte of the Diabetes Care Advisory Committee of Diabetes UK; The Implementation of nutritional advice for people with diabetes, Diabetes Medicine, 20: 786-807, 2003

[48] Nuttall FQ: Diet and the diabetic patient. Diabetes Care, 1983 6: 197-207,

[49] Orchard TJ, Forrest KY, Kuller LH, Becker DJPittsburgh Epidemiology of Diabetes Complications Study. Lipid and blood pressure treatment goals for type 1 diabetes: 10-year incidence data from the Pittsburgh Epidemiology of Diabetes Complications Study. Diabetes Care 2001; 24: 1053–1059

[50] Rudolph A.M. Hoffman J.I.E, Rudolph C.D, Rudolph's Pediatrics,Diabetes mellitus in children 1996,22:1803-1818

[51] Sacks FM, Svetkey LP, Vollmer WM, Appel LJ, Bray GA, Harsha D, Obarzanek E, Conlin PR, Miller ER III, Simons-Morton DG, Karanja N, Lin PH: Effects on blood pressure of reduced dietary sodium and the Dietary Approaches to Stop Hypertension (DASH) diet: DASH-Sodium Collaborative Research Group. N Engl J Med, 2001: 344:3–10,

[52] Salmeron J, Ascherio A, Rimm EB, Colditz GA, Spiegelman D, Jenkins DJ, Stampfer MJ, Wing AL, Willett WC: Dietary fiber, glycemic load, and risk of NIDDM in men. Diabetes Care 20:545–550, 1997

[53] Salmeron J, Manson J, Stampfer M, Colditz G, Wing A, Willett W: Dietary fiber, glycemic load, and risk of non-insulin-dependent diabetes mellitus in women. JAMA 1997:277:472–477

[54] Salmeron J, Manson JAE, Stampfer MJ, Colditz GA, Wing AL, Jenkins DJ, Wing AL, Willett WC: Dietary fiber, glycemic load, and risk of non-insulin-dependent diabetes mellitus in women. JAMA, 1997: 277: 472–477,

[55] Schrroeder HA: Chromium deficiency in rats : a syndrome stimulating diabetes mellitus with retarded growth. J. Nutr: 88: 439-445, 1966

[56] Simopoulos A: Omega-3 fatty acid in healzh and disease and in growth and development. Am J Clinnatur: 1991: 54:438-463

[57] SoltaniNepton, Prevention of Diabetes Complications; Type I Diabetes; complications; 2011, 16: 353-366

[58] Stamler J, Vaccaro O, Neaton JD, Wentworth D for the Multiple Risk factor Intervention Trial Research Group: Diabetes, other risk factors, and 12-yaer cardiovascular mortality for men screened in the Multiple Risk Factor Intervention Trial, Diabetes Care, 1993:

[59] Standards of Medical Care in Diabetes—2012, Diabetes Care, vol. 35, sup. S11-S63

[60] Stepanović R., Nestorović B. I sar. : Ishrana u Pedijatriji :Ishranadeceoboleleodšećernebolesti . Medicinskaknjiga Beograd- Zagreb 1991.,218-221

[61] Stern L, Iqbal N, Seshadri P, Chicano KL, Daily DA, McGrory J, Williams M, Gracely EJ, Samaha FF: The effects of low-carbohydrate versus conventional weight loss diets in severely obese adults: one-year follow-up of a randomized trial. Ann Intern Med 140:778–785, 2004

[62] Thom L.DiabetesAssociates.Nutritional management of diabetes., 1993 Mar;28(1): 97-112.

[63] U.S. Department of Health and Human Services: 2008 Physical Activity Guidelines for Americans.[articleonline],2008.Availablefrom http://www.health.gov/paguidelines/guidelines/default.aspx. Accessed December 2010.

[64] Wheeler ML, Fineberg SE, Fineberg NS, Gibson RG, Hackward LL: Animal versus plant protein meals in individuals with type 2 diabetes and microalbuminuria: effects on renal, glycemic, and lipid parameters. Diabetes Care 25:1277–1282, 2002

[65] Wolever TMS, Mehling C: Long-term effect of varying the source or amount of dietary carbohydrate on postprandial plasma glucose, insulin, triacylglycerol, and free fatty acid concentrations in subjects with impaired glucose tolerance. Am J ClinNutr. 2002, 76: 5–56

[66] Wolscroft J. Barbosa J: Analysis of chromium induced carbohydrate intolerance in the rat. J. Nutr.107: 1702-1706, 1977.

[67] Yu-Poth S, Zhao G, Etherton T, Naglak M, Jonnalagadda S, Kris-Etherton PM: Effects of the National Cholesterol Education Program's Step I and Step II dietary intervention programs on cardiovascular disease risk factors: a meta-analysis. Am J Clin Nutr1999: 69:632–646

[68] ZergollernLj., Reiner Ž. I sar. Pedijatrija 2, 1994: Dijabetes mellitus 17: 1319-1330

Section 6

Therapies in the Pipeline

Chapter 20

Immune Intervention in Type I Diabetes Mellitus

Johnny Ludvigsson

Additional information is available at the end of the chapter

http://dx.doi.org/10.5772/52801

1. Introduction

In many countries Type 1 diabetes [T1D] is the most common life-threatening disease in children, and nobody can be cured. For long time the incidence has increased all over the world [1]. The disease causes serious morbidity and increased mortality [2,3] in spite of an intensive treatment with multiple daily injections of insulin, adapted to regular meals with suitable content based on self-monitoring of blood glucose. Many patients do never succed to get good metabolic control because of the complicated treatment and another problem preventing good metabolic control is hypoglycaemia [4]. Modern insulin pumps and glucose sensors have made it possible to improve insulin treatment [5]. The simplest approach to reduce severity of hypoglycemia when treatment is intensified is to interrupt insulin delivery. There are insulin pumps with an integrated continuous glucose monitoring, which automatically suspends insulin delivery for up to 2 hours when hypoglycemia is detected even when the hypoglycemia alarm is not acknowledged by the patient [6,7]. Closed-loop insulin delivery [artificial pancreas] is aiming to achieve near normal blood glucose without increasing the risk of hypoglycemia [8]. Thus a disposable sensor measures interstitial glucose levels, which are fed into an algorithm controlling delivery of a rapid-acting insulin analog into the subcutaneous tissue by an insulin pump. So far research has focused on closed loop insulin delivery during night, and this technique is improving [9]. However, also in the future there will be need for the patient to learn how to handle also these devices, not least during infections, longer exercise, and several other situations and changes of life.

2. Introduction

Even though patients with T1D need insulin, the primary goal of novel therapies is to preserve residual insulin secretion, in best case to cure diabetes or at least to make the disease milder and facilitate treatment. Patients with residual insulin secretion usually get lower HbA1c, and residual insulin secretion facilitates the treatment, decreases the risk for serious hypoglycaemia and the risk of keto-acidosis [10]. Already very modest beta cell function, with peak stimulated C-peptide above 0.2 nmol/L seems to reduce long-term complications [11]. Furthermore, C-peptide per se has been proposed to decrease the risk of complications, especially neuropathy. There is increasing evidence that C-peptide is not just a connecting peptide to keep the two insulin chains in in a certain structure, but a hormone with several important effects [12]. The relevance of saving beta cells and improving their function has become even more evident when studies suggest that beta cells may regenerate [13, 14]. If this is the case an end of the destructive process might lead to cure of T1D [15].

3. The immunological disease process

The generally accepted opinion is that the majority of the pancreatic beta cells are lost at the diagnosis of Type 1 diabetes. The beta cells are supposed to be killed by an autoimmune process precipitated and promoted by genetic and environmental factors. In recent years the dogma saying that most beta cells are dead has been questioned, and regeneration of the beta cells seems not only possible but quite plausible. Actually that was discussed as a possibility already several decades ago(Fig 1). Thus, many beta cells may still be living in pancreas although they do not respond normally to stimulus with insulin secretion. Auto-antibodies are usually found, but regarded as markers of the process, rather than causing beta cell death. The auto-antibodies react against the islet cells (Islet Cell Antibodies; ICA) [16] or against specific auto-antigens such as Insulin Auto-antibodies against Insulin (IAA) [17], against Glutamic Acid Decarboxylase (GADA) [18], against Tyrosin Phosphatase (IA-2A) [19] or against ZincTransport Antigen (ZnTA) [20]. These antigens are attacked by the own immune system. Dysregulation of the immune system is thought to allow a self-destructive process. Mononuclear cells, mainly T-cells, seem to play the most important role for the killing of the beta cells.

4. Immune interventions

Several immune interventions have been tried since the 1970ies we tried plasmapheresis in Linköping, Sweden, with the aim to preserve residual beta cell function, but so far all different approaches have shown insufficient efficacy and/or given unacceptable adverse effects [21-28]. Broad immunosuppressive or immunoblocking therapies with steroids, cytostatics, high doses of immunoglubulins, anti-lymphocyte globulins have shown some but unfortunately limited efficacy, and adverse events have lead to restrictions both in dose and time. Our studies using photopheresis did show some efficacy, and although the treatment was very laborious it has regained some interest. However, most encouraging is the use of monocloncal antibodies, especially against CD-3 [29-31] but also against CD-20 [32]. Unfortunately treatment with monoclonal antibodies in doses large enough to give efficacy also cause rather common and occasionally serious adverse events.Therefore such therapies are rarely justified as preventive interventions in healthy children with increased risk of developing T1D except for children with extremely high risk of developing T1D close in time.

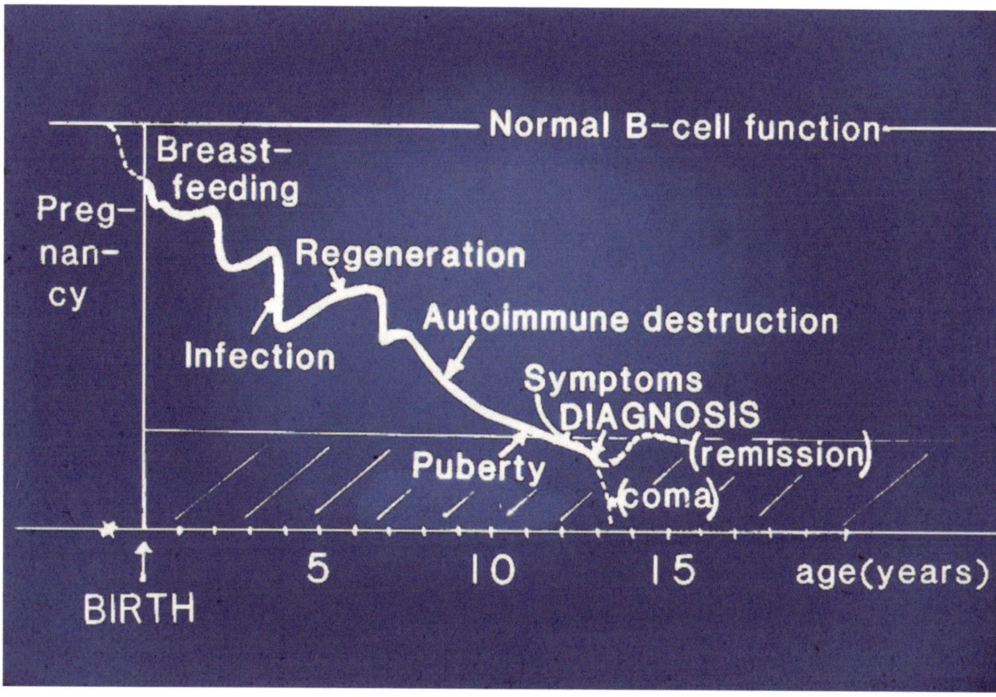

Figure 1. At a Nordic symposium in connection with Annual meeting of Scandinavian Society for the Study of Diabetes, Linköping 1981, the author showed this slide. Type 1diabetes was proposed to develop after a long autoimmune process destroying the beta cells. Events during pregnancy and the importance of breast-feeding was suggested, and later shown to be relevant, and regeneration of beta cells was proposed as a possibility.

After encouraging Phase II trials two different Phase III trials using antiCD3 failed to reach their primary endpoints [33,34], but one of them, the Protégé study, did show efficacy in younger patients age 8-18 years when a reasonably high dose of antiCD-3 was used [34]. This was especially true in certain patient populations (mainly patients in USA, but also in Europe) who had rather well preserved C-peptide, often near-normal HbA1c and low insulin requirement. Further studies are needed to learn what doses are efficient without severe adverse events, and in what patient populations the treatment works best. The old policy defended by many diabetologists to treat all so called T1D in the same way irrespective of age, ethnic background, severity of disease at diagnosis etc may probably have to be left.

5. Vaccines against infections

Traditional vaccinations could either contribute to the development of T1D, or T1D could be prevented by vaccination. Already in the 1920ies mumps infection was shown to be a possible cause of insulin dependet diabetes [35]. A general vaccination against mumps might then either decrease the incidence of T1D, or vaccination with living virus might on the contrary initiate an autoimmune process leading to an increased incidence of T1D. None of these associations have been proven [36, 37]. Neither have there been any associations between vaccinations against other microbes and the development of diabetes [38]

Entero virus infections are most suspected to cause T1D. Epidemiological studies have provided evidence of coxsackie virus (CVB) infections in subjects who later develop T1D [39]. A CVBB4 strain E2 was isolated from pancreas of a diabetic child, and the virus was then passed into islet cells and found to cause diabetes in mice, which was taken as a proof of the concept that coxsackievirus can cause T1D [40]. So far vaccination against these types of infections to preserve beta cells has been disappointing,

The hygiene hypothesis suggests that the immune system would deviate less often towards an autoimmune process if the immune system was occupied by an ongoing defence against serious enemies. In accordance with this hypothesis, Calmette vaccination has been tried to preserve beta cell function but no clinical effect has been seen [41].

6. Immune intervention by probiotics

Several findings indicate that the gut is involved in the development of the disease process leading to T1D [42]. The intestinal barrier may be disturbed. This might facilitate passage of proteins which could contribute to the autoimmune process. Cows milk [43], and bovine insulin in cows milk has been suggested as a possible cause of an autoimmune reaction against insulin [44]. Maturation of the immune system may also be influenced by the gut flora. Probiotics can probably influence immune function through effects on antigen-presenting cells, regulatory T cells and effector T and B cells [45] and probiotics may prevent autoimmune diabetes in NOD mice [46,47]. However, although use of probiotics would be attractive as the adverse events can be expected to be minimal, there are so far no studies proving any effect

7. Heat shock protein used in immune intervention

Studies in experimental animals have shown that use of a 65-kDa heat shock protein can prevent diabetes [48]. A specific peptide, Diapep 277, seems to be the active component and this peptide has been tried with interesting effects.

Clinical trials in humans have shown that sc administration of Diapep 277 may preserve beta cell function in adults [49]. Thus 35 patients with type 1 diabetes and basal C-peptide above 0.1 nmol/L were assigned to subcutaneous injections of 1 mg Diapep277 and 40 mg mannitol in vegetable oil The primary endpoint was glucagon-stimulated C-peptide production. At 10 months, mean C-peptide concentrations had fallen in the placebo group (n=16) but were maintained in the DiaPep277 group (n=15; p=0.039). Need for exogenous insulin was higher in the placebo than in the DiaPep277 group. There were no o adverse events. The treatment of newly diagnosed T1D adults with DiaPep277 seemed to preserve residual insulin secretion through induction of a shift from Thr-1 to Thr-2 cytokines. However, the efficacy seen in adults could not be confirmed in children and adolescents with T1D [50,51] in spite of interesting immunologcval results [52]. In a recent Phase III trial no immunological difference could be found between adults treated with Diapep 277 or those treated with placebo [53]. Treatment with Diapep 277 seemed to preserve C.peptide but only C-peptide after Glucagon stimulation, but not after Mixed Meal Tolerance Test [54]. Thus it is still unclear whether Diapep 277 has a place or not as future intervention to preserve residual insulin secretion in adults.

8. "Inverse vaccination "to reduce the immune response

Traditional vaccination is strengthening the immune reaction against an antigen, usually an infectious microbe. Methods of reducing a pathological specific immune response eg in autoimmune diseases like T1D can be regarded as a sort of "inverse" vaccination. In allergy tolerance against the allergens is created by presenting the antigen/allergen/s in gradually increasing doses. Such Immunotherapy has become quite efficacious [55] and the adverse events are rare.

It would be reasonable to try to reduce an autoimmune process in an analogue way, by administration of auto-antigen/s. Thus, instead of suppressing the immune system, the immune response should be modulated by presenting antigen/s in a way that the immune system shifts from a destructive process to tolerance [56].

If self-reactive T-cells directed against auto-antigens cause some cases of Type 1 diabetes a major question is why such self-reactive T-cells occur. Two mechanisms seem to be necessary for self-tolerance: Clonal deletion of self-reactive T-cells issued from the random recombination of genes (negative selection), and generation of self-antigen-specific natural regulatory T-cells (Tregs) which can inactivate self-reactive T-cells in the periphery when they have escaped intra-thymic negative selection [57]. In T1D auto-reactivity against insulin is a common and early phenomenon. The important role of thymic insulin for development of self-tolerance has been demonstrated in transgenic mice [58], but there is still no technique to use this knowledge in clinical practice.

9. Auto-antigen treatment

9.1. "Vaccination" with insulin

Proinsulin and insulin and its different chains are so far the only known auto-antigens that are specific for the beta cells. Insulin has been used in trials to prevent diabetes among first degree relatives with increased risk of T1D. In Diabetes Prevention Trial-Type 1 Diabetes (DPT-1) human ultralente insulin of 0.25 units x kg/day, or placebo, was given to subjects with >50%

5-year risk of getting T1D. To give such large doses of insulin sc every day can not be regarded as immune intervention, but rather as beta cell support. In any case this type of treatment failed to reach the end-point [59].

Oral insulin is not supposed to be absorbed enough to affect blood glucose or to support remaining beta cells, but such an administration can be regarded as immune intervention. The DPT-1 trial randomized 372 relatives of subjects with T1D, positive for IAA and with normal intravenous and oral glucose tolerance test (IVGTTs and OGTTs), to oral insulin 7.5 mg daily or placebo. Although the result was negative when comparing the groups with the pre-specified inclusion criteria, subanalyses suggested that Type 1 diabetes was significantly delayed in those individuals who had higher concentrations of IAA [60]. This suggests that auto-antigen therapy may be most efficaceous in patients whose immune system reacts strongly against a certain antigen.

The first diabetes-related auto-antibodies in young children are usually IAA and therefore insulin has been tried to prevent diabetes in high risk individuals. Intranasal proinsulin had effect in experimental animals [61] but intranasal administration of insulin in high risk children had no effect [62]. Administration of the insulin B-chain can prevent diabetes in experimental animals [63]. A combination of the insulin B-chain fragment with Freunds adjuvant has been tried also in newly-diagnosed T1D adults [64]. There was effect on T-regulatory cells but no significant effect on C-peptide.

9.2. GAD-vaccination

During our studies with plasmapheresis [21] we discovered a new diabetes-related antigen, 64kD [65], which later on was found to be glutamic acid decarboxylase (GAD [66]. Auto-antibodies towards GAD are common in T1D and there are convincing results from studies of experimental animals that treatment with GAD can prevent autoimmune diabetes [67, 68]..

An adjuvanted formulation, based on Alhydrogel®, a product of Aluminum hydroxide (alum),was developed to provide a drug (Diamyd®) used for evaluation in clinical trials. Alhydrogel® is used as adjuvant in vaccines for children eg DTP, Pneumococcal conjugate, Hepatitis B, Hepatitis A vaccines. Aluminum salts are inducing a humoral (Th2) rather than cellular immune response. As the T1D autoimmune process is deviated towards Th1 (or cellular) response to autoantigens, alum is used to counteract this deviation and "steer" the response induced by GAD away towards a Th2 response. Inclusion of adjuvant is also a way to minimize the quantity of antigen required for treatment.

Diamyd® preclinical safety studies were done and caused no concerns for clinical safety. Evaluation of the effects of Diamyd® in several different animal models of autoimmune disease did not indicate any undesirable effects on the immune system. Phase 1 studies in humans were performed 1999.A randomized, double-blind and placebo-controlled dose-finding Phase IIa study in 47 LADA demonstrated efficacy in beta cell preservation in the 20-μg group [60] There were no Serious Adverse Events (SAEs)) and even though the number of patients was very small, this result was encouraging. Follow-up after five years completed 2008 still showed

http://dx.doi.org/10.5772/52801

a significantly beneficial effect of the 20μg dose of Diamyd®, and there had been very few AE, none of them considered to be treatment related [70]

A Phase IIb, randomized, double-blind, placebo-controlled multicenter Diamyd® study in 160 LADA-subjects was then performed in Sweden. Subjects received 20 μg of GAD65 or placebo on 2 occasions 4 weeks apart. The trial had a main study period of 18 months and was scheduled for unblinding in June 2007. Unfortunately, the study had to be invalidated due to concerns regarding the labeling process of the investigational product. No safety concerns were raised and no SAEs had been observed during 30 months observation.

9.3. GAD vaccination in children and adolescents

To investigate safety and efficacy of Diamyd® in T1D, a Phase II clinical trial in 70 recently diagnosed T1D children and adolescents was performed [71]. The study was a randomized, double-blind, placebo-controlled multicenter study using the same dose regimen as in the successful group of the previous LADA trial. The main study period of 15 months was completed and the trial partly unblinded for sponsor and statistician but continued blinded for all other investigators for another 15 month follow-up. Outcomes from this study provided support for clinical safety and efficacy after administration of Diamyd®. The treatment was very well tolerated and there were no treatment-related adverse events reported still after more than 4 years follow-up. Both treatment groups showed a gradual decline from baseline of both fasting and stimulated C-peptide secretion. There was no significant effect of treatment on change in fasting C-peptide after 15 months (primary endpoint). However, there was a significant efficacy seen on change in fasting C-peptide after 30 months ($p=0.045$), which remained signficant when change in C-peptide/plasma glucose ratio was taken into account ($p=0.02$). Furthermore, stimulated C-peptide secretion, as measured by area under the curve (AUC), decreased significantly less in the GAD-alum treated group compared to the placebo group, both after 15 months ($p=0.01$) and after 30 months ($p=0.04$). The significant effect of treatment as change in fasting and stimulated C-peptide at month 30 remained when adjusting for duration of diabetes, age, gender, and baseline GADA levels.

However, although the c-peptide preservation was evident the insulin requirement in both treatment groups increased in the course of the study, and HbA1c, and plasma glucose levels increased during the study. HbA1c did not differ between the groups.

Duration of diabetes was very important for the efficacy of treatment ($p=0.05$ for fasting at month 30 and $p=0.03$ for stimulated C-peptide area under the curve at month 15 and 30). In patients treated within 6 months of diagnosis both fasting and stimulated C-peptide secretion (AUC), decreased significantly less in the GAD-alum treated group as compared to the placebo group over 30 months (fasting, $p=0.03$, and stimulated $p=0.04$) while no such difference was seen in patients with a longer duration of diabetes (Fig 2). The treatment effect in the short duration was still seen after more than 4 years follow-up [72] in patients with < 6 months duration of diabetes at treatment. There were no treatment-related adverse events.

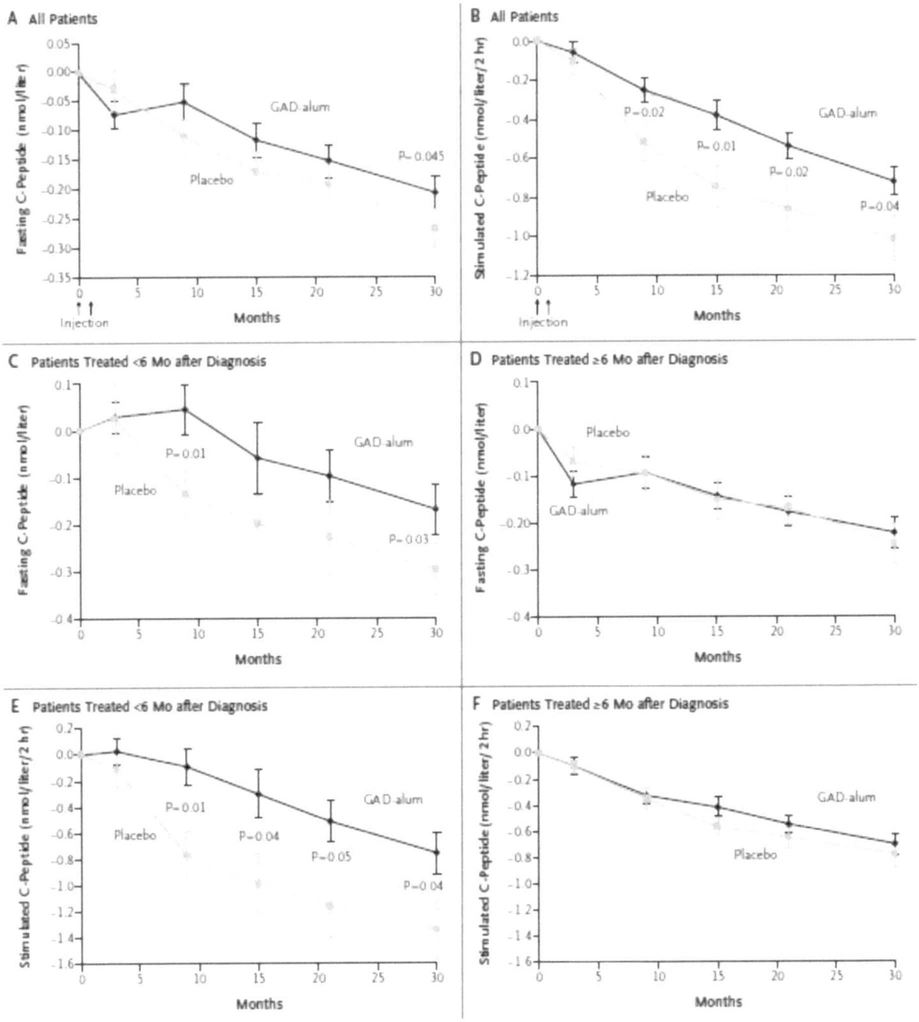

Mean changes from baseline in fasting (panelA) and stimulating (Panel B) c-peptide are fiven for all patients included in intention to treat analyses in the group receiving the recombinant human 65-kD isoform of glutamic acid decarboxulase in a standard vaccine formulation with alum (GAD-alum. 35 patients) and in the group receiving placebo (34 patients). Mean changes from baseline in fasting (Panel C) and stimulated (Panel E) C-peptide levels are also shown for those patienst treated less then 6 month after receiving the diagnosis of diabetes (11 patients in GAD-alum group and 14 patients in the placebo group). Finally, mean changes from baseline in fasting (Panel D) and stimulated (Panel F) C-peptide levels are shown for those treated 6 months or more after diagnosis (24 patients in the GAD-alum group and 20 patients in the placebo group). Stimulated C-peptide level was measured on the basis of areas under the curve in response to the mixed-meal tolerance test. I bars indicate standard errors. To convert values for C-peptide to nanograms per milimeter, devided by 0.33.

Figure 2. Mean Changes from Baseline Levels of Fasting and Stimulating C-Peptide, According to Treatment Group and Time of Treatment Relative to Diagnosis.

The Phase II trial was followed by aPhase III trial in Europe. 334 patients age 10- 20 years were included, with diabetes duration < 3 months at screening, fasting C-peptide >0.1 nmol/l and pos GADA. In this study the two arms of the Phase II study (placebo resp 20 μg of GAD65 (Diamyd®) with 30 days interval, were the same, but in addition there was a third arm where the patients got 20 μg of GAD65 (Diamyd®) sc also at Day 90 and 270 when the patients in the other arms got placebo injections. The primary endpoint was difference in C-peptide AUC after a Mixed Meal Tolerance Test. Surprisingly the study failed! [73]. The difference in AUC was only 16-18 % between the actively treated patients and the placebo group ($p= 0.10$) and the difference in fasting C-peptide was similar ($p= 0.07$). However, in several prespecified subgroups the efficacy was quite pronounced (around 30-40%), and significant.. When combining Phase II and that arm in Phase III in which the patients received 2 doses of GAD-alum, then theefficacy measured both as fasting C-peptide and AUC after MMTT seems quite impressive after 30 months.

The question arises why the results in Phase III was so much weaker than in Phase II. There are some possible explanations: In Phase III the patients who received active drug by chance were more often 10-11 years old whereas patients in the placebo group more frequently were 16-20 years old than in the actively treated arms. It is well known that younger patients loose their residual insulin secretion more rapidly and therefore this difference in ages might have influenced the result. There are also other facts which may have played a role. Thus, in the Phase II trial the patients were treated in March –April and when looking at patients in Phase III who were treated in March-April there was in fact also significant effect of GAD-treatment. Finally, in the Phase II trial no vaccinations were accepted, but in Phase III Influenza-vaccination was allowed. Unfortunately an epidemic of H1N1-flu lead to that almost all patients were vaccinated, many of them in connection with the GAD-vaccinations. In Sweden and Finland the vaccine contained squalen, suspected to influence the immune system towards auto-immunity, and in these two countries there was no efficacy of GAD-treatment, while there was efficacy in other European countries. Patients in Sweden, who did not get the influenza vaccination close to the GAD-treatment, had better effect of the GAD-treatment [73].

9.4. GAD-vaccination and the immune system

In both the Phase IIb and the European Phase III patients treated with two doses of GAD-alum got increasing GADA levels with a a maximum after 3 months and then a gradual decrease even if the concentrations of GADA remained significantly higher than in the placebo group. Four doses given in the Phase III trial lead to even higher GADA levels. Increase of GADA had neither relationship to efficacy of the vaccination, nor to adverse events. There was no change of epitopes related to development of Stiff Person Syndrome, but a rather small but significant shift in isotypes with reduced percentage of IgG1 and increased IgG3/IgG4 detected in GAD-alum treated patients[74], in agreement with a Th2 deviation. Spontaneous/non-stimulated and PHA-induced secretion of all cytokines was similar in samples from children receiving GAD-alum and placebo, both before and 15 months after the first injection. Cytokine secretion of IL-5, IL-10, IL-13, IL-17, IFN-γ and TNF-α, but not of IL-6 and IL-12, in response to in vitro stimulation with GAD65 increased in GAD-alum treated patients from baseline to month 15, but a continuous increase was only seen in IL-5, IL-10 and IL-13 while other cytokines remained elevated but at a stable concentration [75]. This indicates that the treatment caused a Th2-

deviation. The immunological effects were long lasting immune responses, as they remained still 48 months after the first injection [75].

As a sign of increase of T-regulatory cells we noticed an increased GAD65-induced expression of FOXP3 and TGF-β at month 15 in cells from GAD-alum treated patients compared to placebo, and the expression of FOXP3 and TGF-β correlated positively in the GAD-alum group but not in the placebo group[77]. Still after 48 months there were clear effects on the immune system suggesting both a Th2 deviation, a decrease of activated T-cells (CD4+CD25+high) but increase of FoxP3-positive regulatory T-cells. Thus, our interpretation is that Diamyd® treatment deviated the immune system towards tolerance against the auto-antigen GAD.

9.5. Other trials with GAD vaccination

Beside the European phase III trial discussed above [73], a similar trial was started a bit later in USA (US Phase III ClinicalTrials.gov Identifier: NCT00751842 ;Jerry Palmer, PI), with the same design. The recruitment was not so fast as initially only patients >16 years old were accepted, and therefore the recruitment had just finished when the negative results of the European Phase III trial was found. This lead to that the American trial was stopped, before it can give any results. In addition another intervention trial in newly-diagnosed Type 1 diabetic patients aged 3-45 years was performed by TrialNet (TrialNet Intervention ClinicalTrials.gov Identifier: NCT00529399). Patients were randomized in a double-blind controlled study into three arms, one with subcutaneous injections of 20 μg GAD65-alum (Diamyd®) at day 1,30 and 90, a second arm with subcutaneous injections of 20 μg GAD65-alum (Diamyd®) at day 1,30 and placebo at day 90, and a third arm with placebo at all time points The study failed. No effect on C-peptide preservation was found [77]. So far little has been presented from this trial with regard to effects on the immune system. It is difficult to know what the wide age range, variation in ethnic groups, BMI etc meant for the result.

9.6. Ongoing or planned GAD-alum studies

Because of the positive results in the Swedish Phase II study and the positive results in some prespecified subgroups in the European Phase III trial, new studies are planned. As the Phase III trial failed, GAD-alum will be given as part of combination therapy, which hopefully will give a better effect on the disease process. Thus a new pilot trial is just on its way when GAD-alum is combined with Vitamin D, which is supposed to positively influence the dendritic cells, contribute to Th2 deviation, but also influence directly beta cell survival and insulin sensitivity. In addition a third drug, anti-inflammatory, will be given to dampen the inflammation, which might play an important and negative role beside the autoimmune process.

In addition to interventional trials at onset of Type 1 diabetes a pilot trial with the aim to prevent T1D is ongoing in southern Sweden. High risk children have been identified as part of the so called DiPiS (Diabetes Prevention in Skåne) study, in which newborn children in the general population have been screened for auto-antibodies. Children positive for GADA, plus at least one more diabetes-related autoantibody, have been treated with either 20 μg GAD65-alum

http://dx.doi.org/10.5772/52801

(Diamyd®) or placebo subcutaneous at day 1 and 30. As the study is not powered for efficacy the main aim is to study safety.

10. DNA vaccines

T-cells respond to antigens presented by antigen presenting cells (APCs).DNA-vaccines can be used to present the antigen instead of delivering intact proteins. A protein encoded by a plasmid DNA can either be produced outside the APCs if the pasmidDNA is administered into a muscle, or the plasmidDNA may be taken up by the APCs where the encoded protein is presented [78]. Proteins encoded by DNA vaccines can induce different types of antigen-specific immune responses, and perhaps also some non-specific reactions.

Most common routes of administration are either intramuscular, which is thought to favour Th1 responses, or intradermal, which is thought to favour Th2 response. For treatment of Type 1 diabetes intradermal injection should be most interesting. Another way of skewing the response towards Th2 may be to co-administer plasmids encoding Th2 cytokines.

Promoters from virus, eg Cytomegalovirus, can be used. Certain sequences seem to stimulate Th1 response and should therefore be avoided in treatment of T1D.

So far DNA-vaccines to create tolerance in autoimmune disease have been tried mainly in experimental animals. Plasmid DNA encoding for proinsulin [79] as well as for the insulin B chain [80] have been used for prevention of diabetes in experimental animals. Injection of plasmidDNA encoding for GAD has been shown effective in preventing diabetes in NOD-mice [81], while similar effect have been seen by combining plasmidDNA encoding for a fusion protein consisting of both GAD, IgG and IL4 [82]. Treatment with a recombinant vaccinia virus expressing GAD (rVV-GAD65) has also shown to be effective in prevention of autoimmune diabetes in NOD mice by induction of active suppression of effector T-cells [83]. IgG1 antibodies and IL-4 increased and the IgG2 was unchanged, suggesting a Th2 deviation.Before clinical use there are several problems which need to be solved. Correct dosing is necessary as wrong dose might give increased immune response and a more aggressive disease process In addition it is important to be sure that the DNA is not integrated in the host chromosome. Another problem might be production of antibodies against DNA.

11. Beta cell regeneration

The traditional generally accepted view is that when a patient gets Type 1 diabetes there is no longer any capacity of the beta cells to regenerate. However, there are almost no studies on beta cell regeneration in humans. In recent years some studies suggest that the old paradigm may be wrong and that beta cells in fact can regenerate. GLP-1 might stimulate beta cell regeneration.and GLP-1 agonist (Exenatide) in combination with monoclonal antibodies interfering with IL-2 (Daclizumab) was given to patients with longstanding Type 1 diabetes with some residual insulin secretion, to see whether the treatment could increase C-peptide, but in this study the result was negative [84].

Administration of INGAP (islet neogeneis associated protein)in anaimals has caused increased beta cell mass and reversal of hyperglycemia, and hopefully INGAP has regenerating capacity in humans. Daily introductionf of INGAP or placebo has been tried in a double-blind randomized trial in both Type 1 and Type 2 diabetic patients [85], and it showed increased arginin-stimulated C-peptide during the treatment period, but the effect was very short. Already after 30 days the effect was lost, which does not indicate any influence on beta cell mass as such an effect should have been much longer

12. Vitamin D and type 1 diabetes

Experimental studies suggest that vitamin D may play a role in the defence against type 1 diabetes as well as type 2 diabetes. Epidemiological data suggest that there is a link between vitamin D deficiency and an increased incidence of Type 1 diabetes. A multinational case-control study and a birth cohort follow-up study from Finland [86] have concluded that vitamin D3 supplementation at birth protects against type 1 diabetes later in life, and a meta-analysis supports similar conclusions [87]. Low serum levels of 1α,25-dihydroxyvitamin D3 [1,25(OH)2D3, calcitriol] has been found in patients with recently diagnosed type 1 diabetes. The protective effects of vitamin D against diabetes are mediated through the regulation of several components such as the immune system and calcium homeostasis. Thus, mechanistic studies show that 1,25(OH)2D3 modulates dendritic cell maturationand facilitates a shift from a Th1 to a Th2 immune response. There is also ncreasingevidence suggesting that vitamin D also affects beta cells directly thereby rendering them more resistant to cellular stress. There are results indicating that Vitamin D may also improve insulin sensitivity, which in turn decrease beta cell stress.

Vitamin D has been used in patients with recent onset Type 1 diabetes in an effort to preserve residual insulin secretion. However, so far Vitamin D alone has not been efficacious [88. 89]. It seems resaonable to try Vitamin D, both in higher dose, and in combination with other therapy.

13. Anti-inflammatory treatment

In diabetes, both Type 1 and Type 2, there are signs of inflammation, partly related to glucotixicity, partly to other traits of the disease. Thus also in Type 1 diabetes there is an inflammatory componenent in addition to the autoimmune process. IL-1 has been proposed to be of special importance for the destruction of pancreatic beta cells [90], and blocking IL-1 in experimental animals has shown important effects on the disease process. Use of IL-1 inhibitor in Type 1 diabetes has shown reduced serum interleukin 8 (IL-8) levels and reduced CD11b integrin expression on monocytes associated with increased CXCR1 expression. These effects suggest that blocking the IL-1beta pathway results in a reduced ability of mononuclear cells

http://dx.doi.org/10.5772/52801

to go to sites of inflammation. However, there is a great gap between studies in animals and and in vitro mechanistic studies, to clinical studies in humans. Recently at the Congress of American Diabetes Association and at the Immunology Diabetes Society the results of two trials blocking the effect of IL-1 in Type 1 diabetes failed. Thus, the use of IL-1r-antagonist showed no effect on preservation of C-peptide or any related clinical parameter[91], and the same was unfortunately the case in another Phase II trial using a IL-1 antagonist, Anakinra [92]. Furthermore blocking IL-1 caused adverse events. Thus, as single therapy using anti-inflammatory drugs is not good enough, but should be tested in combination with other therapies.

14. Future perspectives of immune intervention

No single therapy has shown to be an effective immune intervention in manifest Type 1 diabetes for preservation of residual insulin secretion. As well as successful treatment of childhood leukemia and cancers needed combination of several drugs, it will most probably be necessary to use combination therapies also for Type 1 diabetes. Auto-antigen treatment will probably be part of such future clinical treatment and/or prevention of Type 1 diabetes. Even though GAD-alum so far has not shown any stable efficacy, and Diapep 277 has shown slight efficacy only in adults with good C-peptide preservation, future studies will tell us how to use auto-antigen therapy more effectively, and then in combination with other therapiesIt may be so that treatment with GAD may be useful in patients with immune recognition of GAD, and treatment with proinsulin or insulin/insulin chains may be useful in patients whose immune system recognizes these auto-antigens. Furthermore, the effect might be improved by combination therapies with eg Vitamin D, anti-inflammatory drugs, perhaps also in combinations with monoclonal antibodies. New ways of administration may be important and/or DNA-vaccines may be found to be another effective way of creating tolerance against auto-antigens,. In spite of recent failures of some immune interventions in clinical trials knowledge is growing and there may soon be a breakthrough.

15. Disclosure

Diamyd Medical was sponsor for the Phase II/III GAD-alum trials and has also given financial support for the investigator-initiated mechanistic studies of this type of therapy. Honorarium for lectures has been received from NovoNordisk, Lilly and SanofiAventis. The author is also member of Advisory Board of LifeScan.

Acknowledgements

In addition to the author the Linköping Diabetes Immune Intervention study group consists of Ass.professor Rosaura Casas, PhD, Stina Axelsson PhD, Mikael Cheramy PhD,and PhD students Mikael Pihl and Linda Åkerman.

We are grateful to excellent technical assitance from Ingela Johansson and Gosia Smolinska, and from research nurses Eva Isacson and AnnMarie Sandström. All pediatricians involved in our studies are also gratefully acknowledged.

Our studies on immune intervention have been generously supported by Barndiabetesfonden (Swedish Child Diabetes Foundation), Swedish Research Council, Research Council of South-east Sweden (FORSS), and the mechanistic studies are supported by Juvenile Diabetes Research Foundation (JDFR).

Author details

Johnny Ludvigsson

Dept of Clin Exp Med, Linköping university, Linköping, Sweden

References

[1] Aanstoot HJ, Anderson BJ, Daneman D, Danne T, Donaghue K, Kaufman F, Réa RR, Uchigata Y.The global burden of youth diabetes: perspectives and potential. Pediatr Diabetes. 2007 Oct;8 Suppl 8:1-44.

[2] The Diabetes Control and Complications Trial Research Group. The effect of intensive treatment of diabetes on the development and progression of long-term complications in insulin-dependent diabetes mellitus. N Engl J Med 1993;329:977-86.

[3] Bojestig M, Arnqvist HJ, Hermansson G, Karlberg BE, Ludvigsson J. Declining incidence of nephropathy in insulin-dependent diabetes mellitus. N Engl J Med 1994;330:15-8

[4] Wild D, Von Maltzahn R, Brohan E, Christensen T, Clauson P, Gonder-Frederick L. A critical review of the literature on fear of hypoglycemia in diabetes: Implications for diabetes management and patient education. Patient Educ Couns. 2007;68:10–15

[5] Tamborlane WV, Beck RW, Bode BW, Buckingham B, Chase HP, Clemons R, Fiallo-Scharer R, Fox LA, Gilliam LK, Hirsch IB, Huang ES, Kollman C, Kowalski AJ, Laffel L, Lawrence JM, Lee J, Mauras N, O'Grady M, Ruedy KJ, Tansey M, Tsalikian E, Weinzimer S, Wilson DM, Wolpert H, Wysocki T, Xing D. Continuous glucose monitoring and intensive treatment of type 1 diabetes. N Engl J Med. 2008;359:1464–1476.

[6] Choudhary P, Shin J, Wang Y, Evans ML, Hammond PJ, Kerr D, Shaw JA, Pickup JC, Amiel SA. Insulin pump therapy with automated insulin suspension in response to hypoglycemia: reduction in nocturnal hypoglycemia in those at greatest risk. Diabetes Care. 2011;34:2023–2025.

[7] Danne T, Kordonouri O, Holder M, Haberland H, Golembowski S, Remus K, Blasig S, Wadien T, Zierow S, Hartmann R, Thomas A. Prevention of hypoglycemia by using low glucose suspend function in sensor-augmented pump therapy. Diabetes Technol Ther. 2011;13:1–6

[8] Hovorka R. Closed-loop insulin delivery: from bench to clinical practice. Nat Rev Endocrinol. 2011;7:385–395.

[9] Hovorka R, Allen JM, Elleri D, Chassin LJ, Harris J, Xing D, Kollman C, Hovorka T, Larsen AM, Nodale M, De PA, Wilinska ME, Acerini CL, Dunger DB. Manual closed-loop insulin delivery in children and adolescents with type 1 diabetes: a phase 2 randomised crossover trial. Lancet. 2010;375:743–751

[10] Madsbad S, Alberti KG, Binder C, Burrin JM, Faber OK, Krarup T, and Regeur L: Role of residual insulin secretion in protecting against ketoacidosis in insulin-dependent diabetes. Br Med J 2: 1257-1259, 1979.

[11] Steffes MW, Sibley S, Jackson M, Thomas W. Beta-cell function and the development of diabetes-related complications in the Diabetes Control and Complications Trial. Diabetes Care 2003;26:832-6.

[12] Wahren J, Ekberg K, Jörnvall H. C-peptide is a bioactive peptide. Diabetologia. 2007 Mar;50(3):503-9.

[13] Jun HS. Regeneration of pancreatic beta cells. Front Biosci. 2008 May 1;13:6170-82

[14] Gonez LJ, Knight KR. Cell therapy for diabetes: stem cells, progenitors or beta-cell replication?Mol Cell Endocrinol. 2010 Jul 8;323(1):55-61.

[15] Ludvigsson J. C-peptide an adequate endpoint in type 1 diabetes. Diabetes Metab Res Rev. 2009 Nov;25(8):691-3.

[16] Bottazzo GF, Florin-Christensen A, Doniach D. Islet-cell antibodies in diabetes mellitus with autoimmune polyendocrine deficiencies. Lancet 1974:2:1279-82.

[17] Palmer JP, Asplin CM, Clemons P, Lyen K, Tatpati O, Raghu PK, Paquette TL. Insulin antibodies in insulin-dependent diabetics before insulin treatment. Science. 1983 Dec 23;222(4630):1337-9.

[18] Baekkeskov S. Immunoreactivity to a 64,000 Mr human islet cell antigen in sera from insulin-dependent diabetes mellitus patients and individuals with abnormal glucose tolerance. Mol Biol Med. 1986 Apr;3(2):137-42

[19] Savola K, Bonifacio E, Sabbah E, et al. IA-2 antibodies - a sensitive marker of IDDM with clinical onset in childhood and adolescence. Diabetologia 1998:41:424-9.

[20] Wenzlau JM, Juhl K, Yu L, et al. The cation efflux transporter ZnT8 (Slc30A8) is a major autoantigen in human type 1 diabetes. Proc Natl Acad Sci U S A. 2007;104:17040-5.

[21] Ludvigsson J, Heding L, Lieden G, Marner B, Lernmark A. Plasmapheresis in the initial treatment of insulin-dependent diabetes mellitus in children. Br Med J (Clin Res Ed) 1983;286:176-8.

[22] Dupre J, Stiller CR, Gent M, et al. Clinical Trials of Cyclosporin in IDDM. Diabetes Care 1988;suppl 1:37-44

[23] Eisenbarth GS, Srikanta S, Jackson R, et al. Anti-thymocyte globulin and prednisone immunotherapy of recent onset type 1 diabetes mellitus. Diabetes Research 1985;2:271-6

[24] Chase HP, Butler-Simon N, Garg S, McDuffie M, Hoops SL, O'Brien D. A trial of nicotinamide in newly diagnosed patients with type 1 (insulin-dependent) diabetes mellitus. Diabetologia 1990;33:444-6

[25] Pozzilli P, Visalli N, Signore A, et al. Double blind trial of nicotinamide in recent-onset IDDM (the IMDIAB III study). Diabetologia 1995;38:848-52.

[26] Coutant R, Landais P, Rosilio M, et al. Low dose linomide in Type I juvenile diabetes of recent onset: a randomised placebo-controlled double blind trial. Diabetologia 1998;41:1040-6.

[27] Ludvigsson J, Samuelsson U, Johansson C, Stenhammar L. Treatment with antioxidants at onset of type 1 diabetes in children: a randomized, double-blind placebo-controlled study. Diabetes Metab Res Rev 2001;17:131–6.

[28] Ludvigsson J, Samuelsson U, Ernerudh J, Johansson C, Stenhammar L, Berlin G. Photopheresis at onset of type 1 diabetes: a randomised, double blind, placebo controlled trial. Arch Dis Child 2001;85:149-54.

[29] Herold KC, Gitelman SE, Masharani U, et al. A single course of anti-CD3 monoclonal antibody hOKT3gamma1(Ala-Ala) results in improvement in C-peptide responses and clinical parameters for at least 2 years after onset of type 1 diabetes. Diabetes 2005;54:1763-9.

[30] Keymeulen B, Vandemeulebroucke E, Ziegler AG, et al. Insulin needs after CD3-antibody therapy in new-onset type 1 diabetes. N Engl J Med 2005;352:2598-608.

[31] Keymeulen B, Walter M, Mathieu C, Kaufman L, Gorus F, Hilbrands R, Vandemeulebroucke E, Van de Velde U, Crenier L, De Block C, Candon S, Waldmann H, Ziegler AG, Chatenoud L, Pipeleers D. Four-year metabolic outcome of a randomised controlled CD3-antibody trial in recent-onset type 1 diabetic patients depends on their age and baseline residual beta cell mass. Diabetologia. 2010 Apr;53(4):614-23.

[32] Pescovitz MD, Greenbaum CJ, Krause-Steinrauf H, Becker DJ, Gitelman SE, Goland R, Gottlieb PA, Marks JB, McGee PF, Moran AM, Raskin P, Rodriguez H, Schatz DA, Wherrett D, Wilson DM, Lachin JM, Skyler JS; Type 1 Diabetes TrialNet Anti-CD20 Study Group Rituximab, B-lymphocyte depletion, and preservation of beta-cell function. N Engl J Med. 2009 Nov 26;361(22):2143-52.

[33] Gottlieb et al Abstract Annual Meeting of ADA, 2011.

[34] Sherry N, Hagopian W, Ludvigsson J, Jain SM et al Teplizumab for treatment of type 1 diabetes (Protégé study): 1-year results from a randomised, placebo-controlled trial. Lancet. 2011 Aug 6;378(9790):487-97

[35] Gundersen E: Is Diabetes of Infectious Origin? The Journal of Infectious Diseases, Vol. 41, No. 3 (Sep., 1927), pp. 197-202..

[36] Hiltunen M, Lönnrot M, Hyöty H. Immunisation and type 1 diabetes mellitus: is there a link? Drug Saf. 1999 Mar;20(3):207-12.

[37] Lindberg B, Ahlfors K, Carlsson A, Ericsson UB, Landin-Olsson M, Lernmark A, Ludvigsson J, Sundkvist G, Ivarsson SA. Previous exposure to measles, mumps, and rubella--but not vaccination during adolescence--correlates to the prevalence of pancreatic and thyroid autoantibodies. Pediatrics. 1999 Jul;104(1):e12

[38] Hviid A, Stellfeld M, Wohlfahrt J, Melbye M.. Childhood vaccination and type 1 diabetes. N Engl J Med. 2004 Apr 1;350(14):1398-404

[39] Hyöty H, Hiltunen M, Knip M, Laakkonen M, Vähäsalo P, Karjalainen J, Koskela P, Roivainen M, Leinikki P, Hovi T, et al. A prospective study of the role of coxsackie B and other enterovirus infections in the pathogenesis of IDDM. Childhood Diabetes in Finland (DiMe) Study Group. Diabetes. 1995 Jun;44(6):652-7

[40] Yoon JW, Austin M, Onodera T, Notkins AL. Isolation of a virus from the pancreas of a child with diabetic ketoacidosis.N Engl J Med. 1979 May 24;300(21):1173-9

[41] Allen HF, Klingensmith GJ, Jensen P, Simoes E, Hayward A, Chase HP. Effect of Bacillus Calmette-Guerin vaccination on new-onset type 1 diabetes. A randomized clinical study. Diabetes Care. 1999 Oct;22(10):1703-7

[42] Vaarala O. The role of the gut in beta-cell autoimmunity and type 1 diabetes: a hypothesis. Pediatr Diabetes. 2000 Dec;1(4):217-25

[43] Virtanen SM, Knip M. Nutritional risk predictors of beta cell autoimmunity and type 1 diabetes at a young age. Am J Clin Nutr. 2003 Dec;78(6):1053-67

[44] Vaarala O. Is it dietary insulin? Ann N Y Acad Sci. 2006 Oct;1079:350-9.

[45] Benno Y, Mitsuoka T. Development of intestinal microflora in humans and animals. Bifidobacteria Microfl 1986;5:13-25.

[46] Matsuzaki T, Nagata Y, Kado S, et al. Prevention of onset in an insulin-dependent diabetes mellitus model, NOD mice, by oral feeding of Lactobacillus casei. APMIS 1997;105:643-9.

[47] Calcinaro F, Dionisi S, Marinaro M, et al. Oral probiotic administration induces interleukin-10 production and prevents spontaneous autoimmune diabetes in the non-obese diabetic mouse. Diabetologia. 2005;48:1565-75

[48] .Elias D, Cohen IR Treatment of autoimmune diabetes and insulitis in NOD mice with heat shock protein 60 peptide p277. Diabetes. 1995 Sep;44(9):1132-8

[49] Raz I, Elias D, Avron A, Tamir M, Metzger M, Cohen IR. Beta-cell function in new-onset type 1 diabetes and immunomodulation with a heat-shock protein peptide (DiaPep277): a randomised, double-blind, phase II trial. Lancet. 2001 Nov 24;358(9295): 1749-53

[50] Lazar L, Ofan R, Weintrob N, et al. Heat-shock protein peptide DiaPep277 treatment in children with newly diagnosed type 1 diabetes: a randomised, double-blind phase II study. Diabetes Metab Res Rev 2007 May;23(4):286-91

[51] Schloot NC, Meierhoff G, Lengyel C, Vándorfi G, Takács J, Pánczél P, Barkai L, Madácsy L, Oroszlán T, Kovács P, Sütö G, Battelino T, Hosszufalusi N, Jermendy G. Effect of heat shock protein peptide DiaPep277 on beta-cell function in paediatric and adult patients with recent-onset diabetes mellitus type 1: two prospective, randomized, double-blind phase II trials. Diabetes Metab Res Rev. 2007

[52] Huurman VA, van der Meide PE, Duinkerken G, Willemen S, Cohen IR, Elias D, Roep BO. Immunological efficacy of heat shock protein 60 peptide DiaPep277 therapy in clinical type I diabetes. Clin Exp Immunol. 2008 Jun;152(3):488-97.

[53] Schloot N et al: Abstract IDS, Victoria 2012

[54] Raz I et al Abstract ADA 2012

[55] Theodoropoulos DS, Lockey RF. Allergen immunotherapy: guidelines, update, and recommendations of the World Health Organization. Allergy Asthma Proc. 2000 May-Jun;21(3):159-66.

[56] Ludvigsson J. Adequate doses of autoantigen administered using the appropriate route may create tolerance and stop autoimmunity. Diabetologia 2009;52 (1):

[57] Castermans E, Baron F, Willems E, Schaaf-Lafontaine N, Meuris N, Gothot A, Vanbellighen JF, Herens C, Seidel L, Geenen V, Cheynier R, Beguin Y. Evidence for neo-generation of T cells by the thymus after non-myeloablative conditioning. Haematologica. 2008 Feb;93(2):240-7.

[58] Klein L, Hinterberger M, Wirnsberger G, Kyewski B. Antigen presentation in the thymus for positive selection and central tolerance induction. Nat Rev Immunol. 2009 Dec; 9(12):833-44.

[59] Pozzilli P. The DPT-1 trial: a negative result with lessons for future type 1 diabetes prevention. Diabetes Metab Res Rev. 2002 Jul-Aug;18(4):257-9

[60] Skyler JS, Krischer JP, Wolfsdorf J, Cowie C, Palmer JP, Greenbaum C, Cuthbertson D, Rafkin-Mervis LE, Chase HP, Leschek E. Effects of oral insulin in relatives of patients with type 1 diabetes: The Diabetes Prevention Trial--Type 1. Diabetes Care. 2005

[61] Every AL, Kramer DR, Mannering SI, Lew AM, Harrison LC. Intranasal vaccination with proinsulin DNA induces regulatory CD4+ T cells that prevent experimental autoimmune diabetes. J Immunol. 2006 Apr 15;176(8):4608-15

[62] .Näntö-Salonen K, Kupila A, Simell S, Siljander H, Salonsaari T, Hekkala A, Korhonen S, Erkkola R, Sipilä JI, Haavisto L, Siltala M, Tuominen J, Hakalax J, Hyöty H, Ilonen J, Veijola R, Simell T, Knip M, Simell O. Nasal insulin to prevent type 1 diabetes in children with HLA genotypes and autoantibodies conferring increased risk of disease: a double-blind, randomised controlled trial. Lancet. 2008 Nov 15;372(9651):1746-55.

[63] Song HY, Abad MM, Mahoney CP, McEvoy RC. Human insulin B chain but not A chain decreases the rate of diabetes in BB rats. Diabetes Res Clin Pract. 1999 Nov;46(2):109-14)

[64] Orban T, Farkas K, Jalahej H, Kis J, Treszl A, Falk B, Reijonen H, Wolfsdorf J, Ricker A, Matthews JB, Tchao N, Sayre P, Bianchine P. Autoantigen-specific regulatory T cells induced in patients with type 1 diabetes mellitus by insulin B-chain immunotherapy. J Autoimmun. 2010 Jun;34(4):408-15 Use of auto-antigens may be a way to modulate the immune process and increa<se T-cell regulation and tolerance.

[65] Baekkeskov S, Nielsen JH, Marner H, Bilde T, Ludvigsson J, Lernmark A. Autoantibodies in newly diagnosed diabetic children immunoprecipitate human pancreatic islet cell proteins. Nature 1982;298:167-9.

[66] Baekkeskov S, Aanstoot HJ, Christgau S, Reetz A, Solimena M, Cascalho M, Folli F, Richter-Olesen H, De Camilli P. Identification of the 64K autoantigen in insulin-dependent diabetes as the GABA-synthesizing enzyme glutamic acid decarboxylase. Nature. 1990 Sep 13;347(6289):151-6

[67] Tian J, Clare-Salzler M, Herschenfeld A, et al. Modulating autoimmune responses to GAD inhibits disease progression and prolongs islet graft survival in diabetes-prone mice. Nature Medicine 1996;2:1348-53.

[68] Tisch R, Liblau RS, Yang XD, Liblau P, McDevitt HO. Induction of GAD65-specific regulatory T cells inhibits ongoing autoimmune diabetes in non-obese diabetic mice. Diabetes 1998;47:894-9.

[69] Agardh CD, Cilio CM, Lethagen A, et al. Clinical evidence for the safety of GAD65 immunomodulation in adult-onset autoimmune diabetes. J Diabetes Complications 2005;19:238-46.

[70] Agardh C-D, Lynch K, Palmér M, Link K et al. GAD65 vaccination significantly reduces insulin dependence at five years follow-up in a dose escalating study in adult-onset autoimmune diabetes patients. Diabetologia 51 2008;(suppl.1):S230.

[71] Ludvigsson J, Faresjo M, Hjorth M, Axelsson S, Cheramy M, Pihl M, et al. GAD treatment and insulin secretion in recent-onset type 1 diabetes. N Engl J Med. 2008;359(18): 1909-20.

[72] Ludvigsson J, Hjorth M, Chéramy M, Axelsson S et al Extended evaluation of the safety and efficacy of GAD treatment of children and adolescents with recent-onset type 1 diabetes: a randomised controlled trial. Diabetologia. 2011 Mar;54(3):634-40.

[73] Ludvigsson J, Krisky D, Casas R, Battelino T et al GAD65 antigen therapy in recently diagnosed type 1 diabetes mellitus. N Engl J Med. 2012 Feb 2;366(5):433-42

[74] Chéramy M, Skoglund C, Johansson I, Ludvigsson J, Hampe CS, Casas R. GAD-alum treatment in patients with type 1 diabetes and the subsequent effect on GADA IgG subclass distribution, GAD(65) enzyme activity and humoral response. Clin Immunol. 2010 Jun 25.

[75] Axelsson S, Chéramy M, Hjorth M, Pihl M, et al Long-lasting immune responses 4 years after GAD-alum treatment in children with type 1 diabetes. PLoS One. 2011;6(12):e29008.

[76] Hjorth M, Axelsson S, Rydén A, Faresjö M, Ludvigsson J et al GAD-alum treatment induces GAD65-specific CD4+CD25highFOXP3+ cells in type 1 diabetic patients. Clin Immunol. 2011 Jan;138(1):117-26

[77] Wherrett DK, Bundy B, Becker DJ, et al. Antigen-based therapy with glutamic acid decarboxylase (GAD) vaccine in patients with recent-onset type 1 diabetes: a randomised double-blind trial. Lancet. 2011 Jul 23;378(9788):319-27.

[78] von Herrath MG, Whitton JL DNA vaccination to treat autoimmune diabetes. Ann Med. 2000 Jul;32(5):285-92.

[79] Zhang W, Jin H, Hu Y, Yu Y, Li X, Ding Z, Kang Y, Wang B. Protective response against type 1 diabetes in nonobese diabetic mice after coimmunization with insulin and DNA encoding proinsulin. Hum Gene Ther. 2010 Feb;21(2):171-8.

[80] Bot A, Smith D, Bot S, Hughes A, Wolfe T, Wang L, Woods C, von Herrath M. Plasmid vaccination with insulin B chain prevents autoimmune diabetes in nonobese diabetic mice. J Immunol. 2001 Sep 1;167(5):2950-5.

[81] Tisch R, Wang B, Weaver DJ, Liu B, Bui T, Arthos J, Serreze DV.Antigen-specific mediated suppression of beta cell autoimmunity by plasmid DNA vaccination. J Immunol. 2001 Feb 1;166(3):2122-32

[82] Weaver DJ Jr, Liu B, Tisch R. Plasmid DNAs encoding insulin and glutamic acid decarboxylase 65 have distinct effects on the progression of autoimmune diabetes in nonobese diabetic mice. J Immunol. 2001 Jul 1;167(1):586-92.

[83] Jun HS, Chung YH, Han J, Kim A, Yoo SS, Sherwin RS, Yoon JW. Prevention of autoimmune diabetes by immunogene therapy using recombinant vaccinia virus expressing glutamic acid decarboxylase. Diabetologia. 2002 May;45(5):668-76

[84] Rother KI, Spain LM, Wesley RA, Digon BJ 3rd, Baron A, Chen K, Nelson P, Dosch HM, Palmer JP, Brooks-Worrell B, Ring M, Harlan DM. Effects of exenatide alone and in

combination with daclizumab on beta-cell function in long-standing type 1 diabetes. Diabetes Care. 2009 Dec;32(12):2251-7.

[85] Dungan KM, Buse JB, Ratner RE. Effects of therapy in type 1 and type 2 diabetes mellitus with a peptide derived from islet neogenesis associated protein (INGAP). Diabetes Metab Res Rev. 2009 Sep;25(6):558-65.

[86] Hyppönen E, Läärä E, Reunanen A, Järvelin MR, Virtanen SM.: Intake of vitamin D and risk of type 1 diabetes; a birth-cohort study. Lancet 2001; 358: 1500–1503.

[87] Zipitis CS, Akobeng AK.: Vitamin D supplementation in early childhood and risk of type 1 diabetes: a systematic review and meta-analysis. Arch Dis Child 2008; 93: 512–517

[88] Markus Walter, MD,1 Thomas Kaupper, MD,1 Kerstin Adler, PHD,1 Johannes Foersch, 1 Ezio Bonifacio, PHD,2 and Anette-G. Ziegler, No Effect of the 1α,25-Dihydroxyvitamin D3 on β-Cell Residual Function and Insulin Requirement in Adults With New-Onset Type 1 Diabetes. Diabetes Care. 2010 July; 33(7): 1443–1448

[89] .Carla Bizzarri, MD,[1] Dario Pitocco, MD,[2] Nicola Napoli, MD,[3] Enrico Di Stasio, MD,[2] Daria Maggi, MD,[3] Silvia Manfrini, MD,[3] Concetta Suraci, MD,[4] Maria Gisella Cavallo, MD,[5] Marco Cappa, MD,[1] Giovanni Ghirlanda, MD,[2] Paolo Pozzilli, MD,[3] and the IMDIAB Group[*] No Protective Effect of Calcitriol on β-Cell Function in Recent-Onset Type 1 Diabetes.The IMDIAB XIII trial. Diabetes Care. 2010 September; 33(9): 1962–1963

[90] Pickersgill LM, Mandrup-Poulsen TR. The anti-interleukin-1 in type 1 diabetes action trial--background and rationale. Diabetes Metab Res Rev. 2009 May;25(4):321-4. Review

[91] Greenbaum C. Abstract IDS 2012

[92] Mandrup-Poulsen T: Abstract IDS 2012

Chapter 21

Immunotherapies for Type 1 Diabetes

Werner Gurr

Additional information is available at the end of the chapter

http://dx.doi.org/10.5772/54717

1. Introduction

This chapter introduces some of the concepts that underlie the approaches to immunotherapy in type 1 diabetes (T1D) and provides examples of clinical trials that are based on these concepts as well as problems arising in this process.

That immunotherapy is an appropriate approach in T1D is convincingly supported by findings that point to a pathogenesis with close involvement of the immune system. Autoantibodies and T-cells reactive to islet-derived self-antigens in humans and in animal models, HLA alleles that are associated with susceptibility to the disease and partial amelioration after systemic immune suppression all indicate that a therapy for T1D will need to have a component that focuses on the immune system.

The aim of any immunotherapy is to influence or reset pathogenic components or processes in the immune system. Fulfillment of this aim requires targeting of these components and an ideal therapy will minimize the impact on the healthy necessary aspects of the immune system while maximizing the effect on its aberrant aspects. This is a demanding and perhaps not fully achievable goal since we are dealing with a system where intervention directed at any one component will not necessarily remain localized but will have the potential to extend to other components.

Immunological interventions may be divided into two basic groups, namely active and passive. In the latter approach the experimenter or clinician provides the targeting reagents, for example antagonists or monoclonal antibodies binding surface receptors of immune cells. In this case the effects usually last as long as the experimental compound is present to block or dampen the targeted processes. However, there are examples where effects are induced that persist beyond the withdrawal of the targeting compound. In the former approach targeting is achieved by indirect means. Here the experimental compound, for example a potential autoantigen is administered as a vaccine either together with an adjuvant or via a specific 'tolerogenic' route. As a consequence the immune system itself generates the targeting response. In contrast to passive approaches effects induced by vaccination take longer to become manifest and it is possible that they persist far beyond the point of vaccine administration because immunological memory may have been generated.

From the definition and characterization of aberrant immune processes to preclinical studies on new therapeutics, the NOD mouse model and its derivatives remain the most important tool for the development of the basic concepts that underlie the understanding of T1D. That human and mouse T1D must differ in important aspects is obvious simply by comparing the lifespan of a human with that of a mouse as well as the fact that NOD mice are inbred while humans are not. The importance of the NOD mouse model lies in its usefulness to generate the essential conceptual understanding that allows comparison and identification of how the disease process in humans differs from that of the mouse. In this regard the NOD mouse model acts as a reference point and guidepost. Where the aim is to understand the pathogenic process that manifests as T1D, insight into the differences between the disease in the human and in the mouse is itself important scientific knowledge. Furthermore, given the relative ease with which mouse models can be genetically manipulated it is not necessary to proceed from mouse to human. The direction can be reversed by introducing human genetic susceptibility elements into mouse models allowing the investigation of how these elements contribute to T1D.

What are the possible targets for an immune intervention? Systemic immune suppression represents a very broad targeting approach and thus causes the most pronounced 'collateral damage'. Since T1D is survivable without any immunotherapy at all this approach is problematic because of its side effects. Nevertheless studies testing these therapies have been performed. On the next level of specificity therapies exist that do not target the entire immune system but rather its major components. Therapies directed against T- or B-cells have been successfully tested in mouse models and are now in the process of clinical evaluation. Here initial findings indicate that some of these therapies have positive effects without inducing pronounced adverse responses. Increasing specificity further, we reach the area of the so-called antigen specific therapies. Here not all T- or B-cells are targeted but only those that recognize a given islet autoantigen. This is the area where active immunotherapy is applied by vaccinating with an islet autoantigen. It is hoped that exposing the immune system in a 'tolerogenic' way to autoantigens induces effects that suppress or re-regulate T-cells with specificity for the appropriate self-antigen. This approach has had some success in the NOD mouse model, however clinical trials in patients with recent onset of T1D conducted so far have had less promising outcomes. The lack of success may have to do with observations coming from the NOD mouse model where the majority of the tested autoantigens and routes of administration are only clinically effective if the antigen is administered well before T1D has become overt. It appears therefore that this type of intervention should be undertaken preventively to fully exploit its potential. There is a further level of specificity where targeting is directed against T-cell receptors of autoreactive T-cells. In this approach the vaccine antigen is the recombinant receptor of the self-reactive T-cell and the resulting immune response blocks activation of, or possibly eliminates, that T-cell. This approach has not been tested in T1D but has proved to be partially successful in models of other autoimmune diseases. Therapies that apply a different perspective of the immune system include administration of reagents that can block certain cytokine receptors or administration of cytokines presumed to exert dampening effects. Here specificity is defined by the targeted cytokine receptor, which does not need to be restricted to a particular cell type and consequently the question of unwanted side effects becomes relevant. These therapies also represent one approach that allows targeting of the innate component of the immune system, which like the adaptive part plays a role in the pathogenesis of T1D.

These diverse therapeutic approaches demonstrate that it is possible to develop useful means of targeting immune dysfunction in T1D on all levels of specificity. However, it is our view that currently available therapies represent only a small fraction of what is possible because our understanding of the pathogenesis of T1D is still in its infancy, despite the vast increase in knowledge gained over recent decades. The review below focuses on interventions that have been translated -mostly from the NOD mouse model- to humans either at risk of developing T1D or already suffering from the disease. It does not discuss the large number of potential interventions that have shown promise in preclinical studies of T1D performed again mostly in NOD mice.

1.1. The constraints of immunotherapies applied after diagnosis of T1D

It must be kept in mind that pancreatic islets are not simply an aggregation of specialized cells that produce insulin and other endocrine hormones. Rather each islet represents a micro organ with well-developed anatomical structure, innervation and, as an endocrine gland, a sophisticated blood supply. As with any other organ in the body there is a large margin of safety allowing for considerable functional impairment and damage to occur before the onset of overt clinical signs of organ failure. This margin of safety is of course a great benefit for the individual. However, in terms of immune therapeutic intervention this also means that once organ failure has become overt (i.e when diabetes is diagnosed clinically) a large proportion of the organ has been destroyed and the residual mass can restore euglycemia only under ideal conditions - that is the restoration of complete and lasting immune tolerance to islets. In other words an immune therapy that begins after the diagnosis of T1D is unlikely to be sufficient on its own to restore euglycemia. If permanent restoration of euglycemia is the aim then therapies that are initiated after diagnosis of T1D will need to contain a component that addresses regeneration/re-growth of pancreatic islets. If the view of pancreatic islets as (micro) organs is adopted then the chances of successful re-growth of human islets may be limited. This also means that for immune therapies that are initiated after diagnosis of T1D the aims need to be set lower than full restoration of euglycemia and permanent insulin independence. These therapies therefore aim at maintaining residual islet mass that still exists after diagnosis of T1D and that can persist for years or even decades after disease onset. Parameters such as improved glycemic control, a decrease in the dose of exogenous insulin needed and maintenance or slower decrease of C-peptide levels measure success of these therapies. Although these aims are less glorious than independence from exogenous insulin they are nevertheless worthy of pursuit and can mean significant improvement in the quality of life of the treated patients.

2. T or B-cell targeting

2.1. Therapy with anti-CD3 antibodies

That treatment with antibodies directed against CD3, a component of T-cell receptor complex, might have potential in the treatment of autoimmune disease was evident since the discovery *in vitro* that immobilized anti CD3 antibody could render T-cells non-responsive or anergic to subsequent stimulation by antigen [1]. Studies in NOD mice revealed that treatment with a hamster antibody against CD3 could reverse diabetes even when it was given at a stage when the mice were already hyperglycemic. This was an important feature in light of the constraints of immunotherapy applied in human patients as outlined above. It was also in contrast to many other promising therapy approaches tested in the NOD mouse that needed to be administered preventively before the onset of overt clinical signs of T1D in order to be effective. Adding to the attractiveness of this approach was the observation that a single course of treatment lasting for 5 days was sufficient to reverse hyperglycemia for several months and that treated NOD mice were resistant to the induction of disease by spleen cells from diabetic donors [2; 3]. This indicated that rather than a passive mechanism such as a blockade of the CD3 receptor some kind of active mechanism of regulation must have been involved in the generation of the clinical effect. Over the years this mechanism has been studied in great detail in mouse models and it has become clear that rather than induction of non-responsiveness in the T-cells a complex cascade of effector mechanisms is initiated by the anti CD3 treatment. It was discovered that binding of the antibody to the CD3 receptor transmits a strong activation signal to the T-cell, which triggers a 'cytokine storm' and then death of T-cells. The ensuing cellular debris is 'cleaned up' by macrophages, which release IL-6. The increased levels of IL-6 together with TGFβ create an environment that favors the development of a subset of T-cells characterized by the secretion of the cytokine IL-17. As these T-cells circulate through the body they pass the small intestine. Epithelial cells at this site respond to the presence of IL-17 with the increased expression of the chemokine CCL20. Since the IL-17 releasing T-cells have a receptor for this chemokine they accumulate in the small intestine. It appears that once these IL-17 releasing T-cells have reached the small intestine they assume a phenotype that allows them to suppress the proliferation of other T-cells and consequently to also attenuate self-reactive T-cells [4]. Thus the impact of a short treatment with anti CD3 antibodies can induce immune suppression that lasts much longer than the presence of the antibody in the system.

Among immune therapies with broader specificity applied to patients with T1D the treatment with anti CD3 antibodies has been tested most extensively despite side effects such as 'cytokine storm' and a selection of recently evaluated trials is summarized below.

All anti CD3 treatments have been given to patients with recent onset of T1D and in accordance with the constraints outlined above, statistically significant increases in the reversal of disease i.e. full independence from exogenous insulin within the study time frame are not observed. However, differences between treatment and placebo groups have been observed and most prominently where results of patient subpopulations are analyzed. This was shown in a trial that observed treated patients and the placebo group for up to four years after treatment with a humanized anti CD3 antibody which was given over a period of six consecutive days.

Statistically significant reduction in daily insulin needs vs. the corresponding placebo group were reported for patients whose residual beta cell function at baseline was above the median of all patients as well as for patients whose age was below the median age. These patients also had a slower decrease in C-peptide levels than the placebo group i.e. their residual beta cell function was maintained for longer than that of the placebo group. Levels of HbA_{1c} (glycated hemoglobin) were also positively affected by the treatment but this occurred again only in younger patients [5; 6]. The dependency of treatment efficacy on age and on the residual beta cell mass (correlated to the time interval between diagnosis of T1D and treatment start) was also observed in a recent published study that compared different dose regimens of an anti CD3 antibody [7]. The fact that anti CD3 treatment was more effective in younger patients was explained by the age-dependency of the insulitis process. Islet inflammation was detected in children but rarely in adolescents and adults. Furthermore, late onset T1D patients are presumed to suffer from a less severe form of the disease. Therefore a more pronounced loss of residual beta cell function was observed in the younger placebo subgroup compared to the older placebo subgroup and the effect of the anti CD3 treatment consequently became more clearly visible in younger patients[6].

Side effects induced by the treatment with anti CD3 antibody occurring in most patients are transient and are in accordance with the mechanism of action of this approach. Fever, which might be explained by the 'cytokine storm' triggered by the antibody treatment, a syndrome similar to acute mononucleosis correlating with an increase in EBV copies which may be a result of the activation-induced T-cell death upon anti CD3 administration are some of the adverse events reported for this treatment. Lymphomas as consequence of the anti CD3 treatment have not been observed.

2.2. B-lymphocyte depletion in patients with recent onset of T1D

While it has been established in the mouse that T-cells are necessary and sufficient to cause the disease the role of B-cells in the pathogenesis of T1D is more indirect. Islet antigen self-reactive T-cells both of the helper and cytotoxic type from diabetic NOD mice can transfer the disease to NOD-SCID recipients whereas B-cells are unable to do so. The contribution of B-cells to the pathogenesis of human T1D is likely also to be more indirect. This is suggested by a report of a child with X-linked agammaglobulinemia who developed T1D [8]. Nevertheless, B-cells must participate in the pathogenesis of T1D because it is possible to prevent the disease by B-cell depletion and it has been shown that B-ells are necessary for the initiation of insulitis in the NOD mouse [9; 10]. B-cells are very efficient antigen presenting cells particularly after they have been activated, which could occur in the accumulation of inflammatory cells in the islets during the pathogenesis of T1D. The rationale for the use of B-ell depletion in humans would therefore be a reduction of antigen presentation, which would result in less T-cell activation and an attenuated inflammatory process. It could also include the elimination of cytokines produced by B-cells that might be damaging to the islets and reduce further recruitment of immune cells to the islets. It is also possible that depletion of B-cells with an antibody initiates complex mechanisms similar to those thought to underlie the effects of treatment with anti CD3 antibody.

Targeting of B-cells is achieved by an antibody against the CD20 molecule, a cell surface phosphoprotein that is expressed during the mid-stages of B-cell development but which does not occur on hematopoietic stem cells or normal plasma cells [11]. Anti CD20 antibody is approved for the treatment of B-cell lymphomas and was used in a study of patients with recent onset of T1D (median time interval between diagnosis of T1D and first infusion 81 days). Four consecutive infusions were given over an interval of 22 days. The results of this trial assessed 12 month after study begin resemble those obtained by anti CD3 treatment- slower decrease of C-peptide levels, lower levels of glycated hemoglobin and lower requirement for exogenous insulin in the treated vs. the placebo group. Although not statistically significant, subgroup analysis again tended to suggest a better response in children and adolescents. Side effects included fever, rash and pruritus as consequence of the 'cytokine storm' (or cytokine release syndrome) triggered by the first injection of the antibody. Again these effects were transient and did not reappear when subsequent doses of the anti CD20 antibody were administered [12].

It is not known whether the effects of T- or B-cell targeting with antibodies can be prolonged or increased if the treatment is given repeatedly or if T-and B-cell targeting are combined. The guess here is that an increased risk of adverse side effects might counterbalance positive effects gained by repeated or combined administration of T or B-cell depleting antibodies and/or that repeated administration become less efficient because the immune system activates counter-acting mechanisms.

3. General immunosuppression

3.1. Autologous nonmyeloablative stem cell transplantation and treatment with cyclosporin

Before reviewing antigen specific immunotherapies two studies with very broad targeting of the immune system shall be mentioned. In one study peripheral hematopoietic stem cells of patients with recent onset of T1D were mobilized, harvested and frozen before immune ablation was achieved by administration of high dose cyclophosphamide and anti thymocyte globulin. The previously harvested hematopoietic stem cells were then infused. During the time needed for the immune system to regenerate extensive supportive care including antibacterial, antiviral and antifungal prophylaxis as well as patient isolation in rooms equipped with air filters was required. This approach resulted in reversal of T1D in the majority of the patients. 12 of the 23 patients participating in this trial became independent from exogenous insulin and this state lasted for 14 to 53 months while 8 patients relapsed and resumed insulin use at low doses [13]. In the insulin-independent group C-peptide levels at 24 and 36 months post transplantation of stem cells had increased while values of glycated hemoglobin had decreased significantly compared to pre transplantation values. The rationale for this study was the possible reconstitution of immune tolerance after an 'immunologic reset' by high dose immunosuppression followed by autologous hematopoietic stem cell transplantation [14]. However, it is known from the NOD mouse that the self-reactive tendency of the immune system cannot be eliminated permanently by this approach. Once the immune system has regenerated autoimmune responses are eventually re-established and islet destruction resumes. This process is reflected by the prolonged but not permanent state of independence from exogenous insulin experienced by the majority of the treated patients in this trial. The results of this study raise the questions whether the increase in C-peptide levels and independence from exogenous insulin was due to a process of regeneration of islets or due to an attenuation of the inflammatory environment the islets were exposed to. Since the majority of the insulin-free patients discontinued insulin use between 3 days before stem cell transplantation (i.e. during the process of immune ablation) and 34 days after transplantation of stem cells it is reasonable to assume that the latter mechanism was dominant at least initially because this time span would appear to be too short to allow extensive regeneration of islets. There was however one patient who achieved insulin independence 610 days after stem cell transplantation and in this case regeneration of islets may have played a role and it is possible that this process also contributed during later stages to the increased C-peptide levels observed in the patients with long term independence from exogenous insulin. If attenuation of the inflammatory environment that islets are exposed to is an important early effector mechanism and if insulitis in humans is predominantly found in children but seldom in adolescents and adults then this approach would be expected to work best in children with recent onset of T1D. However none of the patients in this study was younger than 14 years and therefore the best possible effect might not have been achieved.

The above-mentioned trial could not have been designed as a controlled and blinded study and it is possible that that some of the remissions observed were not related to the treatment but represent spontaneous remissions. However, the close correlation of the observed remissions with the immune ablative treatment and their duration argued for a genuine effect of the treatment. There are results from a double blind and placebo- controlled study applying broad targeting of the immune system with cyclosporine. They show a statistically significant increase in complete as well as complete and partial remissions at the 9th month in the treated vs. placebo group with the effects being more pronounced in the subgroup with whole blood cyclosporine levels of ≥300ng/ml [15].

Certainly immune ablation followed by autologous stem cell transplantation even if it has to be performed only every 3-4 years is not something that could be considered suitable for repeat administration. This also holds in regards to the continued administration of cyclosporine to patients with T1D especially since even a short lasting course of the drug (12.5 +/- 4 months) accelerated the rate of progression of the urinary albumin excretion rate and tended to induce a loss in kidney function [16].

4. Antigen specific therapies

4.1. Insulin

Although it appears from the approaches presented above that the more severe the therapeutic intervention the better its success antigen specific therapies remain attractive conceptually because they allow for an intervention that is more precisely targeted. Rather than targeting all T-cells (or the immune system in its entirety) the idea is to apply an approach that controls only those T-cells that are self-reactive. Here an important question concerns the specificity of the self-reactive T-cells that 'merit' control. It is obvious that insulin is considered a major self-antigen as it is the defining protein of the beta cells that are impaired and destroyed during the pathogenesis of T1D. There are many experimental findings that confirm this view such as the presence of anti-insulin autoantibodies as a proven prediction tool for the assessment of diabetes risk in the pre-clinical state. Furthermore, among the group of beta cell proteins that have been studied to date as potential self-antigens insulin is one of the few that fulfills a formal requirement for a beta cell protein to be considered a self antigen: insulin specific T-cell clones and lines derived from NOD mice can reliably transfer diabetes to NOD-SCID recipients. Another question concerns how these self-reactive T-cells can be targeted and here the mechanisms that mediate oral or nasal tolerance offer a possible approach. Oral or nasal tolerance is defined as the specific suppression of cellular and/or humoral immune responses to an antigen by prior administration of the antigen via the oral or nasal route. The mechanisms of oral tolerance are thought to have evolved in order to generate peripheral tolerance to external agents that gain access to the body via a natural route (the digestive or respiratory tract). As consequence these external agents are 'seen' by the immune system as internal components that become part of self. Two different but not mutually exclusive mechanisms have been defined that can mediate oral tolerance, depending on the amount of antigen administered orally: Induction/activation of regulatory T-cells has been reported to occur when low doses are given whereas induction of anergy or deletion of T-cells appears to be the main mechanism involved when higher doses are administered [17]. According to this schematic, if insulin specific self-reactive or autoaggressive T-cells were to be targeted, feeding of insulin would result - upon presentation of insulin by specialized gut-associated antigen presenting cells - in the activation of insulin-specific regulatory T-cells in the gut. These T-cells then migrate to the pancreatic lymph nodes where they encounter epitopes derived from endogenous insulin and become reactivated. This leads to the secretion of IL-10 and TGFβ-cytokines, which can attenuate the ongoing inflammatory process. Because it is mediated by cytokines this mechanism would not only target insulin reactive T-cells but would suppress T-cells with other specificities as well. A degree of specificity would be generated because both types of T-cells -autoagggressive and regulatory- would become activated in the same location (pancreatic lymph nodes or islet infiltrates) but not in other sites. This is one reason why antigen specific therapies thought to rely on T-regulatory cells might be better applied before the onset of T1D. Once islets have been destroyed the pancreatic lymph nodes can no longer activate T regulatory cells because beta cell antigens are no longer presented.

Anergy or deletion of insulin reactive T-cells might also be achieved by oral administration of insulin with the latter mechanism potentially leading - through the presence of debris from apoptotic insulin specific T-cells - to the generation of T regulatory cells according to the process discovered to be activated by i.v. administration of anti CD3 antibodies. It should be mentioned in advance, that in the studies administering oral or nasal insulin presented below, parameters that would indicate which, if any, of the proposed mechanism (tolerance/anergy/activation of T-regulatory cells) had been triggered were not acquired.

Oral administration of insulin has been tested as intervention in patients with recent onset of T1D [18] and oral as well as nasal insulin have been given to persons at risk of developing T1D in order to assess the potential of this approach to prevent or delay the onset of the disease. The 'Diabetes Prevention Trial-Type 1' (DPT1) screened first and second-degree relatives of patients with T1D for the presence of islet cell antibodies. Relatives who had anti islet cell and anti insulin antibodies but a normal glucose tolerance and first phase response to intravenous insulin were projected to have a 5-year risk of 26-50%. 372 of these individuals were randomized in the oral insulin study. (DPT1 also included a group of individuals classified as having a risk of greater than 50% who received intravenous instead of oral insulin [19]). The follow-up in the oral insulin study was 4.3 years. During this time there appeared no differences between placebo and control groups. The average proportion of subjects who progressed to diabetes was 6.4% per year in the oral insulin group and 8.2% per year in the placebo group. However, upon subgroup analysis there appeared to be a beneficial effect in those individuals who had a higher anti insulin autoantibody titer (≥80nU/ml, n=263). In this group the proportion who developed diabetes was 6.2% per year in the oral insulin group and 10.4% in the placebo group [20]. This effect became even more pronounced if analysis was confined to those with an anti insulin autoantibody titer of >300nU/ml (n=132] with a projected delay of the disease of almost 10 years [21]. These findings were encouraging but since the subgroup analyses had not been prespecified they could not be considered a positive outcome. Another important result this trial yielded was the confirmation that the parameters used to predict development of T1D in relatives of individuals with the disease were sufficient and accurate. Risk was projected to be 26-50% whereas the actual observed value was 35% over 5 years. Accurate risk prediction is essential for the design of further prevention trials, one of which is currently ongoing and builds on the hypotheses generated by the evaluation of the oral insulin DPT1 trial (better efficiency of the treatment in individuals with higher anti insulin autoantibody titers).

A second prevention trial used nasal instead of oral insulin and a screening and staging approach different from the DPT1. In this case cord blood samples of infants were tissue typed for the presence of the T1D susceptibility allele HLA-DQB1. Carriers of this allele and an additional cohort consisting of their siblings were repeatedly tested for the presence of T1D-associated autoantibodies. Individuals of the two cohorts who were positive for two or more autoantibodies but free of clinical diabetes were invited to participate in the prevention trial. Individuals enrolled in this trial were younger than those in the DPT1 (1.6-5.2 years vs. 7-14 years in the DPT1). 224 individuals of the HLA-DQB1$^+$ cohort and 40 individuals of the sibling cohort were randomized to receive intranasal insulin or placebo with a median duration of the intervention of 1.8 years. This trial failed to demonstrate a positive effect of intranasal insulin in all analyzed groups. The annual rate of progression to diabetes in the HLA-DQB1$^+$ cohort was 16.8% for the group receiving intranasal insulin vs. 15.3% for the placebo group. In the sibling cohort these values were 10.8% vs. 6.0% respectively. In contrast to DPT1 a subgroup analysis of individuals with high anti insulin autoantibody titers did not show any benefit of intranasal administration of insulin. Although this trial failed to demonstrate positive effects of intranasal insulin it showed that by screening for HLA risk alleles a cohort with a disease risk similar to that of first-degree relatives could be identified from the general population [22].

Thus even if these two trials largely failed in their primary aim they nevertheless clearly demonstrated the ability to accurately predict disease risk, which is essential to optimize the timing of preventative therapies.

4.2. Glutamic acid decarboxylase

Besides oral or nasal administration of an autoantigen there is in T1D models another approach to induce tolerance. In this case a candidate autoantigen is injected subcutaneously together with the adjuvant alum. Although using an islet autoantigen as a vaccine to prevent or ameliorate disease might appear strange it has nevertheless been shown in the mouse model of T1D that this approach can be effective. The idea is that such a vaccination either activates regulatory T-cells or that it converts autoaggressive T-cells to a non-destructive phenotype. This approach has been tested in humans with GAD65, which is the 65 kd isoform of the autoantigen glutamic acid decarboxylase. In contrast to the prevention studies with oral and nasal insulin the trials with GAD65 have been conducted in individuals with recent onset of T1D. A phase II trial tested the safety and efficacy of vaccination with human GAD65 in alum (two subcutaneous vaccinations with 20μg GAD one month apart) in patients with recent onset of T1D (n=70). Results of this study were reported 30 months and again 4 years after treatment. Of the subgroups prespecified in the protocol (HLA classification, age, sex, baseline GAD autoantibody levels) only duration of T1D had a significant influence on the efficacy of the vaccination. In the patients vaccinated less than 6 month after diagnosis of T1D both fasting and stimulated C-peptide secretion decreased significantly less in the GAD-alum group than in the placebo group by month 30 and this positive effect was retained at 4 years after treatment. There was no significant difference between the GAD-alum and the placebo group for patients treated 6 month or more after diagnosis. As expected, vaccination with GAD-alum lead to strong increase of the GAD autoantibody titers, which was sustained to month 30 and a neurological assessment was performed because of concerns that this might lead to stiff-man syndrome. However, there were no notable neurological differences between treatment and placebo group. In accordance with the B-cell responses anti GAD cytokine responses assessed in PBMCs of treatment and control groups at 15 months showed a significantly increased release of most of the tested cytokines (IL-5, 10, 13, 17, IFN-γ and TNFα) in the GAD-alum group. Furthermore increased GAD-induced levels of FOXP3, a transcription factor associated with T regulatory cells, was found in the GAD-alum group [23] [24]. Given the findings of this trial a second study (phase III) was conducted, which enrolled patients within 3 month of the diagnosis of T1D. Patients were randomly assigned to receive one of three study treatments: either two (n=108) or four vaccinations with GAD-alum (n=111) or a vaccination with the adjuvant alum alone (placebo group, n=115). This trial with a follow up time of 15 months failed to show improvements in stimulated C-peptide levels after either the two or the four-dose vaccination when compared to the placebo group. Pooling of data from both groups with GAD vaccinations failed to show a significant effect on stimulated C-peptide levels compared to the control group [25].

4.3. 60kDa heat shock protein (DiaPep277)

A third antigen tested for its therapeutic value in human T1D, is the 60kDa heat shock protein (hsp60). While GAD and especially insulin are specifically expressed in pancreatic islets this is not the case for hsp60, which is expressed throughout the body. Although anti hsp60 autoantibodies can be detected in patients at the onset of T1D they are not useful as predictive markers for disease beyond what can be achieved by measuring anti insulin or anti GAD titers. If hsp60 is an autoantigen in T1D and is widely expressed throughout the body one would expect to find inflammation driven by hsp60-reactive T-cells in other organs as well. However this is not the case and raises the question as to whether there are beta cell/islet intrinsic factors that set this site apart immunologically from other parts of the body.

In therapeutic applications hsp60 is not given as a whole protein but as a peptide derived from the native sequence of human heat shock protein 60. The sequence of this peptide was first identified in the NOD mouse with the help of diabetogenic T-cell clones responding to the *M. tuberculosis* hsp60. Heat shock proteins are highly conserved proteins and it was discovered that these T- cell clones cross-reacted with the human - and presumably with the mouse form - of hsp60 and specifically recognized an epitope in the C-terminal part of hsp60, which was termed peptide277. Vaccination of NOD mice with peptide277 in mineral oil delayed T1D [26]. Since the sequence of this peptide contained two cysteine residues a more stable form was subsequently generated in which the cysteine residues were replaced by valine. The more stable form of peptide277 was also effective in delaying T1D in NOD mice and was termed DiaPep277 [27]. These studies suggested that the mechanisms mediating the effects of vaccination with DiaPep277 might be similar to the ones proposed for vaccination with GAD (e.g. induction of T regulatory cells). It has become evident however that DiaPep277 (and hsp60) can also exert direct effects on the immune system. Hsp60 can activate B-cells via the Toll like receptor 4 (TLR4), which respond by producing IL-10 [28]. Furthermore, TLR4 activation by hsp60 also occurs in macrophages and dendritic cells promoting pro-inflammatory effectors. At the same time hsp60 can also induce anti-inflammatory effects promoted through TLR2. It is reported DiaPep277 does not engage TLR 4 but only TLR2, which leads to the generation of a T-cell mediated anti-inflammatory environment [29].

Several phase II trials have been conducted with DiaPep277 in patients with T1D. In one of these trials that focused on the changes in immunological parameters after treatment, Dia-Pep277 was administered subcutaneously in a 10% lipid preparation with the placebo group receiving mannitol in 10% lipid preparation. Three different doses of DiaPep277 were tested (0.2mg, 1mg and 2.5mg). Four injections of the drug or the placebo were given over a timeframe of 12 months and a total of 48 patients were enrolled with onset of T1D between 200 and 800 days before start of treatment. Glucagon-stimulated C-peptide production significantly decreased over 12 months in all groups except the group receiving Diapep277 at 2.5mg. The decrease in C-peptide production over 12 months was significantly less in the 2.5mg than in the placebo group. Absolute daily insulin dosage did not decrease over time in any of the groups [30]. These results are in accordance with an earlier trial that found a significantly higher stimulated C-peptide concentration in the treatment vs. placebo group at 6 and 10 months after start of treatment. This earlier trial also found a significantly reduced insulin requirement at 10 months and observed that individuals with higher C-peptide concentration at the time of initiation of treatment showed better preservation of C-peptide concentrations 10 months later [31]. Therefore the rule that the earlier treatment is started the more efficient it tends to be also applies to this approach. The former study was accompanied by an extensive evaluation of immunological parameters before, during and after treatment. As expected, it was observed that immunological responses were quantitatively and qualitatively highly diverse among the subjects. Nevertheless, after development of new methods to evaluate the results obtained from proliferation and cytokine release experiments, some interesting information could be derived. An IL-10 response but not a proliferative response to DiaPep277 before initiation of treatment, and a decrease or loss of proliferative response subsequent to treatment, appeared to provide a correlate for clinical efficiency. These biomarkers might reflect some kind of tolerance to DiaPep277 (hsp60) and appear to be associated with improved clinical outcome. These findings imply that the status of the immune response prior to therapy may be predictive for treatment outcome. Proliferative responses after treatment with DiaPep277 were frequently specific for hsp60 in that responses to GAD or tetanus toxoid were not or only weakly altered [32]. Treatment with DiaPep277 therefore appeared immunologically effective and specific. One phase III trial with DiaPep277 was recently concluded and awaits publication of the results and another phase III trial is currently underway.

What could be reasons for the limited success of the antigen specific therapies presented above? From a conceptual point of view there is a concern that in these therapies there is always a risk that administration of the candidate autoantigen does not lead to attenuation of the autoimmune reaction but rather leads to its exacerbation. This is especially the case when autoantigens are administered with an adjuvant such as was done in the GAD-alum trials. We have observed while studying the Reg proteins as potential autoantigens in T1D that vaccination of NOD mice with an N-terminal fragment of RegII in alum leads to acceleration of T1D instead of prevention [33]. A similar observation was made in BB rats, which like the NOD mice spontaneously develop T1D. Here insulin given orally with an *E.coli*-derived endotoxin-free bacterial adjuvant containing acidic glycolipoproteins lead to an acceleration of the disease compared to the group receiving oral insulin alone [34]. Although the GAD-alum studies did not show any acceleration of T1D in the treated groups, it is noteworthy that in the T1D prevention trial with nasal insulin the subgroup of children who presented with three or four types of autoantibodies before the start of the treatment had an unadjusted hazard ratio of insulin vs. placebo of 1.50. This hazard ratio implied a possible risk of an accelerated effect on the onset of T1D in this cohort. It should also be noted that mechanisms involving the activation of regulatory T-cells such as suggested by the findings of the GAD-alum study and considered to be an important factor in oral tolerance generation may not necessarily have only beneficial effects on T1D. Regulatory T-cells are thought to exert their effects via cytokines (e.g. IL-10 or TGF-β), which might on the one hand attenuate self-reactive effector T-cells. But on the other hand these cytokines might also negatively impact beta cell biology and accelerate beta cell destruction by enhancing insulitis through modulation of the release of other cytokines and the islet microvasculature [35]. Cytokines are molecules with a broad range of effects that may differ depending on the target cells. Therefore a therapy that relies on the alteration of cytokine profiles as important effector mechanism carries the risk that these alterations although beneficial to some systems (e.g. T-cells) might be detrimental to other affected cells (e.g. beta cells, endothelia). The clinical outcome might thus depend on the sum of all these effects and might not be predictable.

5. Conclusion

The analysis of the trials presented here suggests that treatment efficacy can differ from subgroup to subgroup. This indicates that there might not be a single therapeutic approach that fits all. Rather the observations suggest that it may be necessary to establish an individual profile that goes beyond the standard parameters such as sex, age, family history, time of diagnosis of T1D, HLA type, and autoantibody profile for each person intending to undergo an immune therapeutic intervention. These parameters might include the spectrum of T-cell responses to beta cell autoantigens (in terms of proliferation as well as of cytokine release), characterization of the gut flora [36; 37], imaging of islet inflammation [38] type and time of prior vaccinations and infections, season [25], and might even include psychological parameters such as familial stress levels [39]. As new approaches are translated from the pre clinical stage to individuals at risk of developing T1D or to patients already suffering from the disease the palette of possible interventions will grow more diverse. Obtaining highly differentiated profiles may refine the process of matching the time point and the type of immune intervention to an individual and thus optimize outcome.

Author details

Werner Gurr*

Address all correspondence to: Werner.gurr@yale.edu

Yale University, Dept. of Internal Medicine/Endocrinology, New Haven, USA

References

[1] Jenkins MK, Chen CA, Jung G, Mueller DL, Schwartz RH: Inhibition of antigen-specific proliferation of type 1 murine T cell clones after stimulation with immobilized anti-CD3 monoclonal antibody. *J Immunol* 144:16-22, 1990

[2] Chatenoud L, Thervet E, Primo J, Bach JF: Anti-CD3 antibody induces long-term remission of overt autoimmunity in nonobese diabetic mice. *Proc Natl Acad Sci U S A* 91:123-127, 1994

[3] Chatenoud L, Primo J, Bach JF: CD3 antibody-induced dominant self tolerance in overtly diabetic NOD mice. *J Immunol* 158:2947-2954, 1997

[4] Esplugues E, Huber S, Gagliani N, Hauser AE, Town T, Wan YY, O'Connor W, Jr., Rongvaux A, Van Rooijen N, Haberman AM, Iwakura Y, Kuchroo VK, Kolls JK, Bluestone JA, Herold KC, Flavell RA: Control of TH17 cells occurs in the small intestine. *Nature* 475:514-518, 2011

[5] Keymeulen B, Vandemeulebroucke E, Ziegler AG, Mathieu C, Kaufman L, Hale G, Gorus F, Goldman M, Walter M, Candon S, Schandene L, Crenier L, De Block C, Seigneurin JM, De Pauw P, Pierard D, Weets I, Rebello P, Bird P, Berrie E, Frewin M, Waldmann H, Bach JF, Pipeleers D, Chatenoud L: Insulin needs after CD3-antibody therapy in new-onset type 1 diabetes. *N Engl J Med* 352:2598-2608, 2005

[6] Keymeulen B, Walter M, Mathieu C, Kaufman L, Gorus F, Hilbrands R, Vandemeulebroucke E, Van de Velde U, Crenier L, De Block C, Candon S, Waldmann H, Ziegler AG, Chatenoud L, Pipeleers D: Four-year metabolic outcome of a randomised controlled CD3-antibody trial in recent-onset type 1 diabetic patients depends on their age and baseline residual beta cell mass. *Diabetologia* 53:614-623, 2010

[7] Sherry N, Hagopian W, Ludvigsson J, Jain SM, Wahlen J, Ferry RJ, Jr., Bode B, Aronoff S, Holland C, Carlin D, King KL, Wilder RL, Pillemer S, Bonvini E, Johnson S, Stein KE, Koenig S, Herold KC, Daifotis AG: Teplizumab for treatment of type 1 diabetes (Protege study): 1-year results from a randomised, placebo-controlled trial. *Lancet* 378:487-497, 2011

[8] Martin S, Wolf-Eichbaum D, Duinkerken G, Scherbaum WA, Kolb H, Noordzij JG, Roep BO: Development of type 1 diabetes despite severe hereditary B-lymphocyte deficiency. *N Engl J Med* 345:1036-1040, 2001

[9] Noorchashm H, Lieu YK, Noorchashm N, Rostami SY, Greeley SA, Schlachterman A, Song HK, Noto LE, Jevnikar AM, Barker CF, Naji A: I-Ag7-mediated antigen presentation by B lymphocytes is critical in overcoming a checkpoint in T cell tolerance to islet beta cells of nonobese diabetic mice. *J Immunol* 163:743-750, 1999

[10] Noorchashm H, Noorchashm N, Kern J, Rostami SY, Barker CF, Naji A: B-cells are required for the initiation of insulitis and sialitis in nonobese diabetic mice. *Diabetes* 46:941-946, 1997

[11] Pescovitz MD: Rituximab, an anti-cd20 monoclonal antibody: history and mechanism of action. *Am J Transplant* 6:859-866, 2006

[12] Pescovitz MD, Greenbaum CJ, Krause-Steinrauf H, Becker DJ, Gitelman SE, Goland R, Gottlieb PA, Marks JB, McGee PF, Moran AM, Raskin P, Rodriguez H, Schatz DA, Wherrett D, Wilson DM, Lachin JM, Skyler JS: Rituximab, B-lymphocyte depletion, and preservation of beta-cell function. *N Engl J Med* 361:2143-2152, 2009

[13] Couri CE, Oliveira MC, Stracieri AB, Moraes DA, Pieroni F, Barros GM, Madeira MI, Malmegrim KC, Foss-Freitas MC, Simoes BP, Martinez EZ, Foss MC, Burt RK, Voltarelli JC: C-peptide levels and insulin independence following autologous nonmyeloablative hematopoietic stem cell transplantation in newly diagnosed type 1 diabetes mellitus. *JAMA* 301:1573-1579, 2009

[14] Voltarelli JC, Couri CE, Stracieri AB, Oliveira MC, Moraes DA, Pieroni F, Coutinho M, Malmegrim KC, Foss-Freitas MC, Simoes BP, Foss MC, Squiers E, Burt RK: Autologous nonmyeloablative hematopoietic stem cell transplantation in newly diagnosed type 1 diabetes mellitus. *JAMA* 297:1568-1576, 2007

[15] Feutren G, Papoz L, Assan R, Vialettes B, Karsenty G, Vexiau P, Du Rostu H, Rodier M, Sirmai J, Lallemand A, et al.: Cyclosporin increases the rate and length of remissions in insulin-dependent diabetes of recent onset. Results of a multicentre double-blind trial. *Lancet* 2:119-124, 1986

[16] Parving HH, Tarnow L, Nielsen FS, Rossing P, Mandrup-Poulsen T, Osterby R, Nerup J: Cyclosporine nephrotoxicity in type 1 diabetic patients. A 7-year follow-up study. *Diabetes Care* 22:478-483, 1999

[17] Weiner HL, da Cunha AP, Quintana F, Wu H: Oral tolerance. *Immunol Rev* 241:241-259, 2011

[18] Pozzilli P, Pitocco D, Visalli N, Cavallo MG, Buzzetti R, Crino A, Spera S, Suraci C, Multari G, Cervoni M, Manca Bitti ML, Matteoli MC, Marietti G, Ferrazzoli F, Cassone Faldetta MR, Giordano C, Sbriglia M, Sarugeri E, Ghirlanda G: No effect of oral insulin on residual beta-cell function in recent-onset type I diabetes (the IMDIAB VII). IMDIAB Group. *Diabetologia* 43:1000-1004, 2000

[19] Effects of insulin in relatives of patients with type 1 diabetes mellitus. *N Engl J Med* 346:1685-1691, 2002

[20] Skyler JS, Krischer JP, Wolfsdorf J, Cowie C, Palmer JP, Greenbaum C, Cuthbertson D, Rafkin-Mervis LE, Chase HP, Leschek E: Effects of oral insulin in relatives of patients with type 1 diabetes: The Diabetes Prevention Trial--Type 1. *Diabetes Care* 28:1068-1076, 2005

[21] Skyler JS: Update on worldwide efforts to prevent type 1 diabetes. *Ann N Y Acad Sci* 1150:190-196, 2008

[22] Nanto-Salonen K, Kupila A, Simell S, Siljander H, Salonsaari T, Hekkala A, Korhonen S, Erkkola R, Sipila JI, Haavisto L, Siltala M, Tuominen J, Hakalax J, Hyoty H, Ilonen J, Veijola R, Simell T, Knip M, Simell O: Nasal insulin to prevent type 1 diabetes in children with HLA genotypes and autoantibodies conferring increased risk of disease: a double-blind, randomised controlled trial. *Lancet* 372:1746-1755, 2008

[23] Ludvigsson J, Faresjo M, Hjorth M, Axelsson S, Cheramy M, Pihl M, Vaarala O, Forsander G, Ivarsson S, Johansson C, Lindh A, Nilsson NO, Aman J, Ortqvist E, Zerhouni P, Casas R: GAD treatment and insulin secretion in recent-onset type 1 diabetes. *N Engl J Med* 359:1909-1920, 2008

[24] Ludvigsson J, Hjorth M, Cheramy M, Axelsson S, Pihl M, Forsander G, Nilsson NO, Samuelsson BO, Wood T, Aman J, Ortqvist E, Casas R: Extended evaluation of the safety and efficacy of GAD treatment of children and adolescents with recent-onset type 1 diabetes: a randomised controlled trial. *Diabetologia* 54:634-640, 2011

[25] Ludvigsson J, Krisky D, Casas R, Battelino T, Castano L, Greening J, Kordonouri O, Otonkoski T, Pozzilli P, Robert JJ, Veeze HJ, Palmer J: GAD65 antigen therapy in recently diagnosed type 1 diabetes mellitus. *N Engl J Med* 366:433-442, 2012

[26] Elias D, Reshef T, Birk OS, van der Zee R, Walker MD, Cohen IR: Vaccination against autoimmune mouse diabetes with a T-cell epitope of the human 65-kDa heat shock protein. *Proc Natl Acad Sci U S A* 88:3088-3091, 1991

[27] Elias D, Cohen IR: Peptide therapy for diabetes in NOD mice. *Lancet* 343:704-706, 1994

[28] Tuccinardi D, Fioriti E, Manfrini S, D'Amico E, Pozzilli P: DiaPep277 peptide therapy in the context of other immune intervention trials in type 1 diabetes. *Expert Opin Biol Ther* 11:1233-1240, 2011

[29] Zanin-Zhorov A, Cahalon L, Tal G, Margalit R, Lider O, Cohen IR: Heat shock protein 60 enhances CD4+ CD25+ regulatory T cell function via innate TLR2 signaling. *J Clin Invest* 116:2022-2032, 2006

[30] Huurman VA, Decochez K, Mathieu C, Cohen IR, Roep BO: Therapy with the hsp60 peptide DiaPep277 in C-peptide positive type 1 diabetes patients. *Diabetes Metab Res Rev* 23:269-275, 2007

[31] Raz I, Elias D, Avron A, Tamir M, Metzger M, Cohen IR: Beta-cell function in new-onset type 1 diabetes and immunomodulation with a heat-shock protein peptide (DiaPep277]: a randomised, double-blind, phase II trial. *Lancet* 358:1749-1753, 2001

[32] Huurman VA, van der Meide PE, Duinkerken G, Willemen S, Cohen IR, Elias D, Roep BO: Immunological efficacy of heat shock protein 60 peptide DiaPep277 therapy in clinical type I diabetes. *Clin Exp Immunol* 152:488-497, 2008

[33] Gurr W, Shaw M, Li Y, Sherwin R: RegII is a beta-cell protein and autoantigen in diabetes of NOD mice. *Diabetes* 56:34-40, 2007

[34] Bellmann K, Hui L, Radons J, Burkart V, Kolb H: Low stress response enhances vulnerability of islet cells in diabetes-prone BB rats. *Diabetes* 46:232-236, 1997

[35] Almawi WY, Tamim H, Azar ST: Clinical review 103: T helper type 1 and 2 cytokines mediate the onset and progression of type I (insulin-dependent) diabetes. *J Clin Endocrinol Metab* 84:1497-1502, 1999

[36] Vaarala O, Atkinson MA, Neu J: The "perfect storm" for type 1 diabetes: the complex interplay between intestinal microbiota, gut permeability, and mucosal immunity. *Diabetes* 57:2555-2562, 2008

[37] Giongo A, Gano KA, Crabb DB, Mukherjee N, Novelo LL, Casella G, Drew JC, Ilonen J, Knip M, Hyoty H, Veijola R, Simell T, Simell O, Neu J, Wasserfall CH, Schatz D, Atkinson MA, Triplett EW: Toward defining the autoimmune microbiome for type 1 diabetes. *ISME J* 5:82-91, 2011

[38] Gaglia JL, Guimaraes AR, Harisinghani M, Turvey SE, Jackson R, Benoist C, Mathis D, Weissleder R: Noninvasive imaging of pancreatic islet inflammation in type 1A diabetes patients. *J Clin Invest* 121:442-445, 2011

[39] Dube SR, Fairweather D, Pearson WS, Felitti VJ, Anda RF, Croft JB: Cumulative childhood stress and autoimmune diseases in adults. *Psychosom Med* 71:243-250, 2009

Chapter 22

DNA Immunotherapies for Type 1 Diabetes

Alice Li and Alan Escher

Additional information is available at the end of the chapter

http://dx.doi.org/10.5772/55727

1. Introduction

As per the American Diabetes Association, 2-3 million individuals in the United States have type 1 diabetes (www.medicinenet.com/script/main/art.asp?articlekey=159355), with 1 in every 400 to 600 children and adolescents affected by the disease in 2007. Furthermore, similar to other autoimmune diseases, allergies and asthma, the incidence of type 1 diabetes is on the increase at an alarming rate in industrialized countries for unknown reasons. Information released by the American Diabetes Association shows 23% and 21% increased rates of type 1 and 2 diabetes, respectively, from 2001 to 2009. The increase in incidence of type 1 diabetes is especially apparent in young children and has generated an urgent need for novel treatments that can safely control diabetes-causing inflammation, and alleviate the need for administration of exogenous insulin. Indeed, type 1 diabetes has been treated for almost a century in the same fundamental manner using daily insulin injections. Although it is a life-saving treatment and one of the most remarkable accomplishments of medicine, administration of exogenous insulin is still not a cure because it does not address the underlying autoimmunity that targets insulin-secreting beta cells. Because it is currently impossible to mimic regulation of physiological insulin levels faithfully, many type 1 diabetic individuals receiving standard of care are exposed to acute and chronic complications that cause increased morbidity and mortality. As a result, there have been intense efforts to develop immunotherapies that can eliminate or at least alleviate the need for exogenous insulin. In this case the goal is to arrest pathological autoimmunity that destroys beta cells so that the cells can regain function, and possibly proliferate and regenerate.

Two major immunotherapeutic paths have been taken. The first path relies on different forms of systemic suppression of inflammation that inhibit effector T lymphocytes in a non-specific manner. Serious side effects associated with the use of systemic immunotherapies are increased risks of cancer and infection resulting from the decreased activity of effector cells involved in beneficial destructive immune responses against cancer cells and pathogens. These side effects have been observed with broadly acting immunosuppressants used to prevent organ transplant rejection, which have been also investigated for treating type 1 diabetes [1, 2]. Serious side effects can also be seen, albeit to a lesser degree, with more specific agents like antibodies that target specific molecules involved in inflammation [3, 4]. In contrast, the second immunotherapeutic path is based on administration of a self-antigen synthesized by pancreatic beta cells that is a target of pathological autoimmunity, i.e., an autoantigen. This path is thought to be safer because it aims to induce a regulatory immune response that targets the inflamed islets. Here the goal is to manipulate endogenous immune mechanisms of homeostasis that can re-establish some form of tolerance to the chosen autoantigen, as well as to other neighboring beta cell autoantigens through a mechanism known as "by-stander suppression" [5]. Accordingly, it is anticipated that pathological autoimmunity and inflammation of islets can be stopped in an organ-specific manner that does not impair the immune system.

In this chapter, we will review how plasmid deoxyribonucleic acid (DNA) has been used as an immunotherapeutic vector platform to treat type 1 diabetes through each immunotherapeutic path. For the purpose of this review, we have called the first path "gene-based immunotherapy", meaning that plasmid DNA does not encode a known autoantigen, and the second path "DNA vaccine immunotherapy" meaning that a beta cell autoantigen is encoded by plasmid DNA (Figure 1). In other words, gene-based immunotherapy relies on the inherent function of a product encoded by plasmid DNA that can in turn affect cell function. In contrast, DNA vaccine immunotherapy relies on the tolerogenic immune response induced directly by the autoantigen after its processing by immune cells. As we shall see, some DNA vaccine immunotherapies have also a gene-based immunotherapy component that acts as a molecular adjuvant to promote tolerogenic immune responses. Nevertheless, in all cases synthesis of the molecule encoded by plasmid DNA, which is almost always a protein, starts after delivery of the plasmid DNA and its uptake by cells.

Plasmid DNA has several notable advantages compared to other vectors and therapeutic molecules. For example, it consists of relatively low molecular weight circles of double stranded DNA that can be readily isolated from bacteria in a generic and cost-effective manner. In addition, plasmid DNA permits rapid turnaround when developing new candidate products, refrigeration-free storage, and synthesis over time of a chosen antigen in its native conformation. Furthermore, plasmid DNA can be given in repeat doses within short periods of time without inducing an immune response to vector and other side effects. This is in contrast with viral-based vaccines that can induce immune responses to vector and protein/peptides that can cause anaphylaxis [6, 7].

Plasmid DNA can be delivered either as "naked" DNA or packaged into molecular scaffolds like liposomes, cationic lipids, virosomes, and polymer-based nano- and micro-particles to increase efficacy of delivery to cells [8]. Although they may sometime have pro-inflammatory properties that can be detrimental to controlling inflammation, these particles have been used to induce immune tolerance with plasmid DNA. For example, chitosan-DNA nanoparticles encoding an ovalbumin antigen are tolerogenic when delivered orally [9].

Indeed, route of delivery can play a significant role in the type and strength of immune responses induced by DNA vaccines in animal models [10, 11]. In humans, two microgram of a DNA vaccine for treatment of melanoma delivered with gold particles into skin was found to be as efficacious as 1000 microgram injected intramuscularly [12]. These results illustrate the significant impact that choice of route and method of delivery of a DNA vaccine can have not only on efficacy, but also on cost of treatment. Other delivery routes like intravenous, nasal, and sublingual have also been investigated [13]. Post delivery, expression of coding sequences in plasmid DNA results in significant levels of protein production that may persist for six weeks and longer without serious side effects in human patients [14, 15].

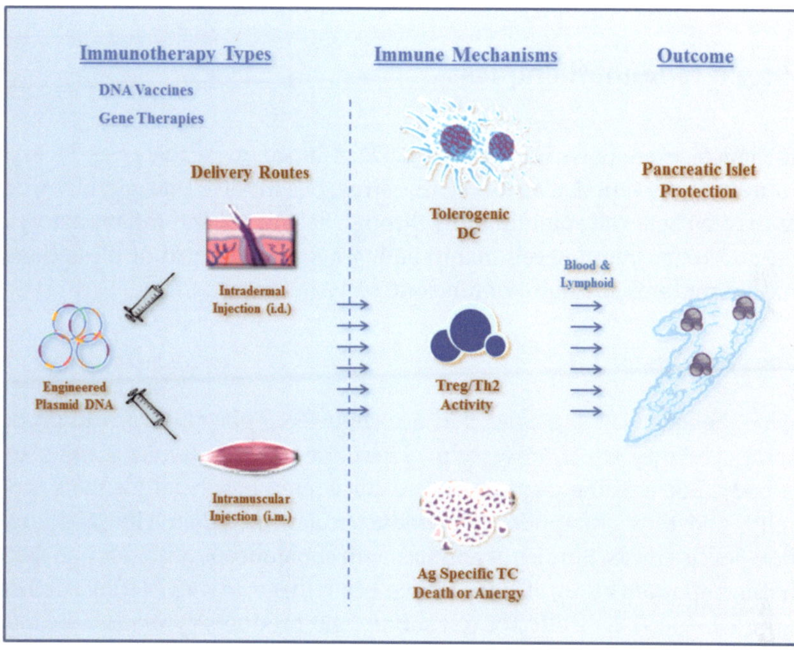

Figure 1. Plasmid DNA Immunotherapy for Type 1 Diabetes. Plasmid DNA immunotherapy for type 1 diabetes can be divided into two categories: DNA vaccines and gene therapies. Plasmid DNA can be delivered using different routes, for example, the intradermal and intramuscular routes. The therapies can induce tolerogenic dendritic cells (DC), T regulatory cells (Treg), and death/anergy of T effector cells (Teff) which are the main cause of pancreatic islet destruction.

DNA vaccination was originally investigated to induce immunogenic responses to pathogens and cancer cells, but it has increasingly been applied to the induction of immune tolerance for treatment of autoimmune diseases like type 1 diabetes. DNA vaccines and other gene-based vaccines belong to a third generation of vaccines after live and attenuated whole organism vaccine and recombinant protein vaccines. These vaccines can be used to either prevent (prophylactic vaccine) or treat (therapeutic vaccine) disease depending on their potency, in which prevention is generally easier to achieve than treatment. Recent reports of beneficial results in different clinical trials using delivery of autoantigens indicate that DNA vaccination is reaching a stage where we are likely to see accelerated development of a therapeutic future for vaccines targeting a variety of autoimmune diseases. In the case of type 1 diabetes, early results using a DNA vaccine encoding insulin have shown promise in humans. In addition,

DNA vaccines encoding human heat shock protein 60 and glutamic acid decarboxylase 65 have also shown efficacy in preclinical trials and are reviewed in this chapter.

In contrast to DNA vaccine immunotherapy, gene-based immunotherapy involves delivery of genetic material by a plasmid vector into a cell, tissue or organ with the aim of improving the clinical status using the function of the encoded product, instead of its properties as an antigen. Gene-based immunotherapy includes delivery of anti-inflammatory cytokines, chemokines, and other factors to modulate the activity of immune cells [16, 17].

2. Gene-based immunotherapies

Several pre-clinical trials have used plasmid DNA-based gene therapies in experimental models of autoimmune type 1 diabetes. These strategies involve plasmid DNA designed to weaken pre-existing beta-cell autoimmunity through delivery of anti-inflammatory cytokines, chemokines, and other immune cell manipulating agents. The goal of these therapies is to reduce clinical symptoms and autoimmune outcome.

2.1. Cytokine gene therapies

Cytokine gene therapies are strategies that use engineered plasmid DNA to produce therapeutic immune cytokines, which are a group of immune active molecules secreted by different cells of the body. Some of these cytokines are considered beneficial for the suppression of autoimmunity, and thus are applied to disease models to reduce clinical symptoms and improve therapeutic effects. Studies of animals with spontaneous autoimmune diabetes have revealed that an important group of autoreactive T cells that mediates islet beta-cell destruction belongs to the T helper-1 type effector cell subset, and produces cytokines like interleukin-2 and interferon-gamma. On the other hand, regulatory T cells that control effector cells can secrete interleukin-4, interleukin-10, and transforming growth factor-beta.

One of the earliest applications of cytokine-engineered plasmid DNA was gene-gun delivery of murine interleukin-4 to prevent spontaneous type 1 diabetes [18]. The plasmid DNA was delivered as three times two microgram within 4 weeks into 3-week-old nonobese diabetic mice, which is the animal model system closest to human type 1 diabetes. Type 1 diabetes incidence was reduced from 90% in controls to 20% at 34 weeks of age, and was associated with T helper-2 type immune responses in the periphery and pancreas of mice. Two other reports have shown that systemic delivery of plasmid DNA constructs coding for interleukin-4 can prevent insulitis, which is an inflammatory sign of immune cell infiltrating pancreatic islets in nonobese diabetic mice [19, 20]. However, contradictory results have been reported. For example, a report indicates that intramuscular electroporation delivery of 50 μg plasmid DNA encoding interleukin-4 accelerated spontaneous type 1 diabetes in nonobese diabetic mice [21].

In addition to interleukin-4, interleukin-10-encoded plasmid DNA alone was also tested for its diabetic suppressive effects. The plasmid DNA was delivered intramuscularly twice for a total of 200 microgram into 3 and 5 week old female nonobese diabetic mice [22]. Although the severity of insulitis at 13 weeks of age was not improved, the incidence of diabetes was markedly reduced to 50% at 35 week old compared to 90% with control mice. These results show that the progression of autoimmune disease in mice can effectively be suppressed by intramuscular DNA injection coding for anti-inflammatory cytokines alone. When the same interleukin-10 encoded plasmid DNA was combined with a cationic polymeric carrier, systemic administration could reduce the severity of insulitis in NOD mice markedly (15.7%) compared with that of naked DNA injection (34.5%) and non-treated controls (90.9%), suggesting an increased protective effect of the polymeric carrier in vivo [23].

Another report investigating the immune effects of interleukin-10 DNA showed that systemic intramuscular administration of 200 microgram interleukin-10 plasmid DNA could alleviate blood glucose and insulitis in a streptozotocin induced diabetic mouse model up to day 28 post injection [24]. In this model, pancreatic interleukin-1b and tumor necrotic factor-alpha gene expression, serum interferon-gamma concentration, and the numbers of CD4+ and $CD8^+$ lymphocytes were decreased on day 28. A similar interleukin-10 construct was modified by introducing nuclear factor kappa-B (NF-kB) binding sites into plasmid DNA to facilitate nuclear transport of the plasmid after delivery into the cell [25]. A single injection of 50 microgram of the plasmid using polyethylenimine as a gene carrier in 5 week old mice reduced the degree of insulitis and serum glucose levels in 100% of mice compared to 40% of the control mice at 32 weeks of age. These results illustrate how plasmid DNA can be easily modified in a generic manner to improve therapeutic efficacy.

As mentioned previously, nanoparticle technology has been used to condense plasmid DNA into nanometer-size complexes to improve delivery. An interleukin-10 encoding plasmid DNA was assembled into a cationic nanoparticle complex, and a single dose of 50 microgram DNA was delivered intramuscularly into streptozotocin-induced diabetic mice [26]. Animals showed higher serum levels of interleukin-10, suppression of interferon-gamma level, reduction of islet insulitis, and lower blood glucose levels compared to those treated with interleukin-10 plasmid alone or the nanoparticle alone up to week 6 post injection. Histology of muscle showed that nanoparticles were biocompatible and did not cause a chronic inflammatory response.

In addition to their use alone, delivery of both interleukin-4 and interleukin-10 DNA has also been investigated. Combined delivery into nonobese diabetic mice of the two plasmid DNA constructs encoding interleukin-4 and interleukin-10 (25 μg each) was done intravenously using a degradable, cationic polymeric carrier, poly (alpha-(4-aminobutyl)-L-glycolic acid) [27]. Overexpression of the two cytokine messenger RNAs was confirmed in the liver of mice 5 days after delivery. Six weeks after injection, 75% of observed islets were intact compared with less than 3% in the control group, and development of diabetes was prevented in 75% of treated animals at 30 weeks of age, compared to 20% in control mice receiving plasmid DNA coding for a single cytokine or vector control alone. The results indicated that the interleukin-4 and interleukin-10 plasmid DNAs had synergistic effects on the prevention of autoimmune diabetes. A report from the same research group showed that a 'chimeric' plasmid expressing both of the interleukin-4 and interleukin-10 under controls of two CMV promoters could also reduce insulitis in the same system [28].

More recently, a research group also reported packaging plasmid DNA constructs coding for interleukin-4 and interleukin-10 into cationic nanomicelles to prevent type 1 diabetes [29]. A single intramuscular dose of 50 microgram of the complex reduced levels of blood glucose and insulitis up to 6-week post delivery in 5-week-old streptozotocin-induced diabetic mouse. It was found that levels of diabetes-associated cytokines like tumor necrotic factor-alpha and interferon-gamma were also reduced, which suggested suppression T helper-1 effector cells by the cytokine/cationic nanomicelle complex therapy. Notably, plasmid DNA coding for interleukin-4 and interleukin-10 has also been used as adjuvant to promote the therapeutic effect of DNA vaccines in a murine model for type 1 diabetes, which will describe later in this chapter in the 'Glutamic Acid Decarboxylase DNA Vaccines' section.

In addition, a number of studies have reported that injection of plasmid DNA coding for cytokines normally considered pro-inflammatory can prevent diabetes. These results reflect the multifaceted role of cytokines on immune response [30], which could be dependent on dosage and time of administration. For example, administration of interleukin-18, also known as interferon-gamma inducing factor, can prevent diabetes in NOD mice [31, 32]. However, it was also shown that intramuscular electroporation of 2 x 100 microgram plasmid DNA coding for interleukin-18 into 4-6-week-old nonobese diabetic mice aggravates diabetes [33]. Another report showed that intraperitoneal administration of 30 microgram of plasmid DNA encoding interferon-gamma promotes insulitis in reovirus type-2 induced diabetic mice compared to controls [34]. This is in contrast with another report showing that injection of interleukin-12 induces interferon-gamma that prevents diabetes in NOD mice [35]. Together, these results suggest that there is risk associated with direct delivery of cytokines for the treatment of type 1 diabetes. This possibility is suggested by a phase I clinical trial where new onset patients with type 1 diabetes received a combination treatment of interleukin-2 and the immunosuppressant rapamycin. The treatment had shown efficacy in preventing disease in mice, but it accelerated disease in humans [2].

2.2. Chemokine gene therapies

Chemokines are a family of small chemotactic cytokines secreted by cells [36]. Their name is derived from their ability to induce directed chemotaxis, or directed cell migration, in responsive cells. Some chemokines are considered pro-inflammatory and can be induced during an immune response to recruit cells of the immune system to a site of infection, while others are considered homeostatic and are involved in controlling the migration of cells during normal tissue maintenance and inhibiting abnormal inflammation like pathological autoimmune response.

Chemokines are involved in pathogenesis of autoimmune disease because they can selectively recruit various subsets of immune lymphocytes [37, 38]. Based on structural motifs near their N-terminal cysteine residue [C], chemokines are divided into four subfamilies, termed CXC, CX3C, C, and CC. The function of chemokines is modulated by the type of chemokine receptors they bind to as ligands on the surface of cells, and studies have shown that chemokines and chemokine receptors are involved in the pathogenesis of autoimmune diseases like type 1 diabetes. Chemokine gene therapies for type 1 diabetes use anti-inflammatory chemokines as well as inhibitors of pro-inflammatory chemokine binding.

With regard to blocking strategies, CXC ligand-10 is an example of a chemokine associated with the pathogenesis of various T helper-1 dominant responses involved in autoimmune diseases, e.g., experimental autoimmune encephalomyelitis, rheumatoid arthritis, and type 1 diabetes. It was found that, in type 1 diabetic adult patients, elevated levels of serum CXC ligand-10 are associated with high-risk of disease in latent diabetic subjects [39]. This finding was translated in animal models where blockade or neutralization of the CXC ligand-10 can prevent type 1 diabetes in nonobese diabetic mice [40]. In virus-induced diabetic mice, virus infection results in rapid and differential expression of CXC receptor-3 and CXC ligand-10, which plays a dominant role in programming the ensuing autoimmune disease [41]. The blockade of CXC ligand-10 by using anti CXC ligand-10 monoclonal antibodies successfully aborts severity of antigen-specific injury of pancreatic beta cells and abrogates type 1 diabetes. Mechanistically, the blockade impedes the expansion of peripheral antigen-specific T effector cells and hinders their migration into the pancreas. A similar effect of the antibodies was confirmed in a cyclophosphamide accelerated model of type 1 diabetes [40].

Based on these reports, plasmid DNA encoding the CXC ligand-10 was constructed to induce production of anti-CXC ligand-10 antibodies in the host [42]. The aim was to avoid side-effects associated with direct injection of antibodies. Intramuscular electroporation of 100 microgram of the plasmid DNA at 4 and 6 weeks of age induced synthesis of anti CXC ligand-10 antibodies *in vivo*, and suppressed the incidence of spontaneous diabetes which went from 75% in control mice down to 25% in treated mice at 30 weeks of age. Although this treatment did not inhibit insulitis or alter the immunological response, it enhanced the proliferation of pancreatic beta cells and resulted in an increase of beta-cell mass.

A subsequent report from the same research group showed that combining complete Freund's adjuvant with plasmid DNA encoding the CXC ligand-10 could reverse diabetes [43]. Intramuscular electroporation combined with complete Freund's adjuvant was used to treat new-onset female nonobese diabetic mice with blood glucose levels higher than 250 mg/dL. Diabetes incidence was reduced from 70% in control mice to 20% in treated mice 10 weeks after plasmid DNA delivery. In contrast, mice receiving complete Freund's adjuvant and control plasmid DNA did not show disease reversal. In mice that were treated successfully, residual beta-cell mass was significantly increased, and some beta-cells were in a proliferative state. Although systemic cytokine profiles were unaffected, the frequency of regulatory T cells expressing CXC receptor-3 was significantly increased in local pancreatic lesions and possibly associated with the regulation of anti-islet autoimmunity.

Another research group found that intra-pancreatic CC ligand-4 levels are increased in a model of diabetes protection by interleukin-4 treatment in female nonobese diabetic mice [44]. The protective effect of CC ligand-4 was confirmed by abrogation of diabetes suppression after injection of anti-CC ligand-4 antibodies [45]. These result led to studies using CC ligand-4-encoded plasmid DNA therapy which showed that gene-gun delivery of 1 microgram of the plasmid DNA protects against type 1 diabetes in NOD mice, with diabetes rates reduced from 75% in control mice to 30% at 35 weeks of age when treated weekly from week 3 to 14, and from 80% in control mice down to 30% when treated weekly from week 9 to 14 [45]. Data also indicated that plasmid DNA delivery could both prevent and treat type 1 diabetes. This protection was associated with a T helper-2-like response in the spleen and pancreas, decreased recruitment of activated CD8 T cells to islets accompanied by diminished CC receptor-5 expression on CD8 T cells, and increased regulatory T cell activity in the draining pancreatic lymph nodes.

To summarize, plasmid DNA encoding CC ligand-4 and CXC ligand-10 have been tested for their type 1 diabetic suppressive effects in spontaneous diabetic mouse models. Diabetes suppression is associated with decreased CD8 T lymphocyte activity and increased CD4 T regulatory cell activity. These results suggest a possible clinical application of chemokine ligand gene therapies, although they are anticipated to have possible side effects associated with systemic immunotherapies.

2.3. Other cell-manipulating gene therapies

Several immune cell populations have deficiencies in type 1 diabetes, such as CD4 T lymphocytes, CD8 T lymphocytes, B lymphocytes, dendritic cells, macrophages, and NK cells in both nonobese diabetic mice and human patients [46, 47]. The goal of cell-manipulating gene therapy is to increase the diabetic suppressive function of cells like T regulatory or T helper-2 lymphocytes, which are considered important not only for therapeutic purposes, but also for playing a determining role in the development of type 1 diabetes.

As mentioned at the beginning of this chapter, type 1 diabetes is a T helper-1-mediated autoimmune disease and strategies suppressing the function of these cells can be expected to have an impact on disease progression. One of these strategies is the delivery of galectin-9, a carbohydrate-binding protein that regulates T helper-1 cells and induces their apoptosis through the galectin-9 receptor. Apoptosis, or programmed-cell-death, is a constantly ongoing process in steady state *in vivo* and helps maintain tissue and immune homeostasis. Mice treated with plasmid DNA coding for galectin-9 were significantly protected from diabetes: intravenous delivery of 2 x 100 microgram bi-weekly protected 85% of mice from diabetes versus 55% in controls [48]. Analysis of immune responses showed that the T helper-1 cell population was markedly decreased in spleen, pancreas, and pancreatic lymph nodes of treated NOD-T1/2 double transgenic diabetic mice, indicating a suppressive role of galectin-9 on pathogenic T helper-1 cells. Splenocytes from treated mice were also less responsive to mitogenic stimulation than splenocytes from the control group. Data indicated that galectin-9 DNA may downregulate T helper-1 immune response in diabetic mice and could be used as a therapeutic agent in autoimmune diabetes.

In contrast with galectin-9, decoy receptor 3 inhibits apoptosis. The membrane protein is a member of the tumor necrosis factor receptor superfamily, and regulates immune responses by neutralizing apoptotic signals transmitted through CD95 (Fas receptor), lymphotoxin beta-receptor, and death receptor 3 on target cells. As a result, transgenic expression of decoy receptor 3 in pancreatic beta cells protects nonobese diabetic mice from autoimmune diabetes [49]. When decoy receptor 3 is delivered systemically as plasmid DNA, it inhibits insulitis and diabetes by modulating immune responses. For example, four weekly intravenous injections of 100 microgram of plasmid DNA coding for decoy receptor 9 into nonobese diabetic mice was reported to reduce diabetes incidence from 90% in controls to 30% when treated at 4 weeks of age, 45% (started at 7 week old), and 70% (as Fc-fusion form, started at 12 week old) in 35-week-old female nonobese diabetic mice [50]. Treated mice showed less splenocyte proliferation and adoptive transfer of the cells ameliorated diabetes. Treated NOD-T1/2 mice had reduced T helper-1, T helper-17, and increased T helper-2 immune responses *in vivo*. Data also indicated that immune modulation by decoy receptor 3 may have been the result of differentiation and maturation of dendritic cells that subsequently regulated T effector differentiation and function.

Cell migration is another process that plays a role in pancreatic beta cell destruction. In this regard, plasmid DNA coding for CD44, which is a protein associated with cell migration and delivery of apoptotic signals by inflammatory cells, was investigated for the suppression of diabetes. It was found that subcutaneous implants of a silicone tube filled with wound dressing sponge carrying CD44 encoded plasmid DNA could attenuate diabetes in a transfer model [51]. Diabetes was induced in male nonobese diabetic mice by transfer of diabetogenic splenocytes from female diabetic mice and was reduced from 90% in controls to 20-30% 12 weeks after two implants. Here the mechanism of treatment was not thought to be strictly a gene therapy effect, but rather induction of anti-CD44 antibodies that inhibited CD44 function.

An increasing body of evidence points to a possible relationship between the central nervous system and diabetes [52]. For example, the pancreatic autoantigen glutamic acid decarboxylase is an enzyme responsible for synthesis of the neurotransmitter gamma-aminobutyric acid (GABA) in the peripheral and central nervous system. Notably, at least two neurotransmitter-related peptides have been used successfully as plasmid DNA immunotherapies for type 1 diabetes.

The first peptide is calcitonin gene-related peptide (CGRP), which has been found to play an important role in the regulation of T lymphocytes and in protecting cells from reactive oxygen species. It was found that a single injection of 200 microgram plasmid DNA encoding the peptide delivered intramuscularly using electroporation could significantly ameliorate hyperglycemia and insulin deficiency [53]. The treatment decreased diabetes incidence from 73% in controls to 23% at 28 days post delivery in a streptozotocin-induced diabetic model. The gene transfer also significantly inhibited T cell proliferation and secretion of the T helper-1 cytokine interferon-gamma, increased the levels of the T helper-2 cytokine interleukin-10, but had no effect on interleukin-4 and transforming growth factor-beta secretion. Therefore, calcitonin gene-related peptide gene transfer appears to ameliorate streptozotocin-induced diabetes through immune deviation.

The second peptide is named vasoactive intestinal peptide (VIP) and functions as a neuromodulator and neurotransmitter [54]. The peptide is a potent vasodilator that regulates smooth muscle activity, epithelial cell secretion, and blood flow in the gastrointestinal tract. Importantly, a body of evidence points to a significant role of vasoactive intestinal polypeptide in regulating immune responses. The peptide acts as a potent endogenous anti-inflammatory molecule and promotes the activity of T regulatory cells, which makes it a promising candidate for the treatments of inflammatory and autoimmune diseases, such as septic shock, arthritis, multiple sclerosis, Crohn disease, and autoimmune diabetes [55, 56]. For example, a single intramuscular injection of 300 microgram of vasoactive intestinal polypeptide-encoding plasmid DNA significantly reduced the incidence of cyclophosphamide accelerated diabetes in female nonobese diabetic mice, from 70% in control to 30% on day 33 post delivery in 8-10-week-old mice [57]. A subsequent report in a different model system indicated that injection of the peptide could activate $FoxP3^{+}CD4^{+}CD25^{high}$ T regulatory cells and protect against acute graft-versus-host disease in a mouse model of allogeneic bone marrow transplantation [58].

2.4. Summary of Section 2

Section 1 covers plasmid DNA encoding small protein molecules like cytokines, chemokines, peptides and other immune cell-manipulating agents with therapeutic effects on preclinical type 1 diabetes (Table 1). These approaches belong to systemic treatments and inevitably bear the risks associated with nonspecific immune suppression and chronic complications resulting from interference with the host immune system. Nonetheless, if used as adjuvants or supplements to pancreatic autoantigen-targeting therapies like DNA vaccines, these approaches could be used selectively in DNA-based combination therapies. We provide examples of such approaches in Section 2 of this chapter.

3. DNA vaccine immunotherapies

Plasmid DNA vaccine-based immunotherapy is a promising therapeutic field for treatment of type 1 diabetes. Clinical proof of concept has already been provided with results from phase I/II trials where individuals with new-onset type 1 diabetes were treated with proinsulin-encoding plasmid DNA [15]. Nevertheless, although beneficial effects were observed, it is clear that efficacy must be significantly improved. Improving efficacy will be likely dependent on the ability to modulate both the innate immune system, through activation of tolerogenic antigen-presenting cells like dendritic cells, and the adaptive immune system, through activation of various populations of regulatory cells. DNA vaccines are particularly well positioned to achieve this goal because plasmid DNA is information-based, and can encode molecules that affect the immune system in different manners. The challenge is to identify which combination of functions should be delivered together with a pancreatic autoantigen to treat disease with maximum efficacy and safety.

Several beta cell autoantigens have been tested in mice for induction of immune tolerance by DNA vaccines and will be discussed in this section. Immune mechanisms associated with the therapeutic effects of DNA vaccines can be complex because of the variety of cells that can process the information encoded by plasmid DNA. Regardless, the major goals are to induce diabetic suppressive dendritic cells, T regulatory lymphocytes, and the cell death and inactivation of T effector lymphocytes that destroy pancreatic beta cells.

http://dx.doi.org/10.5772/55727

Categories	Encoded Products	Immune Responses	Trials	References
Gene Therapies				
Cytokines	IL-4	T helper-2	Preclinical	[18-21]
	IL-10	T helper-2	Preclinical	[22-26]
	IL-4 + IL-10 as Nanoparticle	T helper-2	Preclinical	[27-29]
Chemokines	C-C Motif Ligand 4	T helper-2, Tregs	Preclinical	[45]
	C-X-C Motif Ligand 10	Tregs	Preclinical	[42,43]
Cellular	Galectin-9	T helper-2	Preclinical	[48]
Manipulations	Decoy Receptor 3	T helper-2, DCs	Preclinical	[50]
	CD44	Antibodies	Preclinical	[51]
	CGRP	T helper-2	Preclinical	[53]
	VIP	Tregs	Preclinical	[57]
DNA Vaccines				
	Insulin B chain	T helper-2	Preclinical	[60,67]
	Insulin B Chain + IL-4	T helper-2	Preclinical	[61]
	Proinsulin + Anti-CD154	$CD25^+$ Tregs	Preclinical	[62]
	Proinsulin DNA + Peptide	$CD25^-$ Tregs	Preclinical	[63]
	Proinsulin + PRP III	$CD25^+$ Tregs	Preclinical	[64]
	Pre-proinsulin + B7-1wa	?	Preclinical	[65]
	Proinsulin	?	Preclinical, Clinical	[15,66,68]
	Proinsulin + Anti-CD3	T helper-2, $CD25^+$ Tregs	Preclinical	[71]
	HSP 60	T helper-2	PreClinical	[79]
	HSP 65	T helper-2, Tregs	Preclinical	[80,81]
	Secreted GAD65, GAD65	T helper-2	Preclinical	[84,85,88,92]
	GAD65-Ig Fc + IL-4/IL-10/IL-4 & IL-10	T helper-2	Preclinical	[86,87]
	GAD65 + Anti-CD3	Tregs	Preclinical	[94]
	Secreted GAD65 + BAX	Tregs, DCs	Preclinical	[97-99]
	IA-2 + IL-4	Tregs?	Preclinical	[101]
	GPI + lysosome	nTregs	Preclinical	[102]

Table 1. Plasmid DNA Based Immunotherapies for Type 1 Diabetes. The table summarizes plasmid DNA based immunotherapies under two categories: Gene therapies and DNA vaccines. Immunotherapies are listed according to their category, type of immune response and trial. Abbreviation: IL, interleukin; CD, cluster of differentiation; PRPIII, pancreatic regenerating protein III; CGRP, calcitonin gene-related peptide; VIP, vasoactive intestinal polypeptide; HSP, heat shock protein; GAD, glutamic acid decarboxylase. IA, insulinoma associated protein; Tregs, T regulatory cells; DCs: dendritic cells.

3.1. Insulin DNA vaccines

Thus far, the only DNA vaccine that has been tested in both preclinical and clinical trials is a plasmid DNA construct coding for intracellular proinsulin, which is a partially processed non-functional form of insulin. Insulin is not only the hormone produced by beta-cells that controls carbohydrate and fat metabolism in the body, it is also a main target autoantigen in autoimmune diabetes and the presence of anti-insulin autoantibodies can be an indication of disease initiation [59]. DNA vaccines coding for different forms of insulin have been investigated for type 1 diabetes immunotherapy since the late 1990's. The first report to demonstrate efficacy used a virus-induced diabetic mouse model system, and showed that intramuscular injection of plasmid DNA encoding the insulin B chain reduces the incidence of diabetes (blood glucose > 350 mg/dL) from 100% down to 50% [60]. The DNA vaccine induced insulin B-chain specific $CD4^+$ T regulatory cells that secreted interleukin-4, and locally reduced autoreactive activity of cytotoxic T lymphocytes in the pancreatic draining lymph nodes. Further work showed that co-delivery of interleukin-4 was required to prevent diabetes onset in male nonobese diabetic mice [61].

Two isoforms of insulin are synthesized in rodent animals, insulin I in islets and insulin II in both islets and thymus while humans have only one form of insulin. The pancreatic beta cells synthesize proinsulin before converting it to functional insulin. In that regard, intranasal delivery of plasmid DNA encoding mouse proinsulin II together with injection of an anti-CD154 (also named CD40 ligand) antibody to prevent T cell activation was reported to prevent type 1 diabetes in nonobese diabetic mice [62]. Delivery of 300 microgram DNA and 50 microgram antibody over a 2-week interval at 4 weeks of age synergistically prevented diabetes, reducing disease incidence from 100% diabetic down to 0% in 40-week old mice. Injection of the anti-CD154 antibody alone reduced the incidence to 50%. However, delivery of the DNA vaccine alone did not reduce diabetes incidence, even though it could induce T regulatory cells and reduce insulitis.

Another report has shown that co-delivery of 50 microgram plasmid DNA encoding human proinsulin together with 100 microgram insulin peptide twice over a 2-week interval could prevent diabetes until 24 weeks of age in 6 week old nonobese diabetic mice. In contrast, DNA or peptide alone did not prevent disease [63]. Results also indicated induction of $CD4^+CD25^-$ islet specific T regulatory cells producing transforming growth factor-beta only in the co-immunization group.

In another study, a DNA vaccine encoding proinsulin and pancreatic regenerating (Reg) III protein resulted in a significant reduction of hyperglycemia and diabetes incidence with increased serum insulin in a streptozotocin- induced mice model [64]. The treatment also restored the balance of T helper-1/T helper-2 cytokines, expanded $CD4^+CD25^+Foxp3^+$ T regulatory cells, and attenuated insulitis by inhibiting activation of nuclear factor-kappa B (NF-κB) in the pancreas, which is thought to promote the regeneration of islet beta cells.

Cytotoxic T lymphocyte antigen 4 (CTLA-4 or CD152) is a strong negative regulator of T cell activity and another example of an immunomodulator that can be co-delivered with an autoantigen. Like CD28 (a positive regulator), CTLA-4 binds to B7-1 and B7-2. It was found

http://dx.doi.org/10.5772/55727

that a single amino acid substitution in B7-1 (denoted B7-1wa) could abrogate specific binding to CD28 but not to CTLA-4. Co-delivery of B7-1wa and preproinsulin I encoded by plasmid DNA abrogated reactivity to insulin and ameliorated type 1 diabetes in nonobese diabetic mice, although delivery of either preproinsulin I or B7-1wa alone did not suppress the disease [65]. Interferon-gamma and interleukin-4 were both depressed, arguing against a T helper-2 bias, but reactivity to glutamic acid decarboxylase 65 was not altered. Suppressor cells were not identified, suggesting induction of tolerance to insulin by either T cell anergy or deletion in this model.

Among the most promising reports of insulin DNA vaccination is a plasmid DNA construct encoding mouse proinsulin II that could reduce the incidence of diabetes in nonobese diabetic mice when administered intramuscularly to prediabetic 8-week old mice (prophylactic setting), and to diabetic mice older than 12-week (therapeutic setting) with blood glucose > 170 mg/dL [66, 67]. The efficacy of the vaccine was improved by increasing the level of expression of insulin, frequency of dosing, dosage, and subcelullar localization modification of the autoantigen to the intracellular compartment instead of being secreted. In the prophylactic setting, 8 weekly injections of 50 microgram of the DNA vaccine decreased the incidence of diabetes from 80% in the control group down to 45% in 25-week old mice. The treatment caused increased numbers of interferon-gamma secreting cells and a decrease in insulin autoantibodies. In the therapeutic setting, the DNA vaccine reduced diabetes from 100% in the control groups down to 25% in treated mice 25 weeks post treatment initiation. The treatment induced increased numbers of insulin-specific interferon-gamma-producing T cells and levels of interleukin-10, which suggested the possible induction of T regulatory-1 cells. Adoptive transfer experiments indicated that the protection was not mediated by the induction of $CD4^+CD25^+$ T regulatory cells.

Most important, a similar DNA vaccine encoding human proinsulin was used in phase I/II clinical trials and has been the only human trial of a DNA vaccine for diabetes conducted to date [68, 69]. Construct BHT-3021 was delivered intramuscularly using four doses of plasmid DNA, i.e., 0.3, 1, 3 and 6 milligram, administered once a week for 12 weeks. The interim results for the 1 milligram dose showed pancreatic beta-cell preservation, demonstrated by a mean 17% increase in C-peptide levels with BHT-3021 by week 15 after enrollment, whereas placebo patients experienced a mean 42% decrease in C-peptide. Evidence for immune tolerance was suggested by a mean 17% reduction in anti-insulin antibodies, and 25% reduction in anti-glutamic acid decarboxylase 65 antibodies by week 15 after enrollment, whereas placebo patients experienced a mean 6% and 4% increase, respectively. The most recent report of the trial claimed that BHT-3021 could preserve C-peptide levels for at least six months and one year in some of the patients from the point of initiation of the therapy [15]. These results together with its favorable side-effects profile appear to be somewhat comparable to those reported with anti-CD3 monoclonal antibody, and the glutamic acid decarboxylase 65 protein vaccines for type 1 diabetes.

However, thus far, no immunotherapy alone has been reported to cause long term remission of clinical type 1 diabetes. This was confirmed with the announcements in 2011 of the failure of three phase III clinical trials for type 1 diabetes that tested two anti-CD3 monoclonal antibodies and a GAD65 protein vaccine. The need to increase therapeutic efficacy has generated an increased interest in combination immunotherapies [70-72]. Indeed, it is reasonable to anticipate that a variety of synergistic and additive effects may be induced by combining different agents. For example, combination treatment with anti-CD3 epsilon specific antibody and intranasal delivery of proinsulin peptide could reverse recent onset diabetes in nonobese diabetic mice as well as in a virus-induced diabetic mouse model with much higher efficacy than monotherapy using anti-CD3 or peptide alone [71]. Protection was associated with expansion of $CD25^{+}$ $Foxp3^{+}$ and insulin specific T regulatory cells producing protective cytokines, such as interleukin-10, transforming growth factor-beta, and interleukin-4. In addition, these cells can transfer dominant tolerance to recent onset diabetic recipients, and suppress heterologous autoaggressive CD8 T cell responses. While animal studies do provide a rationale for combining therapies, there are hurdles that still need to be overcome for translation to the clinic. For example, the possibility of unforeseen drug interactions is not in the interest of pharmaceutical and biotech companies and could stop them from evaluating their drugs in combination trials [72].

3.2. Heat shock protein 60 /65 DNA vaccines

Heat shock protein 60 (HSP60) is a 60-kilodalton mammalian protein that promotes the proper folding of mitochondrial proteins and a possible autoantigen in type 1 diabetic children and murine models [73, 74]. Epitope scanning of heat shock protein 60 with antibodies identified peptide DiaPep277 with the amino sequence VLGGGVALLRVIPALDSLTPANED as an immunodominant epitope in type 1 diabetic child patients [75, 76]. From an immunological standpoint, mammalian heat shock proteins can also act as damage-associated molecular patterns that are released or presented by dying cells and can activate antigen-presenting cells of the innate immune system [77]. Heat shock proteins activate macrophages and dendritic cells through Toll-like receptor 4, which belongs to a class of membrane-bound proteins that act as sensors for immune cell activation, and promote proinflammatory effector immune responses. Paradoxically, heat shock proteins can also mediate anti-inflammatory response through Toll-like receptor 2 on T cells, and DiaPep277 peptide functions through a Toll-like receptor 2-mediated mechanism [78].

Plasmid DNA coding for heat shock protein 60 has been shown to prevent type 1 diabetes in mice. For example, two times 100 microgram intramuscular injections of plasmid DNA coding for mammalian heat shock protein 60 into 4-week old nonobese diabetic mice suppressed cyclophosphamide-accelerated diabetes, with 30% of treated mice developing diabetes compared with 60% in vector treated controls [79]. Disease prevention was associated with reduced T cell proliferation, increased in interleukin-10 and interleukin-5 secretion, and decreased interferon-gamma secretion, which suggested a shift from a T helper-1 like toward a T helper-2 like immune response.

In addition, plasmid DNA encoding mycobacterial 65-kilodalton heat shock protein could also affect diabetes by causing decreased insulitis when injected intramuscularly in three doses (100 microgram each) at 2-week intervals into 6- to 8-week-old, streptozotocin-induced diabetic C57BL/6 mice [80]. The treatment was associated with the appearance of a regulatory cell population in the spleen, with higher production of interleukin-10 in the spleen and islets, and with a decreased infiltration of CD8 T lymphocytes in the islets. The same DNA vaccine with the same dose and delivery reduced the occurrence of diabetes from 100% to 33% in 28-week old nonobese diabetic mice when injected at 4-week of age, and was associated with a reduction in CD4 and CD8 T cells infiltration, appearance of CD25 cells, and increased levels of interleukin-10 in pancreatic islets [81].

3.3. Glutamic acid decarboxylase DNA vaccines

Glutamic acid decarboxylase 65 is an enzyme that catalyzes the synthesis of gamma-amino-butyric acid (GABA) which acts as a neuroinhibitor as well as an immunoregulatory molecule. Evidence indicates that glutamic acid decarboxylase 65 may have a critical early role in mediating islet beta cell destruction and is an important target autoantigen in type 1 diabetes. Detection of anti-glutamic acid decarboxylase antibodies in the sera of prediabetic patients is a reliable predictive marker for the progression to overt diabetes, and anti-glutamic acid decarboxylase reactivity can be detected in nonobese diabetic mice model early in the disease process [82, 83].

Plasmid DNA vaccines coding for glutamic acid decarboxylase 65 are currently at the preclinical stage. The first report of a beneficial effect in nonobese diabetic mice showed that plasmid DNA encoding wild-type intracellular or engineered secreted glutamic acid decarboxylase, i.e., a fusion of the interleukin-2 signal peptide with a truncated form of human glutamic acid decarboxylase 65, caused decreased insulitis compared to plasmid vector alone when delivered intramuscularly, and was accompanied by elevated secretion of interleukin-4 by splenocytes [84]. A subsequent report indicated that only the DNA vaccine encoding secreted glutamic acid decarboxylase could suppress cyclophosphamide-accelerated diabetes in 4-week old female nonobese diabetic mice with a tendency to increase T helper-2 like activity when two times 400 microgram were delivered intramuscularly over 3 days [85].

A report published the same year corroborated the notion that secretion of glutamic acid decarboxylase encoded by a DNA vaccine is important to ameliorate diabetes in mice [86]. In this report, plasmid DNA was engineered to encode a secreted fusion protein of a truncated form of glutamic acid decarboxylase 65 and an IgG Fc fragment as well as interleukin-4. Intramuscular injection of 50 microgram of the vaccine effectively prevented diabetes in nonobese diabetic mice treated at early (4-week old, 3 times weekly) or late (12-week old, 4 times weekly) preclinical stages of diabetes. Diabetic onset reduction went from 75% in controls to 25% in treated animals at week 50. Protection was dependent on interleukin-4 as well as endogenous interleukin-4, and associated with the induction of glutamic acid decarboxylase 65 specific regulatory T helper-2 cells [87]. In addition, the same strategy was used with insulin as the target autoantigen. In this case, the DNA vaccine encoding an insulin B chain/IgG Fc fusion protein and interleukin-4 caused accelerated progression of insulitis and diabetes, which correlated with increased numbers of interferon-gamma secreting T cells in response to insulin B chain specific peptides. On the other hand, a group reported that a DNA vaccine encoding full-length intracellular human glutamic acid decarboxylase 65 alone could prevent spontaneous diabetes in nonobese diabetic mice when delivered at 4 or 10 weeks of age using intramuscular injections of two times 50 microgram DNA [88]. Notably, disease prevention was associated with CD28/B7 costimulation because co-expression of B7-1 or B7-2 and glutamic acid decarboxylase 65 by the same DNA vaccine abrogated protection. Another study investigated the relationship between endogenous expression levels of glutamic acid decarboxylase in beta-cells and the efficacy of DNA vaccination [89]. Injection of plasmid DNA coding for glutamic acid decarboxylase into mice with lower expression levels of the autoantigen resulted in the induction of autosuppressive regulatory cells characterized by increased interleukin-4 production (T helper-2 like). In contrast, higher levels of the autoantigen favored T helper-1-like autoaggressive responses characterized by increased the interferon-gamma generation. Immunization with a DNA vaccine coding the glutamic acid decarboxylase and interleukin-4 reduced the risk of augmenting autoaggression and thus increased the safety of this immune-based therapy.

DNA vaccines encoding secreted glutamic acid decarboxylase combined with anti-inflammatory interleukins have also been applied to pancreatic transplant for type 1 diabetes. Survival of syngeneic neonatal pancreata transplanted under the kidney capsule of nonobese diabetic mice was promoted by intramuscular injection of a DNA vaccine encoding the secreted glutamic acid decarboxylase 65/IgG Fc fusion and interleukin-4 plus interleukin-10 [90]. The treatment consisted of 50 microgram of the vaccine delivered weekly for four weeks from the age of 10 weeks with transplantation performed one week after the final DNA vaccination. DNA vaccination protected syngeneic islet in transplanted mice, with 100% diabetic mice in controls compared to 20% diabetes incidence in treated animals at 30 weeks of age and 15 weeks post transplant. Increased islet survival required co-delivery of both interleukin-4 and interleukin-10 and correlated with a marked reduction in interferon-gamma reactivity as well as an increase in interleukin-10 secreting T cells. These results made apparent the increased difficulty in protecting exogenous syngeneic islet and the need for more stringent conditions of vaccination in the transplantation setting.

Most DNA vaccines for type 1 diabetes have been delivered into muscle tissue. The main rationale for using this route of delivery is that it permits administration of larger amounts of DNA, but other routes may be more advantageous to induce tolerogenic responses. In that regard, a report compared intramuscular, intradermal, and oral delivery of plasmid DNA coding for the intracellular or secreted form of glutamic acid decarboxylase for prevention of diabetes in 4-week-old nonobese diabetic mice [91]. Results indicated that both intradermal and oral deliveries were more effective than intramuscular delivery for delaying the disease. Cytokine-specific ELISpot analysis indicated that immune responses induced by the DNA vaccination were generally more dependent on the cellular localization of glutamic acid decarboxylase antigen than on the delivery route, although ELISA indicated that intradermal delivery of DNA is most likely to induce a T helper-2 like response.

In addition to route of delivery, the method used to administer a DNA vaccine can be beneficial by increasing efficacy of DNA uptake and improving immune responses. For example, dermal delivery of plasmid DNA using gene gun technology, which consists in shooting gold microparticles covered with DNA, can improve protection from diabetes. In this regard, gene-gun delivery of 1 microgram of a DNA vaccine encoding the secreted glutamic acid decarboxylase

65/IgG Fc fusion polypeptide into 10-week old nonobese diabetic mice was compared with intramuscular injection of 50 microgram of the same vaccine [92]. Results indicated that, in both cases, gene expression peaked at week 8 post deliveries and was maintained until at least week 35 with more than 40% higher expression from the gene-gun delivery. However, only gene-gun delivery protected mice from diabetes with 90% diabetic animals in controls down to 50% diabetic mice at 35 weeks of age. In contrast, gene-gun administration of plasmid DNA encoding intracellular glutamic acid decarboxylase 65 to 3-week old nonobese diabetic mice did not suppress diabetes in nonobese diabetic mice [93]. The different results might be attributed to the different subcellular localizations of the autoantigen.

As mentioned earlier, combination therapy is being increasingly considered as a means to improve efficacy of immunotherapy for type 1 diabetes. Combining a DNA vaccine coding for intracellular GAD65 with an anti-CD3 monoclonal antibody has been investigated in two different mouse model systems for that purpose [94]. Results indicated that successful treatment was observed in a virus-induced diabetic model (the RIP-LCMV-GP model) but not the nonobese diabetic mouse. Efficacy was associated with an expansion of bystander suppressor T regulatory cells recognizing the C-terminal region of GAD65 and secreting interleukin-10, transforming growth factor-beta and interferon-gamma. These results also showed that efficacy was associated with numbers of antigen-specific T cells available at time of treatment, which was different beween the two animal models. The findings hold important implications to predict the success of antigen-based clinical trials where responsiveness to immunotherapy may vary from patient to patient.

Thus far, we have described in this section how DNA vaccines can be engineered to enhance tolerogenic-like immune responses by co-delivering cytokine-encoding DNA, an antibody, engineering subcellular localization of a target autoantigen, and choosing an effective route and method of delivery. These results obtained by different laboratories illustrate the promising potential of DNA vaccination as a safe, low-cost and patient-friendly means to treat autoimmune diabetes and other immune-mediated inflammatory disorders. Yet, as with all immunotherapies that seek means of improving the life of diabetic individuals, there is a pressing need to improve treatment efficacy through the identification of novel molecular adjuvants for the safe induction of immune tolerance.

Ideally, these adjuvants should attempt to mimic how immune tolerance is maintained in steady state. Here, we briefly discuss plasmid-induced apoptosis as a possible means to mimic physiological immune tolerance and to approach the "Holy Grail" of immunotherapy, namely, the ability to suppress inflammation in a homeostatic manner. Apoptosis is a constantly ongoing form of cell death that produces fifty to seventy billion dead cells on a daily basis in an average human adult [95]. Upon a given intrinsic or extrinsic signal, cells initiate the process of apoptosis and become membrane-bound cellular fragments, or apoptotic bodies, which are rapidly engulfed and processed by surrounding living cells. For many years, it was believed that these apoptotic bodies had little effect on the immune system. Today, it has become clear that apoptosis is an important physiological means to establish and maintain immune tolerance in peripheral tissues. Apoptotic cells play a fundamental role as they not only serve as a source of self-antigens, but also recruit antigen-presenting cells, secrete anti-inflammatory cytokines, and display tolerogenic molecules [96]. The remarkable capacity of apoptotic cells to induce either tolerogenic immune responses or immunogenic responses depending on signals received makes them attractive candidates to intervene in many disorders like infectious diseases, cancer, and autoimmune diseases.

The first report of DNA vaccines designed for pro-apoptotic immunoregulation, i.e., anti-inflammatory, used plasmid DNA coding for the pro-apoptotic BAX protein and intracellular or secreted glutamic acid decarboxylase, to prevent diabetes in the nonobese diabetic mouse [97]. Results indicated that intramuscular injection of the BAX cDNA recruited dendritic cells carrying vaccine-encoded protein in both spleen and lymph nodes. Furthermore, delivery of two times 150 microgram plasmid DNA coding for secreted glutamic acid decarboxylase and BAX at 3 days interval into 4-week old mice prevented diabetes, i.e, reduced the incidence from 93% in controls down to 47% in treated animals. In contrast, the vaccines coding for BAX DNA alone or intracellular glutamic acid decarboxylase and BAX did not prevent diabetes. Notably, ELISA results suggested that co-delivery of BAX suppressed T helper-2 like activity, which indicated that another cell type was responsible for disease suppression. Indeed, a subsequent report showed that delivery of both secreted glutamic acid decarboxylase and BAX were required to induce $CD4^{+}CD25^{+}FoxP3^{+}$ cells with contact dependent regulatory activity [98].

Importantly, additional studies revealed that increased CpG methylation of plasmid DNA together with delivery of secreted glutamic acid decarboxylase and BAX DNA could act synergistically to ameliorate recent onset diabetes in nonobese diabetic mice [99]. A weekly intradermal injection of 50 microgram of the vaccine over eight weeks following early hyperglycemia ameliorated diabetes at 40 weeks of age, from 90% diabetic mice in controls down to 20% in treated mice. Remarkably, DNA hypermethylation caused increased numbers of tolerogenic-like plasmacytoid dendritic cells in lymph nodes. It is hypothesized that increased CpG methylation of plasmid DNA makes the DNA vaccine appear more mammalian-like to the immune system, as it is known that bacterial DNA has low levels of CpG methylation that can act as an inflammatory signal [100]. Taken together these results indicate that apoptosis-inducing DNA vaccination is a promising approach for treatment of type 1 diabetes.

3.4. Other DNA vaccines

DNA vaccines encoding less studied autoantigens have also been investigated. For example, insulinoma-associated protein 2 (IA-2), which is expressed in islets, brain, and neuro-endocrine cells, is a member of the protein tyrosine phosphatase family and targeted by autoimmune T cells in type 1 diabetes. A DNA vaccine encoding insulinoma-associated protein 2 with or without the combination of DNA coding for interleukin-4 and monocyte chemoattractant protein-1 (MCP-1) was injected intramuscularly into pre-diabetic non-obese diabetic mice using 3 x 100 microgram DNA delivered over four weeks [101]. The treatment could protect mice from diabetes, from 60% in controls to 10-20% diabetic animals at 30 weeks of age. There was no difference in efficacy between groups treated with the DNA vaccine alone or combined

http://dx.doi.org/10.5772/55727

with interleukin 4/MCP1, and animals in both groups had fewer CD8 T lymphocyte counts in spleen.

In another example, a DNA vaccine treatment strategy was designed to target an antigenic peptide (glucose-6-phosphate isomerase, GPI) to the lysosomal compartment. A specific T cell population termed 2.5mi$^+$ T cells is known to share reactivity with the diabetogenic T cell clone BDC-2.5 in the NOD mouse [102]. Lysosome targeting of single peptide epitope was sufficient to induce protection against type 1 diabetes which was not the result of antigen-specific T cell anergy. Typical T helper-2 cytokines like interleukin-10 or -4 were undetectable in 2.5mi$^+$ T cells, arguing against a mechanism of immune deviation. Instead, the expanded 2.5mi$^+$ T cell population produced interferon-gamma similar to 2.5mi$^+$ T cells from naive mice. Protection against diabetes induced by DNA vaccination was completely lost in NOD.CD28$^{-/-}$ mice, which are largely deficient of natural T regulatory cells. Furthermore, diabetes onset was delayed in T regulatory-reconstituted and DNA-treated NOD.SCID mice, although antigen-specific Foxp3$^+$ cells did not expand in response to DNA treatment. These findings indicated a T regulatory-mediated protective mechanism that was independent of the expansion or de novo generation of antigen-specific T regulatory cells.

3.5. Summary of section 3

DNA vaccination has been tested in clinical trials for treatment of new-onset type 1 diabetes with encouraging results, but efficacy must be improved. The number and variety of strategies that have been developed to improve efficacy of DNA vaccination for autoimmune diabetes is a testament to the flexibility and potential of DNA vaccine immunotherapy.

4. Conclusion: Plasmid DNA as a promising immunotherapy for Type 1 diabetes

Plasmid DNA is a versatile vector platform permitting the seamless integration of different immune modulators into a product that can be manufactured in a generic manner. As we have seen in this chapter, plasmid DNA has been extensively investigated for the prevention and treatment of type 1 diabetes in different animal model systems. Plasmid DNA-based gene immunotherapies do not encode an autoantigen and act systemically to different degrees, which could result in serious adverse events if used over time. Nevertheless, gene immunotherapies could still be utilized as molecular adjuvants with DNA vaccines that target pancreatic beta cell autoantigens. It is possible that different stages during progression of disease will require different therapeutic agents or combinations thereof according to immune responses to therapy. It is also anticipated that some strategies will be safer and more robust than others, but there is unfortunately no animal model that can predict successful bench-to-bedside translation of a given strategy. In that regard, immunological biomarkers and their pre-clinical and clinical correlates will be needed to determine which strategies are most likely to be effective in humans, and to what extent different immunotherapies might be combined. Combinatorial therapies include co-delivery of DNA vaccines with gene therapy, peptide vaccines, monoclonal antibodies, and other adjuvant agents that have shown synergistic effects. In one possible scenario, autoantigen-specific immunotherapies could be used over the long-term as stand-alone treatments, with the occasional help of systemic immune modulators depending on disease severity. Regardless of the strategy to be chosen, there is a strong case to be made for including plasmid DNA immunotherapy in future treatments of type 1 diabetes.

Author details

Alice Li[1] and Alan Escher[2]

1 Loma Linda University, Loma Linda, California, USA

2 SEKRIS Biomedical Inc., Redlands, California, USA

References

[1] Stiller CR, Dupré J, Gent M, Jenner MR, Keown PA, Laupacis A, Martell R, Rodger NW, von Graffenried B, Wolfe BM. Effects of cyclosporine immunosuppression in insulin-dependent diabetes mellitus of recent onset. Science. 1984;223(4643):1362-7.

[2] Long SA, Rieck M, Sanda S, Bollyky JB, Samuels PL, Goland R, Ahmann A, Rabinovitch A, Aggarwal S, Phippard D, Turka LA, Ehlers MR, Bianchine PJ, Boyle KD, Adah SA, Bluestone JA, Buckner JH, Greenbaum CJ; Diabetes TrialNet and the Immune Tolerance Network. Rapamycin/IL-2 combination therapy in patients with type 1 diabetes augments Tregs yet transiently impairs β-cell function. Diabetes. 2012;61(9):2340-8.

[3] Kasi PM, Tawbi HA, Oddis CV, Kulkarni HS. Clinical review: Serious adverse events associated with the use of rituximab - a critical care perspective. Crit Care. 2012;16(4): 231.

[4] Lichtenstein GR, Feagan BG, Cohen RD, Salzberg BA, Diamond RH, Price S, Langholff W, Londhe A, Sandborn WJ. Serious infection and mortality in patients with Crohn's disease: more than 5 years of follow-up in the TREAT™ registry. Am J Gastroenterol. 2012;107(9):1409-22.

[5] von Herrath MG, Harrison LC. Antigen-induced regulatory T cells in autoimmunity. Nat Rev Immunol. 2003;3(3):223-32.

[6] Liu Y, Huang H, Saxena A, Xiang J. Intratumoral coinjection of two adenoviral vectors expressing functional interleukin-18 and inducible protein-10, respectively, synergizes to facilitate regression of established tumors. Cancer Gene Ther. 2002;9(6): 533-42.

[7] Pedotti R, Sanna M, Tsai M, DeVoss J, Steinman L, McDevitt H, Galli SJ. Severe anaphylactic reactions to glutamic acid decarboxylase (GAD) self peptides in NOD mice that spontaneously develop autoimmune type 1 diabetes mellitus. BMC Immunol. 2003;4:2.

[8] Tyagi RK, Garg NK, Sahu T. Vaccination Strategies against Malaria: novel carrier(s) more than a tour de force. J Control Release. 2012;162(1):242-54.

[9] Goldmann K, Ensminger SM, Spriewald BM. Oral gene application using chitosan-DNA nanoparticles induces transferable tolerance. Clin Vaccine Immunol. 2012;19(11):1758-64.

[10] Gramzinski RA, Millan CL, Obaldia N, Hoffman SL, Davis HL. Immune response to a hepatitis B DNA vaccine in Aotus monkeys: a comparison of vaccine formulation, route, and method of administration. Mol Med. 1998;4(2):109-18.

[11] Hu H, Lu X, Tao L, Bai B, Zhang Z, Chen Y, Zheng F, Chen J, Chen Z, Wang H. Induction of specific immune responses by severe acute respiratory syndrome coronavirus spike DNA vaccine with or without interleukin-2 immunization using different vaccination routes in mice. Clin Vaccine Immunol. 2007;14(7):894-901.

[12] Ginsberg BA, Gallardo HF, Rasalan TS, Adamow M, Mu Z, Tandon S, Bewkes BB, Roman RA, Chapman PB, Schwartz GK, Carvajal RD, Panageas KS, Terzulli SL, Houghton AN, Yuan JD, Wolchok JD. Immunologic response to xenogeneic gp100 DNA in melanoma patients: comparison of particle-mediated epidermal delivery with intramuscular injection. Clin Cancer Res. 2010;16(15):4057-65.

[13] Culina S, Boitard C, Mallone R. Antigen-based immune therapeutics for type 1 diabetes: magic bullets or ordinary blanks? Clinical & Developmental Immunology. 2011;2011:286248.

[14] Abdulhaqq SA, Weiner DB. DNA vaccines: developing new strategies to enhance immune responses. Immunology Reviews. 2008;42(1-3):219-32.

[15] Garren H. DNA vaccines for autoimmune diseases. Expert Review of Vaccines. 2009;8(9):1195-203.

[16] Siatskas C, Chan J, Field J, Murphy K, Nasa Z, Toh BH, Alderuccio F. Gene therapy strategies towards immune tolerance to treat the autoimmune diseases. Current Gene Therapy. 2006;6(1):45-58.

[17] Johnson MC, Wang B, Tisch R. Genetic vaccination for re-establishing T-cell tolerance in type 1 diabetes. Human Vaccine. 2011;7(1):27-36.

[18] Cameron MJ, Strathdee CA, Holmes KD, Arreaza GA, Dekaban GA, Delovitch TL. Biolistic-mediated interleukin 4 gene transfer prevents the onset of type 1 diabetes. Human Gene Therapy. 2000;11(12):1647-56.

[19] Lee M, Koh JJ, Han SO, Ko KS, Ki SW. Prevention of autoimmune insulitis by delivery of interleukin-4 plasmid using a soluble and biodegradable polymeric carrier. Pharmaceutical research. 2002;19(3):246-9.

[20] Hayashi T, Yasutomi Y, Hasegawa K, Sasaki Y, Onodera T. Interleukin-4-expressing plasmid DNA inhibits reovirus type-2-triggered autoimmune insulitis in DBA/1 J suckling mice. International Journal of Experimental Pathology. 2003;84(2):101-6.

[21] Horiki M, Yamato E, Noso S, Ikegami H, Ogihara T, Miyazaki J. High-level expression of interleukin-4 following electroporation-mediated gene transfer accelerates Type 1 diabetes in NOD mice. Journal of Autoimmunity. 2003;20(2):111-7.

[22] Nitta Y, Tashiro F, Tokui M, Shimada A, Takei I, Tabayashi K, Miyazaki J. Systemic delivery of interleukin 10 by intramuscular injection of expression plasmid DNA prevents autoimmune diabetes in nonobese diabetic mice. Human Gene Therapy. 1998;9(12):1701-7.

[23] Koh JJ, Ko KS, Lee M, Han S, Park JS, Kim SW. Degradable polymeric carrier for the delivery of IL-10 plasmid DNA to prevent autoimmune insulitis of NOD mice. Gene Therapy. 2000;7(24):2099-104.

[24] Zhang ZL, Shen SX, Lin B, Yu LY, Zhu LH, Wang WP, Luo FH, Guo LH. Intramuscular injection of interleukin-10 plasmid DNA prevented autoimmune diabetes in mice. Acta Pharmacologica Sinica. 2003;24(8):751-6.

[25] Lee M, Park H, Youn J, Oh ET, Ko K, Kim S, Park Y. Interleukin-10 plasmid construction and delivery for the prevention of type 1 diabetes. Annals of the New York Academy of Sciences. 2006;1079:313-9.

[26] Basarkar A, Singh J. Poly (lactide-co-glycolide)-polymethacrylate nanoparticles for intramuscular delivery of plasmid encoding interleukin-10 to prevent autoimmune diabetes in mice. Pharmaceutical research. 2009;26(1):72-81.

[27] Ko KS, Lee M, Koh JJ, Kim SW. Combined administration of plasmids encoding IL-4 and IL-10 prevents the development of autoimmune diabetes in nonobese diabetic mice. Molecular Therapy. 2001;4(4):313-6.

[28] Lee M, Ko KS, Oh S, Kim SW. Prevention of autoimmune insulitis by delivery of a chimeric plasmid encoding interleukin-4 and interleukin-10. Journal of controlled release. 2003;88(2):333-42.

[29] Mandke R, Singh J. Cationic nanomicelles for delivery of plasmids encoding interleukin-4 and interleukin-10 for prevention of autoimmune diabetes in mice. Pharmaceutical research. 2012;29(3):883-97.

[30] Kovarik P, Sauer I, Schaljo B. Molecular mechanisms of the anti-inflammatory functions of interferons. Immunobiology. 2007;212(9-10):895-901.

[31] Tokui, M., A. Shimada, O. Funae, H. Nomaguchi, H. Okamura, I. Takei, and T. Saruta. 1998. Recombinant IL-18 administration suppresses cyclophosphamide- induced diabetes in NOD mice. Diabetes 47:A9862.

[32] Rothe H, Hausmann A, Casteels K, Okamura H, Kurimoto M, Burkart V, Mathieu C, Kolb H. IL-18 inhibits diabetes development in nonobese diabetic mice by counterregulation of Th1-dependent destructive insulitis. J Immunol. 1999;163(3):1230-6.

[33] Oikawa Y, Shimada A, Kasuga A, Morimoto J, Osaki T, Tahara H, Miyazaki T, Tashiro F, Yamato E, Miyazaki J, Saruta T. Systemic administration of IL-18 promotes diabetes development in young nonobese diabetic mice. Journal of Immunology. 2003;171(11):5865-75.

[34] Hasegawa K, Hayashi T, Maeda K, Onodera T. Plasmid encoding interferon-gamma exacerbates reovirus type-2-induced diabetes in DBA/1 suckling mice. Journal of Comparative Pathology. 2002;127(2-3):203-7.

[35] Zhang J, Huang Z, Sun R, Tian Z, Wei H. IFN-γ induced by IL-12 administration prevents diabetes by inhibiting pathogenic IL-17 production inNOD mice.J Autoimmun. 2012 ;38(1):20-8.

[36] Laing KJ, Secombes CJ. Chemokines. Developmental and comparative immunology. 2004 May 3;28(5):443-60.

[37] Sallusto F, Lenig D, Mackay CR, Lanzavecchia A. Flexible programs of chemokine receptor expression on human polarized T helper 1 and 2 lymphocytes. Journal of Experimental Medicine. 1998;187(6):875-83.

[38] D'Ambrosio D, Iellem A, Bonecchi R, Mazzeo D, Sozzani S, Mantovani A, Sinigaglia F. Selective up-regulation of chemokine receptors CCR4 and CCR8 upon activation of polarized human type 2 Th cells. Journal of Immunology. 1998;161(10):5111-5.

[39] Shimada A, Morimoto J, Kodama K, Suzuki R, Oikawa Y, Funae O, Kasuga A, Saruta T, Narumi S. Elevated serum IP-10 levels observed in type 1 diabetes. Diabetes Care. 2001;24(3):510-5.

[40] Morimoto J, Yoneyama H, Shimada A, Shigihara T, Yamada S, Oikawa Y, Matsushima K, Saruta T, Narumi S. CXC chemokine ligand 10 neutralization suppresses the occurrence of diabetes in nonobese diabetic mice through enhanced beta cell proliferation without affecting insulitis. Journal of Immunology. 2004;173(11):7017-24.

[41] Christen U, McGavern DB, Luster AD, von Herrath MG, Oldstone MB. Among CXCR3 chemokines, IFN-gamma-inducible protein of 10 kDa (CXC chemokine ligand (CXCL) 10) but not monokine induced by IFN-gamma (CXCL9) imprints a pattern for the subsequent development of autoimmune disease. Journal of Immunology. 2003;171(12):6838-45.

[42] Shigihara T, Shimada A, Oikawa Y, Yoneyama H, Kanazawa Y, Okubo Y, Matsushima K, Yamato E, Miyazaki J, Kasuga A, Saruta T, Narumi S. CXCL10 DNA vaccina-

tion prevents spontaneous diabetes through enhanced beta cell proliferation in NOD mice. Journal of Immunology. 2005;175(12):8401-8.

[43] Oikawa Y, Shimada A, Yamada Y, Okubo Y, Katsuki T, Shigihara T, Miyazaki J, Narumi S, Itoh H. CXC chemokine ligand 10 DNA vaccination plus Complete Freund's Adjuvant reverses hyperglycemia in non-obese diabetic mice. Review Of Diabetic Studies. 2010;7(3):209-24.

[44] Cameron MJ, Arreaza GA, Grattan M, Meagher C, Sharif S, Burdick MD, Strieter RM, Cook DN, Delovitch TL. Differential expression of CC chemokines and the CCR5 receptor in the pancreas is associated with progression to type I diabetes. Journal of Immunology. 2000;165(2):1102-10.

[45] Meagher C, Arreaza G, Peters A, Strathdee CA, Gilbert PA, Mi QS, Santamaria P, Dekaban GA, Delovitch TL. CCL4 protects from type 1 diabetes by altering islet beta-cell-targeted inflammatory responses. Diabetes. 2007;56(3):809-17.

[46] Sgouroudis E, Piccirillo CA. Control of type 1 diabetes by CD4+Foxp3+ regulatory T cells: lessons from mouse models and implications for human disease. Diabetes/Metabolism Research and Reviews. 2009;25(3):208-18.

[47] Luczyński W, Stasiak-Barmuta A, Urban R, Urban M, Florys B, Hryszko M. Lower percentages of T regulatory cells in children with type 1 diabetes - preliminary report. Pediatric endocrinology, diabetes, and metabolism. 2009;15(1):34-8.

[48] Chou FC, Shieh SJ, Sytwu HK. Attenuation of Th1 response through galectin-9 and T-cell Ig mucin 3 interaction inhibits autoimmune diabetes in NOD mice. European journal of immunology. 2009;39(9):2403-11.

[49] Sung HH, Juang JH, Lin YC, Kuo CH, Hung JT, Chen A, Chang DM, Chang SY, Hsieh SL, Sytwu HK. Transgenic expression of decoy receptor 3 protects islets from spontaneous and chemical-induced autoimmune destruction in nonobese diabetic mice. Journal of Experimental Medicine. 2004;199(8):1143-51.

[50] Wang YL, Chou FC, Sung HH, Fan PL, Hsueh CW, Lin WC, Chen SJ, Lin WW, Sytwu HK. Decoy receptor 3 protects non-obese diabetic mice from autoimmune diabetes by regulating dendritic cell maturation and function. Molecular Immunology. 2010;47(16):2552-62.

[51] Weiss L, Botero-Anug AM, Hand C, Slavin S, Naor D. CD44 gene vaccination for insulin-dependent diabetes mellitus in non-obese diabetic mice. Israel Medical Association Journal. 2008;10(1):20-5.

[52] Donato J. The Central Nervous System As A Promising Target To Treat Diabetes Mellitus. Curr Top Med Chem. 2012 Nov 12. [Epub ahead of print]

[53] Sun W, Wang L, Zhang Z, Chen M, Wang X. Intramuscular transfer of naked calcitonin gene-related peptide gene prevents autoimmune diabetes induced by multiple

low-dose streptozotocin in C57BL mice. European Journal Of Immunology. 2003;33(1):233-42.

[54] Fahrenkrug J, Emson PC. Vasoactive intestinal polypeptide: functional aspects. Br Med Bull. 1982;38(3):265-70.

[55] Delgado M, Abad C, Martinez C, Juarranz MG, Arranz A, Gomariz RP, Leceta J. Vasoactive intestinal peptide in the immune system: potential therapeutic role in inflammatory and autoimmune diseases. Journal of molecular medicine. 2002;80(1):16-24.

[56] Pozo D, Delgado M. The many faces of VIP in neuroimmunology: a cytokine rather a neuropeptide? Federation of American Societies for Experimental Biology. 2004;18(12):1325-34.

[57] Herrera JL, Fernández-Montesinos R, González-Rey E, Delgado M, Pozo D. Protective role for plasmid DNA-mediated VIP gene transfer in non-obese diabetic mice. Annals of the New York Academy of Sciences. 2006;1070:337-41.

[58] Pozo D, Anderson P, Gonzalez-Rey E. Induction of alloantigen-specific human T regulatory cells by vasoactive intestinal peptide. Journal of Immunology. 2009;183(7): 4346-59.

[59] Bluestone JA, Herold K, Eisenbarth G. Genetics, pathogenesis and clinical interventions in type 1 diabetes. Nature. 2010;464(7293):1293-300.

[60] Coon B, An LL, Whitton JL, von Herrath MG. DNA immunization to prevent autoimmune diabetes. Journal of Clinical Investigation. 1999;104(2):189-94.

[61] Bot A, Smith D, Bot S, Hughes A, Wolfe T, Wang L, Woods C, von Herrath M. Plasmid vaccination with insulin B chain prevents autoimmune diabetes in nonobese diabetic mice. Journal of immunology. 2001;167(5):2950-5.

[62] Every AL, Kramer DR, Mannering SI, Lew AM, Harrison LC. Intranasal vaccination with proinsulin DNA induces regulatory CD4+ T cells that prevent experimental autoimmune diabetes. J Immunol. 2006;176(8):4608-15.

[63] Zhang W, Jin H, Hu Y, Yu Y, Li X, Ding Z, Kang Y, Wang B. Protective response against type 1 diabetes in nonobese diabetic mice after coimmunization with insulin and DNA encoding proinsulin. Human Gene Therapy. 2010;21(2):171-8.

[64] Hou WR, Xie SN, Wang HJ, Su YY, Lu JL, Li LL, Zhang SS, Xiang M. Intramuscular delivery of a naked DNA plasmid encoding proinsulin and pancreatic regenerating III protein ameliorates type 1 diabetes mellitus. Pharmaceutical Research. 2011;63(4): 320-7.

[65] Prud'homme GJ, Chang Y, Li X. Immunoinhibitory DNA vaccine protects against autoimmune diabetes through cDNA encoding a selective CTLA-4 (CD152) ligand. Hum Gene Ther. 2002;13(3):395-406.

[66] Solvason N, Lou YP, Peters W, Evans E, Martinez J, Ramirez U, Ocampo A, Yun R, Ahmad S, Liu E, Yu L, Eisenbarth G, Leviten M, Steinman L, Garren H. Improved

efficacy of a tolerizing DNA vaccine for reversal of hyperglycemia through enhancement of gene expression and localization to intracellular sites. Journal of Immunology. 2008;181(12):8298-307.

[67] Urbanek-Ruiz I, Ruiz PJ, Paragas V, Garren H, Steinman L, Fathman CG. Immunization with DNA encoding an immunodominant peptide of insulin prevents diabetes in NOD mice. Clin Immunol. 2001;100(2):164-71.

[68] Gottlieb P, Eisenbarth G, Kipnes M, Ratner R, Rockell J, Wagner R, Solvason N, Tersini K, Valone F, Woody K, Steinman L, Garren H. Interim Results of a Phase I/II Clinical Trial of a DNA Plasmid Vaccine (BHT-3021) for Type 1 Diabetes. 2008. URL: http://www.bayhilltx.com/abstracts.html

[69] Li L, Yi Z, Tisch R, Wang B. Immunotherapy of type 1 diabetes. Archivum Immunologiae et Therapiae Experimentalis. 2008;56(4):227-36.

[70] Luo X, Herold KC, Miller SD. Immunotherapy of type 1 diabetes: where are we and where should we be going? Immunity. 2010;32(4):488-99.

[71] Bresson D, Togher L, Rodrigo E, Chen Y, Bluestone JA, Herold KC, and von Herrath M. Anti-CD3 and nasal proinsulin combination therapy enhances remission from recent-onset autoimmune diabetes by inducing Tregs. Journal of Clinical Investigation. 2006;116(5):1371-81.

[72] Matthews JB, Staeva TP, Bernstein PL, Peakman M, von Herrath M; ITN-JDRF Type 1 Diabetes Combination Therapy Assessment Group. Developing combination immunotherapies for type 1 diabetes: recommendations from the ITN-JDRF Type 1 Diabetes Combination Therapy Assessment Group. Clin Exp Immunol. 2010;160(2): 176-84.

[73] Birk OS, Elias D, Weiss AS, Rosen A, van-der Zee R, Walker MD, Cohen IR. NOD mouse diabetes: the ubiquitous mouse hsp60 is a beta-cell target antigen of autoimmune T cells. J Autoimmun. 1996;9(2):159-66.

[74] Horváth L, Cervenak L, Oroszlán M, Prohászka Z, Uray K, Hudecz F, Baranyi E, Madácsy L, Singh M, Romics L, Füst G, Pánczél P. Antibodies against different epitopes of heat-shock protein 60 in children with type 1 diabetes mellitus. Immunology Letters. 2002;80(3):155-62.

[75] Eldor R, Kassem S, Raz I. Immune modulation in type 1 diabetes mellitus using DiaPep277: a short review and update of recent clinical trial results. Diabetes/Metabolism Research and Reviews. 2009;25(4):316-20.

[76] Fischer B, Elias D, Bretzel RG, Linn T. Immunomodulation with heat shock protein DiaPep277 to preserve beta cell function in type 1 diabetes - an update. Expert Opinion on Biological Therapy. 2010;10(2):265-72.

[77] Chen W, Syldath U, Bellmann K, Burkart V, Kolb H. Human 60-kDa heat-shock protein: a danger signal to the innate immune system. Journal of Immunology. 1999;162(6):3212-9.

[78] Nussbaum G, Zanin-Zhorov A, Quintana F, Lider O, Cohen IR. Peptide p277 of HSP60 signals T cells: inhibition of inflammatory chemotaxis. Int Immunol. 2006;18(10):1413-9.

[79] Quintana FJ, Carmi P, Cohen IR. DNA vaccination with heat shock protein 60 inhibits cyclophosphamide-accelerated diabetes. Journal of Immunology. 2002;169(10): 6030-5.

[80] Santos RR Junior, Sartori A, Lima DS, Souza PR, Coelho-Castelo AA, Bonato VL, Silva CL. DNA vaccine containing the mycobacterial hsp65 gene prevented insulitis in MLD-STZ diabetes. Journal of Immune Based Therapies and Vaccines. 2009;7(1):4.

[81] Santos Júnior RR, Sartori A, Bonato VL, Coelho Castelo AA, Vilella CA, Zollner RL, Silva CL. Immune modulation induced by tuberculosis DNA vaccine protects non-obese diabetic mice from diabetes progression. Clinical and Experimental Immunology. 2007;149(3):570-8.

[82] Ludvigsson J; Linköping Diabetes Immune Intervention Study Group. The role of immunomodulation therapy in autoimmune diabetes. Journal of Diabetes Science and Technology. 2009;3(2):320-30.

[83] Tisch R, Yang XD, Liblau RS, McDevitt HO. Administering glutamic acid decarboxylase to NOD mice prevents diabetes. Journal of Autoimmunity. 1994;7(6):845-50.

[84] Liu J, Filippova M, Fagoaga O, Nehlsen-Cannarella S, Escher A. Intramuscular injection of plasmid DNA encoding intracellular or secreted glutamic acid decarboxylase causes decreased insulitis in the nonobese diabetic mouse. Gene Therapy and Molecular Biology. 1999; 3: 197-206.

[85] Filippova M, Liu J, Escher A. Effects of plasmid DNA injection on cyclophosphamide-accelerated diabetes in NOD mice. DNA and Cell Biology. 2001;20(3):175-81.

[86] Weaver DJ Jr, Liu B, Tisch R. Plasmid DNAs encoding insulin and glutamic acid decarboxylase 65 have distinct effects on the progression of autoimmune diabetes in nonobese diabetic mice. Journal of Immunology. 2001;167(1):586-92.

[87] Tisch R, Wang B, Weaver DJ, Liu B, Bui T, Arthos J, Serreze DV. Antigen-specific mediated suppression of beta cell autoimmunity by plasmid DNA vaccination. Journal of Immunology. 2001;166(3):2122-32.

[88] Balasa B, Boehm BO, Fortnagel A, Karges W, Van Gunst K, Jung N, Camacho SA, Webb SR, Sarvetnick N. Vaccination with glutamic acid decarboxylase plasmid DNA protects mice from spontaneous autoimmune diabetes and B7/CD28 costimulation circumvents that protection. Clinical Immunology. 2001;99(2):241-52.

[89] Wolfe T, Bot A, Hughes A, Möhrle U, Rodrigo E, Jaume JC, Baekkeskov S, von Herrath M. Endogenous expression levels of autoantigens influence success or failure of DNA immunizations to prevent type 1 diabetes: addition of IL-4 increases safety. European Journal of Immunology. 2002;32(1):113-21.

[90] Seifarth C, Pop S, Liu B, Wong CP, Tisch R. More stringent conditions of plasmid DNA vaccination are required to protect grafted versus endogenous islets in nonobese diabetic mice. Journal of Immunology. 2003;171(1):469-76.

[91] Li A, Escher A. Intradermal or oral delivery of GAD-encoding genetic vaccines suppresses type 1 diabetes. DNA and Cell Biology. 2003;22(4):227-32.

[92] Goudy KS, Wang B, Tisch R. Gene gun-mediated DNA vaccination enhances antigen-specific immunotherapy at a late preclinical stage of type 1 diabetes in nonobese diabetic mice. Clinical Immunology. 2008;129(1):49-57.

[93] Joussemet B, Vu AT, Sai P, Bach JM. Gene-gun biolistic immunization encoding glutamic acid decarboxylase: a model for studying Langerhans cell abnormalities and mimicry in the nonobese diabetic mouse. Annals of the New York Academy of Sciences. 2005;1051:613-25.

[94] Bresson D, Fradkin M, Manenkova Y, Rottembourg D, von Herrath M. Genetic-induced variations in the GAD65 T-cell repertoire governs efficacy of anti-CD3/GAD65 combination therapy in new-onset type 1 diabetes. Mol Ther. 2010 Feb;18(2):307-16.

[95] Reed JC. Dysregulation of apoptosis in cancer. Journal of Clinical Oncology. 1999;17(9):2941-53.

[96] Birge RB, Ucker DS. Innate apoptotic immunity: the calming touch of death. Cell Death and Differentiation. 2008;15(7):1096-102.

[97] Li AF, Hough J, Henderson D, Escher A. Co-delivery of pro-apoptotic BAX with a DNA vaccine recruits dendritic cells and promotes efficacy of autoimmune diabetes prevention in mice. Vaccine. 2004;22(13-14):1751-63.

[98] Li A, Ojogho O, Franco E, Baron P, Iwaki Y, Escher A. Pro-apoptotic DNA vaccination ameliorates new onset of autoimmune diabetes in NOD mice and induces foxp3+ regulatory T cells in vitro. Vaccine. 2006;24(23):5036-46.

[99] Li A, Chen J, Hattori M, Franco E, Zuppan C, Ojogho O, Iwaki Y, Escher A. A therapeutic DNA vaccination strategy for autoimmunity and transplantation. Vaccine. 2010 Feb 23;28(8):1897-904.

[100] Krieg AM. CpG motifs in bacterial DNA and their immune effects. Annual Review of Immunology. 2002;20:709-60.

[101] Guan Y, Zhang M, Li Y, Cao W, Ji M, Liu Y. Vaccination with IA-2 autoantigen can prevent late prediabetic nonobese diabetic mice from developing diabetes mellitus. Diabetes Res Clin Pract. 2012;95(1):93-7.

[102] Rivas EI, Driver JP, Garabatos N, Presa M, Mora C, Rodriguez F, Serreze DV, Stratmann T. Targeting of a T cell agonist peptide to lysosomes by DNA vaccination induces tolerance in the nonobese diabetic mouse. J Immunol. 2011;186(7):4078-87.

Chapter 23

Antibody-Based and and Cellular Therapies of Type 1 Diabetes

Chang-Qing Xia, Yuantao Liu, Qingbo Guan and
Michael J Clare-Salzler

Additional information is available at the end of the chapter

http://dx.doi.org/10.5772/53495

1. Introduction

Type 1 diabetes (T1D) is an insulin-dependent diabetes because of insufficient insulin production by the pancreatic islet β cells. Although the pathogenic mechanism of T1D is not yet completely clear, the current view of T1D pathogenesis is that under certain genetic background, exogenous and/or endogenous factors trigger autoimmunity against islet β cells in the pancreas causing β cell damage and subsequent insufficiency of insulin production [1, 2]. About two decades ago, it was first demonstrated that T cells specific to β cell antigens were activated and participated in the pathogenesis of T1D [3, 4]. A great deal of work following these reports in both animal models and humans has provided convincing data further supporting T1D is a T cell-mediated autoimmune disease. On the other hand, the evidence showing that majority of T1D patients have high titers of autoantibodies against islet β cells [5, 6] suggests that self-reactive B cells must also be involved in the autoimmune process. The role of B cells in the pathogenesis of T1D was further supported by the recent research and clinical data demonstrating B cell depletion by anti-CD20 antibodies delayed the disease process.

The clinical presentation of T1D is preceded by a period of time of active autoimmune response occurring in the pancreatic islets. When overt diabetes occurs, approximately 95% of islets are destroyed. Therefore, tremendous efforts have been pulled in halting or slowing down autoimmune process for the purpose of preventing T1D. Several clinical trials in T1D prevention have been put forward. However, there is, thus far, no effective approach to the prevention of human T1D despite that many have shown promising results in T1D animal models. Further effort is needed to discover new ways to prevent T1D. Importantly, from a practical point of view, reversing overt diabetes is much needed. In this chapter, we will focus on recent research in immune intervention of disease process in T1D including modulation of T cells, B cells by antibodies as well as cellular therapies such as autologous hematopoietic stem cell transplantation (ASCT), treatment with mesenchymal stem cells (MSC) and cord blood transplantation.

2. Antibody-based therapies of type 1 diabetes

In this section, we will discuss antibody-based therapy in T1D including therapies using anti-CD20 and anti-CD3 antibodies as well as anti-thymocyte globulin.

2.1. Anti-CD20 antibody therapy in type 1 diabetes

B cells are immune cells that produce antibodies when stimulated by exogenous or endogenous antigens. Several autoimmune diseases are associated with self-reactive B cells such as systemic lupus erythematosus and idiopathic thrombocytopenia. Reports have shown that depletion of B cells ameliorates such autoimmune conditions [7-9]. CD20 is highly expressed on the surface of mature B cells and is the B cell-specific marker. Thus, anti-CD20 antibody has been employed for the *in vivo* depletion of B cells. The FDA-approved drug, anti-human CD20, Rituximab has been used clinically for CD20+ B cell lymphoma for over a decade and largely improved the survival of patients with B cell lymphoma. Recently, anti-CD20 therapy was tested in several clinical trials for the treatment of B cell-mediated autoimmune diseases and demonstrated promising efficacy including a clinical study for the new onset T1D patients [10]. We will get into details on how anti-CD20 therapy works, its efficacy in treating T1D, the potential adverse effects as well as the issues to be solved in the future.

2.1.1. The mechanisms of action of anti-CD20 therapy

It is generally believed that the effect of anti-CD20 therapy results from the depletion of B cells by the anti-CD20 antibodies *in vivo*. However, the mechanism of action of anti-CD20 therapy is largely beyond B cell depletion. Several mechanisms have been proposed concerning the action of anti-CD20 therapy.

2.1.1.1. Complement activation in anti-CD20 therapy

Complement activation by binding the Fc fragment of the antibody leads to cell lysis, or named complement-dependent cytoxicity (CDC). Complement-dependent cell lysis is controlled by the degree of complement activation and regulated by a series of complement inhibitory proteins, such as CD35, the complement receptor type 1; CD46, the membrane cofactor protein; CD55, the decay accelerating factor; and CD59, the membrane inhibitor of reactive lysis. It appears that the ability of CD20 to move into lipid rafts is needed for CDC to occur [11]. Some protein kinase pathways are also involved in regulating CDC activity, e.g. the activation of PKC, PKA and MEK is associated with B cell resistance to CDC [12]. Furthermore, complement activation has other effects besides cell lysis, such as depositing C3, C3b and additional CD3b breakdown products on the cell surface [13].

2.1.1.2. Antibody-dependent cellular cytoxicity (ADCC)

ADCC effect in anti-CD20 therapy represents killing of target cells (B cells) by the effector cells that are activated by binding the Fc fragment of anti-CD20 antibody bound on B cells. Members of the Fcγ receptor family are expressed on monocytes, macrophages and granulocytes, and include the activating high-affinity FcγRI (CD64) and low-affinity FcγRIIIA (CD16), as well as the inhibitory low affinity FcγRIIB (CD32). FcγRIIB is believed to be a key regulator on B lymphocytes [13-15]. ADCC was recently demonstrated as an important *in vivo* mechanism of anti-CD20 action [13].

2.1.1.3. CD20 binding induces B cell apoptosis

Although the major role of anti-CD20 therapy is cell and complement-mediated cell lysis, there is evidence that anti-CD20 antibody mediates B cell death through inducing B cells to undergo apoptosis [16]. Anti-CD20 antibody, such as Rituximab induces B cell apoptosis through activation of caspase-3 [17], whereas the FAS ligand/FAS death pathway does not seem necessary. Therefore, the mitochondrial-dependent pathway is likely the death pathway induced by anti-CD20. The role of bcl-2-dependent pathways remains unclear.

Most research on the mechanisms of action of anti-CD20 therapy was conducted in B cell lymphoma to study how anti-CD20 therapy kills lymphoma tumor cells but not normal B cells. Anti-CD20 antibody therapy may work differently when used to modulate normal mature B cells. Although the existing evidence shows that anti-CD20 therapy induces regulatory T cells or regulatory B cells in autoimmune settings [18-20], the mechanisms of action of anti-CD20 in modulating normal mature B cells are not fully understood and need to be further addressed. The insight into the mechanisms of action of anti-CD20 therapy in autoimmune settings is of great importance in guiding anti-CD20 therapy in autoimmune diseases.

2.1.2. Animal studies on anti-CD20 therapy in T1D

NOD (nonobese diabetes) mouse is an animal model of human T1D. In this strain of mice, diabetes starts to occur usually around 10 weeks of age. Tremendous measures have been tested for T1D prevention in NOD mice including anti CD20 therapy. Hu reported for the first time that anti-CD20 therapy not only prevented but also reversed T1D in humanized NOD mice (Hu-NOD, CD20 transgenic mice). Furthermore, anti-CD20 therapy-modulated B cells can transfer diabetes-protective effect when co-transferred with diabetogenic spleen cells in NOD-scid mice, suggesting post anti-CD20 depletion the reconstituted B cells might acquire tolerogenic, or regulatory capacity. Additionally, the authors discovered that anti-CD20 therapy significantly induces CD4+CD25+Foxp3+ regulatory T cells [21]. It has been shown that NOD mice deficient for B cells from the birth fail to develop autoimmune diabetes [22]. Xiu, et al [23] directly tested how depletion of B cells influenced T1D pathogenesis in wild-type NOD mice with an intact immune system. NOD female mice at early and late pre-clinical stages of disease were treated with mouse anti-mouse CD20 mAbs. Short-term anti-CD20 mAb treatment in 5-week old NOD female mice reduced B cell numbers by 95%, decreased subsequent insulitis, and prevented diabetes in >60% of littermates. The treatment in 15-week old NOD mice was unable to prevent T1D but significantly delayed the process. In contrast to the study described previously, this study failed to show any changes in T cells and regulatory T cells [22]. The results of anti-CD20 therapy in the above T1D animal models are encouraging. Further clinical studies are needed to determine whether anti-CD20 therapy has the same efficacy in human T1D.

2.1.3. Clinical studies on anti-CD20 therapy in T1D

A randomized, double blind clinical study testing the effect of Rituximab on new-onset T1D was conducted by the T1D TrialNet Anti-CD20 study group. The results were published in New England Journal of Medicine 2009 [10]. In this well-designed clinical study, 87 patients aged 8 to 40 years who had newly diagnosed T1D were assigned to either receive infusions of 375 mg/m^2 Rituximab (57 cases) or placebo (30 cases) on days 1, 8, 15, 22. The primary outcome assessed 1 year after the first infusion, was geometric mean area under the curve (AUC) for the serum C-peptide level during the first 2 hours of a mixed-meal tolerance test. The results showed that at 1 year post treatment, the mean AUC for the level of C peptide was significantly higher in the Rituximab group than in the placebo group. The levels of glycated hemoglobin and requirement of insulin were significantly reduced in Rituximab group as compared to placebo group. Peripheral blood B lymphocytes were quickly depleted in the Rituximab group, and slowly recovered with time. By the end of 1 year observation, the levels of B lymphocytes increased to 69% of baseline. It is noted that the rate of C-peptide loss did not accelerate with recovery of B cells between 6 months and 1 year. Patients in Rituximab group had more incidences of adverse events, displaying mostly grade 1 or grade 2 after the first infusion. The reactions appeared to be minimal with subsequent infusions. No increased frequency of infection or neutropenia with Rituximab was reported. In this study, the authors observed significant reduction of serum IgM but not IgG suggesting Rituximab may selectively deplete sub-populations of B cells. Based on the results of one-year follow-up, anti-CD20 therapy is a promising approach for T1D treatment. Whether repeating the course of anti-CD20 therapy is needed and whether this treatment leads to long-term protection need to be further investigated.

A follow-up study on the patients enrolled in the clinical study described above attempted to address how Rituximab infusion influences the levels of autoantibodies against islet antigens. Autoantibodies to insulin (IAAs), GAD65 (GADAs), insulinoma-associated protein 2 (IA2As), and ZnT8 (ZnT8As) were measured with radioimmunoassays. The results showed that Rituximab markedly suppressed IAAs compared with the placebo injection but had a much smaller effect on GADAs, IA2As and ZnT8As. A total of 40% (19 of 48) of Rituximab-treated patients who were IAA positive became IAA negative versus 0 patient out of 29 placebo-treated patients. In the subgroup (n=6) treated within 50 days of diabetes, IAAs were markedly suppressed by Rituximab treatment in all patients for 1 year and for four patients as long as 3 years despite of continuing insulin therapy. Independent of Rituximab treatment, the mean level of IAAs at study entry was markedly lower for patients who maintained C-peptide levels during the first year of follow up in both Rituximab-treated and placebo groups [24]. The results described above suggest that anti-CD20 therapy differentially suppresses anti-islet autoantibodies. Further studies are needed to investigate whether autoreactive B cell clones against islet antigens are differentially depleted.

As mentioned earlier, mouse studies have demonstrated that anti-CD20 therapy alters T cells. It is of interest to know how Rituximab infusion affects T cell responses in human T1D. This was explored in a follow-up study on patients in the above-described clinical trial Surprisingly, it is noted that Rituximab treatment leads to enhanced proliferative responses of T cells to diabetes-associated islet-specific autoantigens, which are positively correlated with C-peptide levels [25]. It is still unclear why B cell depletion enhances T cell proliferation. It is likely to be related to the refill of immune system post B cell depletion by T cells through homeostatic proliferation. Further studies are needed to characterize those T cells phenotypically and functionally to determine whether those autoreactive T cells are beneficial or harmful for controlling autoimmunity.

Drug resistance is the major reason of failure in the treatment of B cell lymphoma by Rituximab [26, 27]. It had been unknown whether anti-CD20 therapy in autoimmune diseases, such as T1D can also lead to drug resistance until a recent report indicating a potential mechanism for the ineffectiveness of anti-CD20 therapy in T1D [28]. This animal study showed that anti-CD20 efficiently depleted follicular but not marginal zone B cells. Interestingly, the islet infiltrated B cells lost their CD20 expression, which might explain the ineffectiveness of anti-CD20 therapy in late stage of T1D in NOD mice. Gradual recovery of the antibodies against islet antigens further suggests that autoimmune B cells are unable to be completely wiped out by anti-CD20 therapy. New drugs targeting the islet-infiltrated $CD20^{neg}$ B cells, such as anti-CD19 antibodies may be needed to further improve the efficacy of immunotherapy targeting B cells.

One of the most concerned issues regarding anti-CD20 therapy is the potential infection arisen by B cell depletion [29]. Anti-CD20 therapy indeed leads to hypoimmunoglobulinemia [30-32]. However, there is no significant increase in the incidence of infection during anti-CD20 therapy, which is consistent with a recent report demonstrating that anti-CD20 therapy does not deplete memory B cells specific to the antigens previously encountered [33, 34]. Another biggest concern of anti-CD20 therapy is anaphylaxis to anti-CD20 antibodies [35] because the current clinically employed anti-CD20 antibodies like Rituximab are made from animals. Humanized anti-CD20 antibodies are being developed, and are expected to overcome this severe adverse effect.

2.2. Anti-CD3 antibody therapy in type 1 diabetes

Given that T1D is a T cell-mediated autoimmune disease, T cell depletion therapy is expected to be a promising approach in T1D therapy. Much attention to anti-CD3 therapy has been drawn to the researchers and clinicians in the field of T1D. Over the years of basic and clinical studies, enormous progress has been made in terms of mechanism of action and the optimization of anti-CD3 therapy. Several clinical trials in new onset T1D are under way. In the following section, we will discuss T1D anti-CD3 therapy including mechanism of action, animal studies, clinical studies, adverse effects as well as issues to be resolved, etc.

2.2.1. *Mechanism of action of anti-CD3 therapy*

As what has been described in anti-CD20 therapy, anti-CD3 therapy works eventually through non-selective depletion of T cells including CD4+ and CD8+ T cells. Currently, it is believed that the mechanism of action of anti-CD3 therapy is largely beyond T cell depletion. In this section, we will discuss how anti-CD3 therapy works to preserve islet β cells.

2.2.1.1. *Activation-induced cell death in anti-CD3 therapy*

It is known that in the initial stage of anti-CD3 therapy, all T cells including CD4+ and CD8+ T cells are activated as evidenced by the expression of CD69. Activation-induced cell death (AICD) is a major mechanism regulating central tolerance during T cell development in thymus. Yu et al reported that anti-CD3 triggered AICD in activated T cells *in vitro* [36], which might explain anti-CD3 therapy-induced immune tolerance. However, the *in vivo* data are controversial. While accumulating data showed that anti-CD3 therapy is able to induce T cell apoptosis *in vivo* as it behaves *in vitro*, but others provided evidence showing that anti-CD3 therapy does not induce T cell death but induce unresponsiveness to stimuli of mitogens [37]. Therefore, anti-CD3 therapy is not just T cell depletion, but likely other tolerogenic mechanisms participate in this process.

2.2.1.2. *Anti-CD3 therapy promotes regulatory T cells*

In 2003, an elegant study by Belghith, et al [38] reported that anti-CD3 treatment induced TGF-β-producing T cells which was indispensable for the anti-CD3-induced immune tolerance. A later study further confirmed this finding and demonstrated that anti-CD3 therapy induced regulatory T cells through TGF-β released from phagocytes phagocytosing apoptotic T cells induced by anti-CD3 therapy *in vivo* [39]. Neutralizing TGF-β or blocking phagocytosis abrogated the induction of regulatory T cells [39]. Additionally, anti-CD3 therapy might differentially deplete distinct subsets of T cells and preferentially preserve regulatory T cells. Consistent with this concept, a recent report demonstrated anti-CD3 therapy in NOD mice selectively depleted autoantigen-specific effector T cells but preserved regulatory T cells [40]. The increase of regulatory T cells was not due to the conversion of regulatory T cells from conventional T cells because all preserved regulatory T cells expressed helios which is a natural regulatory T cell marker [40]. The resistance of natural regulatory T cells to anti-CD3 depletion is not clear but may be associated with compromised activation of apoptotic pathways in regulatory T cells in response to anti-CD3 therapy. Recently, Bisikirska et al [41] reported that anti-CD3 treatment in human T1D patients expanded CD8+ T cells and induced Foxp3+ CD8+ regulatory T cells, suggesting that this type of regulatory T cells might contribute to immune tolerance induced by anti-CD3 therapy.

2.2.1.3. *Anti-CD3 therapy induces T cell anergy*

Another form of immune tolerance is T cell anergy. To dissect the mechanism of action of anti-CD3 therapy, it is interesting to know whether anti-CD3 therapy induces T cell anergy *in vivo*. There are two forms of anti-CD3 antibodies based on their working principles, i.e.

mitogenic and nonmitogenic antibodies. Nonmitogenic anti-CD3 antibody is thought to induce T cell tolerance mainly through the induction of T cell anergy. Smith reported that nonmitogenic anti-CD3 antibody treatment only delivers partial T cell activation signals thereby inducing T cell unresponsiveness (anergy) [42]. This effect occurs not only in CD4+ T cells but also in CD8+ T cells. Research data from Bluestone's group show that *in vivo* treatment of anti-CD3 antibodies induces long-term CD8+ T cell anergy [43-45]. The mechanism underlying anti-CD3 therapy induced T cell anergy is not known until a recent report from Bluestone's group showing that PD1-PDL1 interaction is required for maintaining long-term T cell anergy and T1D protection [45]. Blocking PD1-PDL1 interaction quickly reverses T cell anergy and the anergic T cells become pathogenic effector T cells. Under blockade of PD1-PDL1 interaction, the protected NOD mice by anti-CD3 treatment quickly develop diabetes [45]. The above data suggest that maintenance of anergic state of autoimmune T cells is essential, and PD1-PDL1 may play a pivotal role in this process.

2.2.2. Anti-CD3 therapy in T1D animal models

There are currently two T1D animal models that spontaneously develop diabetes under genetic susceptibility, NOD mice and diabetes-prone biobreeding (BB) rat. Although these two T1D animal models have some similarities to human T1D, there are many differences between animal and human in terms of disease progression. Nevertheless, studies on animal models will definitely provide very useful information for the immunopathogenesis, prevention and treatment of T1D. Several clinical trials are based on promising results in animal models including anti-CD3 therapy in new onset diabetes.

Anti-CD3 therapy for T1D was first tested in NOD mice. Chatenoud, et al [46] reported that anti-CD3 treatment of adult NOD mice significantly inhibits the autoimmune process. Short-term low-dose anti-CD3 treatment (5 μg/day i.v. for 5 consecutive days) prevented the occurrence of an accelerated form of the disease induced by cyclophosphamide. When this regimen was administered in adult NOD females with newly diagnosed diabetes, 64-80% of treated mice obtained a complete remission of overt diabetes showing permanent normoglycemia. It was noted that this remission was durable (>4 months) and was not associated the disappearance of insulitis. Anti-CD3 treated mice failed to reject syngeneic islet graft but maintained normal response to allogeneic skin grafts, whereas control untreated diabetic NOD females rejected both, suggesting that anti-CD3 therapy reverses diabetes through inducing islet antigen-specific immune tolerance. This study also suggests that diabetes-reversing effect can be obtained by transient targeting of the CD3/T-cell receptor without massive T-cell debulking. As described earlier, this effect may be associated with diabetes-protecting regulatory T cells induced by anti-CD3 therapy.

To improve the effectiveness of anti-CD3 therapy, a strategy of combination with islet antigens has been proposed to more effectively restore self-tolerance to islet antigens. Bresson, et al [47] reported that anti-CD3 and nasal proinsulin combination therapy enhances remission from recent-onset autoimmune diabetes in comparison to monotherapy with anti-CD3 or antigen alone. Further studies demonstrated the expansion of CD25+Foxp3+ and insulin antigen-specific regulatory T cells producing IL-10, TGF-β and IL-4. When adoptively transferred, these cells could transfer immune tolerance to immunocompetent recent-onset diabetic recipients and suppressed autoaggressive CD8+ responsive T cells. This strategy would act more site-specifically thereby reducing the risk for systemic side effects. The same group employed a mathematical disease model, and revealed that preexisting autoantibodies predict efficacy of oral insulin in combination with anti-CD3 antibodies to cure autoimmune diabetes [48]. This study shows that NOD mice with higher pretreatment levels of serum insulin-associated antigens (IAAs) responded with a much higher likelihood to combination therapy but not anti-CD3 monotherapy, indicating that IAAs may be a good biomarker to predict a better capability of the mice in inducing insulin-specific regulatory T cells after oral insulin immunization. Ablamunits, et al [49] reported recently that co-administration of anti-CD3 and IL-1 receptor antagonist had synergistic effect on T1D reversal, which showed that the combinatorial therapy led to persistent remission from islet inflammation. Whether the resolution of islet inflammation leads to regeneration of islet β cells was not addressed in this report.

The outcomes from animal studies have provided very useful information for developing anti-CD3-based therapeutic strategies for human T1D. Although the results of anti-CD3 therapy in human T1D are mixed, the preservation of β cell function in the current clinical trial suggests that anti-CD3 therapy is a viable regimen for human T1D.

2.2.3. Anti-CD3 therapy in T1D clinical studies

The results of the first clinical trial using anti-CD3 therapy for human T1D were reported in New England Journal of Medicine in 2002. Herold, et al [50] studied the effects of a nonactivating humanized mnonclonal antibody against CD3 (hOKT3gamma1 (Ala-Ala) on the loss of insulin production in patients with recently diagnosed T1D. Within 6 weeks after diagnosis, 24 patients were randomly assigned to receive either a single 14-day course of anti-CD3 treatment, or no antibody and, were followed for one year. The results showed that anti-CD3 treatment maintained or improved insulin production after one year in 9 of the 12 patients in the treatment group whereas only 2 of the 12 controls had a sustained response. The treatment effect on insulin response lasted for at least 12 months after diagnosis. Glycated hemoglobin level and insulin dose requiement were reduced in the anti-CD3 treatment group. No severe adverse effect was observed, and the most common side effects were fever, rash, and anemia. Clinical responses were associated with a change of CD4+ T cells to CD8+ T cells ratios at 30 and 90 days after treatment with the responders showing reduced CD4/CD8 ratios. This study provides initial encouraging results. Longer period of follow-up would be needed to establish the long-term effectiveness of this therapy.

A clinical study was conducted using the similar protocol in the above-mentioned study but with different doses at different injection times during the treatment course. The results demonstrated significant improvement in C-peptide response to a mixed meal. The improved C-peptide responses were accompanied by reduced HbA1c and insulin requirements. These results indicate that treatment with anti-CD3 antibody, hOKT3γ1 (Ala-Ala), Teplizumab results in improved C-peptide responses and clinical parameters in T1D for at least 2 years in the absence of continued immunosuppressive medications. In this study, because of severe adverse effect of the increased dose of Teplizumab, the patient enrollment was stopped after 10 patients enrolled [51]. Among these patients, four drug-treated patients were followed up for 5 years. Results showed that C-peptide responses were maintained. During this study, it was found that increased dose of anti-CD3 antibodies caused severe adverse effects without gaining improved therapeutic effect [52]. Thus, the dosing may need to be further modified to gain the best benefit for the patients.

Recently, the results of a randomized and double blind clinical trial (clinicaltrial.gov, number NCT00385697) conducted by multi-centers from different countries on anti-CD3 therapy in treating new onset T1D was reported in Lancet journal [53]. In this 2-year trial, patients aged 8-35 years who had been diagnosed with T1D for 12 weeks or fewer were enrolled and treated at 83 clinical centers in North America, Europe, Israel and India. Participants received one of the three regimens of teplizumab infusions (14-day full dose, 14-day low dose, or 6-day full dose, or placebo). Patients and study staff remain masked through to study closure. 763 patients were screened, of whom 516 were randomized to receive 14-day full-dose teplizumab (n=209), 14-day low dose teplizumab (n=102), 6-day full-dose teplizumab (n=106), or placebo (n-99). Two patients in the 14-day full-dose group and one patient in the placebo group did not start treatment, so 513 patients were eligible for efficacy analysis. The primary outcome did not differ between groups at 1 year. Nonetheless, 5% (19/415) of patients in the teplizumab groups were not taking insulin at 1 year, compared with no patients in the placebo group at 1 year (p=0.03). All groups had similar incidences of adverse effects. The most common clinical adverse event in the teplizumab groups was rash (220/417 [53%] versus 20/99 [20%] in the placebo group). This study suggests that future studies of immunotherapeutic intervention with Teplizumab might have increased success in prevention of a decline in β-cell function and provision of glycemic control at reduced doses of insulin if they target patients early after diagnosis of diabetes and children.

From the results of the above clinical trials, anti-CD3 therapy is a promising regimen for human new onset T1D. However, its efficacy needs to be further improved. For this purpose, combinatorial therapy is a rational approach [54, 55]. As described above, recent animal studies demonstrated that anti-CD3 therapy combined with islet β cell antigens induced islet antigen-specific immune tolerance and significantly improved the effectiveness of anti-CD3 therapy in NOD mice. Anti-CD3 antibody combined with IL-1 receptor antagonist was tested in NOD mice and showed significant improvement of therapeutic efficacy. International multi-center clinical trials have tested the agents, anti-CD3, GAD, diapep227, insulin immunization and IL-1 receptor antagonist, anakinra, separately. There is, thus far, no clinical trial testing the efficacy of combinatorial therapy of the above-mentioned agents in treating T1D. Therefore, a phase 1 clinical trial may be needed in this respect.

2.3. Anti-thymoglobulin (ATG) therapy in type 1 diabetes

Simson, et al reported that ATG treatment (500 μg/mouse) at day 1 and day 3 attenuated T1D development. It was noted that this T1D protection only presented when NOD mice were at disease onset or in the late pre-diabetic phase (12 weeks of age). It was demonstrated that when provided at 12 weeks of age, ATG reversed pancreatic insulitis, improved metabolic responses to glucose challenge, and rapidly increased frequency of antigen-presenting cells in spleen and pancreatic lymph nodes. It was also found that ATG therapy dramatically increased the frequency and functional activity of CD4+CD25+ regulatory T cells. Adoptive transfer/cotransfer studies of T1D support that ATG therapy induces a stable and transferable immunomodulatory repertoire *in vivo*. This study indicates that an induction of immunoregulation, rather than simple lymphocyte depletion, contributes to the therapeutic efficacy of ATG therapy [56]. The same group reported that ATG therapy combined with granulocyte-colony-stimulating factor (G-CSF) was remarkably effective at reversing newly diagnosed diabetes in NOD mice and more efficacious than either agent alone. This combination also afforded durable reversal from disease (>180 days post-onset) in animals having pronounced hyperglycemia (i.e., up to 500 mg/dL). Mechanistically, this combination therapy resulted in both immunological and physiological benefits, showing increased CD4/CD8 ratios and splenic regulatory T cells, as well as increased pancreatic β cell area and attenuated pancreatic inflammation [57].

Our unpublished data show that ATG therapy preferentially depletes naïve T cells, and memory T cells are relatively preserved. In addition, ATG therapy largely spares CD4+CD25+ regulatory T cells. Of interest, ATG therapy does not deplete antigen-specific T cells but alters T cell responses to the previously experienced antigens, showing increased levels of Th2 and IL-10-producing Tr1 cells, which might contribute to ATG therapy-induced T1D protection. In addition, post-ATG therapy CD4+CD25+ regulatory T cells display memory-like T cells phenotypically, suggesting that those regulatory T cells might play an important role in ATG therapy-induced long-lasting T1D protective effect.

Based on the animal studies described above, a couple of clinical trials using ATG, or ATG combined with G-CSF in human T1D are ongoing (www.clinicaltrials.gov/NCT0116157, www.clinicaltrials.gov/NCT00515099). The assessment of the effectiveness of ATG therapy in human T1D await the outcomes from these clinical trials.

3. Cellular therapy of type 1 diabetes

T1D is characterized by the autoimmune destruction of insulin-producing β cells with loss of insulin secretion. Patients with T1D have absolute requirement of insulin for survival. While insulin is effective in lowering blood glucose, hypoglycemia, even life-threatening hypoglycemia, is almost unavoidable with insulin treatment, as exogenous insulin cannot exactly mimic the profile of physiological insulin secretion. Other limitations of insulin therapy include inconvenience of daily life, physical pain and high economic costs caused by recurrent insulin injections.

Therefore, other strategies have been explored to preserve or restore β cell function in the hope that endogenous insulin secretion will achieve better glycaemic control while reducing episodes of severe hypoglycemia. As discussed above, immunotherapy, in particular the use of immunomodulatory drugs has pulled much efforts. Both experimental and clinical data demonstrate that some agents like anti-CD20 and anti-CD3 antibodies are effective in delaying the process of β cell autoimmune destruction. However, no drugs have demonstrated to prevent or reverse human T1D successfully in long-term.

More recently, many efforts have been focused on the use of stem cells as a potential therapeutic strategy for T1D. So far, accumulating data from both experimental and clinical trials have suggested that stem cell-based cellular therapy could be a promising approach for T1D treatment.

3.1. Hematopoietic Stem Cell Transplantation(HST) for T1D

The use of bone marrow transplantation (BMT) as a potential treatment for T1D was first proposed in animal study in 1985 [58], showing that allogenic bone marrow transplantation could prevent insulitis and overt diabetes in NOD mice. This concept was further substantiated by later animal study [59].

The first clinical trial to use hematopoietic stem cell transplantation in T1D patients was reported in 2003 [60]. The objective of the study was to stop autoimmune destruction of β cells with immunosuppressive drugs and to "re-set"the impaired immunologic system with a reconstituted one using autologous HSCs in the expectations of preserving residual β cell mass and facilitating endogenous mechanisms of β cell regeneration. With the above considerations, 15 newly diagnosed T1D patients were enrolled. All received high-dose immunosuppression followed by autologous hematopoietic stem cell transplantation (AHST) within 6 weeks of diagnosis. During a 7- to 36-month follow-up (mean 18.8 months), 14 patients became insulin-free. β cell function was improved as evidenced by the increase in C-peptide levels. No significant adverse effects were observed. The mechanism concerning the beneficial effects of HST is proposed to be associated with the generation of a more tolerant immune system, which blocks the autoimmune destruction of residual β cells. This hypothesis appears to be consistent with a recent clinical observation showing that intra-pancreatic autologous bone marrow infusion has no beneficial effects on long-standing T1D patients with absence of β cell function [61].

To date, it is unclear whether the beneficial effects of HST can be sustained because of the lack of long-term follow-up study. Second, it is not known whether the beneficial effects of HST are due to immune reconstitution *via* stem cell differentiation or modulating the function of existing immune cells. Therefore, randomized controlled trials with prolonged follow-up are needed to confirm the results of current studies and to evaluate the full potential of this regimen as a therapeutic option for T1D.

3.2. Umbilical cord blood (UCB) cell therapy for TID

Bone marrow is a rich source of stem cells, but its application is hampered by the limited availability of bone marrow donors and the invasive procedure for cell collection. Human umbilical cord blood (HUCB) is another source of stem cells. Compared to bone marrow, HUCB has some major advantages such as easy availability, absence of risk to the donor, low risk of graft-vs-host disease and tumorigenicity, high capacity for expansion [62]. UCB has been used successfully in transplantation for diseases like acute anemia, and sickle cell anemia [63]. There have been both animal and clinical studies evaluating the use of UCB cells as a potential therapy for T1D. The rationale is based on experimental studies. *In vitro* cultures of HUCB can yield islet-like structures capable of insulin and C-peptide production [64]. *In vivo,* human cord blood-derived cells is also shown to be able to differentiate into islet cells when transfused into 2 day old NOD-scid mice [65]. A recent report demonstrated that cord blood-derived multipotent stem cells reversed T1D through islet β cell regeneration following immune modulation [66]. Second, UCB contains a population of immature unprimed functional regulatory T cells. Theoretically, these cells could limit inflammatory reaction and anergize effector T cells, which are believed to mediate cellular autoimmune processes. In addition, UCB stem cells may act as nurse cells to stimulate the proliferation of new islets from the remaining viable tissue [67]. Ende et al. [68, 69] reported in two separate studies that infusions of HUCB improved hyperglycemia and diabetic nephropathy in obesity-induced diabetic mice. In addition, nonobese diabetic (NOD) mice can be protected from developing insulitis and diabetes by HUCB dose-dependently. However, the results of available clinical study is disappointing. In a recently completed phase I clinical study [70], 24 children aged 3.4-6.9 years, with new onset T1D received a single autologous UBC infusion within 6 months of diagnosis. After 2 years of follow-up, there was no evidence of reservation of β cell function, as evaluated by the area under the curve C-peptide that was 2% of baseline 2 years after UBC infusion, despite that the numbers of regulatory T cells (Tregs) and naïve Tregs were increased 6 and 9 months after. In that study, there are several possibilities as to why UCB infusion may fail to preserve β cell function. First, the stem cell number is insufficient. Second, there exist memory T cells refractory to regulation by Tregs. Finally, it cannot be excluded that the UCB cells from the T1D patients may have intrinsic defects with compromised biological function. In future, autologous or allogeneic transplantation with expanded UBC Tregs either alone or in combination of immunomodulatory drugs may be worth trying. Importantly, randomized controlled studies are needed before definitive conclusions can be finally reached.

3.3. Mesenchymal stem cell therapy for TID

Mesenchymal stem cells (MSCs) were originally identified by Friedenstein et al. in 1976 [71] in the bone marrow as a fibroblast-like cell population capable of generating osteogenic precursors. MSCs from the bone marrow (BM) are a heterogeneous, stromal population of multipotent non-hematopoietic progenitor cells capable of differentiating into multiple mesenchymal lineages including bone, fat and cartilage. In addition to bone marrow, MSCs have been found to be present in other tissues such as adipose tissue, umbilical cord blood, synovial membrane, skeletal muscle, dermis, deciduous teeth, pericytes, trabecular bone, articular cartilage, umbilical cord, placenta, liver and spleen. It is now known that MSCs are able to differentiate into mesodermal and non-mesodermal cell lineages, including osteocytes, adipocytes, chondrocytes, myocytes, cardiomyocytes, fibroblasts, myofibroblasts, epithelial cells, and neurons [72].

In addition to their pluripotency to differentiate, MSCs have high immunomodulatory capacity. The immunomodulatory property of MSCs are associated with their inhibitory effects on the proliferation and differentiation of both T cells and B cells, as well as dendritic

http://dx.doi.org/10.5772/53495

cell (DC) [73]. Moreover, MSCs can modulate immune response through stimulating the production of $CD8^{+}$ Treg (regulatory T cells) [74]. MSCs are known to secrete a variety of trophic mediators such as growth factors and cytokines (M-CSF, IL-6, IL-11, IL-15, SCF, VEGF) that are involved in the regulation of immune response and hematopoieses. This could be a major mechanism underlying the immunomodulatory action of MSCs. Recently, MSCs have been used in clinical trials for the treatment of acute graft-versus-host disease (GVHD) following allogeneic HSC transplantation [75,76], and for autoimmune diseases such as multiple sclerosis and Crohn disease [77,78]. Another striking characteristic of MSCs is the ability to differentiate into insulin-producing cells (IPCs). *In vitro*, MSCs can be differentiated into IPCs when cultured under proper conditions. The types of MSCs that have been successfully induced to generate IPCs includes BM-MSCs, umbilical cord blood MSCs (UCB-hMSCs), pancreatic MSCs and adipose-derived MSCs,etc. [79].

By now, the use of MSCs for treatment of diabetes have been explored in two animal studies. In a model of murine STZ-induced diabetes, co-administration of BM cells with syngeneic or semi-allogeneic MSCs normalized blood glucose and serum insulin levels. The beneficial effect of this treatment does not seem due to the reconstitution of the damaged islet cells from the transplant since no donor-derived β cells were found in the recovered animals. Instead, the benefits may be due to the immunosuppressive effect of MSCs on the β cell-specific T cell response since MSCs injection caused the disappearance of beta-cell-specific T lymphocytes from diabetic pancreas, which may allow the regeneration of recipient-derived pancreatic insulin-secreting cells [80]. In another study [81], the mechanism underlying the beneficial effects of MSCs on blood glucose was investigated in a diabetic rat model induced by high-fat diet/streptozotocin (STZ) administration. Autologous MSCs were administered either 1 or 3 weeks after STZ injection. Infusion of MSCs during the early phase not only promoted β cell function but also ameliorated insulin resistance, whereas infusion in the late phase merely ameliorated insulin resistance. The improved insulin sensitivity induced by MSCs infusion is associated with an increase of GLUT4 expression and an elevation of phosphorylated insulin receptor substrate 1 (IRS-1) and Akt (protein kinase B) in insulin target tissues.

Taken together, these *in vitro* and *in vivo* experiments suggest that multiple mechanisms may be involved for the beneficial effect of MSCs on blood glucose control in T1D. Thus far, the use of MSCs to treat T1D is limited to animal studies. The efficacy of MSCs to treat patients with T1D needs to be further evaluated in well-designed clinical trials.

In conclusion, both anti-lymphocyte antibody-based and cellular therapies are promising in stopping ongoing autoimmunity against islet antigens and likely leading to a hopeful restoration of self-tolerance. The regimens combining anti-lymphocyte antibodies, islet antigens and cellular therapies could maximize the preventive and/or therapeutic efficacy for T1D.

Acknowledgement

This work was supported by Natural Science Foundation of China (Grant number 81172854 to CQX), and NIH 1R21DK080216-01A2 to CQX

Author details

Chang-Qing Xia[1,2], Yuantao Liu[3], Qingbo Guan[4] and Michael J Clare-Salzler[2]

*Address all correspondence to: cqx65@yahoo.com

1 Department of Hematology, Xuanwu Hospital, Capital Medical University, Beijing, China

2 Department of Pathology, Immunology and Laboratory Medicine, University of Florida, Gainesville, Florida, USA

3 Department of Endocrinology, the Second Hospital of Shandong University, Jinan, China

4 Department of Endocrinology, Provincial Hospital Affiliated to Shandong University, Jinan, China

References

[1] Atkinson MA, Eisenbarth GS: Type 1 diabetes: new perspectives on disease pathogenesis and treatment. Lancet 2001, 358(9277):221-229.

[2] Atkinson MA, Maclaren NK: The pathogenesis of insulin-dependent diabetes mellitus. N Engl J Med 1994, 331(21):1428-1436.

[3] Tisch R, Yang XD, Singer SM, Liblau RS, Fugger L, McDevitt HO: Immune response to glutamic acid decarboxylase correlates with insulitis in non-obese diabetic mice. Nature 1993, 366(6450):72-75.

[4] Kaufman DL, Clare-Salzler M, Tian J, Forsthuber T, Ting GS, Robinson P, Atkinson MA, Sercarz EE, Tobin AJ, Lehmann PV: Spontaneous loss of T-cell tolerance to glutamic acid decarboxylase in murine insulin-dependent diabetes. Nature 1993, 366(6450):69-72.

[5] Miao D, Yu L, Eisenbarth GS: Role of autoantibodies in type 1 diabetes. Front Biosci 2007, 12:1889-1898.

[6] Wang J, Miao D, Babu S, Yu J, Barker J, Klingensmith G, Rewers M, Eisenbarth GS, Yu L: Prevalence of autoantibody-negative diabetes is not rare at all ages and increases with older age and obesity. J Clin Endocrinol Metab 2007, 92(1):88-92.

[7] Virgolini L, Marzocchi V: Rituximab in autoimmune diseases. Biomed Pharmacother 2004, 58(5):299-309.

[8] Sandler SG, Tutuncuoglu SO: Immune thrombocytopenic purpura - current management practices. Expert Opin Pharmacother 2004, 5(12):2515-2527.

[9] Cataland SR, Wu HM: Immunotherapy for thrombotic thrombocytopenic purpura. Curr Opin Hematol 2005, 12(5):359-363.

[10] Pescovitz MD, Greenbaum CJ, Krause-Steinrauf H, Becker DJ, Gitelman SE, Goland R, Gottlieb PA, Marks JB, McGee PF, Moran AM et al: Rituximab, B-lymphocyte depletion, and preservation of beta-cell function. N Engl J Med 2009, 361(22):2143-2152.

[11] Cragg MS, Morgan SM, Chan HT, Morgan BP, Filatov AV, Johnson PW, French RR, Glennie MJ: Complement-mediated lysis by anti-CD20 mAb correlates with segregation into lipid rafts. Blood 2003, 101(3):1045-1052.

[12] Donin N, Jurianz K, Ziporen L, Schultz S, Kirschfink M, Fishelson Z: Complement resistance of human carcinoma cells depends on membrane regulatory proteins, protein kinases and sialic acid. Clin Exp Immunol 2003, 131(2):254-263.

[13] Smith MR: Rituximab (monoclonal anti-CD20 antibody): mechanisms of action and resistance. Oncogene 2003, 22(47):7359-7368.

[14] Clynes RA, Towers TL, Presta LG, Ravetch JV: Inhibitory Fc receptors modulate in vivo cytotoxicity against tumor targets. Nat Med 2000, 6(4):443-446.

[15] Ravetch JV, Lanier LL: Immune inhibitory receptors. Science 2000, 290(5489):84-89.

[16] Byrd JC, Kitada S, Flinn IW, Aron JL, Pearson M, Lucas D, Reed JC: The mechanism of tumor cell clearance by rituximab in vivo in patients with B-cell chronic lymphocytic leukemia: evidence of caspase activation and apoptosis induction. Blood 2002, 99(3):1038-1043.

[17] Alas S, Ng CP, Bonavida B: Rituximab modifies the cisplatin-mitochondrial signaling pathway, resulting in apoptosis in cisplatin-resistant non-Hodgkin's lymphoma. Clin Cancer Res 2002, 8(3):836-845.

[18] Ray A, Basu S, Williams CB, Salzman NH, Dittel BN: A novel IL-10-independent regulatory role for B cells in suppressing autoimmunity by maintenance of regulatory T cells via GITR ligand. J Immunol 2012, 188(7):3188-3198.

[19] Yu S, Ellis JS, Dunn R, Kehry MR, Braley-Mullen H: Transient depletion of B cells in young mice results in activation of regulatory T cells that inhibit development of autoimmune disease in adults. Int Immunol 2012, 24(4):233-242.

[20] Hamel KM, Cao Y, Ashaye S, Wang Y, Dunn R, Kehry MR, Glant TT, Finnegan A: B cell depletion enhances T regulatory cell activity essential in the suppression of arthritis. J Immunol 2011, 187(9):4900-4906.

[21] Hu CY, Rodriguez-Pinto D, Du W, Ahuja A, Henegariu O, Wong FS, Shlomchik MJ, Wen L: Treatment with CD20-specific antibody prevents and reverses autoimmune diabetes in mice. J Clin Invest 2007, 117(12):3857-3867.

[22] Greeley SA, Moore DJ, Noorchashm H, Noto LE, Rostami SY, Schlachterman A, Song HK, Koeberlein B, Barker CF, Naji A: Impaired activation of islet-reactive CD4 T cells

in pancreatic lymph nodes of B cell-deficient nonobese diabetic mice. J Immunol 2001, 167(8):4351-4357.

[23] Xiu Y, Wong CP, Bouaziz JD, Hamaguchi Y, Wang Y, Pop SM, Tisch RM, Tedder TF: B lymphocyte depletion by CD20 monoclonal antibody prevents diabetes in nonobese diabetic mice despite isotype-specific differences in Fc gamma R effector functions. J Immunol 2008, 180(5):2863-2875.

[24] Yu L, Herold K, Krause-Steinrauf H, McGee PL, Bundy B, Pugliese A, Krischer J, Eisenbarth GS: Rituximab selectively suppresses specific islet antibodies. Diabetes 2011, 60(10):2560-2565.

[25] Herold KC, Pescovitz MD, McGee P, Krause-Steinrauf H, Spain LM, Bourcier K, Asare A, Liu Z, Lachin JM, Dosch HM: Increased T cell proliferative responses to islet antigens identify clinical responders to anti-CD20 monoclonal antibody (rituximab) therapy in type 1 diabetes. J Immunol 2011, 187(4):1998-2005.

[26] Maloney DG, Smith B, Rose A: Rituximab: mechanism of action and resistance. Semin Oncol 2002, 29(1 Suppl 2):2-9.

[27] Rezvani AR, Maloney DG: Rituximab resistance. Best Pract Res Clin Haematol 2011, 24(2):203-216.

[28] Serreze DV, Chapman HD, Niens M, Dunn R, Kehry MR, Driver JP, Haller M, Wasserfall C, Atkinson MA: Loss of intra-islet CD20 expression may complicate efficacy of B-cell-directed type 1 diabetes therapies. Diabetes 2011, 60(11):2914-2921.

[29] Furst DE: Serum immunoglobulins and risk of infection: how low can you go? Semin Arthritis Rheum 2009, 39(1):18-29.

[30] Irie E, Shirota Y, Suzuki C, Tajima Y, Ishizawa K, Kameoka J, Harigae H, Ishii T: Severe hypogammaglobulinemia persisting for 6 years after treatment with rituximab combined chemotherapy due to arrest of B lymphocyte differentiation together with alteration of T lymphocyte homeostasis. Int J Hematol 2010, 91(3):501-508.

[31] Guerin V, Yakouben K, Lescoeur B, Pedron B, Dalle JH, Baruchel A, Sterkers G: Prolonged agammaglobulinemia despite unaltered B-cell lymphopoiesis after peritransplant-rituximab administration in a child. Transplantation 2008, 86(9):1322-1323.

[32] Walker AR, Kleiner A, Rich L, Conners C, Fisher RI, Anolik J, Friedberg JW: Profound hypogammaglobulinemia 7 years after treatment for indolent lymphoma. Cancer Invest 2008, 26(4):431-433.

[33] DiLillo DJ, Hamaguchi Y, Ueda Y, Yang K, Uchida J, Haas KM, Kelsoe G, Tedder TF: Maintenance of long-lived plasma cells and serological memory despite mature and memory B cell depletion during CD20 immunotherapy in mice. J Immunol 2008, 180(1):361-371.

[34] Neelapu SS, Kwak LW, Kobrin CB, Reynolds CW, Janik JE, Dunleavy K, White T, Harvey L, Pennington R, Stetler-Stevenson M et al: Vaccine-induced tumor-specific

immunity despite severe B-cell depletion in mantle cell lymphoma. Nat Med 2005, 11(9):986-991.

[35] Biswas G, Parikh PM, Nair R, Bhagwat R, Bakshi A, Prabhash K, Vora A, Gupta S, Pai VR, Menon H et al: Rituximab (anti-CD20 monoclonal antibody) in lymphoproliferative malignancies: Tata Memorial experience. J Assoc Physicians India 2006, 54:29-33.

[36] Yu XZ, Levin SD, Madrenas J, Anasetti C: Lck is required for activation-induced T cell death after TCR ligation with partial agonists. J Immunol 2004, 172(3):1437-1443.

[37] Ben-Amor A, Leite-De-Moraes MC, Lepault F, Schneider E, Machavoine F, Arnould A, Chatenoud L, Dy M: In vitro T cell unresponsiveness following low-dose injection of anti-CD3 MoAb. Clin Exp Immunol 1996, 103(3):491-498.

[38] Belghith M, Bluestone JA, Barriot S, Megret J, Bach JF, Chatenoud L: TGF-beta-dependent mechanisms mediate restoration of self-tolerance induced by antibodies to CD3 in overt autoimmune diabetes. Nat Med 2003, 9(9):1202-1208.

[39] Perruche S, Zhang P, Liu Y, Saas P, Bluestone JA, Chen W: CD3-specific antibody-induced immune tolerance involves transforming growth factor-beta from phagocytes digesting apoptotic T cells. Nat Med 2008, 14(5):528-535.

[40] Penaranda C, Tang Q, Bluestone JA: Anti-CD3 therapy promotes tolerance by selectively depleting pathogenic cells while preserving regulatory T cells. J Immunol 2011, 187(4):2015-2022.

[41] Bisikirska B, Colgan J, Luban J, Bluestone JA, Herold KC: TCR stimulation with modified anti-CD3 mAb expands CD8+ T cell population and induces CD8+CD25+ Tregs. J Clin Invest 2005, 115(10):2904-2913.

[42] Smith JA, Tang Q, Bluestone JA: Partial TCR signals delivered by FcR-nonbinding anti-CD3 monoclonal antibodies differentially regulate individual Th subsets. J Immunol 1998, 160(10):4841-4849.

[43] Fife BT, Bluestone JA: Control of peripheral T-cell tolerance and autoimmunity via the CTLA-4 and PD-1 pathways. Immunol Rev 2008, 224:166-182.

[44] Guleria I, Gubbels Bupp M, Dada S, Fife B, Tang Q, Ansari MJ, Trikudanathan S, Vadivel N, Fiorina P, Yagita H et al: Mechanisms of PDL1-mediated regulation of autoimmune diabetes. Clin Immunol 2007, 125(1):16-25.

[45] Fife BT, Guleria I, Gubbels Bupp M, Eagar TN, Tang Q, Bour-Jordan H, Yagita H, Azuma M, Sayegh MH, Bluestone JA: Insulin-induced remission in new-onset NOD mice is maintained by the PD-1-PD-L1 pathway. J Exp Med 2006, 203(12):2737-2747.

[46] Chatenoud L, Thervet E, Primo J, Bach JF: Anti-CD3 antibody induces long-term remission of overt autoimmunity in nonobese diabetic mice. Proc Natl Acad Sci U S A 1994, 91(1):123-127.

[47] Bresson D, Togher L, Rodrigo E, Chen Y, Bluestone JA, Herold KC, von Herrath M: Anti-CD3 and nasal proinsulin combination therapy enhances remission from recent-onset autoimmune diabetes by inducing Tregs. J Clin Invest 2006, 116(5):1371-1381.

[48] Mamchak AA, Manenkova Y, Leconet W, Zheng Y, Chan JR, Stokes CL, Shoda LK, von Herrath M, Bresson D: Preexisting autoantibodies predict efficacy of oral insulin to cure autoimmune diabetes in combination with anti-CD3. Diabetes 2012, 61(6): 1490-1499.

[49] Ablamunits V, Henegariu O, Hansen JB, Opare-Addo L, Preston-Hurlburt P, Santamaria P, Mandrup-Poulsen T, Herold KC: Synergistic reversal of type 1 diabetes in NOD mice with anti-CD3 and interleukin-1 blockade: evidence of improved immune regulation. Diabetes 2012, 61(1):145-154.

[50] Herold KC, Hagopian W, Auger JA, Poumian-Ruiz E, Taylor L, Donaldson D, Gitelman SE, Harlan DM, Xu D, Zivin RA et al: Anti-CD3 monoclonal antibody in new-onset type 1 diabetes mellitus. N Engl J Med 2002, 346(22):1692-1698.

[51] Herold KC, Gitelman SE, Masharani U, Hagopian W, Bisikirska B, Donaldson D, Rother K, Diamond B, Harlan DM, Bluestone JA: A single course of anti-CD3 monoclonal antibody hOKT3gamma1(Ala-Ala) results in improvement in C-peptide responses and clinical parameters for at least 2 years after onset of type 1 diabetes. Diabetes 2005, 54(6):1763-1769.

[52] Herold KC, Gitelman S, Greenbaum C, Puck J, Hagopian W, Gottlieb P, Sayre P, Bianchine P, Wong E, Seyfert-Margolis V et al: Treatment of patients with new onset Type 1 diabetes with a single course of anti-CD3 mAb Teplizumab preserves insulin production for up to 5 years. Clin Immunol 2009, 132(2):166-173.

[53] Sherry N, Hagopian W, Ludvigsson J, Jain SM, Wahlen J, Ferry RJ, Jr., Bode B, Aronoff S, Holland C, Carlin D et al: Teplizumab for treatment of type 1 diabetes (Protege study): 1-year results from a randomised, placebo-controlled trial. Lancet 2011, 378(9790):487-497.

[54] Waldron-Lynch F, von Herrath M, Herold KC: Towards a curative therapy in type 1 diabetes: remission of autoimmunity, maintenance and augmentation of beta cell mass. Novartis Found Symp 2008, 292:146-155; discussion 155-148, 202-143.

[55] Sherry NA, Chen W, Kushner JA, Glandt M, Tang Q, Tsai S, Santamaria P, Bluestone JA, Brillantes AM, Herold KC: Exendin-4 improves reversal of diabetes in NOD mice treated with anti-CD3 monoclonal antibody by enhancing recovery of beta-cells. Endocrinology 2007, 148(11):5136-5144.

[56] Simon G, Parker M, Ramiya V, Wasserfall C, Huang Y, Bresson D, Schwartz RF, Campbell-Thompson M, Tenace L, Brusko T et al: Murine antithymocyte globulin therapy alters disease progression in NOD mice by a time-dependent induction of immunoregulation. Diabetes 2008, 57(2):405-414.

[57] Parker MJ, Xue S, Alexander JJ, Wasserfall CH, Campbell-Thompson ML, Battaglia M, Gregori S, Mathews CE, Song S, Troutt M et al: Immune depletion with cellular mobilization imparts immunoregulation and reverses autoimmune diabetes in non-obese diabetic mice. Diabetes 2009, 58(10):2277-2284.

[58] Ikehara S, Ohtsuki H, Good RA, Asamoto H, Nakamura T, Sekita K, Muso E, Tochino Y, Ida T, Kuzuya H et al: Prevention of type I diabetes in nonobese diabetic mice by allogenic bone marrow transplantation. Proc Natl Acad Sci U S A 1985, 82(22): 7743-7747.

[59] Mathieu C, Casteels K, Bouillon R, Waer M: Protection against autoimmune diabetes in mixed bone marrow chimeras: mechanisms involved. J Immunol 1997, 158(3): 1453-1457.

[60] Voltarelli JC, Ouyang J: Hematopoietic stem cell transplantation for autoimmune diseases in developing countries: current status and future prospectives. Bone Marrow Transplant 2003, 32 Suppl 1:S69-71.

[61] Esmatjes E, Montana X, Real MI, Blanco J, Conget I, Casamitjana R, Rovira M, Gomis R, Marin P: Regeneration of insulin production by autologous bone marrow blood autotransplantation in patients with type 1 diabetes. Diabetologia 2010, 53(4):786-789.

[62] Fruchtman S: Stem cell transplantation. Mt Sinai J Med 2003, 70(3):166-170.

[63] Lennard AL, Jackson GH: Stem cell transplantation. Bmj 2000, 321(7258):433-437.

[64] Sun B, Roh KH, Lee SR, Lee YS, Kang KS: Induction of human umbilical cord blood-derived stem cells with embryonic stem cell phenotypes into insulin producing islet-like structure. Biochem Biophys Res Commun 2007, 354(4):919-923.

[65] Yoshida S, Ishikawa F, Kawano N, Shimoda K, Nagafuchi S, Shimoda S, Yasukawa M, Kanemaru T, Ishibashi H, Shultz LD et al: Human cord blood--derived cells generate insulin-producing cells in vivo. Stem Cells 2005, 23(9):1409-1416.

[66] Y, Jiang Z, Zhao T, Ye M, Hu C, Yin Z, Li H, Zhang Y, Diao Y, et al. Reversal of type 1 diabetes via β cell regeneration following immune modulation by cord blood-derived multipotent stem cells. BMC Med 2012, 10:3

[67] Brusko T, Atkinson M: Treg in type 1 diabetes. Cell Biochem Biophys 2007, 48(2-3): 165-175.

[68] Ende N, Chen R, Reddi AS: Effect of human umbilical cord blood cells on glycemia and insulitis in type 1 diabetic mice. Biochem Biophys Res Commun 2004, 325(3): 665-669.

[69] Ende N, Chen R, Reddi AS: Transplantation of human umbilical cord blood cells improves glycemia and glomerular hypertrophy in type 2 diabetic mice. Biochem Biophys Res Commun 2004, 321(1):168-171.

[70] Haller MJ, Wasserfall CH, Hulme MA, Cintron M, Brusko TM, McGrail KM, Sumrall TM, Wingard JR, Theriaque DW, Shuster JJ et al: Autologous umbilical cord blood

transfusion in young children with type 1 diabetes fails to preserve C-peptide. Diabetes Care 2011, 34(12):2567-2569.

[71] Friedenstein AJ, Gorskaja JF, Kulagina NN: Fibroblast precursors in normal and irradiated mouse hematopoietic organs. Exp Hematol 1976, 4(5):267-274.

[72] Liu ZJ, Zhuge Y, Velazquez OC: Trafficking and differentiation of mesenchymal stem cells. J Cell Biochem 2009, 106(6):984-991.

[73] Di Nicola M, Carlo-Stella C, Magni M, Milanesi M, Longoni PD, Matteucci P, Grisanti S, Gianni AM: Human bone marrow stromal cells suppress T-lymphocyte proliferation induced by cellular or nonspecific mitogenic stimuli. Blood 2002, 99(10): 3838-3843.

[74] Djouad F, Plence P, Bony C, Tropel P, Apparailly F, Sany J, Noel D, Jorgensen C: Immunosuppressive effect of mesenchymal stem cells favors tumor growth in allogeneic animals. Blood 2003, 102(10):3837-3844.

[75] Le Blanc K, Frassoni F, Ball L, Locatelli F, Roelofs H, Lewis I, Lanino E, Sundberg B, Bernardo ME, Remberger M et al: Mesenchymal stem cells for treatment of steroid-resistant, severe, acute graft-versus-host disease: a phase II study. Lancet 2008, 371(9624):1579-1586.

[76] Ball LM, Bernardo ME, Roelofs H, Lankester A, Cometa A, Egeler RM, Locatelli F, Fibbe WE: Cotransplantation of ex vivo expanded mesenchymal stem cells accelerates lymphocyte recovery and may reduce the risk of graft failure in haploidentical hematopoietic stem-cell transplantation. Blood 2007, 110(7):2764-2767.

[77] Karussis D, Karageorgiou C, Vaknin-Dembinsky A, Gowda-Kurkalli B, Gomori JM, Kassis I, Bulte JW, Petrou P, Ben-Hur T, Abramsky O et al: Safety and immunological effects of mesenchymal stem cell transplantation in patients with multiple sclerosis and amyotrophic lateral sclerosis. Arch Neurol 2010, 67(10):1187-1194.

[78] Ciccocioppo R, Bernardo ME, Sgarella A, Maccario R, Avanzini MA, Ubezio C, Minelli A, Alvisi C, Vanoli A, Calliada F et al: Autologous bone marrow-derived mesenchymal stromal cells in the treatment of fistulising Crohn's disease. Gut 2011, 60(6): 788-798.

[79] Vija L, Farge D, Gautier JF, Vexiau P, Dumitrache C, Bourgarit A, Verrecchia F, Larghero J: Mesenchymal stem cells: Stem cell therapy perspectives for type 1 diabetes. Diabetes Metab 2009, 35(2):85-93.

[80] Urban VS, Kiss J, Kovacs J, Gocza E, Vas V, Monostori E, Uher F: Mesenchymal stem cells cooperate with bone marrow cells in therapy of diabetes. Stem Cells 2008, 26(1): 244-253.

[81] Si Y, Zhao Y, Hao H, Liu J, Guo Y, Mu Y, Shen J, Cheng Y, Fu X, Han W: Infusion of mesenchymal stem cells ameliorates hyperglycemia in type 2 diabetic rats: identification of a novel role in improving insulin sensitivity. Diabetes 2012, 61(6):1616-1625.

Chapter 24

Cell Replacement Therapy in Type 1 Diabetes

Elina Linetsky, Luca Inverardi and Camillo Ricordi

Additional information is available at the end of the chapter

http://dx.doi.org/10.5772/54943

1. Introduction

Type I diabetes (insulin-dependent diabetes mellitus, IDDM) is a chronic autoimmune disease caused by the selective destruction of insulin-producing β-cells in the pancreatic islets of Langerhans, which results in severe insulin deficiency. Insufficient circulating levels of insulin lead to potentially fatal metabolic dysfunction. Although the exact mechanism of islet cell destruction is unclear, a T-cell-mediated autoimmune process seems to be the most likely explanation. Other factors, genetic and environmental, are likely contributing causes, but have not been fully identified as of yet.

Although whole pancreas transplantation has been considered as a therapeutic option for selected patients with IDDM, most individuals with the disease are not likely candidates for this therapy. Since the discovery of insulin in the 1920's, the main therapeutic approach to treating IDDM patients has been insulin replacement [1]. The standard of care for most patients with Type 1 diabetes is based on exogenous insulin therapy delivered through several daily injections. Despite great improvements in insulin delivery systems seen in the last two decades, it's still difficult to provide the precise amount of insulin that is required by the patient at any given time. This results in hypo- and hyperglycemic episodes, potentially leading to cell damage in many tissues, ultimately resulting in the development of severe long-term complications. Therefore, insulin delivery systems which can quickly and continuously respond to constantly changing physiological needs of the organism by adjusting the amount of insulin released into the circulation would be of great benefit.

Due to the fact that IDDM is a disorder in which β-cells in the pancreatic islets of Langerhans are selectively destroyed by an autoimmune attack, cell replacement strategies offer a very attractive treatment option. Recent successes in the field of islet cell transplantation have led to renewed optimism in this area. Clinical trials clearly demonstrated that islet transplantation not only offers a viable option for patients with severe forms of IDDM, but can successfully treat the disease [2,3,4]. It is, however, apparent that islet transplantation is not currently a viable option for the treatment of all potential recipients, due to the limited source of islet cells, i.e. limited number of available donors. Another feature of islet transplantation, as currently performed, is the requirement for life-long immunosuppression that limits the patients' eligibility to individuals with the most severe cases of IDDM. These issues have driven the investigation of alternative cell sources, which include xenografts from other species, embryonic and adult stem cells, and gene therapy products. Such therapies will also likely require immunological protection provided by means such as conventional immunosuppression, administration of immunomodulatory cell subsets or a combination and manipulation of the islets by shielding and/or encapsulation, which can protect transplanted cells from recognition by the immune system and, in particular, from recurrence of autoimmunity.

An adult pancreas contains approximately one million (1 x 10^6) islet cells, which represent a minor part of the organ, i.e. 2-3 % of the pancreatic tissue. Islets designated for transplantation must be isolated from the whole pancreas using the method that combines enzymatic digestion with mechanical disruption. Despite considerable improvements made in the islet isolation process (the process itself, the reagents used during the procedure), that led to improved quantity and quality of islet preparations, it still remains a largely inefficient process. Clinical symptoms of Type 1 diabetes do not develop until 60-80% of the β-cell mass is lost to the autoimmune attack [5]. This means that adequate glycemic control can be maintained with as little as 20-40% of the normal β-cell mass. Intrahepatic islet transplantation is the accepted gold standard at the present time. Ample scientific evidence suggests [4] that a significant number of islets are lost during the immediate post-transplant period, mostly due to the inflammation and thrombosis following initial islet-blood contact and activation of hepatic microenvironment. Thus, if the goal of islet transplantation is to replace 1 x 10^6 islets to achieve long-term normoglycemia, several donors may be requires for each recipient. In fact, it has been previously demonstrated [2,3] that insulin independence is achieved with ≥13,000 islet equivalents (IEQ)/kg of recipient body weight, using more than one islet preparation per recipient, at the same time or in succession. This means that a single islet transplant may require 3-4 donor pancreata. At the present time, the only source of islet cells are pancreata obtained from a deceased, heart-beating, brain-dead donor. This type of donor, especially of suitable age, is rare, making current protocols for human islet transplantation an unlikely candidate for widespread treatment for patients with IDDM. In the US alone, there are approximately 2 million people diagnosed with Type 1 diabetes. This demand is driving the current research trends into alternative functionally competent, i.e. insulin secreting and sensing, β -cell sources as potential replacement therapies for IDDM.

A number of different cell types have been proposed as a starting material to generate sufficient cell mass for transplantation; these include insulin-secreting cell lines, non-β-cell sources engineered through gene therapy, β-cells from non-human species, and β-cells generated from adult (bone marrow, pancreas, liver and neural tissue) and embryonic stem cells [5]. Regardless of the cell source, i.e. β- or non-β cells, many agree that the optimal treatment for Type 1 diabetes should ideally consist of an autologous cell source, which can synthesize, store and release insulin in a highly regulated fashion to maintain glucose homeostasis. Too much or too little is potentially lethal, so the cells must be able to rapidly respond to changes in plasma glucose in either direction.

This chapter will offer a detailed discussion of the latest developments in islet transplantation and its future direction. In addition, attention will be paid to alternative approaches for achieving insulin homeostasis and glycemic control through various novel cell replacement therapies, as well as potential advantages and risks associated with each therapeutic option.

1.1. Allogeneic islet transplantation

Diabetes Mellitus (DM) poses a significant challenge in the United States and around the world. It's increasing in prevalence and, at the present time, affects almost 20 million people in the United States alone [1]. DM is considered to be the sixth leading cause of death in the USA and is a major morbidity hazard [6,7] because of its associated complications that may negatively impact a patient's quality of life. Presently, the disease lowers average life expectancy by about 15 years, increases cardiovascular disease (CVD) risk by about two- to four-fold, and is the main cause of kidney failure, lower limb amputations, and adult-onset blindness. DM is a costly disease: its estimated attributable costs in 2010 were approximately 135 billion dollars [6].

IDDM has an early childhood or young adulthood onset, although it can be diagnosed at any age. It is characterized by profound deficiency in insulin secretion caused by the autoimmune destruction of insulin-producing cells in the pancreas, the pancreatic β-cells. IDDM accounts for approximately 5-10% of all disease cases. Factors that have been associated with the development of Type 1 DM are both genetic and environmental [8-10]. In animal models such as the NOD mouse and BB rat, and in human Type 1 diabetes, there is strong evidence of a role of the class II gene, I-A in NOD mouse (equivalent to human DQ beta gene), most probably in combination with lack of I-E expression (equivalent to human DR) [11]. Although it is entirely possible that the genetic response can be triggered by environmental factors such as infections or drastic change in diet, the clear definition of such factors has been elusive to date [11]. Ultimately, though, it is the autoimmune component of Type 1 diabetes that is responsible for the progressive and selective autoimmune destruction of insulin-producing β-cells in the pancreas. Due to the fact that the disease is the result of the loss of a single cell type, i.e. β-cell, it is considered to be amenable to treatment by cell replacement therapy.

The discovery of insulin in 1922 by the Canadian physician Frederic Banting brought about the realization that it was the pancreas that produced the "sugar-reducing substance" [1], i.e. insulin. Since then scientists have been interested in how this hormone is synthesized and secreted, and the main therapeutic approach to IDDM has been focused on insulin replacement. Until recently, the only available treatment for Type 1 diabetes was the administration of exogenous insulin. The Diabetes Control and Complications Trial (DCCT) [12] demonstrated that, in patients with Type 1 diabetes, intensive insulin replacement therapy can control blood glucose levels to a certain extent [12]. Unfortunately, even intensive care it is not able to mimic normal hormone release that regulates glucose homeostasis [8] and results in the fine-tuned physiological balance [13]. Even in patients with good glycemic control achieved through intensive insulin therapy blood glucose levels can vary greatly outside the normal range [13]. In addition, tight control of blood glucose levels often results in frequent episodes of hypoglycemia. The DCCT trial [12] clearly demonstrated that although intensive insulin therapy is able to delay the onset of diabetes-associated complications, it doesn't result in complete prevention of their development [12,13]. It is also not clear as to how early in the progression of the disease glucose homeostasis must be restored to affect a near-positive outcome.

Thus, the need for alternative or additional therapies has been apparent for some time. Endocrine replacement has been but one approach in the quest for tight glycemic control. Achieved either through transplant of a whole pancreas [14] or allogeneic islet cells [13-15], it has been investigated for quite some time now. There is little doubt that pancreas transplants, especially when performed simultaneously with a kidney, favorably impact metabolic control [14]. Eighty percent of the patients receiving simultaneous kidney-pancreas transplants demonstrate good graft function and insulin independence at one year following surgery, with 50% of the recipients maintaining euglycemia at 5 years [16]. Pancreas transplantation results in independence from exogenous insulin, normalization of glucose levels (both fasting and post-prandial), normal Hemoglobin A1c (HbA1c) levels, and freedom from hypoglycemia [16]. However, pancreas transplantation is still associated with significant morbidity and mortality rates [16-18]. Thus, most patients with Type 1 diabetes are not candidates for pancreas transplantation.

In contrast, islet transplantation requires only a safe interventional radiology technique to implant the graft, and doesn't require general anesthesia, does not call for post-transplant management of pancreatic secretions, and is not associated with post-transplant morbidity and mortality. In addition, in patients with Type 1 diabetes, pancreatic exocrine tissue, which represents the vast majority of the organ, is not affected. These are all factors that contribute favorably toward a wider application of islet cell transplantation.

Of the 159 islet cell allografts reported to the International Pancreas Transplant Registry [18] in 1983, none resulted in insulin independence that could be clearly linked to the implanted graft. These unsatisfactory results could be attributed to the suboptimal islet isolation methods and variable immunosuppressive regiments utilized at the time. It is now apparent that islet isolation methods used at that time - originally developed for the isolation of rat islets by Moskalewski[19] and further improved upon by Lacy [20] - were not entirely adequate for the isolation of human islet cells. The use of unpurified islet preparations was not particularly safe, resulting in reported cases of portal hypertension and even death [21].

Introduction of collagenase through the pancreatic duct during the distension of the organ, and purification of the islet cells from the exocrine tissue using discontinuous Ficoll gradients [22, 23] resulted in the optimization of the islet isolation method, i.e. improved isolation yield and islet purity of up to 90% [9]. These continued improvements in the islet isolation methodology provided a new impetus to continued attempts at islet transplantation during the 1980's. Although none of the islet allografts resulted in insulin independence, clinical trials conducted during this period proved islet cell transplantation to be safe, and for the first time demonstrated a sustained C peptide production [24].

In the 1990's, the International Islet Registry [25] reported that 10% of the patients receiving allogeneic islet grafts could maintain insulin independence at ≥1 year following transplant. Although the majority of transplant recipients continued to require some exogenous insulin, their daily insulin intake was reduced, HbA1c decreased, and they reported fewer episodes of hypoglycemia unawareness. At this point, transplantation of allogeneic islet cells became a reality. However, questions related to partial graft function and eventual graft failure due to recurrence of auto-immunity or rejection - both difficult to predict - remained. Animal studies of glucose metabolism in rat [26], dog [27-29] and cynomolgus monkey [30,31] models demonstrated that long-term normoglycemia could be achieved provided that a sufficient islet mass was transplanted. These studies also showed that, in dog and simian models, the site of implantation did not play a significant role in graft failure. These findings demonstrated that islet transplantation could be successful, and represented a sustainable cell-based treatment for patients with Type 1 diabetes.

Of significant, positive impact was the introduction of the Ricordi automated method for islet isolation [32] which allowed for continuous release of large numbers of islet cells during the digestion phase, protecting them from any further enzymatic action, thereby preventing over-digestion of the islet tissue, and significantly reducing islet cell loss as a result of the isolation process. The digestion process was allowed to proceed until only a fibrous network of ducts and vessels of the pancreas remained. In contrast with previous methods utilized to isolate human islets, the Ricordi method allowed for the digestion of the whole pancreas and a significant improvement in the quantity and quality of the isolated cells [32]. Introduction of more efficient enzyme blends [33,34], development of more effective organ preservation methods [35-37], effective use of semi-automated large-scale purification techniques [38-41], and the introduction of additional reagents during various phases of islet cell processing, all contributed to the improved islet recovery and the utilization of islet preparations for transplantation. Islet preparations can be transplanted fresh, i.e. immediately following isolation, or following culture [2,3], which is of substantial benefit. This window offers sufficient time for both the detailed characterization and quality assessment of the islet preparation, and shipment of the cells to satellite transplant centers, when necessary.

Islet preparations of various degree of purity are normally implanted into the recipient's liver portal vein by transhepatic cannulation using minimally invasive interventional radiological techniques [42-47]. This approach has been demonstrated to be safe, is associated with low morbidity and is well tolerated by the transplant recipients. In fact, when additional islet mass is required to improve recipient's metabolic control, additional preparations of islet cells are delivered using the same route of administration.

New immunosuppressive protocols designed for the recipients of solitary islet allografts, i.e. islet transplant alone (ITA), and the publication of the results of the Edmonton Protocol in the year 2000 [2,3] lead to further improvement in the clinical outcomes reported by a number of centers [42,48-50]. These new protocols moved away from the use of glucocorticoids and calcineurin inhibitors (CNI, cyclosporin A (CyA)) that have diabetogenic effects, and potential islet toxicity [2,3,42,48-50]; and utilized alternative strategies as immunosuppressive therapy. On-going clinical studies clearly demonstrated that allogeneic islet transplantation has the potential to become a viable therapy for patients with severe forms of Type 1 diabetes. However significant challenges need to be overcome before islet transplantation can be considered as the treatment of choice.

Some of the critical questions that remain to be addressed include: (i) definition of an adequate supply of donor organs which can meet the existing need; (ii) isolation of a sufficient number of high quality islet cells from the exocrine tissue, which comprises 98-99% of the pancreas; (iii) improvements in the immunosuppressive strategies that are currently used, by either the development of less toxic drugs or the induction of tolerance; (iv) preventing the recurrence of autoimmunity, demonstrated to have successful outcomes in murine models [5]; (v) identifying the early occurrence of immune rejection, which is quite challenging to monitor given the very small volume of the transplanted tissue and our limited ability to characterize the process.

1.2. Islet cells from xenogeneic sources

At the present time xenogeneic islet cells isolated from pig pancreata offer the most promising alternative to human islets as a treatment for Type 1 diabetes. This is based on a number of observations: (i) there is a large number of facilities in the US with capabilities for high-throughput breeding, rearing and slaughter of pigs; (ii) pig insulin differs from human insulin by just one amino acid and has been successfully utilized as a source of exogenous insulin for many years before the advent of recombinant insulin; (iii) large numbers of islet cells can be isolated from a single pig pancreas using techniques similar to those developed for human islet isolation; (iv) pig donors can be genetically manipulated to increase insulin production, and to protect the islet cells from immune and cytokine assault [5,51].

Several limitations have restricted the use of pig islets in human recipients. The first one is the hyperimmune response, possibly mediated by the galactoseα -1,3-galactose (Gal) epitope. Elimination of this epitope was shown to prevent hyperacute rejection of pig-to-nonhuman primate solid organ xenografts. Immune protection of xenografts utilizing encapsulation techniques resulted in progressive loss of graft viability and insulin secretion over prolonged period of time, during which transplanted islets were expected to function [52]. The second one is the possibility of transmission of porcine endogenous retroviruses (PERV), several copies of which are present in the genome of all pigs and able to infect human cell *in vitro*, with unknown consequences [53]. The possibility of novel viral infections in recipients of porcine islet grafts raised serious safety and ethical concerns, as C-type retroviruses related to PERV have been demonstrated to associate with hematopoietic cell malignancies in the natural hosts [53].

The interest in porcine islets peaked when it was demonstrated that T-cell immunomodulatory therapies which target indirect co-stimulatory pathway, i.e. CD28-CD154, supported prolonged engraftment of unmodified pig islet cells in non-human primates [54, 55] Furthermore, published data drew attention to the fact that, in contrast to human islets that produce copious amounts of islet amyloid polypeptide (IAPP) capable of inducing β-cell apoptosis, pig neonatal and adult islets do not form amyloid deposits. This could be due to the fact that pig IAPP is considerably less amyloidogenic [56]. Recently published data, however, have suggested that the PERV scare may have been overestimated: long-term immunosuppressive regimens and exposure to porcine islet grafts did not result in any detectable PERV transmission. These data clearly showed (a) no expression of PERV in porcine islets in either *in vivo* or *in vitro* studies, and (b) no integration of PERV sequences into recipient cell or organs [55, 57-58]. Additionally, Koulmanda et al successfully demonstrated that, following anti-CD4 treatment, pig islet grafts became resistant to autoimmune destruction in non-obese diabetes (NOD) recipients, suggesting that CD4-mediated autoimmunity, rather than hyper-acute immunological response, might be the cause of the destruction of xenogeneic islet grafts [59].

It is also difficult to overlook the fact that large numbers of porcine islets can be isolated with considerable ease, using protocols similar to those developed for the bulk isolation of human islet cells [32,60]. Since the introduction of highly efficient semi-automated methods for bulk islet isolation of pig pancreatic islets by Ricordi et al [32], the quantity and quality of islet preparations from a pig donor has been consistently higher. Pig donors are healthy and avoid cell senescence due to various co-morbidities, brain death, and cold and warm ischemia injury, as these factors can be controlled and, under normal circumstances, kept to a minimum [60,61]. Using standard purification methods [61] a purity of 70-90% of islet can be achieved. Islet cells isolated from adult pigs are functionally competent, and graft function can be recorded shortly following transplantation [61]. In addition, adult pig islets have appropriate glucose-sensing and insulin release mechanisms, as demonstrated by prolonged diabetes reversal when porcine islets were transplanted into nonhuman primates [534,55]. However, the fragile nature of adult porcine islets leads to significant loss as a result of ischemia and inflammation, during cell culture and early engraftment process. It also makes it challenging to maintain them in culture, and may result in the loss of a significant proportion of cells following isolation. Although a reduction in islet mass and cell viability has been reported when adult porcine islets were maintained in culture, short-term culture is desirable to reduce cell immunogenicity or combine preparations from several donors, prior to transplant [61].

In comparison to adult pig islets, fetal islets have been isolated with even greater ease. Once isolated these require several weeks of culture to facilitate re-aggregation of the endocrine tissue and elimination of exocrine tissue, and to mature to glucose-sensing and insulin production [60]. Additionally, immature cells are much more resistant to the ischemia and inflammation-related injury. Fetal islet isolation is very simple and highly reproducible, and can be accomplished using an exogenous solution of digestive enzymes with minimal loss of immature islet cells [61]. This is due to the fact that fetal islet tissue is not prone to ischemic damage, most probably because of its inherent relative lack of exocrine tissue, capable of inducing damage as a result of the release of proteolytic enzymes from damaged exocrine cells [62,63]. At the same time, there is a relative abundance of endocrine tissue which makes the isolation of fetal islets an easier and more efficient process. Additionally, the copiousness of immature precursor cells in the ductal tissue and their possible presence in the islet-like cell clusters (ICCs) that form during culture, contributes to high capacity of ICC tissue for post-transplant proliferation, a key feature lost in adult pig islets [63]. Thus, small numbers of ICCs can eventually produce large-size grafts, provided that rejection, recurrence of autoimmunity and hyperglycemia can be overcome and controlled [63]. Considering the small size of the fetal pancreas, the capability of a small number of ICCs to mature into a functionally competent graft speaks to the use of this tissue. As mentioned above, a major drawback with using functionally immature cells is their delayed function. ICCs require several weeks, and even months, of development before normal glucose levels in the recipient can be achieved, during which time a poor response to physiological glucose has been observed [64]. This on-going hyperglycemic state during the period of functional maturation can lead to possible damage of the transplanted fetal tissue. Thus, while transplanting immature ICCs in diabetic recipients who are early in the course of their disease might not represent a problem, it is potentially a serious drawback for patients with brittle diabetes and declining kidney function [51,62]. A second disadvantage to using ICCs is the high expression of α-1,3-Gal epitope on the surface of fetal islets, making these cells more susceptible to rejection than adult pig islets, which in contrast express little Gal [62].

Neonatal pancreatic cell clusters (NPCCs) obtained from 1-5 day-old piglets can be also easily procured and successfully isolated in a relatively quick and efficient manner [61,65], using culture media supplemented with collagenase. Due to their availability and inherent capacity to differentiate *in vitro* and *in vivo,* NPCCs represent an attractive source of xenogeneic tissue for clinical transplantation. Although freshly isolated cell clusters contain only 7% endocrine cells, 11% epithelial cells, and ~74% exocrine tissue, this content undergoes dramatic transformation following a 9-day culture [51,61]. Published data indicates that during *in vitro* culture the acinar tissue undergoes apoptosis resulting in the enrichment of the endocrine component to 35% [61] of the total cellular content, with 25% of the cells capable of insulin production. The rest of the tissue is characterized as non-granulated epithelial cells [61]. *In vitro* culture results in the formation of NPCCs [61,65], as well as the proliferation of β-cell as assessed by studies using bromodeoxyuridine (BrdU) [65]. NPCCs have been demonstrated to be more responsive to glucose challenge compared to the fetal ICCs, but not as fully functional as adult islets [61]. Although NPCCs were showed not to correct diabetes immediately following transplantation, the insulin content of the grafts was reported to increase by ~20 fold [61], confirming either NPCCs' capacity for β-cell proliferation, or differentiation of epithelial precursor cells into β-cells, or both. During the period of hyperglycemia, none of the transplanted immunodeficient mice were lost, suggesting that even in the immediate post-transplant period NPCCs are capable of producing small, but sufficient, amount of insulin to keep the recipients alive, stopping short of achieving normoglycemia [61]. This speaks to the fact that compared to the adult porcine islets, NPCCs have an extensive *in vivo* and *in vitro* proliferative capacity [61,65], as well as the ability to acquire endocrine function in a time-dependent manner. In addition, data showing that NPCC can be successfully and reproducibly transfected with a non-immunogenic, non-pathogenic recombinant AAV demonstrated a possible strategy for gene delivery to improve transplantation outcome [65].

On the other hand, NPCCs require long periods of *in vivo* maturation before developing functional competence [65], which represents a potential draw-back with respect to the clinical utilization of this xenogeneic islet cell source.

Small and large animal models to study the potential clinical use of porcine islet transplantation to treat Type 1 diabetes have been developed and success has been reported [54,55,59,61,

62]. Reversal of diabetes with prolonged restoration of insulin independence has been achieved in several porcine-to-nonhuman primate xenogeneic transplant models [54,55] in recipients that developed diabetes as a result of chemical treatment, surgical intervention, i.e. pancreotectomy, or spontaneously. Long-term insulin independence has also been achieved when neonatal and fetal pig pancreatic precursors were implanted intraportaly, subcutaneously, and into the peritoneal cavity [66,67]. The choice of the anatomical implantation site for not only porcine, but human islets is crucial. At the present time, the accepted clinical practice is to deliver islets to the liver, through the portal vein. However, it has been demonstrated that using this route of administration, low oxygen tension, and an active innate immune response that results in complement activation and immediate blood-mediated inflammatory response (IBMIR) contribute to significant islet mass loss in the immediate post-transplant period [68,69]. Different challenges arise when the graft is placed under the kidney capsule, i.e. islets in this case may be damaged by stress as a result of ischemic injury. However, implantation of encapsulated porcine islets under the kidney capsule of non-diabetic Cynomolgus Macaques resulted in low levels of porcine C-peptide, with islet grafts surviving for up to 6 months [70]. Reports of other implantation sites, such as subcutaneous and peritoneal space, have been published, but both have been reported as relatively immunoreactive [51], unless the islets were protected by an immune barrier in the form of a capsule.

Although most of the data regarding the possible use of porcine islets as an alternative treatment modality for Type 1 diabetes became available as a consequence to the extensive effort undertaken in a number of small and large animal models, a number of reports of controversial clinical trials have been published in the last several years. An Australian biotechnology company, Living Cell Technologies Ltd., reported a clinical trial in Moscow where 10,000 encapsulated porcine islet equivalents (IEQ)/kg recipient body weight isolated from adult virus-free pigs (DiabeCell®) were implanted into several adult recipients with brittle form of Type 1 diabetes, leading to reduced insulin requirements and detectable porcine C-peptide 11 months following transplant [71]. Follow-up dose-finding clinical trial conducted in New Zealand, however, produced less optimistic results. Although a statistically significant reduction in hypoglycemic unawareness was demonstrated, insulin requirements and C-peptide were reported to be largely unchanged. Additional dose-finding trials using DiabeCell® are currently in progress. Earlier clinical trials conducted in Mexico utilized neonatal islets co-cultured with Sertoli cells in a collagen-coated device which was implanted subcutaneously into 12 adolescent Type 1 diabetic patients [72]. Although pioneering in nature, this work drew a certain amount of criticism with regard to the ethical implications of conducting clinical trials in countries without strict regulatory oversight, the dearth of relevant pre-clinical data to warrant Phase I clinical trials to assess the safety of the investigational therapy, i.e. porcine islet transplants, as well as the efficacy of the treatment [73].

It's hard to dispute potential clinical and commercial implications of porcine xenotransplantation as a potential therapy for patients with severe forms of Type 1 diabetes. Although not a new idea, recent developments in this field are likely to drive larger, more tightly controlled pre-clinical and clinical studies to explore its enormous potential as a substitute for human islets. However, if xenotransplantation is going to be the way to solve inherent supply problems with allogeneic organs, a much better understanding of the immunological processes involved in the destruction of xenogeneic tissue is necessary.

1.3. Stem cell as β-cell replacement therapy

The most promising cell source for β-cell progenitors is embryonic stem cells (ESCs) derived from the inner cell mass of blastocysts during the early stages of embryogenesis. ECSs offer several notable advantages. First, ESCs differ from adult stem cells in that under the right growth and differentiation conditions they have the potential to differentiate into any cell type *in vitro* and *in vivo*, a potential termed pluripotency. Given the capacity for pluripotency, there is an interest to explore guided *in vitro* differentiation into a desired cell type for the purpose of cell replacement therapy, in this case for the treatment of Type 1 diabetes. Second, ESCs' potential to self-renew while maintaining their stem cell properties is of immeasurable advantage, as it allows for unlimited cell expansion, while the cell differentiation capacity is preserved. Given the need for large number of cells for therapeutic applications, this favors ESCs over the cells at more advanced stages of maturation which, in general, are reported to have a much more limited proliferative capacity [74]. Here, of course, certain precautions are necessary. Directed cell differentiation and proliferation also results in the differentiation of associated cell types, which are not necessarily desired and need to be inhibited. This represents a challenge. It's been previously postulated that to successfully differentiate a cell type such as insulin-producing β-cells, an ideal protocol would involve culture steps that mimic a differentiation process taking place during normal embryonic development. That involves certain signaling pathways and transcription factors necessary to guide the development of undifferentiated progenitor cells into fully mature, metabolically functional insulin-producing β-cells [74-76].

First attempts to generate insulin producing islet-like cells (IPCs) were centered on the selection of cells positive for nestin, an intermediate filament protein which serves as a neural stem cell/progenitor marker [77-79]. The reason behind the focus on nestin-positive cells is that in some species neural cells, namely brain neurons in Drosophila, are the source of circulating insulin. In addition, insulin gene transcription is found in the vertebrate brain, although it's not clear if vertebrate neurons produce or secrete the actual protein [74,78]. Recent reports, however, have demonstrated that selection of nestin-positive cells from ESCs leads to generation of neural cell types [80-82], although differentiation into insulin-producing cells was also achieved. This is consistent with the fact that nestin is a marker of neural and pancreatic exocrine progenitors, but does not indicate endocrine progenitor cells. Attempts to differentiate brain-derived neural ESCs into insulin-producing cells resulted in the formation of glucose-sensing insulin producing cell clusters following the exposure to multiple signals that regulate *in vivo* islet pancreatic development [83]. Following transplantation into immunocompromised mice islet-like clusters were demonstrated to release insulin and C-peptide. However, the C-peptide content of these islet progenitor clusters was estimated to be 0.3% of the normal level found in isolated human pancreatic β-cells [83], suggesting that the resulting islet-like cell clusters were not bona-fide β -cells. In addition, temporal sequence of expression of gene products active during the development of pancreatic islet cells, such as glucokinase,

http://dx.doi.org/10.5772/54943

Glut-2 and Pdx1, did not exactly resemble that observed in the embryonic pancreas; nor was the transcription of other genes normally expressed in β-cells, such as Nkx2-2 and Nkx6-1, detected in the later stage islet-like clusters. Some of these insulin-producing cell clusters [77], while staining positive for insulin, were - in all likelihood - the result of insulin uptake from the culture medium, rather than activation of robust insulin transcription, as demonstrated by other studies [84]. These data pointed to the fact that evidence demonstrating the equivalence of these islet-like cells clusters to mature β-cells was lacking; and that a better understanding of the signaling pathways and transcriptional factors regulating the development of pancreatic β-cell identity during embryogenesis was necessary.

In 2005, D'Amour clearly demonstrated that cells closely resembling fully mature native β-cells could be generated by replicating the culture conditions that closely mimicked embryonic development [85,86]. Utilizing a step-wise approach, ESCs were first directed into definitive endoderm stage, a pre-requisite for all pancreatic cell types, followed by a pancreatic endoderm, and subsequently into β-cells with an insulin content similar to that observed in native islets [86]. However, similar to fetal β-cells, the resulting cells were able to release C-peptide in response to multiple secretory stimuli, but only minimally to glucose. These studies were followed by others [87-89] in which these cells were implanted into immunocompromised mice half way through the differentiation process. When the cells were allowed to mature *in vivo*, the efficiency of the differentiation process was improved, glucose-responsive insulin secretion observed, and chemically induced diabetes reversed [89]. Progress in this area has been rapid and recently, California-based ViaCyte (previously Novocell) has reported positive pre-clinical results with Pro-Islet™, a material based on the technology discussed above, in conjunction with a retrievable encapsulation device. On-going efforts to translate this strategy into pre-clinical and clinical applications were supported by a recent $20 million award from the California Institute of Regenerative Medicine. This works favorably towards ESC-based clinical approaches becoming available in the very near future.

Upon demonstration that the mature state of somatic stem cells can be redirected toward the a progenitor state similar to that of ESCs [90-92], the field of stem cell-based strategies has been further expanded and now includes an attractive alternative to ESCs, i.e. induced pluripotent stem cells (iPSCs). Potentially, iPCSs offer a practical solution to the ethical dilemma posed by the destruction of human embryos necessary for the production of ESCs-based cell therapies. These cells, they are virtually undistinguishable from ESCs in terms of their molecular and biological characteristics. They offer a possibility of generating autologous patient-specific cell therapies directed to treat a variety of medical conditions, including diabetes. This means that depending on the specific illness, desired cells can be differentiated from the patient's own cells. This is certainly attractive as the cells designated for re-transplantation would have the same genetic makeup as those of the patient, and would alleviate the challenges posed by the activation of the recipient's immune system that would occur when allogeneic cells are transplanted.

In 2006, Takahashi et al [90] demonstrated that pluripotent stem (iPS) cells could be generated from mouse fibroblasts by the retrovirus-mediated transfection of four transcription factors, namely Oct3/4, Sox2, c-Myc, and Klf4. Since then, following the main steps of the original β-cell differentiation protocol and retroviral expression of the same four transcription factors, it was reported that differentiation into insulin-producing islet-like clusters was possible. Islet-like clusters were obtained from iPSCs using a serum-free, feeder-free protocol [93]. Following initial reports, a number of modifications to the original protocol have been introduced. These included substituting the originally-described transcription factors with oncogenic potential with stable recombinant proteins [94], episomal constructs [95], DNA minicircles [96], modified mRNAs [97], and small molecule compounds with re-programming properties [98]. Despite these efforts, generation of patient-specific cell lines form iPSCs remains inefficient and expensive, hindering progress in this area. Additionally, there seem to be an inconsistency in the methods utilized for the successful differentiation of insulin-producing islet-like cells, leaving the field open for a much wanted universal protocol utilized to generate a wide variety of patient-specific cell lines, much like that developed by ViaCyte for the Pro-Islet™ technology. Then, of course, the risks inherent to the use of iPSC-and ESC-based approaches must be carefully considered, as these seem to be almost identical.

First, there are the reports of teratoma formation when undifferentiated (cultured *in vitro* for ~12 days) ESCs are utilized in pre-clinical models [89]. Interestingly, when cells cultured under similar conditions for extended period of time were utilized [87], no teratoma formation was observed in recipient animals suggesting that more extensively differentiated ESCs lose their ability for neoplastic transformation. Hence, teratoma formation can probably be controlled through elimination of less differentiated cells via advanced purification techniques, as well as more efficient machinery for cell differentiation.

Another critical aspect that deserves serious consideration is related to the full cell complement present at the final ESC differentiation stages. Transplantation of pancreatic progenitor cells results in the development of not only the endocrine cell types, the full complement of which are probably required for fully functional islet structures, but also the exocrine pancreas, i.e. acinar and ductal cells, albeit at much lower frequency [89]. The presence of these cells that have the ability to produce and release various enzymatically active proteins is worrisome. In addition, under conditions of stress caused by inflammation and injury, acinar cells can develop into cells with progenitor-like activity, able to result in neoplastic lesions as a result of oncogenic mutations. While the possibility of such events is small, detailed investigation into these issues needs to continue to assure that the function of ESC-derived endocrine cells are not compromised by the cancer-related risks associated with exocrine cell populations.

Another issue that needs to be explored is the immune response of the host following transplantation of an allogeneic ESC-derived cellular graft. In the last decade or so sophisticated immunosuppressive regiments have been developed to protect allogeneic islet grafts obtained from deceased donors [46-50] long term, following transplantation. In case of ESC-related therapies, not only the graft must be protected from the immune insult by the recipient's immune system, but the cells with tumorigenic capacity need to be isolated and sequestered. This can be, most probably, achieved with the use of sophisticated immunoisolation / encapsulation devices that have become available in the last few years [4].

Finally, what needs to be ascertained is the fact that stem-cell derived β-cells have the same ability to synthesize, store and release insulin in a highly regulated fashion similar to that of native pancreatic islets. Extensive efforts should be undertaken to understand whether the same regulatory mechanisms are in place in stem cell-derived insulin producing cells to control prolonged and uncontrolled insulin release which would result in sever hypoglycemia. Only when it is clearly and unequivocally ascertained that stem cell-derived insulin producing cells are true equivalents of endogenous pancreatic β-cells, can clinical application of such therapies become a reality.

1.4. Immunotherapy for the prevention and treatment of Type 1 diabetes

As Type 1 diabetes is an autoimmune disease characterized by the selective and progressive destruction of insulin-producing β-cells via the cumulative attack by autoantigen-specific CD4+ and CD8+ T-cells, autoantibodies, and functionally defective bone marrow derived antigen-specific cells, development of various immunotherapeutic options has been the major focus for prevention and treatment of IDDM. Multiple studies in the NOD mouse model demonstrate that islets are attacked in step-wise manner, with benign insulitis being the starting point of this assault. With time and not fully defined qualitative changes, overt diabetes characterized by the efficient destruction of β-cells ensues. It is generally acknowledged that diabetes in animal models and men is strongly associated with the changes in more than 20 genetic loci - with genes encoding MHC class II molecules playing the major role, most probably influenced by a number of environmental factors, although it's been quite challenging to identify either in detail [11].

Animal studies indicate that a number of pathogenic events contribute to the progressive loss of T-cell tolerance to β-cell proteins, and, therefore, expansion of β-cell specific pathogenic CD4+ and CD8+ T-cells. These events seem to take place during the early stages of the pre-clinical IDDM. These include defective negative selection in the thymus, inefficient peripheral tolerance characterized by low frequencies of IL-4, IL-10 and TGF-β secreting CD4+ T helper 2 (Th2) cells, as well as diminished numbers of "natural" immunoregulatory FoxP3 expressing CD4+CD25+ Regulatory T (Treg) cells and invariant natural killer T (iNKT) cells. These events, coupled with reduced frequency / function of immunoregulatory effector cells within the islets, reduced sensitivity of T cells to immunoregulation, and increased levels of pro-inflammatory cytokines produced by macrophages and dendritic cells (DCs), result in the severe loss in the balance between pathogenic effector and immunoregulatory T cells, especially during the later stages of the disease [99-101]. Effective prevention / treatment strategies for Type 1 diabetes must focus on the restoration of this balance..

The progression course of diabetes offers obvious time points for interventional immunotherapeutic strategies. The first opportunity is presented during the pre-clinical stages of diabetes, when the goal is to suppress the on-going β-cell autoimmune process and prevent the development of overt diabetes. Undiagnosed at risk individuals - family members of patients with the previously diagnosed diabetes - can be monitored by screening for autoantibodies specific for several autoantigens found in the serum. These include insulin, glutamic acid decarboxylase 65 (GAD65), and insulinoma–associated tyrosine phosphate (IA-2) [102]. The second time point for intervention is at clinical onset, in an attempt to preserve 10-15% of the β-cell mass that is usually still present at the time of diagnosis.

There is a definite therapeutic potential through the rescue of the residual β-cells, and there are reports that halting autoimmunity at this stage can potentially lead to β-cell regeneration and/or replication and, in ideal circumstances, remission of diabetes [103,104].

Further down the line, when all β-cells are lost, the likelihood of remission through immunoregulation becomes slim, but recent observation in clinical trials performed in patients with undetectable C-peptide suggest that restoration of β-cell function is not impossible in these circumstances. A recent clinical trial conducted in China demonstrated that following treatment with autologous lymphocytes and allogeneic cord blood-derived stem cells, patients with and without residual β-cell function demonstrated improved C-peptide levels, reduced median Glycated hemoglobin A_1C (HbA_1C) values, and decreased daily insulin requirements [105].

The development of specific immunotherapeutic strategies that effectively target pathogenic effector cell populations, promote β-cell tolerance, while maintaining a "normal" immune function, i.e. balance between pathogenic effector and immunoregulatory T-cells, is the ultimate goal. This means that different immunotherapeutic strategies, alone or in combination, must be considered to effectively suppress β-cell autoimmunity at different stages of the disease progression.

There is sufficient information that deals with various immunotherapeutic strategies to prevent / treat Type 1 diabetes, for which both clinical and experimental findings are available. Two major approaches have received most attention, although others have been discussed, namely, antigen- and antibody-based immunotherapies.

1.4.1. Antigen-based immunotherapy

Antigen-based immunotherapy has to do with selectively targeting disease-specific T cells to maintain the normal function of the immune system. β-cell antigen-specific vaccination has proved to be an effective strategy for the induction of the immunoregulatory T cells and suppression of autoimmune pre-clinical diabetes in rodent models and NOD mice. Vaccination of 12-week old NOD mice with GAD65 protein resulted in the inhibition of the progression of insulitis and long-term protection mediated by the GAD65-specific CD4+ T cells [106]. Successful application of antigen-based immunotherapies in the clinical setting has yet to be reported, although some evidence does exist of the successful application of this methodology. The Diabetes Prevention Trial-1 (DPT-1), during which participating pre-diabetic subjects received insulin either orally or parentally demonstrated no significant effect on the development of diabetes or β-cell autoimmunity [107]. Although the reason for why the treatment failed to prevent diabetes in the majority of subjects was never clearly identified, it was thought that insufficient dose of insulin administered to trial participants was the main culprit. One interesting observation had to do with the fact that some effect was observed in subjects receiving oral insulin that presented with high titers of insulin autoantibodies. It is, therefore, entirely possible that success or failure, as well as efficacy, of a given antigen-based immunotherapy is related to the severity of the existing autoimmunity.

http://dx.doi.org/10.5772/54943

It's been demonstrated that treatment with antigen-based therapy can have a dual effect on autoreactive T-cells: induction of T-cell deletion and the induction of immunoregulatory T- cell population [108,109]. The number of immunoregulatory β-cell specific T-cells induced as result of treatment is critical. As diabetes progresses and the pro-inflammatory milieu is established, a relatively high number of immunoregulatory T-cells would be required to effectively suppress β-cell autoimmunity and to restore the balance between pathogenic effector and immunoregulatory T-cell subsets. The number of inducible immunoregulatory effector cells is, at least in part, dependent on the size of the pool of naive precursors for a given β-cell autoantigen [101,106]. As the pool of β-cell specific T-cell precursors actively involved in the autoimmune process is limited, minimizing the pool of immunoregulatory T-cells that can be induced, it is of critical importance to choose the autoantigen utilized for treatment at late stages of the disease wisely. While in experimental models it's been demonstrated that administration of a combination of β-cell autoantigens suppresses β-cell autoimmunity during the late stages of the disease, the same has not been clearly defined in patients [101]. Although some progress has been made towards the development of methods that can be used to detect β-cell specific T-cells, more development is necessary before this approach can become a standard immunotherapeutic approach. In addition, as demonstrated by the DPT-1 [107], the efficacy of a given treatment, i.e. β-cell autoantigen, may vary significantly between individuals, probably based on the extent of autoimmunity, i.e. β-cell specific T-cell precursors. This means that, similarly to the NOD model, immunization with the cocktail of various β-cell specific peptides would be necessary to achieve a measurable degree of success in abating the progress of the autoimmune process taking place during the advanced stages of Type 1 Diabetes.

The number of immunoregulatory β-cell specific T-cells induced as result of treatment also depends on the efficiency of the process involved in the induction of immunoregulatory T-cell population. What complicates matters is the fact that this induction must take place *in vivo*, under the same conditions that favor the expansion of autoreactive β-cell specific T-cell subsets. Hence, strategies that preferentially promote the expansion of immunoregulatory T-cell populations are necessary. Properties of mucosal tissues [110,111], co-administration of various types of adjuvants and cytokines, as well as manipulation of the way the autoantigen is presented have been investigated in both experimental and clinical settings [107], with some degree of reported success. In addition, variety of inducible immunoregulatory T-cell populations has been reported to be of importance as induction of different types of immunoregulatory cells, each with a distinct mode of action, would be expected to increase the overall efficacy of a given immunotherapy [107].

1.4.2. *Antibody-based immunotherapy*

Various monoclonal antibodies have been utilized to target a wide range of immune components actively involved in the progressive autoimmune process. Most of these focus on directly or indirectly targeting the T-cell compartment [101], but also include soluble mediators such as cytokines and chemokines, and antigen presenting cells (APC). Several recent reports suggest that B-cells may also represent a useful target to alter the progression of β-cell autoimmune process.

There is an abundance of literature that discusses the efficacy of monoclonal antibodies targeting T-cells, in a number of experimental models. Following the administration of a short course of depleting CD4 antibody or anti-lymphocyte serum in NOD mice, suppression of β-cell autoimmunity and, in some cases, remission of the recent onset of diabetes is achieved [112,113]. There is, however, a drawback to this approach. Depleting antibody immunotherapy resulted in the indiscriminate depletion of not only the pathogenic, but also non-autoimmune T-cell populations, and induced long-term state of immunosuppression. In addition, after the depleting antibody was cleared from the system the number of T-cells that reappeared was significantly reduced, compared to normal levels. At this same time, the use of non-depleting anti-CD4 and CD8 antibodies resulted in tolerance induction in the antigen-specific manner, with the T-cell numbers intact [114], induction of apoptosis in activated T-cells, and activation of the CD4+CD25+FoxP3+ cell population demonstrated to have a suppressive effect on the differentiation of pathogenic effector T-cells [114].

Studies investigating the efficacy of anti-CD3 monoclonal therapy for the treatment of Type 1 diabetes have been generating a lot of interest ever since they've been first reported [104], Chatenoud demonstrated that a short course treatment of NOD mice with low dose anti-CD3 antibody resulted in long-term remission of recent onset diabetes and β-cell specific tolerance [104]. The mode of action of this therapy proved to be multi-faceted. A critical observation was of the anti-CD3 antibody preferentially affecting activated rather than naïve T-cells by down-regulating the T-cell receptor and reducing TCR signaling, enhancing apoptosis, and altering T-cell trafficking [115]. This treatment was also demonstrated to promote the expansion of the immunoregulatory T-cells with CD4+CD25+ phenotype. Utilization of a non-mitogenic anti-CD3 antibody in a clinical setting, during the first 6 weeks following diagnosis, resulted in the preservation of C-peptide response over a 2-year period in certain patients relative to untreated controls. The fact that residual β-cell function was reported in some patients at the time of treatment speaks to the importance of therapeutic administration at "earlier" stages in the disease progression [116]. Although efficacy with this treatment was observed, the protection offered by the anti-CD3 antibody treatment was nevertheless transient. This suggests that this type of therapy needs to be refined either in terms of schedule or route of the administration, or the therapeutic dose, before it can be applied to a larger patient population.

Studies with monoclonal-based therapies targeting co-stimulatory pathway of immune activation such as CD40-CD40L, and APCs such as DC's and B-cells have also been reported. Blocking the CD40-CD40L pathway proved highly effective in abrogating T-cell responses in autoimmune and transplantation models [117]. However, before this approach could be investigated further the anti-CD40L antibody was withdrawn from use in various clinical trials due to serious adverse events that came into view as a result of treatment.

Targeting B-cells, whose primary role in Type 1 diabetes is that of APCs to T-cells, was never high on the list of targets for potential immunotherapy. The reason behind this is simple: islet-specific autoantibodies have never been considered the primary culprits of β-cell destruction. However, this pathway may prove to be the indirect approach to targeting β -cell autoreactivity [118]. Despite an initial skepticism, some work has been done in this area. Recent studies performed in an experimental setting reported that depleting B-cells with a short course of monoclonal anti-CD20 antibody proved beneficial in abrogating diabetes in young NOD mice, and significantly delaying the onset of the disease in older animals [119]. A recent clinical trial conducted by the TrialNet group confirmed these findings by demonstrating that selective and transient depletion of B-lymphocytes with rituximab, an anti-CD20 monoclonal antibody, partially preserved β-cell function in patients with recent onset of Type 1 diabetes, for a period of 1 year [120].

1.4.3. Regulatory R (Treg) cells

Although this cell subset with unique immunomodulatory properties has been briefly discussed above, these cells deserve special attention and are discussed in more detail in this section. Ever since the realization that Treg cells have an innate capacity to maintain tolerance to self-antigens in peripheral organs under immune assault, this population has attracted great attention with respect to their potential role in the prevention of autoimmune disorders which include Type 1 diabetes. The interest in these immune traffic regulators peaked when it was demonstrated that they represented an inducible population able to halt the progression of IDDM, while curbing autoimmune responses not only to antigens responsible for the induction of autoimmunity but others involved in this process as well. This represents an attractive therapeutic alternative for IDDM as to date no specific antigen(s) has been identified as a causative agent for the diabetogenic response.

As discussed elsewhere in this chapter, autoimmune response aimed at the progressive destruction of pancreatic β-cells can be manipulated through antigen-based manipulation and non-antigen-based treatments, possible though the involvement of Treg cell population. Although immunoregulatory capacity has been demonstrated in several T-cell subsets, the main players in the field are "natural" CD4+CD25+, and "adaptive or induced" regulatory T-cells of various phenotypes. "Natural" CD4+CD25+ regulatory T-cells require a variety of co-stimulatory interactions for their development, and are mainly identified by the FoxP3 transcription factor necessary for the development and function of this cell subset. *In vitro*, natural CD4+CD25+ cells have been demonstrated to have an uncanny ability to inhibit T-cell proliferation and cytokine production, most probably, via cell-cell contact [121]. Despite previously published dissenting reports, there is an agreement that during the development of diabetes, the autoreactive T-cell subsets become unresponsive to CD4+CD25+ mediated suppression mechanism. This could be due to the fact that CD4+CD25+ cell are present in reduced numbers during the development of the IDDM in humans. At the same time, opposing results have been obtained in an NOD model: at the time of diabetes onset, CD4+CD25+ cells exist in equal numbers compared to non-diabetic animals [121]. It's been also demonstrated that while CD4+CD25+ cells are relatively abundant in normal individuals, data obtained from various animal models suggest that antigen-induced Treg cells are present in relatively low numbers. Despite this fact, of most benefit is the data that demonstrated that once induced, Treg cells become activated in the immediate tissue where the given autoantigen is expressed. Of added benefit is the realization that in addition to suppressing the responses of an autoantigen in question, Treg cells are able to modulate other autoreactive T-cell responses as well, most probably via production of anti-inflammatory soluble cytokines such as IL-4, IL-10 and

TGF-β. Pre-clinical studies in non-obese diabetic mice have demonstrated that adoptive transfer of Tregs can slow diabetes progression and, in some cases, reverse new onset diabetes. Clinical trials investigating the effect of natural expanded and patient-specific Treg cells on autoreactive T-cell responses, preservation of β-cell function and other outcomes related to diabetes management are in progress at the present time [122].

The effect of antigen-based immunotherapy has been discussed earlier in this chapter. However, to recapitulate, the available data demonstrates that antigen-based immunotherapeutics probably favor the induction of immunoregulatory T-cell subsets by reacting with endogenous reactive autoantigens, and halting the progression of diabetes. In animal models of IDDM, amplification of Treg cell responses has been achieved using several self-antigens administered using tolerogenic means such intravenous, intranasal or subcutaneous injection, or oral feeding. It has also been shown that Treg cells are able to exert their modulatory effector function through the action of several cytokines, namely IL-4 and IL-10. The situation with TGF-β is much more complex. When administered as a vaccine, it was shown to confer protection from diabetes in NOD mice, but not in other animal models [123].

"Adaptive or induced" Treg cells comprise a group of heterogeneous T-cell subsets that arise as a function of a specific context in which they are generated [120]. These normally go along with antibody-specific approaches to treating IDDM. For example, treatment with CD3 antibody, a potent treatment option for autoimmune disease, has been associated with a marked increase in Treg cell populations, although the mode of action was never elucidated [101,121]. The results of the administration of non-mitogenic anti-CD3 therapy proved to be encouraging [116]. Recent-onset IDDM patients treated with FcR-nonbinding humanized anti-CD3 monoclonal antibody were found to maintain their insulin production for ~2 years following treatment. Although the mechanism of action is well understood, it was thought that the treatment had a direct effect on pathogenic T-cells and resulted in the induction of Treg cell population, or both [116,121]. Data from several other clinical trials seems to indicate that anti-CD3 monotherapy could neither elicit long-term protection, nor protect from adverse effects. Hence, it is possible that combination of immunotherapeutic options might offer a better sustained protection against the disease over time.

1.5. Bone Marrow Chimerism

It was Owen, back in 1945, who made an observation that bone marrow cells have the ability to induce transplantation tolerance to donor histocompatibility antigens. Billingham, Brent and Medawar confirmed and expanded on this idea by transplanting Major Histocompatibility Complex (MHC)-disparate bone marrow cells (BMC) into neonatal recipient mice which resulted in the induction of specific, systemic, stable tolerance to the donor, while preserving immunocompetence required to reject genetically disparate third party grafts [124]. Fetuses and neonates, of course, offer an immunoprivileged state, during which pre-conditioning is not required for the successful BMC engraftment that leads to chimerism. The situation changes after that. Over the last several decades, numerous investigators working in the area of bone marrow (BM) conditioning to reduce the immunogenicity of solid and cellular grafts, demonstrated that adult recipient pre-conditioning is necessary to "make space" for the successful engraftment of donor BMC and induction of donor-specific chimerism.

It was initially thought that lethal recipient conditioning which leads to complete BM ablation was necessary for engraftment of allogeneic BMC. Over time, however, it has become clear that stable engraftment can be achieved using partial pre-conditioning strategies [125,126]. Conditioning approaches to allow for stable engraftment of donor cells have included total body irradiation, total lymphoid irradiation, cytoreductive approaches, low dose irradiation with polyclonal or monoclonal antibodies, single or multiple infusions of large doses of donor BMC with T-cell co-stimulatory blockade, anti-CD4 and anti-CD8 antibodies with local thymic irradiation, and targeted BM ablation using bone seeking ^{153}Samarium-Lexidronam (^{153}Sm) compound with transient T-cell co-stimulatory blockade [125-127]. The fact that hematopoietic chimerism induces donor-specific tolerance, while preserving third-party reactivity, has been established in experimental animal models, i.e. rodents [127,128], large animals [129], primates [130] and in humans [131]. Using conditioning approaches listed above full or mixed chimerism leading to stable, long-term donor-specific tolerance has been achieved. Although both full and mixed chimerism can be achieved in animal models, fully chimeric animals demonstrate immune-incompetence for antiviral activity and antibody production [125,126]. Mixed allogeneic chimerism is much more preferable in tolerance induction protocols, as both donor and recipient antigen presenting cells can be found in the recipient [125].

The realization that BM transplantation represents a credible treatment for diabetes came as a result of animal studies that demonstrated the interdependence between BMC transplantation and autoimmune disease: the disease could be transferred from NOD mice to mouse strains resistant to autoimmunity, while BM from disease-resistant mouse strains could prevent the development of autoimmunity in NOD mice [125,126]. BMC-associated tolerance to islet cell grafts has been achieved in a number of animal models and human subjects [125,126,132]. Donor-specific tolerance has been demonstrated in both animals that were first preconditioned, treated with donor-specific BMC, with the islet graft placed at a later date, and those that received islet grafts 24-48 hours after BMC infusion [125,126]. Over the last several decades a profound contribution has been made to the understanding of underlying processes in the induction of BM-derived tolerance to pancreatic islet grafts in the later stages of diabetes, prevention of recurrence of autoimmunity in the graft, and reversal of overt diabetes once the pre-diabetic state is identified [125,126].

Animal Type 1 diabetes models fall into two groups, which deal with etiology of the disease. Diabetes can be induced chemically or surgically, or developed spontaneously as in BB rat or NOD mouse model. In the first case autoimmunity is not an underlying factor of the disease. In the second case, however, the disease progresses spontaneously, similarly to the clinical course of Type 1 diabetes, which is autoimmune in nature. BMC transfer experiments between the NOD mouse and disease-resistant mouse strains discussed earlier have suggested that it is a BMC-derived stem cell that is associated with the development of the autoimmunity observed in Type 1 diabetes. Both unmodified and T-cell depleted NOD-derived BMC can transfer autoimmunity followed by diabetes development [125,126]. Conversely, BMC from diabetes-resistant mouse strains, when transferred to a lethally, or sub-lethally conditioned

NOD mice and rendering these recipients mixed chimeras, reverses insulitis and the autoimmune process, halting the development of overt diabetes. Ildstad proposed two possible explanations for how allogeneic BMC-derived chimerism can prevent diabetes. First, donor BMC activates a regulatory cell instrumental in suppressing the activation of autoreactive lymphocytes identified as a culprit in the progression of autoimmunity, development of the overt diabetes and fully developed disease. Second, BMC can cause clonal deletion of autoreactive T lymphocytes via donor-specific disease resistant APCs [126].

Taking into an account that it is a BM stem cell that's involved in the development of autoimmune disease, the timing of BMC administration for the treatment of autoimmune diabetes is critical. Due to the fact that autoimmunity results in the progressive destruction of pancreatic β-cells, the ultimate timing for BMC infusion is during the early stages of the disease, when overt diabetes ensues, exogenous insulin is administered, and return to normoglycemia and even production of endogenous insulin are observed. However, the main drawback for the widespread use of BMC therapy to treat Type 1 diabetes is harsh, often lethal, recipient preconditioning regiments. Although non-lethal conditioning protocols, discussed earlier, have been developed, donor-specific chimerism reported under such circumstances is often transient [126]. However, encouraging results in terms of the induction of stable chimerism in kidney transplant recipients have been recently reported by Leventhal et al [132]. He used mobilized cells enriched for hematopoietic stem cells (HSC) in combination with a graft-facilitating cell (FC) population ($CD8^{dim}$, $CD3^{+}/CD45R^{+}/Thy1^{+}/Class\ II^{dim/intermediate}$, $\alpha\beta\text{-TCR}^{-}$ and $\delta\lambda\text{-TCR}^{-}$) and nonmyeloablative conditioning in recipients of MHC mismatched, unrelated kidney grafts. Five out of eight transplant recipients exhibited stable donor-specific chimerism, and were weaned of immunosuppression at 1 year following transplant. None of the transplant recipients were reported to show signs of GVHD. As previously reported by Ildstad [125], the FC is not a stem cell, but this population seems to be necessary to enable successful BMC engraftment in MHC disparate environment. Although the mechanism by which FC aids engraftment is not clear, it was characterized previously and found to be necessary to prevent GVHD and promote engraftment in standard BMC transplant protocols [125,126]. These results are exciting and offer much optimism towards treatment strategies applicable to patients with Type 1 diabetes.

Type 1 diabetes is a multifaceted disease, for which no single arm immunotherapeutic approach is possible. It has been long established that immunotherapies that target early vs. later pre-clinical stages in the disease progression offer a treatment approach with higher likelihood of success. However, even that might not be enough to effectively solve this formidable problem. It is possible that no single immunotherapeutic approach will offer long-term protection from diabetes onset and progressive autoimmune destruction of β-cells, in either prevention or treatment setting. A number of immunological approaches, in combinatorial manner, that exploit the strengths and circumvent the adverse events of potential therapies at the same time, might prove to be the answer. At this point such approaches are still in the development stage, albeit many hurdles have been overcome to move this approach forward. Latest developments in this area do offer much optimism.

1.6. Concluding remarks

Cell replacement strategies offer an enormous potential for the treatment of patients with Type 1 diabetes, in both clinical and economic terms. The availability of unlimited amounts of functionally competent graft material to treat millions of patients suffering from IDDM and its dreadful, debilitating complications can move this field forward from the experimental stage it has found itself in for the last several decades to the forefront of transplantation medicine. The fact that allogeneic islet transplantation offers the most extensively studied and sensible solution to potential cure for IDDM is clear. However, this therapeutic option is far from a perfect solution, and comes hand-in-hand with several problems in the form of serious shortages of the available organs and resulting tissue to satisfy the ever-growing demand, recurrence of autoimmunity and rejection and life-long immunosuppression. Porcine islets offer a viable substitution or addition to the allogeneic islet therapy, offering both a functionally competent adult cell source with already developed insulin-sensing machinery, and sufficient quantities of tissue immediately available for transplant. However, before persistent problems with immune rejection and destruction of the graft can be overcome, porcine islets do not have a hope of replacing or supplementing allogeneic islet cells as a viable treatment option. Embryonic stem cells have the required proliferative potential, with recent studies clearly demonstrating that ESCs provide a definitive platform for differentiation into insulin producing structures. However, it remains to be seen whether (a) current experimental protocols can be scaled-up to generate sufficient number of cells for transplant; (b) current purification methods offer sufficiently stringent protocols to be able to transplant glucose-sensing β-like cells only, all the while unequivocally excluding potentially oncogenic "other types" of cell populations; (c) functional equivalency of the resulting glucose-sensing β-like cells to native β-cells can be clearly confirmed; and (d) the cell graft can be adequately protected to avoid efficient immune surveillance systems of the host. This is where the concept of generating sufficient insulin-producing tissue from an autologous, i.e. patient-specific, source becomes attractive. However, the early promise of this iPSCs has not translated from it early success in the experimental setting to the clinical model, mostly due to the same problems that are associated with ESCs. These, however, are multiplied by the limited proliferative capacity of these cells, as well as issues with inadequate function, i.e. poor insulin expression coupled with very low insulin secretion. The problems that stem from immunogenicity of the graft tissue are intrinsic to cells from various sources, including a tailored patient-specific iPSCs-derived approach. With the number of factors impacting the way β-cell autoimmunity can be manipulated, several key issues might be considered when it comes to the development of immunotherapeutic solutions to diabetes. These include the requirement for the suppression of the diabetogenic response early in the course of the development of the disease, as well as clear understanding of the autoreactive antigen(s) that might be defined by particular genotype and/or environmental exposure. The complexity of IDDM means that immunomodulatory therapies, antigen- and antibody-specific, might offer a solution when utilized in combination. The goal here is to preserve the functional capacity of the cellular graft or innate islet cells, while at the same time attempting to restore the unique balance between the pathogenic effector and the immunomodulatory T-cell population eroded by the autoimmune assault brought forth by the onset of the disease. Combination immunotherapy will likely prove the most effective by exploring the strength of each approach, while limiting the adverse effects associated with each. Despite significant success attained in this area, most progress so far has been made in experimental models, while clinical applications are still relatively early in their development. Although the challenge of bench-to-bedside technology transfer is significant, success of the last few years give much hope and even optimism for future clinical developments.

Various types of cellular therapies discussed in this chapter might offer multi-faceted and practical approaches to the treatment of diabetes. It is entirely possible that a choice of several different therapeutic options is of great benefit, and might provide a platform to avoid frustrating developmental pains towards a "universal cure". While the prospect of developing patient-specific, i.e. personalized, cellular therapy is appealing, it is complicated, quite expensive and, it's tempting to say, unrealistic to develop. Each of the allogeneic cell replacement approaches towards a potential therapeutic option discussed here needs to be carefully studied, dissected, and defined regardless of the costs associated with it. Further development in the area of immunotherapeutic approaches and various immunoisolation methodologies, which are beyond the scope of this chapter, will be able to help move cell replacement therapy to the forefront of transplant science. Given the fact that for almost a century administration of exogenous insulin was the only real available therapeutic alternative to the treatment of IDDM, the developments of the past several decades are exiting. It is quite possible that the following decade will see clinical application of a whole gamut of therapeutic options to treat this devastating disease.

Author details

Elina Linetsky, Luca Inverardi and Camillo Ricordi

Diabetes Research Institute, University of Miami Miller School of Medicine, Miami, Florida, USA

References

[1] Ricordi, C. Preface. In Ricordi C. (ed.) One century of transplantation for diabetes. Pancreatic cell transplantation. Austin: R. G. Landes Company, 1992: XV.

[2] Shapiro AM, Lakey JR, Ryan EA, et al. Islet transplantation in seven patients with type 1 diabetes mellitus using glucocorticoid-free immunosuppressive regiment. New Eng J Med 2000; 323:230-8.

[3] Shapiro AM, Ricordi C, Hering B. Edmonton's islet success has indeed been replicated elsewhere. Lancet 2003; 362:1242.

[4] Marzarati S, Pileggi A, Ricordi C. Allogeneic islet transplantation. Expert Opin Biol Ther 2007; 7:1627-1645.

[5] Jones PM, Courtney ML, Burns CJ, Persaud SJ. Cell-based treatments of diabetes. Cell discovery today 2008; 13:888-893.

[6] American Diabetes Association. All about diabetes, 2012. (Available at www.diabetes.org/risk-test.jsp (accessed July 9, 2012).

[7] US Department of Health and Human Services. Healthy People 2010: Objectives for improving health. Diabetes 2000; 5:2-40.

[8] Zimmet P, Shaw J. Diabetes on six continents – Ethnic and geographic differences: Views on the culture. In Raz I, Skyler J, Shafrir E, eds. Diabetes: From research to diagnosis and treatment. London: Taylor & Francis Group, 2003:1-10.

[9] Centers for Disease Control and Prevention. National diabetes fact sheet: General information and national estimates on diabetes in the United States (Rev Ed.). Atlanta: US Department of Health and Human Services, 2003.

[10] Bottino R, Trucco, M. Multifaceted Therapeutic approaches for a multigenic disease. Diabetes 2005; 54(Suppl 2): S79-S86.

[11] Eisenbarth GS, Nayak RC, Rabinowe SL. Type I diabetes as a chronic disease. J Diabet Complications 1988; 2(2):54-58.

[12] The Diabetes Control and Complications Trial Research Group. The effect of intensive treatment of diabetes on the development and progression of long-term complications of insulin-dependent diabetes mellitus. The New Eng J of Med 1993; 329:977-86.

[13] Gray DWR, Phil D. Islet transplantation and glucose regulation. World J. Surg. 2001; 25:497-502.

[14] Robertson RP. Islet transplantation as a treatment for diabetes: A work in progress. New Eng J Med 2004; 350:694-705.

[15] Weir G, Bonner-Weir S. Scientific and political impediments to successful islet transplantation. Diabetes 1997; 16:1217-56.

[16] Sutherland D, Gruessner A, Bland B. International Pancreas Transplant Registry, 2000. Minneapolis, Minn, University of Minnesota, 2000.

[17] Gaber AO, Shokouh AH, Grewal HP, Britt LG. A technique for portal pancreatic transplantation with enteric drainage. Surg Gynecol Obstet 1993; 177:417-419.

[18] Sutherland D. Pancreas and islet registry statistics. Transplant Proc. 1984; 16:593.

[19] Moskalewski S. Isolation and culture of the islets of Langerhans of the Guinea Pig. Gen Comp Endocrin 1965; 5:342-53.

[20] Lacy P, Kostianovsky M. Method for the isolation of intact islets of Langerhans from the rat pancreas. Diabetes 1965; 16:35-9.

[21] Mehigan DG, Bell WR, Zuidema GD, et al. Disseminated intravascular coagulation and portal hypertention following pancreatic islet autotransplantation. Ann Surg 1980; 191:287.

[22] Gray DWR, McShane P, Gant A, et al. A method for isolation of islets of Langerhans from the human pancreas. Diabetes 1984; 33:1055-61.

[23] Scharp DW, Lacy PE, Finke E, et al. Low-temperature culture of human islets isolated by the distention method and purified with Ficoll or Percoll gradients. Surgery 1987; 5:869-79.

[24] Scharp DW, Lacy PE, Santiago JV, et al. Results of our first nine intraportal islet allografts in type 1, insulin-dependent diabetic patients. Transplantation 1988; 51:76.

[25] Hering BJ. Insulin independence following islet transplantation in man: A comparison of different recipient categories. Inter Islet Registry 1996; 6:5-19.

[26] Leow CK, Gray DW, Morris PJ. The long-term metabolic function of intraportal and renal subcapsular islet isografts and the effect on glomerular basement membrane thickness. Diabetologia 1995; 38:1014.

[27] Alejandro R, Cutfield RG, Shienvold FL et al. Natural history of intrahepatic canine islet cells autografts. J Clin Invest 1986; 78:1339.

[28] Warnock GL, Cattral MS, Rajotte RV. Normoglycemia after implantation of puritified islet cells in dogs. Can J Surg 1988; 31:421.

[29] Merrell RC, Maeda M, Basadonna G, et al. Supression, stress and accommodation of trnapslanted islets of Langerhans. Diabetes1985; 34:667.

[30] Sutton, R, Gray DW, Burnett M, et al. Metabolic function of intraportal and intrascplenic islet autografts in cynomologous monkeys. Diabetes (Suppl. 1) 1989; 38:182.

[31] Leow CK, Shimizu S, Gray DWR, Morris PJ. Successful pancreatic islet autotransplantation to the renal subcapsule in the cynomologous monkey. Transplantation 1994; 57:161.

[32] Ricordi C, Lacy PE, Finke EH, et al. Automated method for isolation of human pancreatic islets. Diabetes 1988; 37:413-20.

[33] Linetsky E, Bottino R, Lehman R, et al. Improved human islet isolation using a new enzyme blend, Liberase. Diabetes 1997; 4 6:1120-3.

[34] Bucher P, Mathe A, Morel P, et al. Assessment of a novel two-component enzyme preparation for human islet isolation and transplantation. Transplantation 2005;79:91-7.

[35] Kuroda Y, Kawamura T, Suzuki Y, et al. A new, simple method for cold storage of the pancreas using perfluorochemical. Transplantation 1988; 46(3):457-460.

[36] Ricordi C, Fraker C, Szust J et al. Improved human islet isolation outcome from marginal donors following addition of oxygenated perfluorocarbon to the cold-storage solution. Transplantation 2003; 75(9):1524-1527.

[37] Noguchi H, Ueda M, Nakai Y et al. Modified two-layer preservation method (M-Kyoto/PFC) improves islet yields in islet isolation. Am J Transplant 2006; 6(3): 496-504.

[38] Alejandro R, Strasser S, Sucker PF, Mintz D. Isolation of pancreatic islets from dogs. Semiautomated purification on albumin gradients. Transplantation 1990; 50(2): 207-210.

[39] Lake SP, Bassett PD, Larkins A et al. Large-scale purification of human islets utilizing discontinuous albumin gradients in IBM 2991 cell separator. Diabetes 1989; 38(Suppl. 1):143-145.

[40] Ichii H, Pileggi A, Molano RD et all. Rescue purification maximizes the use of human islet preparations for transplantation. Am J. Transplant 2005; 5(1):21-30

[41] Van der Burg MPM, Ranuncoli A, Molano R, et al. Efficacy of the novel iodixanol-UWS density gradient for human islet purification. Acta Dibetol, 35: 247, 1998.

[42] Shapiro AM, Ricordi C, Hering BJ et al. International trial of the Edmonton protocol for islet transplantation. N Engl J Med 2006; 355(13):1318-1330.

[43] Alejandro R, Mintz DH. Experimental and clinical methods of islet transplantation. Transplantation of the Endocrine Pancreata. Elsevier Science BV 1988: 217-223.

[44] Tzakis AG, Ricordi C, Alejandro R et al. Pancreatic islet transplantation after upper abdominal exoneration and liver replacement. Lancet 1990; 336(8712): 402-405.

[45] Baidal DA, Froud T, Ferrara JV, et al. The bag method for islet cell infusion. Cell Transplant 2003; 12(7): 809-013.

[46] Goss JA, Soltes G Goodpastor R, et al. Pancreatic islet transplantation: the radiographic approach. Transplantation 2003; 76(1):199-203.

[47] Froud T, Yrizarry JM, Alejandro R, Ricordi C. Use of T-STAT to prevent bleeding following percutaneous transhepatic intraportal islet transplantation. Cell Transplant 2004; 1391): 55-59.

[48] Froud T, Ricord C, Baidal DA, et al. Islet transplantation in type 1 diabetes mellitus using cultured islet and steroid-free immunosuppression: Miami experience. Am J Transplant 2005; 5:2037-46.

[49] Markmann JF, Deng S, Huang X, et al. Insulin independence following isolated islet transplantation and single islet infusions. Ann Surg 2003; 237:741-9.

[50] Hirshberg B, Rother KI, Digon BJ III, et al. Benefits and risks of solitary islet transplantation for type 1 diabetes using steroid-sparing immunosupression: the National Institutes of Health experience. Diabetes Care 2003; 26:3288-95.

[51] Marigliano M, Bertera S, Gruppillo M, at al. Pig-to-Nonhuman primates pancreatic islet xenotransplantation: An overview. Curr Diab Rep 2011; 11:402-412.

[52] Park SJ, Shin S, Koo OJ, et al. Functional improvement of porcine neonatal pancreatic cell clusters via conformal encapsulation using an air-driven encapsulator. Exp Mol Med. 2012; 44(1):20-25.

[53] van der Laan LJ, Lockey C, Griffeth BC, et al. Infection by porcine endogenous retrovirus after islet xenotransplantation. Nature 2000; 407(6800):90-94.

[54] Hering BJ, Wijkstrom M, Graham ML et al. Prolonged diabetes reversal after intraportal xenotransplantation of wild-type porcine islets in immunosuppressed nonhuman primates. Nature Medicine 2006; 12(3):301-303.

[55] Cardona K, Korbutt GS, Milas Z, et al. Long-term survival of neonatal porcine islets in nonhuman primates by targeting costimulatory pathways. Nature Medicine 2006; 12(3): 304-306.

[56] Potter KJ, Abedini A, Amrek P et al. Islet amyloid deposition limits the viability of human islet grafts but not porcine islet grafts. PNAS; 107(9): 4305-4310.

[57] Irgang M, Laue C, Velten F, et al. No evidence of PERV release by islet cells from German landrace pigs. Ann Transplant 2008; 13(4) 59-66.

[58] Denner J, Specke V, Karlas A, et al. No transmission of porcine endogenous retroviruses (PERVs) in a long-term pig to rat xenotransplantation model and no infection of immunosuppressed rats. Ann Transplant 2008; 13(1):20-31.

[59] Koulmanda M, Qipo A, Smith RN, Auchincloss H Jr. Pig islet xenografts are resistant to autoimmune destruction by non-obese diabetic recipients after anti-CD4 treatment. Xenotransplantation 2003; 10:178-184.

[60] Ricordi C, Finke EH, Lacy PE. A method for the mass isolation of islets from the adult pig pancreas. Diabetes 1986; 35:649-653.

[61] Korbutt GS, Elliott JF, Ziliang A, et al. Large scale isolation, growth, and function of porcine neonatal islets cells. J Clin Invest 1996; 97(9):2119-2129.

[62] Mandel TE. Fetal islet transplantation in rodents and primates. J Mol Med 1999; 77:155-160.

[63] Weir GC, Bonner-Weir S, Leahy JL. Islet mass and function in diabetes and transplantation. Diabetes 1990; 39:401-405.

[64] Hardikar AA, Wang XY, Williams LJ et al. Functional maturation of fetal porcine beta-cells by glucagon-like peptide 1 and cholecystokinin. Endocrinology 2002; 143(3): 505-514.

[65] Vizzardelli C, Molano RD, Pileggi A, et al. Neonatal porcine pancreatic cell clusters as a potential source for transplantation in humans: Characterization of proliferation, apoptosis, xenoantigen expression and gene delivery with recombinant AAV. Xenotransplantation 2002; 9:14-24.

[66] Hecht G, Eventov-Friedman S, Rosen C, et al. Embryonic pig pancreatic tissue for the treatment of diabetes in a nonhuman primate model. Proc Natl Acad Sci USA 2009; 106:8659-8664.

[67] Dufrance D, Goebbels R, Gianello P. Alginate macroencapsulation of pig islets allows correction of streptozotocin-induced diabetes in primates up to 6 months without immunosuppression. Transplantation 2010; 90:1054-1062.

[68] Bennet W, Sundberg B, Groth G-G, et al. Incompatibility between human blood and isolated islets of Langerhans. Diabetes 1999; 48:1907-1914.

[69] Bennet W, Bjorkland A, Sundberg B, et al. Expression of complement regulatory proteins om islets of Langerhans: A comparison between human islets and islets isolated from normal and hDAF transgenic pigs. Transplantation 2001; 72(2):312-319.

[70] Dufrance D, Goebbels R-M, Saliez A, et al. Six-month survival of microencapsulated pig islets and alginate biocompatibility in primates: Proof of concept. Transplantation 2006; 81(9): 1345-1353.

[71] Elliott RB, Escobar L, Tan PLJ, et al. Live encapsulated porcine islets from a type 1 diabetic patient 9.5 yr after xenotransplantation. Xenotansplantation 2007; 14(2): 157-161.

[72] Valdes-Gonzalez RA, Dornates LM, Garibay GN, et al. Xenotransplantation of porcine neonatal islets of Langerhans and Sertoli cells: a 4 year study. European J of Endocrinol 1005; 153:419-427.

[73] Sykes M, Cozzi E. Xenotransplantation of pig islets into Mexican children: Were the fundamental ethical requirements to proceed with such a study really met? European J of Endocrinol 2006; 154: 921-922.

[74] Guo T, Hebrok M. Stem cell to pancreatic β-cells: New sources for diabetes cell therapy. Endocrine Reviews 2009; 30(3):214-227.

[75] Hori Y. Insulin-producing cells derived from stem/progenitor cells: Therapeutic implications for diabetes mellitus. Med Mol Morphol 2009; 42:195-200

[76] Efrat S. Prospects for gene therapy of insulin-dependent diabetes mellitus. Diabetologia 1998; 41:1401-1409.

[77] Lumselsky N, Blondel O, Laeng P, et al. Differentiation of embryonic stem cells to insulin-secreting structures similar to pancreatic islets. Science 2001; 292:1389-1394.

[78] Hori Y, Rulifson IC, Tsai BC, et al. Growth inhibitors promote differentiation of insulin-producing tissue from embryonic stem cells. Proc Natl Acad Sci USA 2002; 99:16105-16110.

[79] Blyszczuk P, Czyz J, Kania G et al. Expression of Pax4 in embryonic stem cells promotes differnetiation of nestin-positive progenitor and insulin-producing cells. Proc Natl Acad Sci USA 2003; 100:998-1003.

[80] Delacour A, Nepote V, Trumpp A, Herrera PL. Nestin expression in pancreatic exocrine cell lienages. Mech Dev 2004; 121:3-14.

[81] Esni F, Stoffers DA< Taleuchi T, Leach SD. Origin of exocrine pancreatic cells from nestin-positive precursors in developing mouse pancreas. Mech Dev 2004; 121:15-25.

[82] Lendahl U, Zimmerman LB, McKay RD. CNS stem cells express a new class of intermediate filament protein. Cell 1990; 60:585-595.

[83] Hori Y, Gu X, Xic X, Kim SK. Differentiation of insulin-producing stem cells from human neural progenitor cells. PloS Med 2005; 2(4):E103 347-356.

[84] Rajagopal J, Anderson WK, Kume S, et al. Insulin staining of EX cell progeny from insuloin uptake. Science 2003; 299:363.

[85] D'Amour KA, agulnick AD, Eliazer S, et al. Efficient differentiation of human embryonic stem cells to definitive endoderm. Nat Biotechnol 2005; 23(12):1534-1541.

[86] D'Amour KA, Bang AG, Eliazer S, et al. Production of pancreatic hormone-expressing endocrine cells from human embryonic stem cells. Nat Biotechnol 2006; 24(11): 1392-1401.

[87] Jiang J, Au M, Lu K, et al. Generation of Insulin-producing islet-like clusters from human embryonic stem cells. Stem Cells 2007; 25:1940-1953.

[88] Best M, Carroll M, Hanley NA, Hanley KP. Embryonic stem cells to beta-cells by understanding pancreas development. Molecular and Cell Encrionol 2008; 288:86-94.

[89] Kroon E, Martinson LA, Kadoya K, et al. Pancreatic endoderm derived from human embryonic stem cells generates glucose-responsive insulin-secreting cells in vivo. Nat Biotechnol 2008; 26(4):443-452.

[90] Takahashi K, Yamanaka S. Induction of pluripotent stem cells from mouse embryonic and adult fibroblast cultures by defined factors. Cell 2006; 126(4):663-676.

[91] Takahashi K, Okita K, Nakagawa M, Yamanka S. Induction of pluripotent stem cells from fibroblast cultures. Nat Protoc 2007; 27(12):3081-3089.

[92] Takahashi K, Tanabe K, Ohnuki M, et al. Induction of pluripotent stem cells from adult human fibroblasts by defined factors. Cell 2007; 131(5):861-872.

[93] Tateshi K, He J, Taranova O, et al. Generation of insulin-secreting islet-like clusters from human skin fibroblasts. J Bio Chem 2008; 283(46):31601-31607.

[94] Zhou H, Wu S, Young JK, et al. Generation of induced pluripotent stem cells using recombinant proteins. Cell Stem Cell 2009: 4(5):381-384.

[95] Yu J, Hu K, Smuga-Otto K, et al. Human induced pluripotent stem cells free of vector and transgene sequences. Science 2009; 324(5928):797-801.

[96] Jia F, Wilson KD, Sun N, et al. A non-viral minicircle vector for derived human iPS cells. Nat Methods 2010; 7(3): 197-199.

[97] Warren L, Manos PD, Ahfeldt T, et al. Highly efficient reprogramming to pluripotency and direct differentiation of human cells with synthetic modified mRNA. Cell Stem Cell 2010; 7(5):618-30.

[98] Shi Y, Desponts C, Do JT et al. Induction of pluripotent stem cells from mouse embryo9nic fibroblasts by Oct4 and KLF4 with small-molecule compounds. Cell Stem Cell 2008; 3(5):568-574.

[99] Tisch R, McDevitt, HO. Insulin-dependent diabetes mellitus. Cell 1996; 85:291-297.

[100] Atkinson MA, Leiter EH. The NOD mouse model of type 1 diabetes: As good as it gets? Nature Medicine 1999; 5(6):601-604.

[101] Goudy KS, Tisch R. Immunotherapy for the prevention and treatment of Type 1 diabetes. Int Rev of Immunol 2005; 24:307-326.

[102] Eisenbarth GS. Prediction of type 1 diabetes: The natural history of the pre-diabetic period. Adv Exp Med Biol 2004; 552:268-290.

[103] Nishio J, Gaglia JL, Turvery ES, et al. Islet recovery and reversal of murine type 1 diabetes in the absence of any infused spleen cell contribution. Science 2006; 311:1775-1778.

[104] Chatenoud L, Thervet E, PrimoJ, Bach JF. Anti-CD3 antibody induces long-term remission of overt autoimmunity in nonobese diabetic mice. Proc Natl Acad Sci USA 1994; 91:123-127.

[105] Zhao Y, Jiang Z, Zhao T et al. Reversal of type 1 diabetes via islet beta cell regeneration following immune modulation by cord blood-derived multipotent stem cells. BMC Medicine 2012; 10:1-11.

[106] Tisch R, Wang B, Weaver B, et al. Antigen-specific mediated suppression of beta cell autoimmunity by plasmid DNA vaccination. J Immunol 2003; 171:469-476.

[107] Skyler JS, Krischner JP, Wolfsdorf J, et al. Effects of oral insulin in relatives of patients with type 1 diabetes: The Diabetes Prevention Trial – Type 1. Diabetes Care 2—5; 28:1068-1076.

[108] Tisch R, McDevitt HO. Antigen-specific immunotherapy: Is it a real possibility to combat T-cell mediated autoimmunity. Proc Natl Acad Sci USA 1994; 91:437-438.

[109] Liblau RS, Pearson CI, Shokat K et al. High-dose soluble antigen: Peripheral T-cell proliferation or apoptosis. Immunol Rev 1994; 142:193-208.

[110] Tian J, Atkinson MA, Clare-Salzler M, et al. Nasal administration of glutamine decarboxilase (GAD65) peptides induces Th2 responses and prevents murine insulin-dependent diabetes. J Exp Med 1996; 183:1561-1567.

[111] Harrison LC, Honeyman MC, Steele CE, et al. Pancreatic beta-cell function and immune responses to insuloin after administration of intranasal insulin to humans at risk for type 1 diabetes. Diabetes Care 2004; 27:2348-2355.

[112] Wang Y, Hao L, Gill RG, Lafferty KJ. Autoimmune diabetes in NOD mouse is L3T4 T-lymphocyte dependent. Diabetes 1987; 36:535-538.

[113] Simon G, Parker M, Ramiya V, et al. Murine antilymphocyte globulin therapy alters disease progression in NOD mice by a time-dependent induction of immunoregulation. Diabetes 2008; 57:405-414.

[114] Waldman H, Cobbold S. Regulating the immune response to transplants, a role for CD4+ regulatory cells? Immunity 2001; 14:399-406.

[115] Chatenoud L, Bluestone JA. CD3-specific antibodies: A portal to the treatment of autoimmunity. Nat Rev Immunol 2007; 7:622-632.

[116] Harold KC, Hagopian W, Auger JA, et al. Anti-CD3 monoclonal antibody in the new onset type 1 diabetes mellitus. N Engl J Med 2002; 346:1692-1698.

[117] Molano RD, Pileggi A, Berney T, et al. Prolonged islet allograft survival in diabetic NOD mice by targeting CD45RB and CD154. Diabetes 2003; 52:957-964.

[118] Bour-Jordan H, Bluestone JA. B cell depletion: A novel therapy for autoimmune diabetes? J Clin Invest 2007; 117:3642-3645.

[119] Li L, Zuoan Yi, Tisch R, Wang B. Immunotherapy of type 1 diabetes. Arch Immunol Ther Exp 2008; 56: 227-236.

[120] Pescovitz, MD, Greenboaum CJ, Krauses-Steinrauf H, et al. Rituximab, B-lymphocyte depletion, and preservation of beta-cell function. N Engl J Med 2009; 361:2143-2152.

[121] Putnam AL, Brusko, TM, Lee MR, et al. Expansion of human regulatory T-cells from patients with type1 diabetes. Diabetes 2009; 58:652-662.

[122] Filippe C, Bresson D, von Herrath M. Antigen-specific induction of regulatory T cells for Type 1 diabetes therapy. Int Rev Immunol 2005; 24:341-360.

[123] Homann D, von Herrath M. Regulatory T cell and type 1 diabetes. Clin Immunol 2004; 112: 202-209.

[124] Billingham RE, Brent L, Medawar PB. Actively acquired tolerance of foreign cells. Nature 1953; 172:603-606.

[125] Exner BG, Fowler K, Ilstad ST. Tolerance induction for islet transplantation. Ann Transplant 1997; 2:77-80.

[126] Domenick MA, Ildstad ST. Impact of bone marrow transplantation on Type 1 diabetes. World J, Surg 2001; 25:474-480.

[127] Inverardi L, Linetsky E, Pileggi A et al. Targeted bone marrow radioablation with ^{153}Samarium-Lexidronam promotes allogeneic hematopoietic chimerism and donor-specific immunologic hyporesponsiveness. Transplantation 2004; 77:647-655.

[128] Ildstad ST, Sachs DH. Reconstitution with syngeneic plus allogeneic or xenogeneic bone marrow leads to specific acceptance of allografts or xenografts. Nature 1984; 307:168-170.

[129] Rapaport FT. Immunologic tolerance: irradiation and bone marrow transplantation induction of canine allogeneic unresponsiveness. Transplant Proc 1977; 9:984.

[130] Kawai T Cosimi AB, Colvin RB et al. Mixed allogeneic chimerism and renal allograft teolrance in cynomologous monkeys. Transplantation 1995; 59:256-262.

[131] Sayegh MH, Fine NA, Smith JL et al. Immunologic tolerance to renal allografts after bone marrow transplant from the same donors. Ann Rev Med 1991; 114:954-955.

[132] Leventhal J, Abecassis M, Miller J, et al. Chimerism and tolerance without GVHD or engraftment syndrome in HLA-mismatched combined kidney and hematopoietic stem cells transplantation. Sci Transl Med 2012; 4:1-10.